# The Complete Book
## of
# VITAMINS

# The Complete Book of
# VITAMINS

*By the Staff of Prevention® magazine*

*Compiled and Prepared by:*

## *Charles Gerras*
*Executive Editor*

## *Joseph Golant*
## *E. John Hanna*
Senior Editors

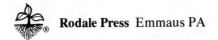 **Rodale Press**  Emmaus PA

**Library of Congress Cataloging in Publication Data**

Main entry under title:

The complete book of vitamins.

    Includes index.
    1. Vitamin therapy.  2. Vitamins.  I. Gerras,
Charles.  II. Golant, Joseph.  III. Hanna, E. John.
IV. Prevention.
RM259.C65    613.2'8    77-1280
ISBN 0-87857-176-0  hardcover

*Printed in the United States of America on recycled paper*

20          hardcover

# Table of Contents

# BOOK III—VITAMIN THERAPY FOR DISEASE

# BOOK I

# VITAMINS
# IN YOUR DAILY LIFE

# CHAPTER 1

# Vitamins: What They Are and What They Do

Despite all the talk about vitamins today, few people actually know what they are and why they are so important. Vitamin research goes on constantly, new discoveries are reported from time to time, but scientists are all too aware that they don't know all of the facts about all of the vitamins. Today 15 vitamins have been recognized and analyzed. Scientists believe that again as many probably exist and are essential for our health.

Vitamins are organic food substances—that is, substances that occur naturally only in living things, plant or animal. They exist in foods in minute quantities; they are absolutely necessary for proper growth and the maintenance of health. Plants manufacture their own vitamins. Animals obtain theirs from plants or from other animals that eat plants. Some animals manufacture in their own bodies some of the vitamins they need.

It was around the turn of the century that someone first suspected there might be more in foodstuffs than fats, proteins, carbohydrates, and minerals. Laboratory experiments showed that even when all those elements were present in the diet, laboratory animals could still die of malnutrition. Scientists began to search for this important missing link. They discovered vitamins. The name comes from *vita* (life) plus *amine* (the chemical compounds that were originally thought to be vitamins).

3

Vitamins are not foods in the sense that carbohydrates, fats, and proteins are foods. They are not needed in bulk to build muscle or tissue. Carbohydrates, fats, and proteins are broken down into other substances which the body uses in the process of metabolism. Not so with vitamins. They retain their original form in the body and are built into body structure, where they are important parts of the machinery of all cells. Just by their presence in the cells they bring about certain changes and processes. For example, the B vitamins do not cause an increase in weight, as large amounts of certain foods might do. But a very thin individual suffering from some digestive complaint might bring about an increase in weight by taking B vitamins because the presence of the B complex in the digestive tract helps to digest and utilize food completely. Like hormones, vitamins regulate body processes. As in the case of trace minerals such as iodine, the presence or absence of vitamins in very small amounts means the difference between good and poor health.

The green leaves of plants are the laboratories in which plant vitamins are manufactured. So the green leaves and stalks of plants are full of vitamins. Foods that are seeds (beans, peas, kernels of wheat and corn, etc.) also contain vitamins which the plant has provided to nourish the next generation of plants. The lean meat of animals contains vitamins; the organs (heart, liver, etc.) contain even more, which the animal's digestive system has stored there. The yolks of eggs contain vitamins which the mother animal provides for the use of her young. Fish store vitamins chiefly in their livers.

Basically there are two classifications of vitamins—fat-soluble vitamins and water-soluble vitamins. These terms refer to a basic structural difference within the two kinds of vitamins which determines some of their properties. Fat-soluble vitamins are soluble in a solution of alcohol and are more easily stored within the body; water-soluble vitamins will dissolve in water, and are lost much more easily by the body through normal elimination.

The fat-soluble vitamins are vitamins A, D, E, and K. The

water-soluble vitamins include all the B vitamins, vitamin C, and the bioflavonoids (also known as vitamin P).

Researchers have established approximate estimates of the daily requirements of most of the vitamins for perfect health. These amounts are usually spoken of in terms of milligrams (A milligram is 1/1000 of a gram. A gram is 1/28 of an ounce.) You may also find daily requirements of vitamin A expressed in terms of International Units, which are a measure of activity, not just quantity (see Chapter 6).

# CHAPTER 2

# Why We Need
# Vitamin Supplements

In the abundance of misinformation on the subject of food and nutrition, there is one steady theme: Modern American food is the best there is. It's nutritious, it's health-giving. No one needs food supplements (vitamins or minerals) as long as he eats a "good diet."

The "good diet" is not spelled out. We are given a list of general categories of food. "Eat some of these every day and you can't help but be healthy," say the nutrition columnists, the syndicated M.D. columns, the women's magazines, and the TV commercials.

If indeed the American diet is everything we need, how can we account for the astounding incidence of chronic disease?

A solid answer to the claim that we don't need food supplements appeared in the *American Journal of Digestive Diseases* (March 1953), written by Morton S. Biskind, M.D., a careful researcher and a practicing physician. In spite of the passage of time, the statement is just as valid, the arguments just as clear and convincing as when they were first presented.

## All Important Food Elements
## Have Not Been Isolated

"Several misconceptions . . . have become increasingly prevalent," wrote Dr. Biskind. "One common misconception is that all the important nutritional elements have already been isolated and indeed, that a number of those currently available are not significant in human nutrition. The extremely conservative attitude of the Federal Food and Drug Administration which requires disclaimers on labels of vitamin preparations for the vitamins they consider not adequately studied in human nutrition has further fostered the assumption that administration only of the pure factors thus far considered 'important' is sufficient for satisfactory nutritional therapy." Consumers want to know why, beside many of the vitamins and minerals listed on their food supplements, this statement appears: "Need for in human nutrition is not established." This is what Dr. Biskind meant. Any substance not studied for years and not officially accepted as being necessary to life in certain minimum amounts must be listed on labels as being "not established" as a necessary part of human nutrition.

## A Single Deficiency Is Impossible

Furthermore, said Dr. Biskind, experts talking about nutrition are inclined to speak of deficiencies of one or another vitamin— "thiamine deficiency," "riboflavin deficiency," etc. This is entirely incorrect, he said, for such a thing simply never happens. In a laboratory an animal may be put on a diet completely free of vitamins. Then all known vitamins except thiamine are added. Whatever symptoms are produced in the animal are then said to be due to deficiency of thiamine. But, of course, they are due to lack of thiamine, and all the other *unknown* vitamins as well.

Once thiamine is lacking, other food elements are lost from the body stores, so the condition finally produced involves the loss of all these known and unknown substances.

"In the human being, how much more unlikely that deficiency of single factors should occur," said Dr. Biskind. "Not only are deficiencies multiple but the administration of single nutritional factors or even of a combination of a few of them may actually lead to serious disturbance of a tenuous nutritional equilibrium and precipitation of new avitaminotic lesions"—that is, new symptoms of deficiency.

For many years, he went on, investigators have stressed the need for complete therapy—which includes, of course, giving the deficient patient a source of all those as yet unidentified essential food factors. Dr. Tom Spies, a famous worker in nutritional fields, suggested many years ago that a "basic formula" be worked out which would include all those B vitamins discovered up to that time, which could be given to patients, along with a natural source of the unknown vitamins. But somehow, according to Dr. Biskind, people began to think of this as a "complete formula" and soon it was given to patients as the only source of nutritional elements aside from their meals. The impression rapidly spread that this basic formula contained *all* the important vitamins. He wrote that, time and again, conditions which do not respond at all to the taking of such a preparation improve overnight when a food source of the other, as yet undiscovered vitamins, is given.

"Simply adding desiccated liver or suitable liver fraction to the regime invariably has resulted in a dramatic and lasting improvement often evident within a few days," he said.

A final misconception occurs, he continued—that the average American diet contains all the necessary nutritional elements; that nutritional deficiency, when it does occur, results only from deficiency in the diet and that all that is necessary to cure such a deficiency is a "good diet."

## We Are Not Getting Full Nourishment From Our Food

Dr. Biskind's answer to the misconception that our diets supply all nutritional needs includes these six points:

1. Depletion of much of the soil on which food is grown has produced crops that are nutritionally inferior.

2. The increasing use on crops of toxic insecticides which leave harmful residues in and on food and further harm the soil by killing necessary microorganisms and earthworms.

3. The increasing tendency to pick and ship produce before it has ripened, so that there is less danger of loss from spoilage. These days, we eat few foods that have been ripened on the vine and this ripening is essential to the full nutritional value of the food.
4. The continuously increasing tendency toward processing and chemicalizing our food—dyes, waxes, detergents, emulsifiers, bleaches, etc.
5. The use of virtually pure, vitamin-free sugar for as much as one-fourth of the average caloric intake.
6. The use of many chemical additives such as artificial fats and things of this kind, which may be toxic and many of which replace essential food elements.

The fact that Americans consume about 100 pounds of sugar per person per year indicates that, here alone, a deficiency of about .25 mgs. of thiamine and riboflavin (B vitamins) occurs. This would be a deficit of about 90 mgs. of each of these two important B vitamins in the course of a year. For niacin, another of the B vitamins, the deficiency would be about ten times this much. "And those who refrain from using sugar in coffee or sprinkling it on cereals and fruit in the belief that the intake is thus reduced to zero, are of course mistaken. Sucrose (sugar) is incorporated in so many staple foods today even including bread, that it can hardly be avoided," said Dr. Biskind.

## There Are Other Reasons for Deficiencies

But even if a person was getting all the vitamins in a daily diet, a nutrition deficiency could still occur. There are many conditions and circumstances which can cause a person either to lose vitamins or to need more than the normal day's requirements. Any difficulty with the digestive tract which impairs our ability to absorb vitamins can result in a deficiency—diarrhea, colitis, liver or gallbladder trouble, or many more disorders. Pregnancy and lactation increase one's need for vitamins, as does hyperthyroidism, excessive physical activity, infections, etc. Antibiotics, sulfa drugs, industrial poisons, inhalation of toxic substances such as lead from polluted air, insecticide residues, and so forth, all cause the destruction of vitamins. Emotional disturbances, especially when they are protracted or severe, can cause extremely serious nutritional difficulties.

For all these reasons, and from his own observations, Dr. Biskind held that "gross lesions (disorders) of nutritional deficiency, easily detectable to the naked eye, are extremely common."

He noted that, once tissues have become deficient, it is necessary to take many times the usual amounts of vitamins to make up for the deficiency—as much as 10, 20, or even 50 times the maintenance amounts adequate for people who have not suffered from any previous lack. It is also unfortunately true, he said, that many times the tissues have been so damaged that no excess amount of vitamin therapy can repair them. He gave as an example laboratory rats who were made deficient in riboflavin. After the damage had been done to the cornea of their eyes, no amount of riboflavin in the diet would restore the eyes to their normal healthy state.

Dr. Biskind questioned how we can speak of some standardized amount of vitamins which each and every one of us must require. Would we insist on giving the same amount of insulin to every diabetic? The consequences might be fatal. So why should we assume that any two humans have the same nutritional requirements? One person may need ever so much more of the various vitamins than another!

Other critics of vitamin therapy insist that getting a certain vitamin in a food supplement is useless, since one may get that amount in daily food. But, said Dr. Biskind, what they seem to forget is that the food supplement does not *substitute* for the food—it simply *adds* vitamins to those already being eaten in food.

The water-soluble vitamins (B and C) are not easily stored in body tissues, so these must be supplied every day. While the fat-soluble vitamins are usually well stored by healthy persons, they are lost readily once a severe deficiency has occurred. This is especially true when severe liver damage has taken place.

To continue with Dr. Biskind's ideas, he stated that there are three basic principles of nutritional therapy. It should be *complete, intensive,* and *persistent.* No half-way measures will succeed. Vitamins, minerals, proteins, phosphates, fats, and trace minerals are forever related like links in a chain, when one is considering the way the body uses them. It is useless to strengthen only one or several of these links. All must be equally strong, or the chain will fail.

It seems evident that the average doctor, asking nothing whatever about his patient's diet or way of life except the routine "Do you eat a good diet?" would fail to promote good health, if he prescribed some isolated, synthetic vitamin and mineral preparations to be taken along with the patient's usual diet. This diet, of course, was at least partly responsible for putting him out of sorts to begin with—probably a typical American diet of which a large part is refined carbohydrates—products made chiefly of white sugar and white flour.

## Factors Which Interfere with Nutritional Therapy

No matter how adequate the source of one's diet supplements, the complete repair of a nutritional deficiency may be impossible under certain conditions. Here are some circumstances of life and health which may impair one's ability to use the vitamins and minerals in one's diet to maintain health: poor appetite, diarrhea, insomnia, muscular tension, and spasm of the digestive tract. In addition, wrote Dr. Biskind, "The list of chemicals and drugs which impair cellular enzyme systems and produce tissue anoxia is very long indeed. An incredible number of them are in such indiscriminate use that daily exposure to them is almost unavoidable for many reasons. These range from a variety of chemicals used in industry to carbon monoxide, lead, and other products of combustion in automobile exhaust, the . . . insecticides . . . paint solvents, and drugs such as sulfonamides, antibiotics and estrogens."

It is essential, said Dr. Biskind, to question any patient very closely about his exposure to these various chemicals when outlining a nutritional program for him.

The next time you read in a newspaper or magazine that Americans are well fed and there is no need for them to eat any special diet or to take food supplements, ask yourself, "Which American is well fed? Doesn't it depend on what his individual body needs are, how well-planned his diet is, where his food comes from, what drugs he is taking, and what poisonous chemicals he is exposed to?" All of these things must be considered with regard to every individual. If he is eating a diet carefully planned to meet each of the nutritional stresses he faces, *that* American might be well fed.

# CHAPTER 3

# There's Nothing Average About *Your* Vitamin Needs

The matter of individuality in nutritional requirements is perhaps the most overlooked and ignored health factor in the practice of medicine in the Western world today. And yet it may be the most important single factor that determines who gets sick and who doesn't!

The distinguished scientist who, for the past quarter of a century, has stressed the connection between susceptibility to disease and the individual's own unique pattern of nutritional needs is Roger Williams, Ph.D., of the University of Texas. Summarizing his findings and thesis in an article appearing in *Perspectives in Biology and Medicine* (Autumn 1973), the Texas investigator suggests that many common noninfectious diseases may develop because susceptible persons have far-from-average requirements for a particular vitamin or mineral or amino acid or essential fatty acid—requirements which the ordinary diet does not adequately provide for them.

In the whole world's population, Dr. Williams calculates, there's probably only a handful who inherit an "average" need for each and every one of the 40-odd known nutrients essential to human life and health. The overwhelming majority of humans (and animals, too, as Dr. Williams' own experiments have shown) inherit a far-from-average need for at least one or two nutrients, and, if this need is not satisfied then body cells will fail to function properly. That's when disease takes over.

## A Missed Opportunity

The discovery of deficiency diseases and the identification of vitamins in the early decades of this century could have led to a radical change in medicine along nutritional lines, Dr. Williams says. Scurvy, beriberi, pellagra, and the other disorders found to be caused not by a microbe but by a missing food factor, might have suggested to the medical world that here was revealed not just a handful of peculiar, "different" diseases but the basic underlying cause of perhaps all disease—a missing (or inadequate) nutritional factor necessary for healthy human physiology.

Instead, the medical establishment was hung up on the doctrine that diseases are caused by microorganisms—microbes and viruses—and that treatment and cure depend on finding the "magic bullet" that kills the infecting agent. Even today, when noninfectious ailments are by far the most prominent in American medical practice, the search for a virus as the cause of such degenerative diseases as cancer, arthritis, and multiple sclerosis continues to be the prestigious, fashionable, and well-funded research approach to these disorders. As for infectious diseases, very little attention is paid to the known role of nutrition in enabling the body's own defenses to function effectively against invading microorganisms.

In today's medical establishment, outright deficiency diseases—that is, the final, fulminating evidence of a dietary lack—are still regarded as being exceptional in that they're diet-caused. Even the treatment with vitamin supplementation is not looked upon in the light of restoring a normal balance of nutrients but as medication—in effect, that "magic bullet" specific for "killing off" the particular causative factor. When the Food and Drug Administration wants to label all vitamins "drugs" if their potency exceeds an arbitrarily established low-level amount, it is acting quite within the medical tradition of this country.

"As a result of decades of neglect of nutritional science by medical science," Dr. Williams writes, "what we would regard as sophisticated, well-rounded, nutritional science does not exist." Because the mainstream of scientific thinking has ignored basic facts about nutrition and health, sophisticated tools for nutritional analysis have yet to be developed, let alone to be put to use in correlating unusual requirement patterns with the incidence of disease.

It is at present possible to test (expensively) for a particular patient's individual requirements in respect to only some of the known essential nutrients. The possibility of computerized mass screening, with quick answers on individual needs for every food factor, has never engaged the interests of medical-scientific engineers. Even the range of human differences in requirements has been established for only 10 nutrients, according to Dr. Williams—these differences, incidentally, ranging from two-fold to ten-fold.

Dr. Williams lists four uncontested basic facts that dictate (or should) a "renaissance of nutritional science."

1. Every individual inherits a distinctive pattern of nutritional requirements. The "average person", for whom the National Academy of Sciences and the Food and Drug Administration and the American Medical Association concoct "average" daily allowances for food factors, is a myth. The "average" concept here is about as helpful as the concept of "average" fingerprints.

2. Every essential nutrient becomes a necessary part of the body's internal environment, as does the water we drink and the oxygen we breathe. Functioning of body cells is totally dependent on these factors.

3. In the body, nutrients work as a team, with cells dependent not on this or that nutrient performing a solo role but on total nutritional teamwork. Scarcity of a single nutrient reduces the efficacy of all the nutrients with which it is teamed.

4. A prevailing fact in the natural world is that living

species—plant and animal—rarely are supplied with optimum nutrition, and, when it comes to humans in industrial societies, such less-than-perfect conditions are worsened by the destruction of nutrients in food processing.

Dr. Williams sees hopeful signs that the significance of this set of facts (whose validity is not challenged) at last is being grasped by a growing number of doctors and medical students. He predicts that "a renaissance in nutritional science is imminent." Let's hope he is right—though medical education, research, and practice are so intimately tied up with the drug industry, and therefore with medication as the "solution" to health problems, that such a change in medical outlook may still be a long way off.

How many diseases which now plague mankind might be countered or even totally prevented if all the inventiveness and know-how of modern medical science were devoted to the nutritional approach? "What medical science needs to ascertain by using expertise that is not generally cultivated," Dr. Williams says, "is whether individuals who are peculiarly susceptible to heart disease, obesity, arthritis, dental disease, mental disease, alcoholism, muscular dystrophy, multiple sclerosis, and even cancer, can be benefited by nutritional adjustments."

In many of these disorders, there is evidence of inherited susceptibility. But it seems likely that the inherited trait is not at all a tendency to acquire a particular disease but rather a pattern of nutritional demands that leads to a particular disease if the diet fails to provide certain nutrients required in nonaverage amounts.

## How To Plot Your Own Nutritional Safeguards

While we wait for medical science to take up Dr. Williams' challenge, we certainly can look around and find at least some answers for ourselves. There are health-promoting nutritional steps every family can take despite the lack of medical concern and expertise.

Eat Whole Foods: Remember that every essential nutrient,

known and unknown, is equally vital—not just that handful arbitrarily selected for "enrichment" of processed foods. So rule out all foods that are not whole natural products. Processing strips nutrients from whole foods, adds often-harmful preservatives, coloring agents, artificial flavors, emulsifiers, binders, etc. When you recognize that the only way your body cells can work properly is by getting the full team of nutrients they need, you will not want any food on your table which has had nutrients removed and nonnutrients added.

Find Supplements for Your Special Needs: You are a unique individual and, just as you inherit distinctive fingerprints, you inherit a distinctive pattern of nutritional requirements. Aware that even the best of foods may provide less-than-optimum nutrition to suit your own particular nonaverage needs, you will see the sense of trying out a variety of concentrated nutrients in natural food supplements.

Nobody can answer, exactly, the commonly asked question about supplements, "How much should I take?" Someday, if Dr. Williams' prediction comes true, your own physician may be able to run a simple test and come up with complete and accurate answers. But, for the time being, this is something you'll have to figure out for yourself as best you can, using the Recommended Daily Allowances (designed for the mythical "average" person) not as a final safe answer but as your starting point.

Keep Up With Nutritional Discoveries: Though the mainstream of medical thinking in the United States is not concerned with nutrition, many individual doctors and researchers are. Other investigators, with primary interests in such popular research areas as cellular enzymes, inevitably contribute information on nutrients which enter into biochemical reactions which they are studying. Through reading you can keep up with some of the new discoveries and apply the knowledge to your own better health. Dr. Williams' book, *Nutrition Against Disease* (New York: Pitman, 1971), summarizes and documents many findings on nutrients proved sometimes helpful in the prevention and treatment of major noninfectious diseases.

Over the years, we have picked up such information as the relationship of marginal vitamin C deficiency to atherosclerosis (hardening of the arteries), the value of vitamin B$_6$ in ameliorating certain types of arthritis, the fact that diabetic symptoms can sometimes occur because of a marginal deficiency of the trace mineral chromium, whose best source is brewer's yeast. Presumably, individuals with higher-than-average need for these nutrients can develop such disease symptoms on a diet that provides adequately for others.

By satisfying our exceptional inherited nutritional needs we can make the difference between life-threatening disease and full and vigorous health. It would be helpful if physicians had the education, research background, and sophisticated equipment to be expert consultants on nutritional inheritance. But, until they do, we'll have to be our own experts.

# CHAPTER 4

# Spotting Vitamin Deficiencies in the Elderly

You've been visiting with your Uncle Lou and he doesn't seem right. He's "slipping" much faster than ever. He doesn't look healthy. His skin is pale and translucent. His eyes seem glassy and he stares as though he doesn't see very well in the dim light of his living room. There's a twinge of forgetfulness which makes conversation a chore for everyone. His mind just seems to wander from subject to subject with little regard for logic.

On the way home, you discuss it between yourselves and chalk it up to the fact that Uncle Lou is getting up in years. Besides, he's lonely, and badly misses his wife who died a few years ago.

The fact that Uncle Lou may be suffering from a vitamin deficiency never enters your mind. Yet, there is a good possibility that he is, and not just a slight deficiency, but a severe one that could be causing or aggravating many of the problems that are pushing him downhill.

Although our Uncle Lou is mythical, he is very real in the sense that most of us have someone in the family, or a friend, who is in a similar situation, where he or she becomes extremely vulnerable to deficiency states. Who are such people?

Like Lou, they are often older people who live alone. They

have poor appetites, and often, poor dietary habits. They are on limited or fixed incomes, so even if they do have an appetite, there may not be much they can do to satisfy it with good food. They often have digestive problems, which also limits the variety and amount of food they eat.

People who drink alcohol to excess, whether or not they are considered "alcoholics," are also highly vulnerable to gross nutritional deficiencies. Other high-risk groups are those with chronic illness, or who have endured long periods of strength-sapping hospitalization.

Typically, the person with severe nutritional problems has a background of several of these problems, and frequently is suffering from more than one specific deficiency.

According to Samuel Dreizen, D.D.S., M.D., professor of pathology at the University of Texas in Houston, the first evidence of malnutrition in the elderly "is a conglomerate of nonspecific complaints . . . ." In other words, you can't expect to find one very specific symptom which will tell you that the person is suffering from a particular deficiency.

Among the most common or prominent of these "nonspecific complaints," according to an article by Dr. Dreizen (*Geriatrics*, May 1974), are:

| | |
|---|---|
| abdominal discomfort | depression |
| loss of appetite | digestive upsets |
| anxiety | fatigue |
| backache | headaches |
| confusion | insomnia |
| irritability | palpitation |
| exhaustion | tingling or numbness in |
| muscle pain or weakness | the extremities |
| nervousness | poor concentration |

Of course, no single symptom guarantees that the person has a nutritional deficiency. But any of them—particularly in a susceptible individual—may well signal a deficiency, even in the absence of clinical signs, including blood tests.

Here is a synopsis of classic vitamin deficiencies and some of their most visible and usual symptoms.

# Vitamin A

Rough, bumpy skin is probably the most obvious sign of vitamin A deficiency. This used to be called "toad skin," but today doctors prefer the term follicular hyperkeratosis. It looks much like goose pimples, except that the bumps don't go away. They are caused by a hardening of the hair follicles along with other skin changes.

The other classic sign of vitamin A deficiency, which may not be noticeable to anyone except the person afflicted, is difficulty seeing in dim light—sometimes called night blindness. Adjusting to dim light after exposure to bright light is particularly difficult for a person with this condition.

A more severe symptom of vitamin A deficiency may develop in which the eye loses its ability to remain moist by secretion. This condition, known as xerophthalmia, can lead to irreversible blindness.

Severe vitamin A deficiency is not something that happens overnight. The liver of a healthy person can store enough vitamin A to take care of body requirements for a year or more. But long-term marginal deficiency, coupled with the stress of disease and poor appetite, can bring on the appearance of outright deficiency.

# Vitamin B Complex

It is beyond the ability of the layman—and of most physicians—to diagnose which component of the B complex of vitamins is causing any given symptom or symptoms. For example, a deficiency of thiamine ($B_1$) can produce several symptoms, one of which is neuritis, usually beginning in the legs. However, this neuritis may manifest itself as tenderness in the calf, muscle weakness, cramping, tingling sensations, or other abnormalities. Thiamine deficiency can also cause severe swelling, beginning in the feet and legs and moving upward.

Deficiency of riboflavin, or vitamin $B_2$, most typically produces pathology of the lips, tongue, eyes, and skin. The lips are either unusually red or whitish. Ulceration and painful fissuring at the corners of the mouth is frequent. The cornea of the eye may develop blood vessels, a condition called vascularization. Scaly lesions may develop around the nose, cheeks, chin, and sometimes on the lobes of the ears. The scrotum or vulva may also be affected.

Niacin deficiency also produces severe skin lesions. But the first signs of deficiency may be mental symptoms, including irritability, forgetfulness, and morbid fears, all of which can be easily mistaken for advanced senility or even psychosis. Diarrhea is another hallmark of severe niacin deficiency.

Folic acid deficiency produces a dangerous form of anemia, but its more obvious symptoms will be ulcers around the lips, tongue, and mouth which are very painful. The tongue typically swells and becomes unusually red and sick-looking, a condition known as glossitis.

Deficiency of vitamin $B_{12}$ is also characterized by glossitis, along with weakness, and tingling in the extremities. However, the most serious effect of vitamin $B_{12}$ deficiency is pernicious anemia, which may not be obvious to the observer except through symptoms such as pallor, weakness, and loss of appetite. Except in the very debilitated, pernicious anemia is usually produced by a malabsorption problem, and must be corrected by $B_{12}$ injections.

It is useful to know that the B complex is plentifully available from foods such as whole-grain wheat, brown rice, liver, beans, brewer's yeast, milk, and other unrefined staples.

# Vitamin C

Although most of us associate a severe lack of vitamin C with scurvy, the first apparent signs may simply be a sallow complexion and bloating of the face. The weakness and irritability that result from other vitamin deficiencies are also produced by a deficiency of vitamin C. By the time capillary hemorrhaging, spontaneous bruises, and bleeding gums develop, the deficiency is advanced and is bringing about the literal disintegration of living tissue.

## Vitamin D

Vitamin D deficiency is usually associated with children, in whom it produces rickets. In adults, it brings about osteomalacia, in which the bones are weak and easily bent or broken. Nutritional osteomalacia is relatively uncommon in the United States, but can be suspected in older people who have not been in the sunlight (which enables the body to make its own vitamin D) for a long time.

## Vitamin E

The reputation vitamin E has as the "sex vitamin" probably comes from the fact that it was first studied in connection with fertility. Researchers discovered that female rats deficient in vitamin E can conceive but cannot carry their young to term. The reason: an abnormality in the blood vessels leading to thrombosis. It is known that vitamin E protects the body's store of two vitamins, A and C, that are both sensitive to the presence of oxygen; presumably, less A and C are required when E is present. Researchers have found this oxygen-preserving characteristic effective in treating reproductive, circulatory, and joint disorders. It is reasonable to assume that a heart working to pump oxygen to the cells has less of a burden when vitamin E is present to make the oxygen last, hence the use of this vitamin as a heart-saver.

## Now . . . What to Do?

There will come a point at which you may have to ask yourself: is nutritional deficiency really a problem in this case? Probably the most reasonable way to proceed is to consider the individual's nutritional history and present situation. Is his appetite impaired? Does he exclude from his diet whole classes of foods, such as citrus fruits, vegetables, grain products, meat, and fish or dairy products? Is he locked into a pattern of eating only a few foods that agree with him, day after day, month after month?

The combination of health deterioration along with this kind of nutritional history should be enough to alert you to the possible presence of serious dietary deficiency. Don't feel that you need to play doctor in this kind of situation. The decision that someone is not eating properly, and may be suffering for it, is a decision which is based more on common sense than on science. And the act of helping such a person to improve his diet is more one of compassion than of medical intervention.

There is a good and very positive side to this grim litany of nutritional problems, though: unless they have progressed to the point of no return, they are always correctable. In some cases, massive doses of nutrients may be called for. In other cases, where there is malabsorption present, injections may be needed. But in one way or another, the important thing to remember is that they *can* be cleared up.

Of course, it may not be all that easy to get the person suffering from nutritional deficiency to improve his diet, or even to take supplements. You have to use your ingenuity, your powers of persuasion, and a lot of tact.

The important thing is to make sure that all your loved ones never get to the point where they become ill and weary of life simply because of dietary inadequacies.

# CHAPTER 5

# Food Enrichment: Fact and Fallacy

People often confuse the nutritional value of vitamin-enriched processed foods with the nutritional value of fresh foods with their natural vitamin complements intact. They have very little in common. Food enrichment is essentially a commercial maneuver. In fact, few of the nutrients lost in the bulk processing of foods are ever returned to the finished product. One reason is that we don't know what all of them are.

This is clear from a statement of policy issued by the Federal Food and Drug Administration on July 1, 1943 (Federal Register, 1943a). At that time the FDA realized that new food processing techniques were destroying important nutrients; hence, they established regulations requiring large commercial food houses to "enrich" their foods. But they acknowledged that enriched processed foods couldn't be expected to measure up to the real thing:

> Even though adequate nutrition could be better assured through the choice of natural foods than through reliance on enrichment, unenriched foods of the kinds and in the quantities necessary for adequate nutrition are not now available to substantial parts of the population and are not likely to be available soon; nor are most consumers sufficiently edu-

25

cated on nutritional questions to enable them to make an intelligent choice of combinations of unenriched foods on the basis of nutritional values.

Because of the lack of adequate production of a number of foods high in certain nutrients and the lack of consumer knowledge of nutrition, appropriate enrichment of a few foods widely consumed by the population in general or by significant population groups will contribute substantially to the nutritional welfare of consumers and to meeting their expectations of benefit.

These regulations were originally intended as corrective measures levied by the federal government on behalf of the American consumers' health. Food manufacturers turned the regulations into a public relations asset. Through carefully controlled advertising, they make it appear that the so-called enrichment of foods is done as an added bonus for the consumer, when they are really complying with federal standards that acknowledge the superiority of natural foods. Worse, consumers are often led to believe that the nutritive value of the original food has been completely restored. Nothing, of course, could be further from the truth.

## Bread: A Classic Case of "Enrichment"

A classic example of this is the case of enriched bread. While four nutrients have been artificially added to the refined product in the approximate quantity in which they appear in the whole grain, others are present "at only a fraction of their original concentration," according to an article in *Nutrition Reviews* (April 1967). Specifically, the journal mentions drastic reductions in the B-complex vitamins biotin, inositol, para-aminobenzoic acid, and pantothenic acid, as well as a lesser reduction of folic acid.

Besides the B vitamins destroyed, vitamin E is totally lost, since it is concentrated in the wheat germ which is discarded in the milling. As for the minerals, iron is restored in part, while the milling process "removes 40 percent of the chromium, 86 percent of the manganese, 89 percent of the cobalt, 68 percent of the copper, 78 percent of the zinc, and 48 percent of the molybdenum—all trace elements essential for life or health," according to the late Dr. Henry A. Schroeder of the Dartmouth Medical School, testifying at Senate hearings in the summer of 1970 (*New York Times,* 27 August 1970).

Dr. Schroeder expressed even less optimism for the fate of essential vitamins at the hands of the food processors in his book *The Poisons Around Us: Toxic Metals in Food, Air and Water* (Bloomington, Ind: Indiana University Press, 1974). "We can make the food refiners and processors put back what they take out. They will do it, too. They want to sell. But that won't work for the unstable vitamins: pantothenic acid, folacin, C, E, B6," Dr. Schroeder reported.

## Vitamin E Loss During Processing

Vitamin E is one of the most vulnerable of vitamins during food processing. A testing firm reported in the early 1970s that as much as 90 percent or more of the natural vitamin E is lost during the flaking, shredding, and puffing of grain for breakfast cereals. Puffed wheat products suffered losses of about 22 percent while wheat flour lost 92 percent of its vitamin E value. The manufacture of oatmeal resulted in relatively little or no decrease, but more extensive processing of oats increased losses to about 95 percent. Rice cereal products consistently suffered more than a 70 percent loss of vitamin E during production, and similar tests on corn showed losses of vitamin E during processing that ranged from 35 percent for white meal to 98 percent for corn flakes.

In a publication entitled "Proposed Fortification Policy for Cereal-Grain Products" (Washington, D.C., 1974) the National Academy of Sciences reported "certain studies have estimated that the majority of the population gets a sufficient intake of vitamin E although 6 to 14 percent may be at marginal levels of consumption." This is a serious problem when you consider that vitamin E was recognized as early as 1944 for its antioxidant properties, according to Arthur F. Wagner and Karl Folers in *Vitamins and Coenzymes* (New York: Interscience Publishers, 1964). These antioxidant properties of vitamin E prevent the destructive oxidation both of fat-soluble nutrients (particularly vitamin A) and of unsaturated fatty acids. Now, in the case of unsaturated fatty acids, vitamin E's antioxidant role inhibits the formation of dangerous peroxides that are believed to be the cause of the aging of cells throughout the body—and hence the aging property itself, according to Dr. A.L. Tappel of the University of California.

"Because the biochemistry of vitamin E deficiency and the aging processes run parallel," Dr. Tappel said in concluding a summary of the scientific findings on destructive peroxides, antioxidants, and aging damage to cells, "it is apparent that research should continue to explore more fully the optimization of vitamin E intake," according to an article in the October 1968 edition of *Geriatrics*.

# Food Processors Base Nutrient Need on Superficial Priorities

The nutrients favored for enrichment or fortification are limited in number, and (aside from protein and calcium fortification) generally are those associated with the frank deficiency diseases. Anemia, pellagra, and beriberi result from lack of (respectively) iron, niacin, thiamine, and riboflavin. Other common fortifiers are vitamin A, whose deficiency shows up overtly in night blindness and impaired mucous membrane function; vitamin C, without which scurvy develops; and vitamin D, which prevents rickets.

These overt diseases—and their causes—have been known for decades. Basing a claim for nutritional improvement solely on amounts of nutrients that prevent such gross manifestations of an impoverished diet is an approach that is half a century out of step with scientific progress. In addition to their obvious and long-known roles in preventing such frank deficiency diseases, the so-called "enrichment" vitamins have many other functions of a far more subtle nature.

## Interdependence, Balance, and the Unknown Factors

It is not only the loss or diminution of known vital nutrients that makes fortification a hollow pretense of restoring natural nourishment. The gravest error lies in the assumption that we can duplicate all the subtleties of interdependence, balance, and hidden trace substances that have evolved in our nutritional environment over millions of years.

There is an interdependence among many vitamins found together in nature. The B vitamins provide a prime example. None of the nutrients known to make up the B complex is ever found isolated in the natural state. We ingest them all together when we eat whole grain, wheat germ, liver, or nutritional yeast. And inside the body, they work together for our better health when we take them in the proportion to which the human species has become adapted through millennia of living on the natural foods provided by the environment.

"Most of the B vitamins act in close synergism on the carbohydrate metabolism," Dr. Henry Schroeder reported in an article in *Munch. med. Wschr.* (20: 1050-1053, 1961). But then he warned; "However, in certain circumstances, they can also compete with each other and supplant one another. Large doses of vitamin $B_1$ (thiamine) may bring to light a latent pellagra ($B_3$ deficiency) or in some instances an increase of its symptoms."

In other words, an unnatural increase in one single member of the B vitamins can cause the diminution of another B vitamin so severe that symptoms of its deficiency disease appear.

Processing foods also destroys unknown factors in natural foods—that is, subtle nutrients that have yet to be discovered, as many of the vitamin B-complex substances have been discovered in quite recent years. You can't "restore" to processed food what you don't know you have stripped.

Obviously, we can't give examples of the unknown. But an article in *Science* (November 1967) points to the kind of nutritional bonus that comes unrecognized in natural foods.

The author of the article, Dr. Howard A. Schneider, started his experiment on diet and infection on this presupposition: "That 'natural' foods contain some important items that are not yet known and so not supplied by the assembled semisynthetic diet." After years of elaborating his experimental model and devising just the right laboratory techniques for sharply revealing the role played by nutrients, Dr. Schneider and his colleagues succeeded in identifying a hitherto unknown nutrient—one which he calls a "pacifarin," because it "pacifies" (but does not kill) the virulent salmonella bacteria.

In the natural diet fed to rats, the pacifarin was present. In the synthetic diet, carefully prepared to include all standard nutrients, it was not. When the pacifarin (a bacteriological by-product found in the outer fraction of the wheat kernel) was fed to the rats in concentrated form, it led to survival of 90 out of 100 rats challenged with the infecting bacteria; the control rats, on a synthetic diet, survived in the exact opposite ratio: 90 out of 100 died.

Is it wrong to enrich foods? Certainly not—putting something back is better than leaving a complete void. What's wrong is the impression, studiously fostered by processors, that processed and enriched foods are as nutritious as their natural counterparts. The best efforts at enrichment result in only a pale imitation of the real thing. If you know that, you know enough for self-protection. The choice is yours: will you eat the fresh food you know has the perfect nutritional package, or will you settle for a machine-mauled product that has a processor's approximation of the nutrients contained in the original?

# CHAPTER 6

# How to Read Your Vitamin Label

If you've ever been bewildered by the information on labels of the vitamin supplements you take, you aren't alone. Most people don't understand why one vitamin, say B₁, is measured in milligrams, while another is sold in International Units and a third in micrograms.

Yet it really isn't so difficult. Once you've mastered the system, you'll be able to compute your vitamin intake quickly, accurately, and confidently.

Very simply, the standards of vitamin measurement fall into two categories: activity-based and quantity-based.

The activity-based measurements are International Unit (I.U.) and the United States Pharmacopeia unit (U.S.P.), which many may recognize as commonly used with vitamins A, D, and E. The reason this form of measurement is used for these vitamins is that although quantities may be the same, there may be variations in the source and type of materials that alter how much of the vitamin you absorb, or how active it is within your system.

For example: crystalline vitamin A alcohol is twice as potent as pure beta-carotene, so one International Unit (I.U.) of vitamin A is equal to the activity of 0.6 micrograms of pure beta-carotene, but only 0.3 micrograms of crystalline vitamin A alcohol. Different forms of vitamins D and E also carry different potencies, and for this reason, they're also rated by their strength, either in International Units (I.U.) or in United States Pharmacopeia units (U.S.P.). Is there a difference between I.U. and U.S.P.? Yes, but it is too slight to affect a person's vitamin intake. All you need to remember is that both terms refer to activity measurements.

The quantity-based measurements are used when the vitamin has a standard strength. They come in two types: metric and apothecary. Many of us learned the metric system in school—liters, meters, and grams—and that same measurement is on vitamin labels. Milligrams (mg), equal to 1/1000 gram, are used to measure vitamins and minerals which we need in moderate doses; micrograms (mcg), equal to 1/1,000,000 gram, are used when we're talking about those nutritious substances that are needed and supplied only in microscopic traces. For example, some vitamin B-complex preparations may contain 14 *milligrams*(mg) of vitamin $B_2$ but only 25 *micrograms* (mcg) of vitamin $B_{12}$. When dealing with smaller quantities, you measure them on the smaller scale—micrograms; moderate quantities, moderate scale—milligrams. In still-larger amounts, we go to the apothecary system. The easiest way to give some idea of the most common measurement there is, the grain (gr), is to say it equals about 65 milligrams, or one-fifteenth of a gram.

Liquids, such as wheat germ oil in capsule form, are often measured in apothecary system, too. The apothecary unit of measurement for them is a minim (min) and is approximately equal in volume to one drop of water.

For quick reference here is a summary:

| Activity-Based Measurements | |
|---|---|
| **Unit of Measure** | **Used to Measure** |
| International Unit (I.U.) | Vitamins A, D, E |
| United States Pharmacopeia Unit (U.S.P.) | Vitamins A, D, E |

The standards for the I.U. and U.S.P. measurements are almost identical. The standard I.U. for vitamin A is defined as the activity of 0.6 micrograms of beta-carotene; the standard for vitamin D is the activity of .025 micrograms pure crystalline vitamin D; the standard for vitamin E is the activity of one milligram of a synthetic racemic alpha-tocopherol acetate.

| Quantity-Based Measurements | | |
|---|---|---|
| **Unit of Measure** | **Equal to** | **Used to Measure** |
| microgram (mcg) | 1/1,000,000 gram | Other vitamins and minerals in smaller amounts |
| milligram (mg) | 1/1,000 gram | Other vitamins and minerals in moderate amounts |
| grain (gr) | about 65 mg | Other vitamins and minerals in larger amounts |
| minim (min) | about 1 drop water | Vitamins and minerals in liquid form |

# Understanding the RDA and the MDR

Once you understand the standards of vitamin measurement, how can you tell what doses of vitamins and minerals you should be taking? Every supplement label has a listing of the amount of each nutrient in the container. Along with the dosage, you will find a column showing what percentage of the MDR or the RDA of that particular nutrient the dosage is. The MDR and the RDA are standards of average nutritional needs established by the federal government.

The MDR, which stands for the Minimum Daily Requirement, is the very smallest amount of a particular nutrient that must be consumed daily by the average person to prevent an actual deficiency disease. The MDR is also sometimes listed as the MDAR, or the Minimum Daily Adult Requirement. The MDR has not been established for all the known essential nutrients, but for only a few of the better-known vitamins and minerals that have been more extensively researched.

| Minimum Daily Requirements | | | | | | |
|---|---|---|---|---|---|---|
| | Infants | Children (1–5) | Children (6–11) | Children (12–over) | Adults | Pregnancy Lactation |
| Vitamin A .... | 1500 I.U. | 3000 I.U. | 3000 I.U. | 4000 I.U. | 4000 I.U. | .... |
| Thiamine (B₁) . | .25 mg. | .50 mg. | .75 mg. | 1 mg. | 1 mg. | .... |
| Riboflavin (B₂) | .6 mg. | .9 mg. | .9 mg. | .9 mg. | 1.2 mg. | .... |
| Niacin (B₄) ... | .... | 5 mg. | 5 mg. | 5 mg. | 10 mg. | .... |
| Vitamin C .... | 10 mg. | 20 mg. | 20 mg. | 30 mg. | 30 mg. | .... |
| Vitamin D .... | 400 I.U. | 400 I.U. | 400 I.U. | 400 I.U. | * | .... |
| Calcium ...... | .... | .75 mg. | .75 grams | .75 grams | .75 grams | 1.50 gr. |
| Phosphorus ... | .... | 75 gr. | .75 gr. | .75 gr. | .75 gr. | 1.50 gr. |
| Iron ......... | .... | 7.5 mg. | 10 mg. | 10 mg. | 10 mg. | 15 mg. |
| Iodine........ | .... | .1 mg. | .1 mg. | .1 mg. | .1 mg. | .1 mg. |

Originally established by the Food and Drug Administration in 1941, the MDRs are now considered obsolete and have been replaced by the more up-to-date RDAs.

When you see RDA on a supplement label, it is referring to the United States Recommended Daily Allowances (U.S. RDA). The U.S. RDAs are amounts of 19 vitamins and minerals established by the Food and Drug Administration in 1973 to replace the MDR. While it is a more complete listing than the MDR, human requirements for many nutrients have still not been officially established. Although the U.S. RDAs are broken down into three age groups and one group for pregnant or lactating women, only one listing of the RDAs appears on supplement labels. This listing refers to the allowances set for adults.

## What Do the RDAs Tell Us?

Just what do these standards mean to the consumer? Many people wrongly assume that the U.S. RDAs are all that anyone needs to fulfill nutritional requirements. Actually, the U.S. RDAs are based on averages of different population groups to determine how much of a particular nutrient is needed to maintain good health in the average healthy person.

However, in a world comprised of individuals, one would be

hard-pressed to find an *average* person. According to the Food and Nutrition Board of the National Research Council, the organization which establishes the more detailed figures on which the U.S. RDAs are based, " . . . it is only within the framework of statistical probability that RDA can be used legitimately and meaningfully. . . . One individual with low requirements might have a high intake of a specific nutrient and another with a high requirement might have a low intake—but the average would give no indication that one of the two had an inadequate diet." *(Recommended Dietary Allowances,* Eighth Revised Edition, National Academy of Sciences, 1974).

Furthermore, the statistical averages of nutritional intakes do not take into consideration nutrient losses due to food storage and processing, the adverse effects of illness or any type of stress which can increase nutritional demands, or what the Food

| United States Recommended Daily Allowances (US-RDA) | | | | |
|---|---|---|---|---|
| | Infants (0–12 mo.) | Children under 4 yrs. | Adults and children 4 or more yrs. | Pregnant or lactating women |
| Vitamin A | 1500 IU | 2500 IU | 5000 IU | 8000 IU |
| Vitamin D | 400 IU | 400 IU | 400 IU | 400 IU |
| Vitamin E | 5 IU | 10 IU | 30 IU | 30 IU |
| Vitamin C | 35 mg | 40 mg | 60 mg | 60 mg |
| Folic Acid | 0.1 mg | 0.2 mg | 0.4 mg | 0.8 mg |
| Thiamine ($B_1$) | 0.5 mg | 0.7 mg | 1.5 mg | 1.7 mg |
| Riboflavin ($B_2$) | 0.6 mg | 0.8 mg | 1.7 mg | 2 mg |
| Niacin | 8 mg | 9 mg | 20 mg | 20 mg |
| Vitamin $B_6$ | 0.4 mg | 0.7 mg | 2 mg | 2.5 mg |
| Vitamin $B_{12}$ | 2 mcg | 3 mcg | 6 mcg | 8 mcg |
| Biotin | 0.05 mg | 0.15 mg | 0.3 mg | 0.3 mg |
| Pantothenic acid | 3 mg | 5 mg | 10 mg | 10 mg |
| Calcium | 0.6 g | 0.8 g | 1 g | 1.3 g |
| Phosphorus | 0.5 g | 0.8 g | 1 g | 1.3 g |
| Iodine | 45 mcg | 70 mcg | 150 mcg | 150 mcg |
| Iron | 15 mg | 10 mg | 18 mg | 18 mg |
| Magnesium | 70 mg | 200 mg | 400 mg | 450 mg |
| Copper | 0.6 mg | 1 mg | 2 mg | 2 mg |
| Zinc | 5 mg | 8 mg | 15 mg | 15 mg |

and Nutrition Board calls the "unrecognized nutritional benefits of foods." These unrecognized benefits include any kind of nutritional program designed for *maximum* health benefits or *preventive* health measures.

If all this is true, of what use are the U.S. RDAs?

They serve as a reference point against which the consumer can compare the amount of a nutrient he is buying. For example, in the sample label shown below, the consumer can readily see that this particular supplement contains relatively large amounts of thiamine and riboflavin, and relatively small amounts of vitamin B₆ and pantothenic acid.

### MULTI-VITAMINS

*Each 2 Capsules Contain:*

| | | *RDA% |
|---|---|---|
| Vitamin-A (Fish Liver Oil) . . . . . . . . . | 10,000 I.U. | 200% |
| Vitamin-D . . . . . . . . . . . . . . . . . . . . . | 400 I.U. | 100% |
| Vitamin-E . . . . . . . . . . . . . . . . . . . . | 75 I.U. | 249% |
| Vitamin-C (with Rose Hips) . . . . . . . | 210.0 mg. | 350% |
| Folic Acid . . . . . . . . . . . . . . . . . . . . | 60.0 mcg. | 15% |
| Thiamine (Vitamin B-1) . . . . . . . . . . | 7.0 mg. | 466% |
| Riboflavin (Vitamin B-2) . . . . . . . . . . | 14.0 mg. | 823% |
| Niacin . . . . . . . . . . . . . . . . . . . . . . . | 4.5 mg. | 22.5% |
| Vitamin B-6 . . . . . . . . . . . . . . . . . . . | 72.0 mcg. | 3.0% |
| Vitamin B-12 . . . . . . . . . . . . . . . . . . | 25.0 mcg. | 415% |
| Pantothenic Acid . . . . . . . . . . . . . . . | 200.0 mcg. | 1.8% |
| Choline . . . . . . . . . . . . . . . . . . . . . . | 6.2 mg. | ** |
| Inositol . . . . . . . . . . . . . . . . . . . . . . | 8.3 mg. | ** |
| L. Lysine Hydrochloride . . . . . . . . . . | 50.0 mg. | *** |
| Nucleic Acid . . . . . . . . . . . . . . . . . . | 75.0 mg. | *** |
| Debittered Brewer's Yeast . . . . . . . . | 100.0 mg. | *** |

*U.S. Recommended Daily Allowance. (U.S. RDA)
**Need in human nutrition established, but no RDA established.
***Need in human nutrition not established.

Many noted nutritionists believe that the U.S. RDAs should be used as a basis for nutritional planning, to which extra amounts and additional nutrients should be added, as dictated by dietary habits, work demands, general physical condition, age, and sex.

The type of vitamins you purchase and the care you take in storing them are also highly significant to their potency. Manufacturers produce their products to keep their potency for at least six months to a year before opening. Once they are opened, they should be refrigerated to maintain potency. The government spot-checks nutritional supplements to be sure they contain the advertised potency. Manufacturers realize potency tends to dwindle with age, and therefore they usually put *more* than the advertised amount of each vitamin in their products. Because the potency does diminish with age, don't "stock up" on vitamins. Why let them lose strength on the shelf? The fresher the better.

# CHAPTER 7

# Guidelines for Choosing a Vitamin Supplement

Hundreds of vitamin supplements are available today, but selecting one that is right for you can present quite a dilemma. The very number and variety leaves many people helplessly confused. While no vitamin supplement can be singled out as the best for everyone, there are guidelines that can make selecting one easier. Knowing what is available and what the differences are can help, too.

No single vitamin or limited group of vitamins is all-important. Vitamins work together with other vitamins, and with proteins, minerals, fatty acids, and probably with other nutritional elements that have not yet been identified.

Unfortunately, many people have a tendency to take only a few of the more popular vitamins. Roger J. Williams, Ph.D., D. Sc., a noted nutritionist and professor of chemistry, discusses this problem in a chapter entitled "The Role of Nutritional Supplements" in his latest book, *Physicians' Handbook of Nutritional Science* (Springfield, Illinois: Charles C. Thomas, 1975):

"Perhaps in no way have people in general exhibited the nutritional illiteracy (to borrow a phrase from H. J. Heinz, Jr.) more consistently than in the way they take their vitamins. One person, a former college president, was reported to me as having taken two tablets of vitamin B6, thinking this was the same as vitamin $B_{12}$. If people start taking a widely publicized brand of vitamins, they are likely to continue (if at all) without reference to new developments or the contents of the preparation, so long as it is well advertised.

"The use of supplements began when only a few vitamins had been discovered, and they were thought of as magic wands. Wand A, wand B, wand C, and wand D gradually became available for waving. With the advent of more knowledge about nutrients, their number, their functioning, and their interrelations, there should have been a revolutionary change in attitude, but there has been a strong tendency to stick by the old favorites.

"In the 1940s the high priests and priestesses of nutrition thought the nutritional situation had settled down, and there were about six major concerns: vitamins A and D, thiamine, riboflavin, niacin, and iron. Calcium, iodine, and ascorbic acid were perhaps minor concerns. All these substances were available candidates for inclusion in nutritional supplements. The fact that four of these—thiamine, riboflavin, niacin, and iron—were being added to bread and flour did not diminish their strong appeal; they were general favorites and were furnished in supplements, often as the principal ingredients.

"Currently the entire list of known nutrients (minerals, trace minerals, amino acids, and vitamins) needs to be brought into view when and if supplements are formulated, because every cog is an essential one, and there is no ruling out the importance of any nutrient."

## Multiple Supplements— What Should They Offer You?

In an effort to get a more complete supplement package, many people take multiple vitamin and mineral supplements every day. Some rely on all-in-one tablets to meet their supplementary needs. Others take multiples in addition to various individual supplements for the maximum degree of nutritional insurance. In either case, most people choose multiples because of their convenience. The idea of wrapping up several nutrients in a common tablet is an appealing one; it helps uncomplicate life a little bit. In addition, a great many people assume that by taking a multiple supplement, they are getting the nutrients they need in a carefully formulated and scientifically balanced form. This is often true, but as we'll see, it's not *always* the case.

When comparing multiple supplements, pay special attention to how complete the supplement is; (does it supply all the vitamins and minerals you need?) and examine the potencies of the nutrients offered carefully. (Potencies should at least be equal to the United States Recommended Daily Allowances.) Most multiples have their strong points and their weak points. A few commit serious sins of omission. Only by taking a close look at the label on your own supplement can you tell exactly where you stand.

A good multiple supplement should contain vitamins A, D, C, the B complex, vitamin E, and a good selection of minerals. Let's take a closer look at each one of these to understand better what to look for.

Almost every multiple does a good job of delivering vitamin A, so valuable for a healthy complexion, good vision, and resistance to infection. More likely than not, the label of a good supplement will list 10,000 I.U. of vitamin A, well above the adult RDA of 5,000 I.U.

Vitamin D is another nutrient whose presence is virtually automatic in a good supplement. In this case, 400 I.U. is the figure to look for. Because of its importance in the bone-building process, vitamin D makes an excellent and logical addition to multiples that also contain minerals.

Vitamin C is one item you should check very closely. Many multiples don't provide this important nutrient in anywhere near the amounts proven effective in resisting colds and other ailments. If you're counting on the multiple to fill your vitamin C needs, it should have no less than 100 to 200 mg. Your best bet here is to find a multiple you like for other reasons and then also take an individual vitamin C supplement if your needs are greater.

# B Complex—Key to a Good Multiple

The key to a really good multiple supplement is how adequately it provides the B complex of vitamins. Some products are not well balanced, offering large doses of certain factors (usually vitamins $B_1$ and $B_2$) while stinting on niacin or other factors. In addition, some parts of the B complex may be left out entirely. Today, new formulas are available which are more complete and potent. Whether you are shopping for a total multiple or simply a multiple B complex product, it pays to inspect the label very carefully.

There's usually no problem getting enough thiamine ($B_1$), the "morale" vitamin. According to the RDAs, most adults need between 1.0 and 2.0 mg. of $B_1$, depending on sex and age. Almost any good multiple will supply that and then some. In fact, it's not uncommon to find supplements containing 10 mg. of thiamine. Like all the B vitamins, thiamine is water-soluble; any excess is simply excreted. There's no danger of toxicity.

Right below thiamine on most labels, you'll find riboflavin, or vitamin $B_2$. The adult RDAs for riboflavin also fall between 1.0 and 2.0 mg., but people generally need slightly more riboflavin than thiamine every day. Most supplements contain adequate to generous amounts of $B_2$, ranging from one to several times the RDA.

It was mentioned earlier that niacin, or vitamin $B_3$, is sometimes undersupplied in multiples. RDAs for niacin range from 10 to 20 mg., or ten times as much as $B_1$ or $B_2$. Yet there is often less niacin in a supplement than there is thiamine or riboflavin. It's true that our bodies can make extra niacin from protein-rich foods (the amino acid tryptophan is a precursor of niacin), but that's no reason to sell yourself short when buying a supplement. Look for at least 10 mg. of niacin in your multiple, preferably more. Disregard completely any niacin potency that falls after a decimal point, such as 0.6 mg.—it's an insignificant amount.

One of the best ways to determine just how complete a multiple you are taking is to check its vitamin $B_6$ or pyridoxine potency. This long-neglected nutrient is gaining new stature among medical researchers and clinicians. Vitamin B6 has been found protective in a wide variety of conditions, ranging from convulsions to arthritic-like swelling to female problems associated with menstruation and menopause. And there is evidence that many Americans aren't getting enough of this nutrient; oral contraceptives, for example, deplete B6 in the body. An adult RDA of 2.0 mg. (2.5 mg. for pregnant and lactating females) has been established, and there are indications that this is a very conservative estimate of our needs. Yet some multiple supplements are still supplying B6 in micrograms (mcg.), not milligrams (mg.). (A microgram is just one-thousandth of a milligram.) Why settle for any B6 potency expressed in micrograms, when there are formulas available containing as much as five to 10 *milligrams*?

Because we need such small amounts, vitamin B12 is one of the few nutrients whose potency should properly be expressed in micrograms (folic acid, biotin, and iodine are others). The RDA for this potent blood-builder is 6.0 mcg. For expectant or nursing mothers it is increased to 8.0 mcg. You should have no trouble finding a multiple supplement supplying at least these potencies of B12.

## Folic Acid and Other Essential B Vitamins

Folic acid is an extremely important part of the B complex, vital for healthy blood, and especially needed by pregnant and lactating women whose stores are usually depleted. Yet, until quite recently, most multivitamins contained very little or no folic acid. Now some of the better multiples on the market contain 300 mcg. or more of folic acid. Women are better off with 400 mcg. (.4 mg.) of folic acid. Products containing less than 100 mcg. of folic acid (and some provide considerably less) really aren't supplying this important B vitamin in anywhere near optimum amounts. Many popular multivitamin formulations sold in drugstores omit folic acid completely!

Pantothenic acid is another essential but relatively unknown member of the B complex. While an official RDA has not yet been set by the Food and Nutrition Board of the National Research Council, that body warns that "marginal deficiencies may well exist in generally malnourished individuals" (*Recommended Dietary Allowances*, Eighth Revised Edition, 1974). Many nutritionists believe we need at least 10 mg. of this nutrient daily. A good multiple will supply that amount or more. On the other hand, you should be aware that some products contain as little as 100 or 200 *micrograms* of pantothenic acid. As with B₆, the use of the abbreviation *mcg.* should serve as fair warning.

No supplement of the B complex would be complete without biotin, inositol, choline, and PABA (para-aminobenzoic acid). Choline and biotin are both essential nutrients, although RDAs have been established only for biotin. The adult RDA for biotin is 300 mcg., but exact requirements in the human diet for both nutrients are still debated. The picture is clouded by the fact that we are apparently able to synthesize both these nutrients to some extent inside the digestive tract. But deficiencies can still occur—a certain type of stubborn dermatitis, for example, has been found to respond only to biotin supplementation. It's estimated that a typical diet supplies from 100 to 300 mcg. of biotin daily. The same amount of food supplies an estimated 400 to 900 mg. of choline. The essentiality of inositol and PABA to human beings has not yet been officially established, but the average diet supplies about 1,000 mg. of inositol and anywhere from 2.0 grams (2,000 mg.) to 6.0 grams of PABA have been used therapeutically.

The point is, as long as you're taking the B complex daily, you might as well be taking the *whole* B complex with all the associated factors found in nature, and in meaningful amounts. Some multiples omit choline, inositol, biotin, and PABA; others provide insignificant amounts. Look for products that express their potency of choline, inositol, and PABA in milligrams, not micrograms.

One final word on the B complex. Many supplements containing the B vitamins are prepared in a base of yeast, and therefore contain tiny amounts of various other nutrients—such as chromium—which naturally occur in yeast. This is good, but you can't depend on multiples to supply anywhere near enough yeast to meet your needs for such trace nutrients. For chromium and other factors naturally inherent in yeast, there's no substitute for taking a brewer's yeast supplement every day.

## Vitamin E Often Inadequate

Vitamin E is often a weak spot in multiple supplement products. For example, some multiples provide only 60 I.U., 40 I.U., or less of vitamin E. And some of the most popular synthetic products marketed by the large pharmaceutical companies supply as little as five I.U. You'll have to search hard to find a multivitamin offering 100 I.U. or more. In this case, probably the best bet is to take additional vitamin E supplements along with your multiple.

## Mineral Content is Critical

Mineral nutrition is one area where the gap between drugstore products and formulas from natural food sources is at its widest. No multiple supplement or nutritional program can be called complete without the addition of minerals. In general, many of the popular drugstore varieties fall down completely, offering pitifully small amounts of certain minerals, illogically selected. Such products just haven't kept pace with scientific findings of recent years highlighting the vital role of minerals in good health.

A good example is calcium. Medical investigators now know that a high intake of this bone-building mineral is absolutely essential if the ravages of osteoporosis are to be avoided in later years. Studies indicate that a daily calcium intake of 1,000 mg. (one gram) or more is most desirable—a difficult goal to reach from food sources alone. For that reason, 600 to 800 mg. or more of supplementary calcium a day makes sense. Some multi-mineral products made with bone meal and other sources do provide such potency. Check the label on a typical drugstore variety multiple, however, and you're liable to find just 30 or 60 mg. of calcium.

Many labels will also list phosphorus among the minerals. Our bodies need phosphorus to help absorb calcium and produce strong new bone. It is generally believed that a calcium-to-phosphorus ratio of two to one is best. A multimineral product derived from bone meal will provide this ratio naturally.

With so many Americans facing the prospect of iron-deficiency anemia at some time in their lives, iron is a very important mineral nutrient. For this reason, virtually every multivitamin supplement contains at least 10 mg. of iron—the RDA for adult males. But most women need even more iron—about 18 mg. daily. So women should read the small print even more closely where iron is concerned.

## Magnesium and Zinc

Magnesium is a major weak spot in many multiple formulations. The RDA for this important mineral is 400 mg. for adults. Yet many products supply magnesium in extremely small amounts—4.0 or 6.0 mg., for example. The best way to get around this shortcoming is by taking a magnesium supplement every day. Either dolomite or magnesium oxide tablets can provide you with hundreds of milligrams of magnesium daily—the kind of potency that makes sense.

A good multiple supplement also contains iodine, and almost certainly in adequate amounts. Most multiples provide from 100 to 150 mcg. (0.1 to 0.15 mg.) of this trace mineral—enough to cover the RDA.

Zinc is another matter. Some multiples contain this important mineral; some don't. Many products now provide a full 30 mg. of zinc (twice the RDA), but others omit it completely or include it in small amounts. A zinc potency expressed in micrograms or even 1.0 or 2.0 mg. obviously isn't worth much. You can get around this by taking an additional zinc gluconate supplement daily.

Other trace minerals such as copper and manganese may also

be listed on the label. These elements are essential to human health, but generally we need them in very small amounts—2.0 mg. each is probably adequate, and at least part of that is supplied by our food.

# Read the Labels Carefully

Always read the labels of supplements carefully, and be just as conscious of what has been omitted as of what is listed. Don't be fooled into thinking that a supplement that supplies "10 essential vitamins, plus iron" is giving you all the nutrients you need. Pay close attention to the potencies, and don't confuse mcg. (micrograms) with mg. (milligrams). A decimal point can also be deceptive—0.6 mg. is a far cry from 6.0 mg.

Other food factors such as bran, desiccated liver, wheat germ oil, pectin, and various amino acids may also be listed at the bottom of multiple supplement labels—often because they are part of the base used in putting together the tablet. However, their presence is generally without nutritional significance since they are not provided in really preventive amounts. To get the benefit of such factors, you would have to take them separately as individual supplements. Only then would you be consuming them in meaningful amounts. Exceptions to this are rutin and other parts of the bioflavonoid complex. If the multiple contains 50 to 100 mg. or more of those factors, it is at least getting into the lower range of therapeutic value. (Clinical investigators have used from 60 to 600 mg. of rutin, for example, to strengthen capillary walls and also to treat bleeding gums.)

Sometimes you will see a list of ingredients resembling this one:

| | |
|---|---|
| Folic Acid, Choline | 880 mcg. |
| Protein | 120 mg. |
| Arginine | 7 mg. |
| Histidine | 3.0 mg. |
| Lysine | 8.5 mg. |
| Tyrosine | 4.1 mg. |

| | |
|---|---|
| Tryptophane | 1.3 mg. |
| Phenylalanine | 3.5 mg. |
| Cystine | 1.2 mg. |
| Methionine | 1.8 mg. |
| Glycine | 4.9 mg. |
| Threonine | 5.7 mg. |
| Leucine | 7.5 mg. |
| Isoleucine | 5.4 mg. |
| Valine | 6.0 mg. |
| Potassium | 4.3 mg. |

While the list may look impressive, it is basically meaningless. Except for the folic acid, choline, and potassium, these are insignificant amounts of amino acids, constituents of protein. Anyone can (and usually does) get much greater amounts of all of these nutrients in a normal meal.

Not all multiple supplements are the one-pill-a-day type. Your multiple's recommended dosage may be one, two, three, or even six tablets daily. Or you may be taking both a multivitamin and a multimineral preparation. This is largely a matter of personal preference. Sometimes it just isn't possible to pack a really complete formula into a single tablet, especially when you're dealing with nutrients from bulkier natural sources such as bone meal, fish liver oil, or yeast. But be sure to check on how many tablets should be taken when comparing prices, since 100 tablets of a supplement that must be taken three times a day is really about the same supply as 30 tablets of a one-a-day supplement.

An alternative to buying a multiple vitamin supplement is putting your own together. By buying individual vitamins and designing your own supplement program, you have the advantage of a multiple supplement that meets your own personal needs. The cost usually will be more than the average multiple supplement, but the advantages may be worth it to some.

Just remember that every multiple supplement must be judged on its own merits. If you want the convenience of this form of supplementation, you must examine, compare, and pick out the one you think is best for you. No multiple formulation is perfect.

Each will have its strong points and its weak points. Vitamin E, magnesium, folic acid, and vitamin B₆ are among those nutrients most likely to be lacking or poorly supplied. A deficiency in one area does not necessarily mean that a particular product is not worthwhile. But you should be able to recognize weak points, and be prepared to compensate for them.

**Editor's Note:**

Potencies suggested in this chapter are appropriate for routine multivitamin/mineral supplementation. They are rough guidelines, not dogma. People with health problems or higher-than-normal requirements of certain nutrients may want to take individual supplements in addition to a multiple. A woman with a tendency to osteoporosis, for instance, should be taking at least 1,000 mg. of calcium, unless otherwise instructed. A person with circulatory problems might be better off with 400-800 or more units of vitamin E than with only 100-200. And many others will want considerably more vitamin C.

Because no multiple vitamin can provide meaningful amounts of fiber, yeast, pectin, and other important food factors, most readers will want to take a number of concentrated food supplements daily, along with their multivitamin. If you take a multiple daily, think of it as just one part of your total preventive health program—albeit a very substantial part, if you select your formulation wisely.

# CHAPTER 8

# Vitamin Antagonists

Many reasonable people are convinced that taking vitamin supplements is a waste of time and money. They believe that a person gets plenty of vitamins in a good regular diet. If not, how did the human race make it to the twentieth century when vitamin supplements were first introduced? Until then people had to get their vitamins from their foods and they got along well enough without having the Harvard Medical School and the United States Department of Agriculture set standards for proper vitamin rations. Why are we complicating everything so?

The problem is that our whole way of life has become complicated, food included. What happens to foods in modern societies between the harvest and the table is antagonistic to original vitamin values. We process most of our foods and any food processing takes its toll in the vitamin content of that food.

But the complexities of modern living go far beyond food processing in limiting our nutrition supply. When we created factories, automobiles, jet planes, and atomic power stations we created air pollutants that systematically erode our vitamin stores. Drugs such as antibiotics, oral contraceptives, and steroids became additional threats to the vitamin stores in our bodies. When white sugar became available to the masses, about a hundred years ago, serious losses of the B vitamins became inevitable for those who consumed excessive amounts of this dietary favorite. Many of us drink alcoholic beverages, smoke cigarettes, and swallow aspirin by the handful. Each one of these is antagonistic toward vitamin stores.

Are you a victim of vitamin antagonists? The following chart will give you a basis for deciding that for yourself. If, through some good fortune, you have managed to side-step many or most of the threats to your vitamin stores, you may be one of the lucky few who can do without supplementary vitamins. If, on the other hand, your daily habits take their toll in nutrition, this chart will help you decide how to meet your basic vitamin needs.

| Vitamins | Prominent Antagonists | Primary Allies |
|----------|----------------------|----------------|
| Vitamin A | mineral oil<br>nitrates from high<br>    nitrogen fertilizers<br>ozone, nitrogen dioxide<br>    (air pollutants) | protein<br>vitamin E |
| Thiamine B$_1$ | heat (cooking)<br>excess sugar consumption<br>antibiotics<br>stress conditions (preg-<br>    nancy, lactation,<br>    fever, surgery)<br>alcohol | entire B complex<br>vitamin C<br>vitamin E |
| Riboflavin B$_2$ | exposure to direct light<br>heat (cooking)<br>antibiotics<br>alcohol<br>oral contraceptives | entire B complex<br>vitamin C |
| Niacin B$_3$ | excess sugar consumption<br>heat (cooking)<br>antibiotics<br>alcohol<br>during illness, niacin<br>    absorption by the<br>    intestines is decreased | entire B complex<br>vitamin C |
| Pyridoxine B$_6$ | steroid hormones<br>    (cortisone and estrogen)<br>aging (after age 50,<br>    pyridoxine levels<br>    decline rapidly) | entire B complex<br>magnesium<br>vitamin C |

| Vitamins | Prominent Antagonists | Primary Allies |
|---|---|---|
| Folic Acid | heat (cooking)<br>food processing<br>high protein diets ($B_6$ intake must also be increased)<br>severe stress situations (surgery)<br>oral contraceptives<br>vitamin C deficiency<br>alcohol | complete B complex<br>vitamin C |
| Vitamin $B_{12}$ | iron-deficiency (prolonged)<br>oral contraceptives<br>stress situations (pregnancy)<br>vegetarianism (if all animal products and by-products are avoided) | complete B complex<br>vitamin C |
| Biotin | heat (cooking)<br>avidin (found in raw egg whites)<br>antibiotics<br>sulfa drugs | complete B complex<br>vitamin C |
| Choline | alcohol<br>excessive sugar consumption | complete B complex<br>vitamin A |
| Inositol | antibiotics (by destroying intestinal bacteria) | complete B complex<br>vitamin E<br>vitamin C |
| Pantothenic Acid | methyl bromide (insecticide fumigant for foods) | complete B complex<br>calcium<br>vitamin C |
| Vitamin C | aspirin<br>corticosteroids<br>indomethacin<br>fatigue<br>stress situations (surgery)<br>smoking<br>alcohol<br>diabetic state | vitamin B complex<br>vitamin P (bioflavonoids) |

| Vitamins | Prominent Antagonists | Primary Allies |
|---|---|---|
| **Vitamin D** | insufficient exposure to ultraviolet light | calcium<br>vitamin A<br>vitamin C |
| **Vitamin E** | oral contraceptives<br>food processing<br>inorganic iron (ferric) compounds<br>rancid fats and oils<br>mineral oil | vitamin A<br>vitamin C<br>B complex<br>selenium<br>manganese |
| **Vitamin K** | antibiotics<br>intestinal illnesses (diarrhea, colitis)<br>anticoagulants<br>mineral oil<br>radiation | |
| **Vitamin P (bioflavonoids)** | | vitamin C |

# CHAPTER 9

# Nutritional Freedom:
# Can the Government
# Limit Your Vitamin Intake?

On 20 June 1962, a notice was published in the *Federal Register* announcing that the Food and Drug Administration was making some basic changes in the existing vitamin regulations which had gone virtually unchanged since 1941.

Among a grab-bag of proposals, two were particularly significant. One provision stated that the label on all supplements could list *only* those nutrients recognized by competent authorities as essential and of significance in· human nutrition. These included vitamins A, B6, B12, C, D, thiamine, riboflavin, niacin, calcium, phosphorus, iron, and iodine.

As for other vitamins and minerals that were regarded as essential in the diet, they were considered so plentiful that no implications should be made that they were of any value in the product by listing them with the other 12 approved vitamins and minerals.

Another proposal called for minimum and maximum amounts of recognized nutrients to be set out on the label for both children and adults as Recommended Daily Allowances (RDA) instead of the Minimum Daily Requirements (MDR). As is the practice with most announcements of this nature that appear in the *Register*, the FDA gave all interested parties a chance to comment on the proposals.

It wasn't long before those comments came in and the FDA found itself being buried under a nation-wide barrage of criticism such as it had never experienced in its long history. An estimated 54,000 pieces of mail—an absolutely astounding number for pre-Viet Nam and pre-Watergate days—landed on bureaucrats' desks in Washington all demanding the same thing: rescind the proposals that threaten to take away the individual's nutritional freedom of choice.

The then FDA commissioner George P. Larrick defended the proposals on the grounds that they protected the consumer who wasn't informed enough to make his own decisions. "The average purchaser of vitamin-mineral supplements is not well informed about his needs for supplementing his usual diet with these nutritional factors. He easily can be led to believe that his diet is likely to be inadequate in one or several of these nutrients, and that a great many conditions of ill health may result from his possibly inadequate diet."

Commissioner Larrick went on to say that the labeling change was necessary to discourage the addition of needlessly large amounts of vitamins and minerals to food supplements simply as a sales promotion device. He maintained, overall, the consumer ought to be protected by the new regulations, not harmed by them.

## FDA Calls "Time Out"

The public was not swayed by these arguments and the criticism continued unabated. Finally, the FDA withdrew the proposals and no public hearings were ever held on them. Although the onerous provisions had become history, the FDA hadn't given up on the plans to introduce them. The agency merely called a "time out" to regroup.

There is no apparent answer to the question of why the FDA decided to go after vitamin consumption just then and in that way. Commissioner Larrick said at that time, that it was an attempt to take advantage of the significant increase in the knowledge of nutrition since the original regulations went into effect in 1941. For one thing, these had been designed to feed a nation going to war. In addition, great changes had taken place in the production and marketing of dietary foods. All of these reasons called for a major overhaul on the regulations, in Mr. Larrick's opinion. But why such a militant antivitamin stance?

There is no record that any single group pressured the FDA to take the antivitamin action. Of course the American Medical Association had always been against those who advocated taking supplements—except under doctor's orders—calling it "quackery." There's no evidence that industry pressured the government. However, both groups surely welcomed the FDA's move, since those who took supplements were inferring that they didn't believe they were being properly nourished by the foods available to them.

The decision to rewrite the vitamin regulations might have been just one of those bureaucratic decisions that surfaces as if by accident. What was astonishing about the whole vitamin question was the amount of protest generated by it and the bulldog determination with which the FDA carried on the fight.

The break in the action lasted almost four years to the day of the first *Federal Register* announcement. Then, on 18 June 1966, the FDA came back on the playing field wih a new set of regulations that were more all-inclusive, far more sweeping, and were of greater critical importance to both the health food industry and consumers than anything the now-retired George Larrick had ever envisioned.

That single announcement, probably more than anything else the FDA has ever done, made an indelible impression on the fabric of American life. It resulted in two years of FDA hearings which cost more than a million dollars in tax money. It stirred bitter debate in the halls of Congress where numerous bills guaranteeing nutritional freedom were introduced. This, of course, meant more lengthy hearings which ran into the early 1970s. Countless informational sessions on the "value" of supplements occurred across the country (and are still taking place).

Indeed, the regulations proved to be sweeping in nature.

They included some provisions for classifying diet foods and again called for the Recommended Daily Allowances to replace the Minimum Daily Requirements. More important, dietary supplements could not exceed the RDAs which had been established by the National Academy of Science—National Research Council.

The regulations also established eight classes of foods that could be fortified such as breakfast cereals and iodized salt and stipulated just what vitamins and minerals in what amounts could go into that fortification. And yet another provision prohibited what the FDA considered extravagant promotion of "shotgun" multivitamin and mineral supplements containing nutrients that the FDA said met no dietary need and tended to deceive the customer.

Under terms of the regulations, the manufacturers would not be able to say on the label that their product was from a natural source rather than from a synthetic one. Manufacturers couldn't say that a food or supplement was effective for the treatment or prevention of any ailment including diseases caused by deficiency of the nutrients contained in the supplement. In addition, advertising could not suggest that deficiencies could develop because ordinary foods lose nutritive value when they are grown in poor soil or because of losses in storage, transportation, processing, or cooking.

## Crepe Label

But probably the biggest outcry arose over the provision that later came to be known as the "crepe label" because of what it obviously would have meant to the consumer. It stipulated that *all* multivitamin and mineral supplements had to bear the following statement: "Vitamins and minerals are supplied in abundant amounts in the foods we eat. The Food and Nutrition Board of National Research Council recommends that dietary needs be satisfied by foods. Except for persons with special medical needs, there is no scientific basis for recommending routine use of dietary supplements."

Almost immediately, the "crepe label" came under fire from

some very important professional nutritionists and scientists around the country. Thomas H. Jukes, Ph.D., of the University of California at Berkeley wrote to the FDA saying that the very first sentence was a generalization that didn't apply to individual cases. "I do not think that any professor of nutrition would give a passing grade to a student who made such a statement." Then he added: "There is a strong basis for recommending routine use of dietary supplements to make sure that overt signs and symptoms do not develop in persons who have unrecognized special needs."

William H. Sebrell, M.D., of the National Academy of Sciences, the man who chaired the Food and Nutrition Board, complained bitterly about the "crepe label," saying it was "objectionable and misleading and uses the authority of the Food and Nutrition Board of the National Research Council to support a statement which, taken out of context, creates a false impression.

"The generalization that vitamins and minerals are supplied in abundant amounts in the foods that we eat has no relevance applied to a particular individual and there is abundant evidence that many individuals in the United States do not get all of the vitamins that they need from the foods that they eat."

George M. Owen, M.D., a pediatrician with Ohio State University Children's Hospital said, "It is mistakenly assumed that most people in this country receive a diet adequate in all respects simply because of the abundant food supply. The fact is, that the nutritional status of the people of the United States is not known and no one has a right to pass laws guessing at it. It is discouraging to see the government forming regulations pertaining to matters for which scientists have not yet provided enough information," he concluded.

Under the withering criticism of experts like Doctors Jukes, Sebrell, and Owen, the "crepe label" was bound to wind up on the cutting room floor—which it eventually did. However, what eventually took its place wasn't much better.

After two years of public hearings, which ran from 21 May 1968 to 14 May 1970, the so-called "final" regulations issued in

January, 1973, contained no "crepe label." However, one of the resulting provisions specified manufacturers could not state on the labels of their products that the nutrients contained in the package could be of any use whatsoever. It was not even permissible to state that the nutrients could prevent or cure a deficiency state of those very nutrients.

## Facts Established

If nothing else, two years of hearings established one startling fact: poor nutrition was widespread throughout the United States. According to the *Hearing Examiner's Report*, the document filed after the lengthy hearings, dietary habits appeared to have worsened. In addition, some foods did not contain abundant or sometimes even adequate amounts of some nutrients due to losses in transportation, storage, processing, and cooking.

Among other statements, the *Hearing Examiner's Report* contained two seemingly unconnected observations. One was that "frank, or obvious, apparent manifestations of vitamin or mineral deficiency disease is extremely rare, and, for deficiencies caused by the lack of some vitamins, non-existent in the United States." In other words, apparent vitamin deficiencies were non-existent.

The other statement noted that "the untrained or lay person is incapable of determining for himself whether he has or is likely to develop a vitamin or mineral deficiency." In other words, most people are not educated enough to know whether or not they need supplements, so they'd be better off just seeing a doctor.

The actual final vitamin regulations that were published in January, 1973, and were scheduled to go into effect that August, forced the consumer to rely heavily on medical authority since one of the provisions stated that any supplement in a dose larger than 150 percent of the RDA was classified as a drug and had to be prescribed by a doctor.

Besides the 150 percent limitation for supplements, the FDA

stated that no mineral or vitamin could be packaged in combination with any other vitamin or mineral unless the combination was one approved by the FDA. All combinations had to contain either all the vitamins, all the minerals, both, or all the vitamins and iron. No other combinations were to be permitted. If a vitamin preparation contained more than one vitamin, it had to contain vitamin A, vitamin E, vitamin C, thiamine, riboflavin, niacin, vitamin $B_6$, and vitamin $B_{12}$. Vitamin D, biotin, and pantothenic acid were considered optional.

If the product contained minerals as well as vitamins, it had to contain the following minerals: calcium, phosphorus, iodine, iron, and magnesium. Copper and zinc were considered optional as was phosphorus if the preparation was to be used for pregnant or lactating women.

Still another provision prohibited vitamins or minerals from being combined with any other associated food factors. It meant, for example, that the bioflavonoid complex could not be packaged in the same supplement as vitamin C, even though these two substances were usually found together in nature. Many others fell into the same category.

While the FDA was, in fact, holding a trial on vitamins and sitting as the judge and jury, pressure began building up on the U.S. Congress to thwart the FDA's efforts. Among those who immediately responded to the call were now-retired Congressman Craig Hosmer from California and Senator William Proxmire from Wisconsin.

## FDA Opposed

When it became apparent that the FDA was going through with its plans severely to limit nutritional freedom, in 1966 Rep. Hosmer introduced a bill to prevent just such a move. In a speech on the floor of the House before his colleagues, Rep. Hosmer said, "I have been told there has never been an accidental death due to vitamin overdosage, but it is said that one person dies every three days from taking lethal doses of aspirin which the FDA permits to go unlabeled.

"People may not generally have a physical need for food supplements, but if they feel that they are helped, then the FDA should leave them alone. No one, neither the FDA nor medical practitioners, should have a monopoly on a simple therapy where no danger is involved. Freedom of choice should be routine in a healthy society," he said.

Hosmer quickly gained the support for his bill from his colleagues and before long it had a number of co-sponsors. Across Capitol Hill in the U.S. Senate, Senator Proxmire was gathering support for his version of the Hosmer Bill. However, before either of the bills had a chance to pass, the courts intervened.

The FDA's January, 1973, action had been subject to legal action in addition to the violent criticism. On 15 August 1974, Judge Henry J. Friendly, of the United States Court of Appeals for the Second Circuit in New York, dealt the FDA a serious setback when he invalidated a number of the FDA regulations.

In the first place, he delayed the implementation of any regulations for at least six months. Perhaps more important, he completely disallowed the provision that any supplement over 150 percent of the RDA was to be classified as a drug. Instead, it remained classified as a food or mineral supplement. Judge Friendly also directed the FDA to allow supplement manufacturers to market additional combinations which the FDA had previously disallowed.

Judge Friendly's decision did not apply to vitamins A and D. In a separate case, the court broadly construed the FDA's power to classify these as prescription drugs because of toxicity, and indicated that there was ample basis to classify the two vitamins at higher potencies as prescription drugs. As the regulations now stand, prescriptions are needed to buy vitamin A capsules at levels higher than 10,000 International Units and vitamin D in supplements greater than 400 International Units because of potential toxic effects. However, a suit seeking to nullify this regulation is still winding its way through the court system and may eventually wind up before the Supreme Court.

While Judge Friendly's decision may have forced the FDA to

back down from its hard-line stand against health food supplement, Congressional critics aren't taking any chances. Action is expected on a bill which would write into law many of the safeguards needed to insure that nutritional freedom remains a fact and not just a temporary measure that the FDA can regulate away in some future issue of the *Federal Register*.

Following months and months of parliamentary maneuvering, a nutritional freedom bill passed both houses and was signed into law by President Gerald Ford in April, 1976. The bill specifically guarantees the right of the American public to take nutritional supplements by prohibiting the Food and Drug Administration from classifying them as drugs subject to prescription.

In addition, the bill permits a broader selection of combinations to be sold.

The bill changes very little as far as the FDA's power goes. It is still charged with the responsibility of insuring wholesomeness, safety, and accurate labeling of all nutritional products. However, the FDA does assume the power to act jointly with the Federal Trade Commission in reviewing the advertising of nutritional supplements, a power it didn't have before.

# CHAPTER 10

# Why Are Vitamins a Touchy Topic in the Doctor's Office?

You may have been stymied in your efforts to get your doctor to take any interest in your nutrition beyond advising you to "eat a balanced diet" and to "get all the vitamins you need with your knife and fork." You may have been unable to find a dentist who not only fills the holes in your children's teeth but fills you in on dietary do's and don'ts that will prevent the need for the dentist's drill.

No matter how well you get along with the physician who watches your blood pressure and appraises the systolic beat of your heart, you have learned that vitamins are a "touchy" point in your relationship. The very mention of them makes the conversation take on an edgy tone.

Either you become annoyed because the doctor simply dismisses the notion that vitamins are worth talking about, or he gets upset because he interprets your interest in vitamins as a lack of faith in him!

The most prestigious journals published by and for the medical profession regularly carry reports of studies showing the wide gap between the average person's need for certain nutrients and his actual supply. Other journal articles demonstrate the values of vitamins as preventives or treatments for specific physical problems. Government health agencies frequently assail the nutritional status of the average citizen. Obviously nutritional concern is not synonymous with faddism. Yet most doctors seem to think of it in that way.

It may fall to those outside of the medical profession to foster a change in the doctors' negative attitude toward using nutrition as a specific weapon against disease. In recent years government agencies have become aware of increased nutritional inadequacies in the general population and the relationship of this situation to rising disease rates. Several presidential committees have formally recognized the need for change and Senator Richard S. Schweiker, Republican of Pennsylvania, has been particularly active in advocating a more realistic and useful approach to nutrition by medical men. In 1972 he wrote:

*Many diseases are related directly or indirectly to nutritional factors. In a follow-up report to the White House Conference on Food, Nutrition, and Health, the panel on Advanced Academic Teaching of Nutrition pointed out that:*

*"Atherosclerosis (including coronary heart disease), obesity, diabetes mellitus, hypertension, and osteoporosis are representative of many disorders in which nutritional factors are either of principal or contributory importance. In addition, new trends in food processing and environmental concerns require a great expansion of research in the area of trace minerals, 'secondary vitamins', pollutants, and involuntary and voluntary food additives. Much of the research directed toward these problems must be conducted by individuals who have received (or should receive) advanced academic training in nutrition."*

*Because of the importance of sound nutritional practices to the maintenance of health and prevention of medical disorders, doctors must have enough knowledge of the relationship between nutrition and good health to advise his patients how to help prevent medical problems from occurring. As the ranking minority member of the Health Subcommittee, I am very conscious of the great need for much more emphasis on preventive medicine in our health care system today. We should not just* treat medical problems after they have already become serious, but should use nutritional dietary practices as a key means of preventing these medical problems from arising in the first place.

In addition, many doctors today have not been given sufficient knowledge of nutrition to deal with the nutritional aspects of diseases patients already have. The White House panel said, for instance:

"The effectiveness of physicians in providing optimal care for the many patients who have diseases with an important nutritional component, is dependent in considerable part on the kind of nutrition teaching offered them at medical school and thereafter. At the present time, nutrition teaching in medical schools and in teaching hospitals is woefully inadequate."

Therefore, I believe it is essential that the fundamentals of nutrition be taught early in the medical school educational program, with follow-up courses which are more detailed and sophisticated.

A study by one medical school indicated that physicians questioned were more knowledgeable about theoretical aspects of nutrition than practical uses of nutrition in our daily lives. The study indicated that younger doctors did not know as much about nutrition as they should, but would like to know more. In contrast, many older doctors did not know much about nutrition, but did not feel that education in this area was needed.

Food faddism and "folk medicine" are becoming more popular today, and many people are turning away from physicians to obtain information about nutrition. I believe part of the problem is that many doctors simply are not in a position to provide nutritional information patients need and desire for the maintenance of good health. We urgently need more scientific information about nutrition and health. We need more and better nutrition research but we will not get it unless our medical schools are able to provide nutritional training and can impress upon young doctors the need for emphasizing good diets to help prevent illness or disease.

## Nutrition Needs Top Priority

*Only a few medical schools have separate divisions or departments of nutrition. Special courses in nutrition are rare, particularly in applied nutrition as opposed to the biochemical aspects of nutrition. There is a significant shortage of trained people in this field, and grants to stimulate the teaching of nutrition education in medical schools will help to develop an adequate supply of medical personnel who can help people become aware of the importance of good nutrition to their health and well-being.*

*The White House Conference Panel on Advanced Academic Teaching of Nutrition made the following recommendation about teaching nutrition:*

*"In each of the professional schools in a university such as medicine, dentistry, and dental hygiene, nursing, public health, food science, and technology or applied health sciences, an individual or committee should be assigned responsibility for the surveillance of nutrition-teaching in that school. In some professional schools, it will be desirable to teach nutrition in a designated course dealing with basic scientific principles of nutrition and their application to human health. In many schools, nutrition-teaching will be incorporated in courses such as biochemistry, physiology, and certain clinical specialties. Regardless of the plan of instruction, basic nutrition should be part of the required, or core, curriculum. In schools where trained nutrition personnel are not available because of financial restrictions, grants should be established to support nutrition for teaching in the categories listed above."*

*In 1972 I introduced legislation toward meeting that goal: The "Nutritional Medical Education Act of 1972" provided for five million dollars for each of the next five fiscal years for grants by the Secretary of HEW to public or nonprofit private schools of medicine to plan, develop, and implement a program of nutrition education; the grants to be structured by HEW to assure that properly trained faculty members are available. The purpose of the program is to provide a single focus on applied nutrition education in our medical schools.*

*Our national health is at stake. Each person's individual health and life are at stake. We must take every step possible to insure that all citizens are aware of the importance of their diet and of maintaining a proper nutritional balance in their food on a regular basis. By educating our future doctors about nutrition, we are helping to insure that future generations grow up knowledgeable about the great importance of nutrition. Our doctors hold the key to our health and that key must include nutrition. Nutrition must become a top health priority.*

# CHAPTER 11

# Three Approaches to Vitamin Use

There are almost as many ways of using vitamin supplements as there are people, which is the way it should be. We are all different, not only in the way our faces and bodies look but also in the structure and function of our internal organs. Each one of us has a pattern of metabolism that differs in significant ways, causing us to react uniquely to food, to exercise, to threats of disease, to vitamins, minerals, and other aspects of environmental exposure. So to say that there is one vitamin program that suits everyone would be going against natural principles. It would be almost like saying that there is one dress or suit of clothes or dinner menu that would please everyone all the time.

Yet despite our built-in diversity, there is need for some pattern of vitamin usage. While we have our differences as individuals, we also have important similarities. We need to consider basic principles of nutrition that apply to everyone in developing personal plans for improving and supplementing our diet.

## Insurance Approach

Most people follow one or the other of three basic vitamin-use plans: NUMBER ONE might be called the "insurance" approach. The general underlying idea is to take only enough of each important vitamin per day to insure against deficiency disease. Users of that method tend to choose supplements that contain dosages that are usually modeled closely after the Recommended Daily Allowances of each nutrient. The amounts of each vitamin and mineral contained in these formulas are somewhat in excess of what you would get in a typical diet containing a good selection of natural foods.

The insurance approach was born out of the conviction that vitamins are primarily important as substances that prevent scurvy, pellagra, rickets, beriberi, and other horrible examples of total nutritional breakdown. Getting one of those diseases is no picnic, and preventing them by taking insurance doses of food supplements costing pennies a day makes good sense. That insurance concept of vitamin use is the oldest. In fact, the vitamin pioneers espoused supplementation as insurance against disease, especially when there was doubt about the quality of food.

Starting about 30 years ago another point of view on vitamin usage began to be expressed. A subtle but extremely important switch in the outlook of some nutrition scientists was at the root of this change. Instead of looking at vitamins only in a negative way—as the cause of terrible disease when they were absent— these research workers began focusing on vitamins as tools for creating greater human efficiency. The evidence that vitamins were central to the structuring of a healthful diet was so apparent to these people that they could not rule out the possibility that vitamins served a much greater function in our welfare than the prevention of deficiency disease. They began looking for positive effects of greater-than-normal vitamin usage.

A step toward the recognition of that new vitamin concept was the discovery of the effects of *subclinical* vitamin deficiencies. Scurvy is the very bad effect of an almost total lack of vitamin C in the diet, and for years that was thought to be the only result of inadequate vitamin C intake. But as nutritional science and medicine became more sophisticated, other effects of less serious vitamin C lack were noted. Wounds didn't heal as fast when the vitamin C level was low—even though it wasn't low enough to cause scurvy. Infections didn't heal rapidly in experimental animals kept on slightly low C levels. From those and many similar observations, not only with C but other vitamins, a much broader concept of vitamin need began to be recognized in the scientific literature. To this day, many questions about subclinical vitamin deficiencies remain to be answered, but the door has been opened to a view of vitamin need and function that was almost totally ignored a few decades ago.

## Maximum Positive Benefits

Awareness of the positive value of larger amounts of vitamins led to other approaches to vitamin supplementation.

NUMBER TWO plan for vitamin supplementation calls for the use of vitamins and other food supplements to produce maximum *positive* benefits. This plan focuses on the positive (improved health and efficiency) rather than the negative (insurance against outright deficiency disease). This suggests an intake of vitamins considerably in excess of the Recommended Daily Allowances. These amounts are needed to be sure of getting most of the benefits of supplement use—particularly the extra efficiency and health mentioned earlier. People taking these amounts of vitamins really do feel better and enjoy many benefits, especially if they also cut down on refined foods.

Much of the benefit achieved by this program is long-range as well. Preventing degenerative disease is a long-time proposition, and is the fruit of years of wise living and enlightened nutrition.

Scientists are just waking up to the tremendous importance of the long-term view of nutrition. For years they were handicapped by the fact that there was no money available to support experimental work that lasted for more than a few years. They themselves didn't want to hamper their career possibilities by working on a project that might take several decades to begin to produce results. So they kept busy on the abundant short-term challenges of nutritional science.

Now they have suddenly realized that all of human life for the past 40 or 50 years in the United States has been a gigantic experiment in nutrition. Over that time there have been very significant changes in the kinds and amounts of food that most people eat. According to Jean Mayer, Ph.D., of Harvard's School of Public Health (*Science,* 21 April 1972), in 1941 only 10 percent of our foods were highly processed. "Today," he wrote, "that amount has risen to 50 percent." And while processing of food has increased so drastically, chronic, degenerative disease has increased too.

Refining of foods is only one of the changes that has affected our diet on a national scale, but it is extremely important to long-term health. When food is processed, there is almost always a change in the amount of nutrients it contains. Usually the recognized and important nutrients, such as protein, are preserved. But other facets of food that contribute to its nutritional value, including vital trace elements, are sacrificed in the name of such values as shelf-life, cost, appearance, and flavor. And since not all of the nutrients that are of value have been discovered, it is almost a certainty that processing of food takes out things that will someday be found to be of value over the long term.

The obvious solution to that problem is to avoid eating processed foods. But that's not always easy, or even possible. Many people choose processed foods for some of their meals because they're in a hurry, because they can't unhook themselves from the taste of foods they're used to, or because nothing else is conveniently available. More and more, the answer to getting the vitamins and minerals you need for long-term health points toward food supplements.

The experiment in long-term nutrition that the American diet has become has already attracted scientists who have begun to tabulate results, draw up charts and graphs, and make recommendations for corrective action. One of the most significant of such efforts is reported in a publication titled *Human Nutrition: Report No. 2, Benefits from Nutrition Research,* authored by C. Edith Weir, Ph.D., for a joint task group of the U.S. Department of Agriculture and the State Universities and

Land Grant Colleges. The book, issued in August 1971, lists all the diseases and conditions that can be prevented by improved nutrition, and is a real eye-opener. It states in blunt terms that almost all of the health problems of our day can be corrected to some degree by better nutrition—especially if that improved nutrition is maintained for many years.

Concerning cancer, Dr. Weir writes: "There is a small but growing body of data suggesting that chronic, low-level intake of some nutrients is a factor in the incidence of cancer in man. There is evidence that vitamin deficiency plays a role in the occurrence of cancer of the oral cavity and the esophagus.

"Chronic vitamin B complex deficiency, due to inadequate supply of vegetables in the diet, appears to be incriminated. There is recent evidence, March 1970, that dietary iodine deficiency may contribute to breast cancer, at least in rats. Demographic studies reveal that human breast cancer incidence is high in iodine-deficient areas."

Dr. Weir concludes in another section of her report that if everyone improved his or her diet, getting the right amount of nutrients, there would be a 20 percent reduction in the incidence of cancer. She also lists similar figures for other diseases. Here are her estimates:

| Health Problem | Potential Savings |
|---|---|
| Heart and vasculatory | 25 percent reduction |
| Respiratory and infectious disease | 20 percent fewer incidents |
| Mental health | 10 percent fewer disabilities |
| Infant mortality and reproduction | 50 percent fewer deaths |
| Early aging and lifespan | 10 million people without impairments |
| Arthritis | 8 million people relieved of afflictions |
| Dental health | 50 percent reduction in incidence, severity, and expenditures |
| Diabetes and carbohydrate disorders | 50 percent of cases avoided or improved |
| Osteoporosis | 75 percent reduction |

| Health Problem | Potential Savings |
|---|---|
| Obesity | 80 percent reduction in incidence |
| Alcoholism | 33 percent reduction |
| Eyesight | 20 percent fewer people blind or with corrective lenses |
| Allergies | 20 percent people relieved (90 percent for milk and gluten allergies) |
| Digestive | 25 percent fewer conditions |
| Kidney and urinary | 20 percent reduction in deaths and acute conditions |
| Muscular disorders | 10 percent reduction in cases |
| Cancer | 20 percent reduction in incidence and death |
| Improved work efficiency | 0.5 percent increase in on-the-job productivity |
| Improved growth and development | 25 percent fewer deaths and work days lost |
| Improved learning ability | Raise I.Q. by 10 points for persons with I.Q. of 70 to 80 |

That is a spectacular listing of health benefits, all predicted to result from better nutrition. No wonder-drug could approach that kind of record for health improvement. In fact, many of the benefits on that list are beyond the reach of drug medication as we know it today, and as it is likely to be in the future.

Of course, it would be wrong to imply that the use of food supplements, even the best natural kinds, could achieve all the benefits that Dr. Weir and her coworkers list for improved nutrition. In many cases, she says, these benefits will result only if you *don't* eat certain things, and food supplements can't help you there. But a great many of the improvements she lists are within the power of food supplements to achieve, because they require only the assurance of adequate amounts of nutrients over a long period of time.

The long-term necessity for good nutrition is stressed emphatically by Dr. Weir. "Major health benefits are long-range," she says. "Minor change in diet and food habits instituted at an early age might well avoid the need for major change, difficult to adopt in later life." The best course of all is to start an improved diet routine with young people, even small children, but a start at any age is better than ignoring the importance of these nutritional findings.

## Megavitamin Therapy

NUMBER THREE approach to vitamin supplementation is best labeled megavitamin therapy. Another less-familiar name is orthomolecular medicine. This branch of healing, used primarily by physicians, is rapidly gaining in popularity and use, and will probably become a major influence on health in the future, if the promise indicated by present research is realized.

The phrase megavitamin means the use of large amounts of vitamins—so large, in fact, that they bear little reference at all to the quantities normally found in foods. In this approach, vitamins are used to get the effect drugs might normally achieve. Some megavitamin concepts are preventive, but many are curative. If you take large amounts of vitamin C when you have a cold, you're using megavitamin therapy. Some people have said that when you cross over from milligrams of vitamin C to a gram or more per day, you're moving into the area of megavitamins.

Mental illness has been the first great testing ground for megavitamin therapeutic concepts. There are important and obvious reasons for that. First, the need for a new approach was painfully apparent. Increasingly, psychoanalysis was being attacked as an elitist technique that pays no attention to the human organism's greatest environmental exposure, food. The drugs being so widely used to treat mental illness don't cure, they merely put patients into a state bordering on suspended animation. Finally, the vast number of victims of mental illness was itself a major factor in the move toward megavitamin concepts. There are in this country today at least 10 million people considered mentally ill who are not treated. They are a source of serious trouble to their families, friends, and to society. Ultimately, many become a burden on the state. And worst of all, the number of mentally ill appears to be expanding.

Schizophrenia was the first target of large-scale megavitamin therapy. Abram Hoffer, M.D., Ph.D., and Humphry Osmond, M.R.C.P., D.P.M., in 1952 began using high levels of niacin and other vitamins, especially vitamin C, to treat patients suffering from what was then called the "split-personality" disease. They reported that about three-quarters of these sufferers from schizophrenia were improved, and their book *How to Live with Schizophrenia* (Secaucus, New Jersey: University Books, 1974) became an important introduction to their unique techniques of treatment.

Many articles have been published about the work of Doctors Hoffer and Osmond, Allan Cott, M.D., David Hawkins, M.D., and others who have made important contributions to the treatment of mental illness with vitamin therapy. One of the most important people on that scene is Linus Pauling, Ph.D. He's important not only because of his advocacy of megadoses of vitamin C for prevention and treatment of the common cold, but he has coined the phrase "orthomolecular psychiatry" to describe an even broader effort to attack mental problems using natural methods. Dr. Pauling says his concept involves "the treatment of mental disease by the provision of the optimum molecular environment of the mind, especially the optimum concentrations of substances normally present in the human body."

Those last six words are important. Most drugs are "abnormal" substances, synthetic compounds created in laboratories and factories and totally foreign to the natural scheme. To use those substances in large amounts to try to treat disease creates large risks. Seeking to create a healthful environment within the body is a far safer procedure. It is also eminently logical.

Clearly, the megavitamin concept is attractive, and not only to people with schizophrenia or other mental illness. Rapidly accelerating work in the field is opening up other areas, ranging from treatment of learning disabilities in children to treatment of alcoholism, depression, a wide range of heart problems, and possibly even cancer, which may be shown someday to be preventable through regular use of moderate dosages of vitamin A. Considerable research work is already pointing in that direction.

The potential for the use of larger-than-normal amounts of vitamins and minerals to *prevent* disease logically far exceeds their potential as curative agents. We know—almost everyone today knows—that the most troublesome diseases of modern life have their origin in a lifetime of wrong living and eating habits. Problems like heart disease, cancer, arthritis, and similar failures of the human organism don't just happen suddenly when you get to be a certain age. Unfortunately, they are being programmed into many people's lives by habits and actions that start early in life and have continued for decades.

It is even more unfortunate that each year fewer people are able to live the kind of totally natural life which is the best preventive of chronic disease. We are exposed to pollutants of constantly expanding variety. Each year hundreds of new and entirely different kinds of chemicals are created and introduced by industry. Self-inflicted pollutants like tobacco and alcohol take a bigger toll of health each year. Widespread use of drugs is a very important cause of long-range insult to the health integrity of the human body, and this does not refer primarily to the use of drugs for thrills, which is a problem all its own. What is doing the most damage is the routine use of tranquilizers, antibiotics, pain killers, sleeping pills, laxatives, and literally hundreds of other types of drugs, each dragging the body down with side effects.

The standard, old-time advice on health is not enough to combat those mounting insults. The "balanced diet," if there ever was such a thing, has been lost for most people among a welter of convenience foods packed with sugar, white flour, colorings, preservatives, and other additives. Eating normal food and getting enough sleep are not going to prevent the serious diseases which right now are getting a toehold in the bodies of many millions of Americans. We are, in fact, facing a crisis in future disease that has the potential to wreck our society.

Can vitamins, in large amounts, really be our salvation? Of course, there is no absolute guarantee that you will never get sick even if you come from the healthiest family, eat the best food, never smoke or drink, and follow a good vitamin plan your whole life. But it is also true that people who do those things, on the average, have a much better record of health. They also report subjectively that they feel better, are "more alive," and generally enjoy life more than those who move hardly a finger to try to improve their health on their own.

To some, vitamins are still controversial. The main problem is that almost all doctors still adhere to old ideas about vitamins, thinking of them only as preventers of those terrible deficiency diseases which are seen today primarily in the pockets of poverty. Doctors are also reluctant to embrace vitamins as a basic health-building tool, perhaps because they lack the mystery and exclusiveness of the prescription drug. Gradually that will change and vitamin supplements will become accepted as a desirable and even necessary part of life in our modern world.

# CHAPTER 12

# Good Nutrition for the Good Life*

*by Linus Pauling*

I believe that it is possible by rather simple means, essentially nutritional, to increase the length of life expectancy for young people and middle-aged people (and to some extent, perhaps, old people, too) by about 20 years. Not only can the life expectancy be increased, I believe, but also the length of the period of well-being can be increased by the same amount, or perhaps even a little longer; because it is likely that, as long as the process of aging goes on, the process of deterioration that culminates in death will proceed more rapidly at a late age than an earlier one.

The principal procedure to use is that of introducing nutrient substances into the human body in the optimum amounts. Take the vitamins, for example. We have in the United States a committee called the Food and Nutrition Board that is described as consisting of outstanding nutritional scientists, which makes recommendations to the people about the intake of vitamins and minerals. These recommendations are made for vitamins in the amounts that will prevent overt manifestations of avitaminosis for most people—95–99 percent of the people.

*Reprinted with permission of Engineering & Science Magazine, California Institute of Technology, June, 1974

For example, for vitamin C, the studies that have been made with a rather small number of human subjects show that 10 mg. a day is enough to prevent overt manifestations of scurvy from developing over a period of several months, or years even—the time it takes scurvy to develop for people on a scorbutic diet—and 45 mg. might be enough for most adults, even taking into account their biochemical individuality. It is true that Roger J. Williams—who discovered one of the B vitamins, pantothenic acid—has suggested, on the basis of studies with guinea pigs, that the amount required for good health varies by a factor of 20, probably even among guinea pigs, and by even a greater factor among human beings, who are more heterogeneous genetically than the guinea pigs that he was using. There may well be some people who will become prescorbutic with only 45 mg. per day.

About 40 years ago, Albert Szent-Gyorgyi, who in 1928 made the first preparations of ascorbic acid, which turned out to be vitamin C, asked the question: What is the amount of vitamin C that would lead to the best of health for human beings—not just the amount that prevents them from dying of scurvy, but the amount that would lead to the best of health? He apparently decided that 1,000 mg. a day might be a reasonable estimate, because he started taking 1,000 mg. a day himself, and I think rather recently has increased his intake to 2,000.

This is a question that has been essentially ignored by the Food and Nutrition Board, not only for vitamin C but for all other vitamins, too. It has been pretty much ignored by nutritional scientists as well; yet it is an important question. One way in which we might try to answer it is to ask: What amounts of various vitamins did human beings or their predecessors receive from the natural foods they were eating? It may be that at some time our predecessors were vegetarians rather than meat eaters, or catholic eaters—meat, vegetables, and so on. But in checking raw natural plant foods for the average amount of vitamin C in them, I found that for 110 foods the average amount in a day's ration of the various vitamins came out between two and five times the recommended daily allowance of vitamin A and thiamine and riboflavin and pyridoxine.

This, I think, suggests that the optimum intake of these vitamins might be two to five times the recommended daily allowances, but it is no more than a rough suggestion. On the other hand, for vitamin C the amount came out 55 times 45 mg., the currently recommended daily allowance. I think that this calculation is significant, and it may well be that the daily recommended allowance of vitamin C should be much larger than the present value, and that the optimum intake is in the neighborhood of several grams a day, rather than a few tens of milligrams a day.

In 1949, G.B. Bourne, an English biochemist, was engaged in discussing the question of what the British recommended daily allowance of vitamin C should be—10 mg. per day or 20 mg. per day. Bourne pointed out that the bamboo shoots and other foods eaten by gorillas in the wild state contain about five grams of vitamin C, corresponding to something like two grams (2,000 mg. per day) for a human being, taking the smaller body weight into consideration, and he asked the question: Should we not, instead of discussing whether 10 mg. or 20 mg. is the right amount to recommend, be discussing whether 1,000 or 2,000 mg. is the right amount?

Irwin Stone, a biochemist from Staten Island, who now lives in Mountain View, California, collected information about vitamin C over the years and in 1965 and 1966 published four papers on "Hypoascorbemia, a Genetic Disease." He contended that the human race as a whole has been suffering from a deficiency in the intake of ascorbic acid and from a disease that he named hypoascorbemia, too small a concentration of ascorbic acid in the blood.

He gave several arguments to support his contention. For one thing, plants manufacture vitamin A, vitamin $B_1$ (thiamine), vitamin $B_2$, $B_6$, and other vitamins for themselves. Animals require these substances exogenously, and we can ask why. I think the answer is this: In the early days of the existence of animals, they had inherited from their plant ancestors the machinery for making these important substances. But they were eating plants, and the plants manufactured these substances, so they were getting a supply of them in their food. It may well be that the amount of vitamin A that animals were getting was just about as much as they needed—close to the optimum. Now if a mutant came along that had suffered a genetic deletion, losing the genes that are involved in producing the enzymes that catalyze the reactions leading to the synthesis of vitamin A, the mutant would still have vitamin A from his food, but he would be a streamlined animal, not burdened by the machinery for *making* vitamin A, and in the competition with a more slowly moving competitor who was handicapped by this machinery, he would win out. The situation would be the same with thiamine, riboflavin, pyridoxine, and other vitamins. I believe that this is what happened, and that this is why all animals require the vitamins.

But this didn't happen with vitamin C. The dog, the cat, the rat, the mouse, and other animals make their own vitamin C. Only human beings and their close relatives require exogenous vitamin C, and a few other animals such as guinea pigs. The reason, I would say, is that there isn't enough vitamin C in the plant food. For one thing, vitamin C is required for the synthesis of collagen, the connective tissue in animals. Plants don't synthesize collagen, so far as I am aware. They use cellulose for connective tissue. There's an extra need for ascorbic acid among animals. The fact is that these animals did not give up the power to make ascorbic acid—and I calculated 2,300 mg. per day as the amount available in a diet for man of raw natural plant foods. This, I would say, surely means that the optimum intake for man is greater than 2,300 mg. a day.

But human beings and anthropoids all require exogenous vitamin C. What happened? I think with little doubt that these are not separate mutations for human beings and gorillas and rhesus monkeys and other primates, but rather a single mutational loss—a common ancestor 25 million years ago, living in a tropical valley where the fruit foods were especially rich in vitamin C (providing 10 or 15 grams per day for a body weight of 70 kilograms), underwent a mutation. The mutant lost the machinery for making the vitamin C and was correspondingly streamlined and able to compete and as a result the mutant won out and we are all descended from this mutant, who suffered this unfortunate accident. As long as our ancestors stayed in this area they were getting enough vitamin C. When they moved into temperate and sub-arctic regions, the food available contained less vitamin C, and they began to suffer from scurvy.

One measure of good health is resistance to disease. There have been about a dozen carefully controlled studies carried out on a comparison of vitamin C tablets and placebo tablets in blind trials, with respect to the incidence and severity of the common cold. Every one of these studies carried out with people exposed to cold viruses by casual contact with other people has shown that vitamin C has protective value. There is no doubt about it. In fact, if, in addition to taking regular doses of vitamin C, you carry a supply with you and increase the intake at the first sign of a cold, or even other illness, taking 10 to 20 grams during the first day, and then tapering off, you can stop the cold. Many cold medicines make you feel better, but they don't prevent the cold from developing. Vitamin C will do this. Not only that, but vitamin C prevents other diseases.

In 1965 it was reported by Claus W. Jungeblut, working in the College of Physicians and Surgeons at Columbia University, that concentrations of vitamin C that you can produce in the blood plasma by taking the substance in good amounts will inactivate poliomyelitis virus, so that when this virus is exposed to the solution for half an hour and then injected into the brains of monkeys the monkeys do not become paralyzed, although monkeys treated with virus that has not been inactivated in this way get paralysis. Also, monkeys given large doses of vitamin C did not become paralyzed, and those receiving small amounts did. Jungeblut and others also reported that inactivation of other plant and animal viruses be effected by treatment with vitamin C, and Japanese workers have published a half-dozen papers during the last three or four years on inactivation of bacterial viruses by vitamin C.

In 1973, Hume and Weyers in Scotland reported in the *Scottish Medical Journal* on the protection against bacterial diseases by vitamin C. It had been known for several decades that the white cells, leucocytes, are effective phagocytes (that is, with the ability to engulf bacteria) only if the leucocytes contain 20 micrograms per 100 million cells or more of vitamin C. Hume and Weyers found that people in Scotland eating an ordinary Scottish diet with perhaps 15 or 20 mg. per day of vitamin C had an average of 20 micrograms in their white cells. When they caught cold, the value dropped in the first day to 10 micrograms and stayed that way for three days, and then began slowly to rise. That's below the limit at which the leucocytes have phagocytic activity. By giving extra vitamin C—1,000 mg. per day, and eight grams per day when the person caught cold—this effect was averted. The concentration was 30 micrograms per 100 million cells and it dropped to no less than 24, so that the phagocytic activity was retained. This explains why people who take vitamin C, even if they catch cold—a viral cold—do not get a secondary bacterial infection, in general.

Vitamin C seems to be valuable in many different ways. Constance Spittle, a pathologist in England, reported that she had been monitoring her own serum cholesterol, which ran about 210 mg. per deciliter. Then she began taking about one gram a day of vitamin C and found that her serum cholesterol dropped to 130 micrograms per deciliter. She found a similar effect in over 50 subjects.

Edme Regnier, a physician in Salem, Massachusetts, wrote some papers about vitamin C and the common cold and then got out a book, *You Can Cure the Common Cold*. In this book he describes the studies he carried out with his friends and patients. He decided some 15 years ago that vitamin C in proper doses had value against the common cold, and he gave tablets to his friends and patients, sometimes a vitamin C and sometimes a placebo, with instructions that they were to take a tablet every hour at the first sign of a cold and continue throughout that day and the next day. He reported that 90 percent of the colds were averted by the simple procedure of taking only a few grams of vitamin C per cold.

After five years Regnier had to give up his study because his telephone began ringing in the middle of the night and one of these people would be saying, "You gave me the wrong tablets," because the cold didn't go away as it had before.

I don't know why it is that there has been so much opposition by the establishment to vitamin C as a way of controlling the common cold and other diseases, but there has been. Several years ago I wrote a paper with Ewan Cameron on "Ascorbic Acid and the Glycosominoglycans: A Contribution to the Orthomolecular Treatment of Cancer." Cameron is a cancer surgeon in Scotland. We talked about where we would publish the paper, and I said, "Why don't I send it to the *Proceedings of the National Academy of Sciences?*" So I did, and it was turned down. The policy of the NAS had then been for 58 years, since it was started, that a member had the right to publish papers, but they decided to change the policy and turn this paper down.

When word of this leaked out—I didn't say anything, but an article was published in *Science* about it—I got a telegram from the editor of *Oncology*, saying that their policy was that papers were not accepted for *Oncology* until they had been refereed and examined thoroughly, but in this case they would accept the paper sight unseen. So it was published in 1973, and although many people have written for reprints, it hasn't caused any great stir so far as I am aware, and the dangers stated by the editorial board of the NAS that we would be raising false hopes in people haven't materialized.

I think there's no doubt that ascorbic acid is helpful in preventing and treating cancer, but there is still doubt as to how great its benefit is. There are good arguments. You know ascorbic acid is required for the synthesis of collagen; connective tissue contains collagen fibrils, and the tissues are strengthened by an increased intake. It's valuable for wound healing. There is little doubt that the proper intake of ascorbic acid strengthens the tissues enough to permit them to offer increased resistance to infiltration by a growing malignant tumor. There is also evidence that ascorbic acid works against the enzyme hyaluronidase, probably by facilitating the synthesis of hyaluronidase inhibitor. Many cancerous growths produce this enzyme, which attacks the hyaluronic acid in the intercellular cement of the surrounding tissues and weakens these tissues in such a way as to permit infiltration by the cancer.

When I spoke at the dedication of the Ben May Laboratory for Cancer Research at the University of Chicago in November 1971, I said that with the proper use of ascorbic acid the mortality from cancer could be reduced by about 10 percent. I am now willing to make an estimate that the age-specific incidence of this disease might well be decreased by 50 percent. In fact, I think it may well be that with ascorbic acid alone, a proper intake—getting people back to the level of animals that manufacture their own ascorbic acid; perhaps we might say to the natural level—the age-specific morbidity and mortality in general can be decreased by 50 percent. This means an extension of the period of well-being by eight years, and an extension of the life expectancy by eight years.

I am now director of the Institute of Orthomolecular Medicine in Menlo Park, a new institution just across from the Stanford campus; the assistant director is a former Caltech student, Arthur B. Robinson, who received his BS in chemistry in 1963. I invented the word "orthomolecular" in 1968. It is from the Greek "ortho," meaning right or correct, as in "orthodox"; and "molecular," meaning molecular. "Orthomolecular" means the right molecules in the right amounts—having the right molecules in the right amounts—having the right molecules in the right concentrations. The right molecules are those that are normally present in the human body. Many of them are required for life—such as the vitamins and essential amino acids. Orthomolecular medicine is the prevention and treatment of disease, the preservation of good health, by varying the concentration of these molecules in the human body. The powerful drugs that are used by doctors, who treat crises with these crisis drugs, do the job, but they usually have serious side effects and you have to be careful about them. In particular they shouldn't be taken day after day, whereas the vitamins can be taken day after day for the rest of your life.

The paper in which I introduced the word orthomolecular had

the title "Orthomolecular Psychiatry." In 1954 I began work here at Caltech with the support of a grant from the Ford Foundation and later from the National Institute of Mental Health on the molecular basis of mental disease. After some time I learned about the work of Doctors A. Hoffer and D. Osmond in Saskatoon, Saskatchewan. Hoffer had observed that large doses of one of the B vitamins, the antipellagra vitamin nicotinic acid, niacin, seemed to be beneficial to schizophrenic patients. Hoffer and Osmond carried out the first double-blind test done in psychiatry, and they concluded from the results of this test that, taken in amounts of several hundred times the amount that will prevent pellagra, the substance did have value for many schizophrenic patients—especially young, acute schizophrenics who were hospitalized for the first time.

I wrote a paper in 1968 in which I presented a number of arguments about why megavitamin therapy should be especially valuable for mental disease. This argument appealed to people who were using this therapy to such an extent that there is now a journal named *Orthomolecular Psychiatry*, an International Academy of Orthomolecular Psychiatry, and a book, *Orthomolecular Psychiatry*, (San Francisco, California: W.H. Freeman, 1973)—of which a psychiatrist, David Hawkins from Long Island, and I are coeditors—about the basis of megavitamin orthomolecular treatment.

I believe there's no doubt that the statements made by the orthomolecular psychiatrists are right. The ordinary treatment with the use of phenothiazines mainly for acute schizophrenics leads to about 35 to 45 percent success. This means that 35 to 45 percent of these acute schizophrenics are released from the hospital and do not suffer a second hospitalization. But if they also receive orthomolecular treatment in addition to the phenothiazine and whatever else the psychiatrist wants to give them, it is said that 80 percent of them are released and not hospitalized a second time. They are to continue the vitamins the rest of their lives. The phenothiazine they stop taking quickly.

In my paper, I pointed out that the brain is probably the most sensitive of all organs to its molecular composition, and that it is not surprising that the megavitamin therapy should have been developed first of all for mental disease. But it is valuable also for physical disease.

The amounts given these schizophrenic patients vary—they are not the same for individual patients, but they usually run about four to eight grams of ascorbic acid, about eight to 20 grams a day of niacin or niacinamide, and about 400 to 800 mg. of pyridoxine and sometimes 400 to 800 units of vitamin E and thiamine. These all vary, but usually with emphasis on ascorbic acid and niacinamide.

Vitamin E is an important substance. Early in 1974 the Food and Nutrition Board brought out a statement to the effect that they have reduced the daily recommended dosages of vitamin E from 30 mg. to 15 units. It's hard to know why they have reduced it, but I believe it would have been wiser to increase it. Perhaps one reason for reducing it is that the big food companies have begun stripping the cooking fats, the oils, of their vitamin E so that the fats you eat don't contain as much vitamin E as they used to. Then they sell the vitamin E, and it's rather high priced—nearly $100 per kilogram. (Vitamin C can be purchased for $7.50 per kilogram as pure crystals, and it is cheapest this way.)

Well, about vitamin E—in the Food and Nutrition Board report they said that there is no evidence that any disease, except one rare disease among infants, is benefited by taking large doses of vitamin E. So I wrote to Jean Mayer, professor of nutrition at Harvard, who has a newspaper column in which I first saw this reported, and asked him why he made the statement (he is a member of the committee) in light of the report by Knut Haeger of Sweden about peripheral occlusive arterial disease, and the other reports on this disease. And he replied by a letter in which he said that he was asking the Food and Nutrition Board to send me a copy of the statement, and that was all. The statement arrived, and it was just as he had quoted it. So I wrote to the chairman of the Food and Nutrition Board three months ago asking why they made this statement in the light of Haeger's results, and I haven't gotten an answer from them.

Knut Haeger published a paper in 1968 about a seven-year study he had made of patients with peripheral occlusive arterial disease. He had 220 patients under observation—people perhaps with diabetes or prediabetic conditions who have hardening of the peripheral arteries with a decreased flow of blood to the extremities; sometimes they get gangrene in the foot. He gave half of them 300 units a day of vitamin E and the other half a placebo. They were age-matched so that the average ages were the same in these two groups. During the seven years of the study, one of the vitamin E patients had to have a leg amputated because of gangrene, and 11 of the control group had to have legs amputated; this difference has high statistical significance. It's not a statistical fluctuation—one chance in a thousand of that. Nine of the vitamin E patients died during the seven years, and 19 of the control patients. This difference has borderline statistical significance—about 10 percent chance of its being a statistical fluctuation.

These people have what is called intermittent claudication—that's a highbrow name for limping occasionally. They can start out walking at a good rate; after they have walked a while, they develop angina in the calves of the legs. The work of the muscles uses up the oxygen so that they have to stop walking because of the pain caused by anoxia. It takes about six months for them to get in a stable state. After about six months, though, the vitamin E subjects could walk on average about twice as far as the control subjects before they developed claudication, and this is statistically significant, too—the standard deviations are such that the difference is statistically significant. There are a number of other studies that report essentially the same thing.

Haeger asked the question, who is it who believes that angina in the calves of the legs is different from angina in the heart muscle caused by anoxia? There have been no good double blind studies made of vitamin E in relation to heart disease. But Wilfrid and Evan Shute in Canada treated 30,000 heart patients by giving them large doses of vitamin E, and they report that there is no doubt they are benefited. For example, a Dr. George wrote them about himself. He had diabetes and had a leg amputated because of gangrene—poor circulation—and then after that he heard of the work the Shutes were doing and he started taking vitamin E. He was scheduled to have the other leg amputated, but it healed when he took the vitamin.

And yet the medical profession as a whole has rejected this evidence in the same way that they have rejected the evidence about the value of vitamin C for the common cold and other diseases.

Now I don't know just what the optimum intake of vitamins is. I take 1,200 units of vitamin E per day, which gives an indication of what I judge to be the sensible thing to do. And I take super-B vitamins every day which contain 50 mg. (that's about 25 to 30 times the recommended daily allowance) of thiamine, and 50 mg. of riboflavin and 50 mg. of pyridoxine, and 100 mg. of niacinamide (though I usually take 300 to 400 mg. of nicotinic acid separately too), and a multivitamin tablet that gives me 4,000 units of vitamin A plus other vitamins and minerals, and sometimes I take 25,000 units of vitamin A. I am trying to see if I can discover what the optimum intake of vitamin A is. But this is a hard problem. I think there should be hundreds of millions of dollars expended on finding out what the optimum nutrition is for a human being.

I think that vitamin E has great value, and that these other vitamins have value, and I'm willing to estimate that the morbidity and mortality of various diseases and the rate of aging can be decreased by another factor or two in this way.

There's one more nutritional orthomolecular treatment that I'll mention. This is a negative one involving sugar—sucrose. John Yudkin was professor of biochemistry and nutrition at the University of London in 1959, and he published a paper on his research on sucrose in relation to heart disease. He studied the incidence of heart disease as a function of the amount of sugar ingested, and he concluded that people who take 120 lbs of sugar per year have six times the chance at a given age of coming down with coronary heart disease as people who take 60 lbs per year or less. Those who take 150 lbs or more a year have 15 times the chance at a given age of developing coronary heart disease as those who take 60 lbs or less.

I believe that if people were to avoid sucrose—hardly ever spoon out a spoonful of sugar from the sugar bowl onto anything, avoid sweet desserts except when you're a guest somewhere, avoid buying foods that say "sugar" as one of the contents—they could cut down on the incidence of disease and increase life expectancy. Take a fair amount of vitamins. Stop smoking cigarettes. And you'll have a longer and happier life—more vim and vigor and a better time altogether.

# CHAPTER 13

# An Important New Theory on Why Extra Vitamins Provide Happy Surprises

Sometimes a dietary modification, the addition of a food supplement, or a boost in intake of a specific vitamin brings beneficial changes which seem to defy logic. You may know someone who has experienced such an effect. Or it may have happened to you. These unexpected results can be as confusing as they are delightful, but they are not uncommon.

For example, a young woman starts taking vitamin B-complex supplements including desiccated liver and brewer's yeast. Her long-standing severe acne problem begins to clear. A woman with a 10-year history of bad nerves and tranquilizer dependency begins taking zinc three times daily. "In two weeks I was a new person," she reports.

Another person with a heart condition embarks on a daily food supplement regimen, hoping for more energy—and finds cataracts disappearing! A lady begins using lecithin and draws the curtain on 27 years of migraine misery. A mother and her three-month-old baby take vitamin C, and their hiccups go away. "I don't understand the logic behind it," she admits.

Actually, none of the occurrences cited above make any sense at all. You won't find an explanation in any medical or nutritional textbook. Even the most open-minded and nutritionally oriented physician would be at a loss to pinpoint a cause-and-effect mechanism in those examples. Yet the individuals involved did obtain relief. Is this just the power of suggestion at work, or is something more happening?

A new theory advanced by a leading authority in the field of nutrition goes a long way toward explaining how many beneficial "side effects" can be not only legitimate, but even logical responses. According to biochemist Roger J. Williams, Ph.D., the key to understanding can be found under the microscope, at the level of the cell. Dr. Williams, who for over 20 years directed the University of Texas' Clayton Foundation Biochemical Institute in Austin, is convinced that many disorders in both animals and human beings occur because the cells do not get adequate nutrition. In his latest book, *Physicians' Handbook of Nutritional Science,* (Springfield, Illinois: Charles C. Thomas, 1975) he calls this generalized condition of cellular malnutrition *cytopathy.*

Because every cell in the body requires virtually every nutrient, Dr. Williams explains that a deficiency of any given nutrient in our diets can lead to symptoms *anywhere* in the body.

## Deficiencies More Than Skin Deep

Usually, we associate certain vitamins and minerals with various "target" areas. For example, vitamin A ensures healthy skin, B vitamins influence mental temperament, magnesium helps regulate heartbeat, etc. But the concept of cytopathy suggests that each nutrient has a much broader role.

By way of illustration, Dr. Williams describes an experimental study he conducted in which chickens deprived of pantothenic acid developed a condition called "chick dermatitis." (Pantothenic acid, a part of the B vitamin complex, was first discovered by Dr. Williams.) Birds suffering from this vitamin deficiency developed obviously unhealthy skin and feathers. Probing further, however, Dr. Williams and his colleagues in the laboratory found that the disease was far more than "skin deep." Pantothenic acid deficiency had also affected the blood, muscles, liver, kidneys, and brains of the birds. Livers and kidneys, for example, were found to be less than half their normal size.

"Since every tissue examined was more or less severely diseased biochemically, it seems a reasonable extrapolation to conclude that every other tissue in the entire animal would have exhibited some deficiency if it had been examined," Dr. Williams speculates.

"If this conclusion is valid, chick dermatitis, in addition to being a disease of the blood, liver, kidney, muscle, brain, and spinal cord, is also a disease of the heart, lung, gizzard, intestines, spleen, endocrine glands, the organs of the special senses, the reproductive system, and, in fact, of every cell and tissue in the body of the chicken. Correspondingly, pantothenic acid deficiency in mammals would also cause biochemical lesions in every cell and tissue."

Dr. Williams goes on to present evidence that similar wide variations in symptoms may occur in human beings, again using pantothenic acid deficiency as an example. In one instance, a retired army nurse paid a personal visit to the famous biochemist to relate how extra pantothenic acid had helped her in unexpected and, at the time, totally unexplainable ways. She had begun taking the vitamin simply because it was newly available. To her surprise, her graying hair began to darken and her faltering memory seemed to improve.

This latter effect was particularly remarkable because the nurse had been forced to retire from the army early because of her memory problems. She would often fail to report for duty or report at the wrong hour, simply because she had forgotten. After taking supplemental pantothenic acid, however, her memory came back strongly. So strongly, in fact, that when appearing in court as a passenger involved in an auto accident, she was complimented on the clear-cut and decisive testimony she presented. Her memory was now able to retain almost every detail.

Another acquaintance told Dr. Williams that his lifelong constipation problem disappeared completely and quite by accident when he began taking pantothenic acid regularly. If he discontinued the vitamin, bowel sluggishness returned.

# Why Deficiency Symptoms Vary So Much

So far, for purposes of illustration, much of this discussion has centered mainly on one nutrient: pantothenic acid. But many other nutrients are absolutely essential to healthy cell function, and deficiencies of any of them might be expected to cause cytopathy also. Dr. Williams lists thiamine, riboflavin, niacin, folic acid, biotin, vitamins $B_6$ and $B_{12}$, essential amino acids found in protein, calcium, and the trace minerals as other nutrients needed by each and every cell of the body. Vitamins A, C, E, and D are also needed for a wide range of functions, he adds, although the dependence of *every* cell on those nutrients has yet to be absolutely confirmed.

Assuming that a person is suffering from a deficiency of any one or more of these nutrients resulting in a generalized cytopathy, what determines which part of the body will be affected? According to Dr. Williams, symptoms emerge first wherever the body's cells are weakest and most susceptible to impaired nutrition. For many people, the skin is the first organ to be affected.

"The skin, partly because the circulation does not supply it with copious nutrition, is notoriously sensitive to nutritional lacks," says Dr. Williams. "In the oral cavity—the tongue, lips, and the gums—we find a favorite region where nutritionists look to detect evidence of malnutrition." Dry, flaky patches around the mouth, for example, are a classic response to riboflavin deficiency. Biotin shortage leads to a characteristic facial dermatitis. Inadequate vitamin A often results in rough, scaly skin.

But in other individuals, the cells of the skin are not always the first to "crack." In pellagra, caused by severe niacin deprivation, dermatitis is a common symptom—but so are diarrhea and mental derangement. "Niacinamide is an essential part of the energy-metabolism machinery of every cell in one's body,"

Dr. Williams points out. "When one is deficient in niacinamide, the functioning of every cell must be impaired to a greater or lesser degree. Whether the overt symptoms show up on the skin or in a pathological intestinal tract or in the brain is somewhat incidental to the probability that pellagra exemplifies a generalized cytopathy, incapacitating each and every tissue."

## The Key Concept of Biochemical Individuality

Dr. Williams believes that the real key to understanding the myriad manifestations of cytopathy, and why they occur where they do in whom they do is biochemical individuality. This is a concept based on the scientific observation that every person is unique internally as well as externally. The phenomenon of biochemical individuality tells us that there is no such thing as an "average" human being, but rather, as Dr. Williams puts it, only "*hard facts* regarding how *real people* are constituted."

Numerous scientific observations have confirmed, for example, that various organs, including the stomach, heart, liver, etc., vary in shape and size from individual to individual. Different people secrete different amounts of digestive juices and enzymes. So, depending on the efficiency of their own metabolic systems, different people will require differing amounts of any given nutrient. The amount of calcium, for example, that satisfies the bone-building requirements of one individual may result in a bone-eroding negative calcium balance in another person.

You might say that everyone has his or her own special metabolic profile, as unique as a set of fingerprints.

Once we are aware of biochemical individuality and Dr. Williams' theory of cytopathy, some of the unusual fringe benefits some people derive from improved nutrition become easier to understand. Dr. Williams himself has seen many such instances. In one case, a woman doctor came to his office to discuss what appeared to be an outlandish effect of generous doses of thiamine. After taking the vitamin, her eyesight improved to the point where she was able to use her eyes once again for long stretches of continuous reading. No medical text would suggest taking thiamine for vision impairment, yet this woman could not dismiss the obvious results of her supplementation program. Dr. Williams suspects that the retinal cells within the woman's eyes responded to the extra thiamine.

A young science professor's eyes were so painfully irritated by bright fluorescent lighting that he was forced to wear a protective eyeshade to keep out the glare. His condition was disturbing enough that he actually considered moving to a less developed country where fluorescent lights were still not widely used.

At Dr. Williams' suggestion, he began taking five mgs. a day of riboflavin, simply as an experiment, expecting no result. But surprisingly, his sensitivity disappeared and he was able to throw away his eyeshade. "It seems probable that this young man had an inborn need for riboflavin that is higher than average," Dr. Williams concludes.

Another professor told Dr. Williams that in an attempt to cure a skin problem diagnosed as psoriasis, he began taking rather large doses of vitamin A—about 25,000 I.U. every day. In a few months, his rash went away and stayed away. Later he was sent on a mission to a foreign country where he could not obtain vitamin A. His skin condition returned. Upon his return to the United States, continued trials convinced him that vitamin A did indeed control his skin problem. With an understanding of cytopathy, "this observation becomes credible," Dr. Williams says, even though there is no evidence in the medical literature that vitamin A will cure psoriasis in most patients.

"The most bizarre observation in the area of nutrition that I have encountered was relayed to me by an officer of one of our largest New York foundations," Dr. Williams says. It seems that a man undertaking a comprehensive program of nutritional supplementation—involving several vitamins and minerals—was surprised to discover that as a side effect, a long-standing problem of foot odor disappeared. Such a connection is not as far-fetched as it seems, he points out, since body odors are the product of metabolism.

A similar bizarre effect was reported a few years ago by a man who began taking zinc at the age of 59 because of published evidence that the trace mineral is intimately involved in the health of the prostate. "The big surprise was in another area, however," he said. A body odor problem that had troubled him for more than five years suddenly disappeared.

Not everybody can expect that zinc supplementation will have the same effect in terms of body odors. The whole point of these so-called illogical nutritional benefits is that they don't work for everybody. But if Dr. Williams' theory of cytopathy is correct, there may be almost as many fringe benefits to improved nutrition as there are people with special nutritional needs. If this is true, and if enough of these people begin taking supplements, then as Dr. Williams predicts, "there are no limits to the kinds of benefits that can accrue."

# BOOK II

# A GUIDE TO THE
# INDIVIDUAL VITAMINS

# VITAMIN A

## CHAPTER 14

# Vitamin A: The Growth Vitamin

Several thousand years ago, the Egyptian physicians were prescribing various forms of liver, the best source of preformed vitamin A, as a treatment for night-blindness, today one of the most commonly recognized symptoms of vitamin A deficiency. But it was only through laboratory research that began in full force at the turn of this century that vitamin A (known simply as the "A factor" in early experiments) was identified as a distinct nutrient. It was soon shown to have salutary effects in treating such diseases as conjunctivitis and in promoting healthy animal growth patterns.

Dr. Elmer V. McCollum, then a biochemist at the Farm Experiment Station at Madison, Wisconsin, and his associates reported in 1926 that food substances such as butterfat, cod-liver oil, and egg yolks were instrumental in promoting growth in laboratory test animals after their growth had been deliberately stunted on experimental diets of pure starch, sugar, and fats. Professor McCollum and his team of researchers called the biologically active, colorless substance they found in these foods "fat-soluble vitamin A." The extraordinary progress in growth patterns exhibited by the test animals prompted several of the researchers of the day to refer to vitamin A as the "growth vitamin," a name which is still used.

Later Professor McCollum and his colleagues discovered that green vegetables, such as spinach, cabbage, and various leguminous plants also contained a property which had a similar stimulating effect on the growth of laboratory animals. Unlike the fat-soluble extracts which were colorless, this substance had a greenish yellow hue. These classic experiments were the first indication that vitamin A was derived from two different sources.

Preformed vitamin A, or retinol, is found in foods such as eggs, milk fat, fish liver oils, and organ meats, especially liver. The advantage of preformed vitamin A is that the body can use it as it comes. Plants, as Professor McCollum later discovered, supply us with a precursor, or provitamin, of vitamin A called carotene. Deep red in its pure form, carotene is the bright yellow or orange pigment found in carrots and other vegetables. Its true color is masked in part by chlorophyll, nature's protection against harmful oxidation, which explains the greenish yellow hue described by Dr. McCollum in the early experiments.

When taken into the body the carotene is converted by the liver and intestinal wall into usable vitamin A. Once absorbed, vitamin A flows through the bloodstream to cells throughout the body. The liver stores excess vitamin A, releasing it when necessary. Under normal conditions, the liver can store the vitamin for long periods of time.

## Daily Requirements of Vitamin A

There are several conditions that prohibit the body from absorbing vitamin A. Gastrointestinal or liver diseases or infections of any kind limit our capacity to use vitamin A. Intake of mineral oil (as a laxative, for example) mixes with the vitamin A in the body and carries it away before it can be absorbed.

Since vitamin A is stored in your body, it is not absolutely necessary to eat some of it every day. However, since there is no way of checking how much reserve you have, you may find that all your vitamin A has been exhausted and you are suddenly showing symptoms of deficiency, unless you're faithful about getting enough of the vitamin over a period of time. The daily recommended allowances of vitamin A have been set as follows:

| | |
|---|---|
| Moderately active adults ........ | 5000 International Units per day |
| Children up to 12 years old ....... | 1500-3500 International Units per day |
| Children over 12 ............... | 4500-6000 International Units per day |
| Pregnant women .............. | 6000 International Units per day |
| Nursing mothers .............. | 8000 International Units per day |

Many nutritionists believe that these amounts are too low. The easiest way to obtain vitamin A without much attention to diet is to take fish liver oil. Halibut liver oil contains about a hundred times as much as cod liver oil. These oils are sold with the number of units of vitamins A and D that they contain specified on the label, standardized so that you cannot make a mistake in dosage. Buy the oil in the most economical form, for the amount you want to take.

## Is Vitamin A Ever Toxic?

In Sebrell's and Harris's authoritative work, *The Vitamins, Vol. 1* (New York: Academic Press, 1967), Dr. Thomas Moore of the Dunn Nutritional Laboratory, Cambridge, England, wrote the chapter on "Pharmacology and Toxicology of Vitamin A." The adult human liver, Dr. Moore says, can absorb and store "at least 500,000 I.U." of this vitamin.

That doesn't mean that you can (or should) take 500,000 I.U. daily, for under ordinary circumstances you don't use up anywhere near that much, and the surplus is not harmlessly excreted as is the case with vitamin C and the B vitamins. But when an adult—whether because of malnourishment or extreme trauma—has become overtly vitamin A-deficient, then, Dr. Moore says, physicians should make this high amount available to the patient within the first few days of treatment.

Under ordinary circumstances, when there is no reason to believe a vitamin A deficiency is present or threatening, Dr. Moore offers these "hard" figures as a guideline: In adults, "doses of 200,000 I.U. daily incur the danger of chronic hypervitaminosis A if continued over prolonged periods." Doses of 20,000 I.U., he says, "should be harmless even over indefinite periods." When it comes to a single dose, you would have to take as much as 2,000,000 I.U. to induce acute hypervitaminosis A. For infants, Dr. Moore adds, all these dosage rates "should probably be divided by 10."

According to Dr. W.H. Stimsom reporting in the *New England Journal of Medicine* (265:369, 1961), the principal symptoms of hypervitaminosis of vitamin A include "bone or joint pain that tended to be intermittent, fatigue, insomnia, loss of hair, dryness and fissuring of the lips and other epithelial involvement, anorexia and weight loss and hepatomegaly." However, the antidote is simple. If symptoms occur, merely reduce the intake of the vitamin.

You will have to be your own judge about how much vitamin A you need under varying circumstances. Relying on Dr. Moore's guidelines, supplement your diet with natural vitamin A (found most conveniently in fish liver oil) as you believe your body requires it.

## Symptoms of Vitamin A Deficiency

Just as the symptoms of vitamin A poisoning are clearly defined, so are the symptoms of a deficiency of this important nutrient. Vitamin A can be stored in the body (in the liver, chiefly). The supply may be considerably depleted before symptoms of deficiency become obvious. The eyes are a well-known barometer of vitamin A deficiency. Night blindness, the inability to see well in a medium-dim light, is a major symptom. There may also be itching and burning in the eyes, or a slight redness of the eyelids.

Skin diseases, especially in children, suggest the possibility of vitamin A deficiency. In adults, a serious shortage of vitamin A leads to a dry condition of the mucous membranes of the mouth, the respiratory system, and the genitourinary system. Inability to store fat is a symptom of too little vitamin A. Bladder stones appear in rats deprived of vitamin A, as do diseases of the nerves, somewhat akin to sclerosis in human beings. In many cases, a diet abundant in vitamin A appears to improve the condition of a person suffering from hyperthyroidism or goiter.

Vitamin A helps to fight infection, not by killing off the disease germs, but by providing for the defense of the mucous membranes which the germs attack. Because of this property, it is powerful protection against colds, sinus trouble, and pneumonia. Scientists have observed that, especially in children, symptoms of very serious vitamin A deficiency are generally preceded by colds and other respiratory troubles.

# CHAPTER 15

# Is It Necessary to Take Supplementary Vitamin A?

Preformed vitamin A does not occur in vegetable foods. Carotene, which does occur in these foods (yellow and green foods, chiefly), is made into vitamin A by the body. If, through any disorder, you are not able to convert carotene into vitamin A and you are not taking any food supplement that contains vitamin A itself, then you are likely to suffer from a deficiency.

Two New York physicians reported that diabetics are unable to transform carotene into vitamin A. In their studies they experimented with laboratory rats fed carotene rather than vitamin A. The studies indicated that these diabetic rats then had only one-fourth as much vitamin A in their bodies as the nondiabetic ones. But when they were fed preformed vitamin A, as in fish liver oil, both the diabetic rats and their healthy controls showed an equal store of vitamin A. Drs. Albert E. Sobel and Abraham Rosenberg, who were then at the Polytechnic Institute of Brooklyn and conducted these experiments, reported, "These studies carry the clear indication that the diabetic rat must receive some source of preformed vitamin A, such as fish liver oils, rather than the usual carotene source, such as vegetables. The discovery that the conversion of carotene to vitamin A is impaired in experimental diabetes can be regarded as the first step toward the discovery of an agent to control the premature aging of the arteries found in individuals suffering from diabetes mellitus.''

It is apparent that anyone who suffers from diabetes should consider taking some type of vitamin A supplement to maintain good health and a youthful vigor. Those who suspect there is anything wrong with the function of their liver should also be getting fish liver oils, or any other source of preformed vitamin A, because liver disorders also interfere with conversion of carotene (in food) into vitamin A.

The type of vitamin A used as a supplement is important in its effect. In a letter to the *Journal of the American Medical Association* (December 1962), Robert A. Peterman, M.D., reminded the physician-readers that "conversion of provitamin A carotenoids to vitamin A in vivo is very inefficient and is influenced by many factors. Extensive testing for toxicity done on pure beta-carotene, the most potent and important of the provitamin A carotenoids, has provided compelling proof of the lack of toxicity of this compound and of its inability to cause a hypervitaminosis.

"Fifteen human subjects received daily oral dosages of beta-carotene equivalent to 100,000 I.U. of vitamin A for three months. Serum carotene values rose from an initial 128 to 308 after one month, but did not rise above this level during the remainder of the observation period. Serum vitamin A levels of these subjects were not elevated. There were no clinical signs of vitamin toxicity, indicating that excessive amounts of beta-carotene are not absorbed after oral administration and that conversion to vitamin A does not automatically follow absorption," reported Dr. Peterman. He went on to state that he knew of no diet anywhere in the world too high in carotenoids, but if there were, "our experience would not indicate that this would raise any question of hypervitaminosis A. The most that could happen would be widespread, but harmless, carotenemia (yellowing of the skin)."

Dr. Peterman appeared convinced that provitamin A, as it occurs naturally in foods, rarely presents a problem. Every vitamin works best and is safest in its natural combination. For this reason, the fish liver oil supplements, which contain vitamin A, as well as vitamin D and other important nutritive elements, can work together for the best effect. Even doctors who are most concerned about a possible overdose of vitamin A are aware of its necessity, and would urge that any patient make certain of a sufficient supply.

## Vitamin A Deficiency in the United States

Annually, almost 80,000 children around the world fall victim to permanent blindness as a direct result of vitamin A deficiency, according to a statement by the Western Hemisphere Nutrition Congress (*Miami Herald,* 31 August 1971). Most of these children live in undeveloped countries where malnutrition is common, and many go on to die due to a deficiency of this important nutrient. Although the effects of vitamin A deficiency in the United States rarely reach the point of causing blindness, the number of Americans deficient in stores of vitamin A is surprisingly large. One-third of the population of the United States consumes less than the "Recommended Daily Allowance of vitamin A," according to the Congress.

A 1955 survey by the United States Department of Agriculture (USDA) indicated that, despite the fact that 60 percent of the people were eating a "good" diet, vitamin A was the principal nutrient lacking in the diet. Another USDA survey taken ten years later showed that the number of people found to have "good" diets had decreased to 50 percent. According to this expanded study, vitamin A was deficient in every age group. The official government position: "Vitamins and minerals are supplied in ample amounts in the average American diet."

The Citizen Board of Inquiry into Hunger and Malnutrition in the United States in 1968 reported that up to 40 percent of all Americans were deficient in vitamin A, and that largely as a result of this, as many as 46 percent of the children in some states suffered from stunted growth. Evidence from human and animal studies has long indicated that vitamin A status is affected by disorders of malabsorbtion, parasitic diseases, certain liver maladies, infectious diseases, sustained fever, renal disease, and interference with the conversion of raw carotene to vitamin A. But the extent to which this deficiency is present among humans was graphically depicted by Canadian researchers at a Symposium on Metabolic Functions of Vitamin A at the Massachusetts Institute of Technology in 1969.

The Canadian study involved liver samples taken during autopsies of 100 subjects from five major Canadian cities. All had died from either disease or accidents. The study indicated that in excess of 10 percent of the people examined had no store of vitamin A left in their liver.

As T. Keith Murray, Ph.D., Chief of Nutrition Research Division of the Canadian Food and Drug Directorate, pointed out, "About 90 percent of the body's store of vitamin A is in the liver. Determination of the concentration of the vitamin in the liver, therefore, provides a convenient index of vitamin A status. . . . We were astonished to find that a significant number of Canadians die with little or no reserves of vitamin A. . . . I see no reason why the same would not be as likely to occur in the United States as well." A further 21 percent, according to Dr. Murray and his colleagues, had vitamin A stores which they described as "typical of the newborn" (*Journal of the Canadian Medical Association,* 13 December 1969).

Dr. Murray concluded that "We can no longer assume that vitamin A's status in North America is satisfactory." And little, if anything, has happened during the intervening years to change Dr. Murray's thought-provoking conclusion.

In 1972, a study by Nicholas Raica, Jr., Ph.D., and coworkers, published in the *American Journal of Clinical Nutrition* (March 1972), concluded that depending upon which region of the United States is surveyed, vitamin A stores are low in 12 percent to 37 percent of all people. Dr. Raica further warned that the picture is probably worse than mere paper statistics indicate, because in certain disease states, vitamin A supplies of the liver become unavailable for protective action in the rest of the body.

And, unless the individual is getting liberal amounts of vitamin A every single day, he or she will definitely suffer the effects of a vitamin A deficiency.

# Vitamin A Intake from Fresh Food Decreasing

One reason why an estimated 50 million Americans are dangerously deficient in vitamin A showed up when a recent survey disclosed that Americans are eating 31 fewer pounds of fresh fruits and 20 fewer pounds of fresh vegetables than they did in 1950. Calculating the average vitamin A content of an assortment of 10 varieties of fruits and vegetables, including those which are rich in vitamin A (e.g., broccoli and apricots) and those which are notably lacking in vitamin A (e.g., pears and beets) you discover that a pound of these foods averages slightly less than 5,000 I.U. of vitamin A. This is just about the amount which government nutrition publications say we need every day in order to avoid vitamin A deficiency. Now, multiply this deficit by 51 pounds of fruits and vegetables which we aren't eating, and you get an annual deficit of over 225,000 I.U. of vitamin A, or 51 days worth of vitamin A intake!

You might think that this deficit is filled by other dietary sources, but this hardly seems to be the case. Consumption of dairy products peaked a long time ago, and the industry has been in a slump for years. What we do eat more of today is beef and pork, but except for the organs, which few people eat, the vitamin A content of beefsteak and pork is almost negligible. We also eat a lot more processed foods today, and eat more in restaurants, where food is often prepared long before we eat it. Processing losses of vitamin A can be as high as 40 percent.

It was thought that vitamin A, because it withstands high temperatures, is not destroyed to any great extent by cooking when the food is not permitted to come into contact with the air. However, a study published in the *Journal of the American Dietetics Association* (59,238, 1971) by Dr. J. E. Sweeney and A. G. Marsh, revealed that although the carotene in vegetables may not be destroyed by cooking, biological activity—which is to say its ability to do us any good—is dramatically reduced. The actual value of the vitamin A in green vegetables is reduced by 15 to 20 percent after cooking, and that of yellow and red vegetables reduced between 30 and 35 percent! So a very substantial part of the vitamin A which nutritionists had assumed people were getting is actually being destroyed in the cooking pot.

## Nitrates Ravage Vitamin A Supply

Among the worst threats to our store of vitamin A, both before and after we ingest it, is the widespread use of commercial fertilizers high in nitrogen. The nitrites that develop from them interfere with the body's ability to convert raw carotene into usable vitamin A. The plant foods that we eat and those fed to commercial livestock are saturated with these compounds, and so is the tap water in most areas of the country.

Commercially raised plant crops contain very high amounts of inorganic nitrogen. As soon as the plants are harvested, the nitrate begins turning to nitrite, a dangerous chemical. The longer these plants are stored, the more nitrates turn to nitrites.

For the average American consumer there is literally no way to avoid these compounds in the diet. The animals that are the source of the fresh meats in the commercial marketplace are saturated with nitrates at the end of a lifetime of ingesting commercial livestock feed. Nitrate compounds, such as sodium nitrate and sodium nitrite, are used to preserve and color all types of processed, canned, and cured meats such as frankfurters, salami, bologna, and sausages. They even appear in popular baby foods.

Extensive experiments carried out by Dr. R. J. Emerick and his colleagues at South Dakota State College proved that nitrite destroys vitamin A (*Feed Age*, April 1963). When nitrite was placed in an acid environment such as the stomach, it destroyed the precursor of vitamin A, raw carotene. Ironically, leafy greens such as spinach, which theoretically are very rich in vitamin A, also pick up huge amounts of nitrates when commercially grown. So unless you eat spinach right out of your own garden, you lose much of the vitamin A the nutrition charts promise in spinach.

Another researcher, E.E. Hatfield, Ph.D. *et al.,* showed in a study reported in 1961 (*Proc. Soc. Animal Prod.*) that the addition of nitrite to the diet of rats acted to reduce their liver's vitamin A content.

In April of 1964 W. M. Beeson, Ph.D., of the Department of Animal Sciences at Purdue University cited 64 different research studies showing that the plant foods eaten by us and by livestock contain far less provitamin A (carotene) than they should. And worse yet, these nitrate-loaded foods destroy the already depleted stores of vitamin A within our bodies.

## Today's Environment Threatens Our Vitamin A Supply

With every breath we take, air passes through nasal passages which are lined with hairs and mucus, both of which trap foreign particles. What reaches our lungs should be only filtered air containing the oxygen which will dissolve into the bloodstream in exchange for carbon dioxide waste. The vitamin A-dependent mucous lining of the nasal passages, while it is there for our protection, is also a potential source of infection. In either case, the more pollutants these mucous membranes must fight off, the more vitamin A they use up in the process. Looking at it that way, we see that air pollution uses up vitamin A.

No longer just a danger in specified regions such as cities and industrial areas, pollution now pervades our entire land. When we breathe, we draw it into our bodies, where it attacks our nasal mucous membranes and even our lungs with poisonous gases, irritating particles, and carcinogenic matter. Air pollution wears down our mucous lining and lungs and makes them easier prey for invading organisms.

The pollutants, ozone and nitrogen dioxide, both destroy vitamin A by oxidation, according to a report by doctors from the Battelle-Northwest Institute presented at a symposium on pollution and lung biochemistry in Richland, Washington. Without this vitamin, glycoprotein synthesis in lung tissue may be affected and, instead of the body's normal production of mucus-secreting cells in the bronchial tubes, it forms thin layers of hard cells. Dr. Luigi M. De Luca, of the Massachusetts Institute of Technology, observed that when vitamin A is added to the diet, the rate of synthesis increases and healthy tissue is once again formed.

Under normal conditions, the body is able to take care of itself, but the relentless aggression of pollution is taking its toll. Besides ozone and nitrogen dioxide, the air is filled with hydrocarbons, lead, sulphur dioxide, carbon monoxide, and dozens of other poisons, all of which are alien to our breathing apparatus and every other facet of our bodies, internal organs and external parts as well. Vitamin A is one of the foremost safeguards against this ever-present onslaught upon our health. The demands on the respiratory system alone, and the consequent need for more vitamin A, are increasing daily.

If the obstacles to keeping an adequate supply of vitamin A stopped with air pollution, that would be enough to cause concern, for a certain amount of vitamin A is needed just to keep the body working at its normal pace. However, it is reasonable to expect the body to demand more of the vitamin since there are many ways that vitamin A can be used up, or simply wasted.

# CHAPTER 16

# Infectious Illnesses and the Vitamin A Response

Vitamin A concentrates in the retina of the eye and in the liver. It also flows through the bloodstream, which gives tissues throughout the body access to the vitamin. The chances of maintaining a healthy reserve of vitamin A are good provided no one part of the body overtaxes the supply. However, should an actual or threatened infection demand the lion's share of it, the blood plasma content of vitamin A may drop considerably.

According to the book, *Foundations of Nutrition*, by Dr. Clara Maye Taylor and Dr. Orrea Florence Pye (New York: Macmillan Publishing Company, 1966), infections cause a decrease in the plasma levels of vitamin A even though the liver maintains its own supply. The authors say that "infection tends to interfere with utilization of the vitamin and to cause depletion of body reserves." Furthermore, "Organisms usually harmless may become harmful if the subject already has a low resistance to infection."

Several simultaneous emergency demands from infections could deplete the blood's supply of vitamin A, even though the eyes and liver retain enough to keep them working properly. It can work the other way, too. That is, the liver's supply might drop precariously while the bloodstream gives no indication of the deficiency. Consequently, a vitamin A deficiency may defy diagnosis until the nutrient is practically exhausted. This condition is rare, but the steps leading up to it may be undetectable, and even a partial depletion is enough to give trouble.

When vitamin A stores drop below the safe level, it is usually at the expense of the epithelial cells throughout the body. They are included in the skin, glands, and mucous membranes and also the lining of the hollow organs and passages of the respiratory, alimentary, and genitourinary tracts.

The main value of vitamin A lies in its ability to prevent rather than cure infectious illnesses. According to statistics, people who maintain high levels of vitamin A in their systems are less susceptible to colds than others, and the ones they do contract are usually less severe.

## Antiinfection Action

The medical profession does not emphasize the role that vitamin A plays in maintaining our body health and preventing disease. However, one leading nutritional authority has attempted to reverse this trend. In 1968, Dr. George Wolf, a professor at the Massachusetts Institute of Technology, surprised an audience of doctors at an international medical symposium at MIT with the assertion that the human being cannot effectively resist many kinds of infection unless his or her vitamin A status is high.

According to Dr. Wolf, vitamin A helps the body fight off infection by maintaining cell-wall strength so that viruses cannot penetrate. Viruses can't reproduce on their own, so they must enter the body cells and take over the cells' reproductive mechanism to produce more viruses.

Viruses rarely succeed in overcoming the body, since it is capable of producing antibodies which can destroy these hostile organisms. The body also produces interferon, a natural substance which works to prevent the viruses from utilizing cell reproductive mechanisms. Vitamin A's effect on the cell walls provides still another means of protection—perhaps the most important of all because it keeps viruses from invading the body in the first place.

Scientists should have recognized vitamin A's importance in combating infection long ago. Researchers know that as soon as laboratory animals develop a severe deficiency of this nutrient, they become susceptible to serious infection and often die in a matter of days.

Drs. J. G. Bieri, E. G. McDaniel, and W. E. Rogers, Jr., at the Laboratory of Nutrition and Endocrinology, National Institute of Arthritis and Metabolic Diseases, showed that vitamin A-deficient rats quickly fall victim to even the simple infectious organisms normally present in the conventional animal room. By contrast, their litter mates, kept germ-free on the same diet, lived as long as 272 days—five to 10 times as long.

According to *Science* (February 1969), all of the rats suffered the usual symptoms of vitamin A deficiency: slower rates of weight gain, development of nervous symptoms characterized by head wobble, slow gait, and hind leg weakness, a loss of color around the eye (so-called spectacled eye). All the rats had urinary bladder stones, and most eventually died of urinary blockage and intestinal strangulation. The researchers demonstrated that vitamin A-deficient rats can survive—though not comfortably nor with normal function—for prolonged periods only if they are protected from the germ-ridden atmosphere we all live in. Control rats with proper vitamin A rations enjoyed the normal life span in an uncontrolled atmosphere.

Dr. Thomas Moore of Dunn Nutritional Laboratory in Cambridge, England, found the same results. In his chapter "Effects of Vitamin A Deficiency in Animals," in *The Vitamins* (ed. By W. H. Sebrell, Jr., and Robert S. Harris, second edition, New York and London Academic Press, 1967), he noted that a vitamin A deficiency weakened the outer layer of tissue so that bacteria and viruses were able to take hold and produce diseases in experimental rats. Dr. Moore's work on rats indicated that lesions originating in such tissues of the respiratory and urinary tracts, and in the intestine, were the commonest cause of death in vitamin A deficiency. "Thus in one experiment most of the rats may develop pneumonia, in another, urinary infections, in a third, enteritis (intestinal inflammation)," he reported.

# Vitamin A and Respiratory Infections

In a paper, "The Antiinfectious Action of Vitamin A," written in the early 1950s, Dr. M. Comel reported that animals that appeared close to death were able to recuperate when supplied with high doses of vitamin A. It was also shown that vitamin A helped animals successfully to fight reinfection with tuberculosis. "From those and many other observations," concluded Dr. Comel, "it was established eventually that vitamin A has marked antiinfectious action."

After carefully examining all existing literature on the subject, he said that "The deficiency in vitamin A might be one of the chief sources in an increase in the number of infectious processes as has been stated repeatedly in the observation of human pathology and in experiments as well. Thus, organisms lacking in vitamin A may become less resistant to infections. Such a lack might further deplete the organic deposits in vitamin A as an accompaniment to diminished resistance. Other authors have been able to relate a lack of vitamin A in infants to an increased susceptibility to infections, such as skin infections, colitis with chronic diarrhea, bronchitis, etc."

About 1952 Dr. Max Odens, of London, began a long-term clinical trial in which 17 patients, aged 48 to 67, suffering from chronic bronchitis, were given daily doses of vitamin A in addition to their usual therapy. After 15 years Dr. Odens reported in the German medical publication *Vitalstoffe* (December 1967) that all 17 patients showed "considerable improvement, in spite of the unfavorable English climate—and luckily all of them are still alive, including the oldest, aged 79 years. Even in the severe winter of 1952/53, when there was continuous dense fog and thousands of elderly people suffering from chronic bronchitis died, my patients continued to respond to treatment and were not unduly affected."

Dr. Luigi M. DeLuca explained vitamin A's resistance-building powers, speaking at a 1968 symposium on pollution and lung biochemistry held at the Massachusetts Institute of Technology. The professor postulated that the vitamin helps your body ward off infection by promoting the growth of mucus-secreting cells in the epithelial tissue (also called the mucous membrane) which lines your respiratory, alimentary, and genitourinary tracts.

Mucus production is especially important in our respiratory system. The mucous membrane, which lines the nose, mouth, throat, and bronchial tubes, contains protective devices that guard against invading substances such as bacteria or the common cold virus. Attached to the mucous membranes are large numbers of ciliated cells, each containing about eight microscopic hairlike structures known as cilia. Each nostril has literally millions of cilia. According to Dr. Noah D. Fabricant and Groff Conklin in *The Dangerous Cold* (New York: Macmillan Publishing Company, 1965), the mucous glands secrete mucus, a film of moisture kept in constant motion by the cilia which "whip back and forth about 250 times a minute and operate in such a sequence that they form waves, very much like those you can see in a field of grain or tall grass when a wind passes over it."

The motion of the cilia sweeps the unwanted substances back from the nose into the mouth, where they are expectorated or swallowed (the gastrointestinal system has its own protective devices to deal with such substances). Other cilia in the respiratory system perform a similar task when the viruses manage to get past the nose, which is the respiratory system's first line of defense.

## The Thymus—Organ of Immunity

There is another way that vitamin A strengthens and improves the body's ability to resist disease. It is an important and probably essential factor in maintaining a healthy and functioning thymus gland. The thymus is a small but vital part of the body's immunity system. As described in *Scientific American* (July 1973) by Dr. Niels Kaj Jerne, the blood cells that produce antibodies, while produced in the bone marrow, reproduce themselves to the necessary number in the thymus and other organs of the lymph system. Known as lymphocytes, these blood cells have the remarkable ability to recognize the structure of a particular invader of the bloodstream, bacterial or otherwise, and produce an antibody that will recognize and attack just that invader and no other. When we become immune to any particular disease, it is because we have been invaded by the agent that causes that disease and our lymphocytes have formed antibodies against that particular agent. Thereafter, we are protected.

The role of the thymus is particularly important in childhood when the blood has not yet constructed its antibodies against the host of invading diseases. As a person grows older, the need for antibody formation diminishes and the thymus dwindles in size. Ultimately it may become totally inactive, which is never desirable but has long been accepted as one of the inevitable consequences of aging. However, there are indications that the atrophy of the thymus may result less from aging than from the inadequacy of the body's stores of vitamin A. It is well known that when people are under unusual stress, whether it be psychic anxiety, a polluted environment, or physical damage like a broken bone, they become more vulnerable to disease generally.

At Albert Einstein Medical College in New York, Dr. Ely Seifter has been studying the relationship between vitamin A and the size of the thymus. His particular concern has been stress and the way that stress interferes with the body's ability to protect itself. Studying mice that were stressed by being put into a partial body cast which did not injure them in any way but kept them from moving normally, Dr. Seifter and his colleagues found on sacrificing his mice that the abnormal strain had caused their thymus glands to shrink (*Federation Proceedings*, March 1973).

It was a significant indication of how it is that great anxiety, overwork because of excessive ambition, and other stressful psychological conditions can render us vulnerable to illnesses that we would otherwise be able to throw off.

In a way, Dr. Seifter's work thus far was a repetition and confirmation of the classic studies of stress made by Dr. Hans Selye. Dr. Selye had, many years ago, postulated shrinkage of the thymus as a major signpost of excessive stress. Another was enlargement of the adrenal gland, and Dr. Seifter has linked these two by showing that excessive production of cortisone by the adrenal (connected with its enlargement) destroys lymph cells, presumably depriving the thymus of what it needs in the way of nourishment and stimulation.

But Dr. Seifter and his associates at Einstein Medical College have made another extremely important step forward. They have found that by administering large doses of vitamin A to mice under the same stressful condition with which they induced the thymus shrinkage, they were able to reduce the amount of shrinkage. In addition, they discovered that when they removed the stress, vitamin A was an invaluable aid in restoring the thymus to its normal size.

To summarize as simply as possible, what Dr. Seifter has found is that stress, through its influence on our glands, makes us more vulnerable to all sorts of unrelated diseases that may just happen to invade our bodies at the time of stress. The best protection we have against disease during periods of stress is to take extra quantities of vitamin A at such times.

# CHAPTER 17

# Protein Synthesis is a Basic Vitamin A Function

For protein to function efficiently in the body, vitamin A is required. The reverse is equally as true. New knowledge indicates that a protein shortage often results from the body's failure to absorb the protein properly due to a vitamin A deficiency. Sufficient protein is essential to build and repair cells, tissues, and organs, defend against infection, and maintain the delicate balances inside tissues and blood.

Scientists now know that without vitamin A, the protein being fed to undernourished and malnourished persons actually does more harm than good. Writing in *Nutritional Metabolism* (vol. 15, 1973), a group of Israeli researchers from the Hebrew University in Rehovot determined that a vitamin A deficiency caused increases in the activities of kidney arginase and liver xanthine oxidase in young chicks, reactions which are extremely important in the metabolism of protein in the body.

The researchers from the university's Department of Animal Nutrition and Agricultural Biochemistry, raised a number of chicks on various diets ranging from one that had absolutely no vitamin A to one which was very high in the vitamin. All diets had the same amount of protein in them.

After 19 days, the chicks were tested for their vitamin A stores. Those fed adequate protein but no vitamin A had only a very low amount of vitamin A in their blood plasma. None could be detected in their livers, usually the main storage point for the vitamin. Those raised on a marginal amount of vitamin A (40 I.U. per 100 grams of weight) had some liver stores remaining. In addition, the plasma level was low, but not dangerous.

Taking a close look at the animals who received absolutely no vitamin A, the researchers noted that both liver xanthine oxidase and kidney arginase levels were raised. They speculated that the increase was caused by the vitamin A-deficient diet and may indicate "a failure in the amino acids utilization for protein synthesis." Apparently vitamin A is intimately involved in the process of converting dietary protein into living flesh. If the vitamin is in scarce supply, it will preferentially be used for protein synthesis at the expense of its other functions. If there is no vitamin A, even the protein synthesis stops.

It has been known for several years that protein and vitamin A are in some way related, and that kwashiorkor, the protein deficiency disease, is frequently accompanied by vitamin A deficiency. Kwashiorkor affects thousands of youngsters in Indonesia, Brazil, and other countries where complete protein foods are in short supply.

The logical way to relieve the distress of protein malnutrition would seem to be by adding protein to the diets of these starving children. But when UNICEF (United Nations International Children's Emergency Fund) with the best of intentions distributed a protein supplement in the form of dry skimmed milk to these children, a strange and distressful situation occurred. There was an epidemic of eye diseases, the kind that frequently lead to blindness (*Tropical and Geographical Medicine*, 16, 271, 1964). It is perfectly obvious that milk does not cause eye lesions, but what does cause eye lesions? Vitamin A deficiency. In 1968 the non-fat milk used in the food donation programs was fortified with vitamin A because it was now clear that *increased protein intake increased the need for vitamin A*. This dependency of protein on vitamin A was cited by Dr. Oswald A. Roels of Columbia University and Dr. James P. Mack of City University of New York in a study of "Vitamin A and Protein

Metabolism" (*Journal of Agricultural Food Chemistry,* vol. 20, No. 6, 1972).

Drs. Roels and Mack reported that it is clear that in man, vitamin A deficiency and protein malnutrition frequently occur simultaneously. The absorption of dietary vitamin A is impaired in acute protein malnutrition, and adequate serum and dietary proteins are necessary for the mobilization of vitamin A from the liver and its transport in the blood. Increased protein intake results in greater vitamin A requirement, and both protein and vitamin A are required for growth.

A landmark study by T. R. Varnell, Ph.D., of the Division of Animal Science, University of Wyoming, provided insight into the interaction between vitamin A and protein. Dr. Varnell has determined that vitamin A enters into the synthesis of protein in the liver. Therefore, according to his report in the *International Journal of Vitamin Nutrition* (3 October 1972), when this vitamin is deficient, protein is not fully synthesized.

The liver has many important jobs to do. One of them is to assemble the amino acids delivered by the bloodstream into the orderly chains that constitute the protein molecule which is then carried by the bloodstream back to wherever it is needed to carry on the business of life.

The finding that vitamin A is necessary to this process elevates this vitamin to a position of even more importance than has heretofore been recognized. Besides all the many well-known functions of vitamin A—for the eyes, for the skin, for the health of the mucous membranes, to guard against infection—to mention a few, we must now add another vital function to the list: vitamin A is necessary to the synthesis of protein.

It means that if our diets are low in protein, we need vitamin A to effect full utilization of every single amino acid. But, the more protein we consume, the more vitamin A we need to get those amino acids lined up for action. Which means that a high protein diet can actually bring about a vitamin A deficiency—with dire consequences.

In Dr. Varnell's experiment, laboratory rats were subjected to four different dietary regimens: a basal diet devoid of vitamin A;

a basal diet pair-fed with deficient animals, plus a daily oral dose of 250 I.U. of vitamin A; a basal diet, fed *ad libitum* (at will), plus daily oral vitamin A; or the basal diet fed *ad libitum* including a source of vitamin A.

When Dr. Varnell examined the livers of these rats, he found a strange thing happening. In those animals deficient in vitamin A, there were high levels of free amino acids, particularly alanine, valine, isoleucine, leucine, proline, threonine, serine, methionine, and tyrosine. "The hepatic (liver) accumulation of free amino acids was primarily due to a lack of vitamin A," Dr. Varnell reported.

Dr. Varnell determined that where vitamin A is deficient in the diet, there is a concentration of free amino acids in the liver. In other words, these amino acids have no way of getting together into the protein chain which the bloodstream then supplies to the cells where it becomes the body's building blocks. When these protein factors are not available, we cannot build and repair cells, tissues, and organs, defend against infection, or maintain all the delicate balances inside tissues and blood that are so vital to every single life process.

In fact, this new finding which implies that you can be protein-deficient on a diet that is adequate in protein has far-reaching implications. Is it, for instance, possible to suffer loss of hair because of a shortage of methionine even though you are eating methionine-rich eggs, milk, and meat, if you are not getting enough vitamin A to participate in the job of lining up methionine into the protein chain?

Is it possible that this pile-up of amino acids playing havoc in your liver instead of playing their role in the protein chain is seriously hampering the effectiveness of your liver and slowing down its job-order rate at a time when toxins in the air, water, and food demand peak efficiency from this detoxifying organ?

This "togetherness" of protein and vitamin A probably accounts for the fact that vitamin A deficiency and protein malnutrition frequently occur together because just as the absorption of protein is impaired when there isn't enough vitamin A, so also is the absorption of dietary vitamin A impaired when there is acute protein malnutrition. Vitamin A is necessary in order to synthesize protein in the liver but dietary proteins are also "necessary in order to mobilize the vitamins from the liver into the bloodstream," reported Drs. Roels and Mack. "Increased protein intake results in greater vitamin A requirement, and both protein and vitamin A are required for growth."

This partnership was apparent in Dr. Varnell's study which demonstrated that the decrease in the growth rate of vitamin A-deficient rats was accompanied by a decrease in protein utilization. He also noted a severe depression of the serum albumin (blood protein) level in a vitamin A-deficient steer. Serum albumin was increased when vitamin A was administered—but not when carotene was administered.

# CHAPTER 18

# More Vitamin A Required in Winter

If the action of vitamin A comes through general health, why is it so much more effective against the winter diseases like colds and bronchitis than against warm weather infections? A study, described in the *Journal of Nutrition* (October 1967), was made at the U.S. Army Research Institute of Environmental Medicine (Natick, Massachusetts) and it dealt with the effect of low temperatures in the environment on the vitamin A metabolism.

It was found that as the weather or the external temperature gets colder, the body becomes less able to utilize its supply of vitamin A. This lower level of utilization sets up an increased requirement for vitamin A, in order to maintain a normal metabolic activity of that vitamin through a period of low temperature.

The researchers studied the question by taking young male rats and feeding them for four weeks on a diet that was rounded and balanced in every respect except that it was deficient in vitamin A. Then they were given uniform amounts of vitamin A and kept under various environmental temperatures.

It was found that at a temperature of five degrees F., the rats gained little weight and did little growing. At a temperature of 25 degrees F., on the other hand, there was a significantly higher level of growth and weight gain. At the end of this particular experiment, when the rats were sacrificed and examined, it was found that a rat kept at the low five-degree temperature had stored most of the vitamin A received in the liver, but had not utilized it for growth. (It is well known that vitamin A is one of the indispensable components in the growth of bones.) The rats kept at the milder temperature of 25 degrees F., on the other hand, had significantly greater increases in growth and weight, and on *post mortem* examination proved to have far less vitamin A stored in their livers, demonstrating that more of it had been used in the metabolic process of growing.

The researchers then investigated the question of why a drop in the outside temperature should reduce the ability of the animal to utilize vitamin A. The obvious area to investigate was that of the relationship to the production of thyroid and adrenal hormones, since it is by stimulation of these two glands, which leads to a faster rate of oxidation of food, that a body manages to keep its temperature constant as the outside temperature drops. Testing with the administration of antimetabolites that prevented these glands from speeding up, the research scientists found, sure enough, that in this way the vitamin A metabolism could be encouraged. Naturally enough, however, when their glands were unable to respond to the stimulation of a drop in temperature, the rats quickly died of cold exposure.

The final aspect of the study involved simply leaving the glands alone but administering larger quantities of vitamin A to rats that were exposed to the five-degree temperatures. It worked!

There was a definite proportional relationship between the amount of vitamin A injected into the rats and the number that were able to survive the five-degree cold. At 2.5 micrograms, none of them survived. At 10 micrograms, one out of six survived. At 100 micrograms, two out of four survived, and at the 100 microgram-per-day injection level, the rats actually grew and gained weight, which was not true of any of those receiving less vitamin A.

This study is of prime importance. It answers so many questions. Why do children grow faster in summer than they do in winter? Because their diets contain approximately the same amount of vitamin A, but as the temperature drops they utilize the vitamin A less effectively. Give them more of this vitamin and they should grow faster. Why do vitamin A supplements increase our resistance to colds? Because when the cold weather comes, we use a smaller proportion of the vitamin A in our systems and keep more of it stored in the liver. It takes the supplements to provide equivalent vitamin A activity. The effect is caused by the stimulating effect the cold has on the thyroid and adrenal glands, and this is necessary if our bodies are to keep warm. Yet the reduced utilization of vitamin A when no supplements are taken, means a reduced level of health, lowering our ability to resist colds and other respiratory diseases.

As the weather gets colder, the consumption of vitamin A should increase to help maintain the same level of health during the winter as in the warmer months.

In addition to an adequate intake of vitamin A, the healthy functioning of the respiratory system's mucous membrane should be guarded from abuse. Those who smoke are actually paralyzing the cilia for as long as 30 to 40 minutes with each cigarette. A heavy smoker must do without this valuable defense against infection entirely—and heavy smokers demonstrably get heavier colds and get them more frequently.

# CHAPTER 19

# Vitamin A and the Senses

Many people regard some hearing loss, the inability to smell (or anosmia), and night blindness as normal occurrences of aging and never bother to seek relief. They are often unaware that adequate stores of vitamin A are indispensable in keeping these senses in balance and staving off some degrees of sensory malfunction.

## Sense of Smell and Vitamin A

If you are unable to savor the aroma of baking bread, of blooming roses or expensive perfume, it may be that you are deficient in vitamin A.

Drs. M. H. Briggs and R. B. Duncan of Victoria University of Wellington, New Zealand, reported in the British publication, *Nature* (191: 1310, 1969), that animals raised on diets free of carotenoid (that's the group of yellow, orange, red, and purple pigments) had an impaired sense of smell. It has been known, for instance, that the soft membranes of the olfactory areas are yellow whereas areas not related to the sense of smell are not. These yellow areas are known to contain carotenoids, which, in experiments, can be liberated from their combination with proteins. The fact that patients treated with vitamin A recovered their sense of smell is probably related to interaction of carotenes and simple carotenoids to vitamin A in the olfactory area. A lost sense of smell was recovered by 48 of 53 patients given large intramuscular injections of vitamin A, according to an article in *Science Newsletter* (7 October 1961).

## Vitamin A Deficiency and Hearing Loss

Otosclerosis, a conductive type of deafness in the aged, blocking the sound waves from entering the inner ear, is a major cause of hearing impairment. In this process, explains Dr. Robert E. Rothenberg in his book, *Health in the Later Years* (New York: New American Library, 1964), "the bones surrounding the middle and inner ear tend to become hardened and overgrown; this will result in interference of the transmission of sound waves."

Because otosclerosis is a disease that fixes the middle ear bones so that they cannot vibrate sound, some doctors rely on surgery for improvement. A stapedectomy either removes the malfunctioning stapes, which is then replaced by a stainless steel or plastic filament, or frees the stapes of adhesions so it can vibrate normally. A fenestration—an operation in which a hole is drilled into the bone so that sound waves can pass through to the inner ear—might also restore hearing.

Once otosclerosis is diagnosed, surgical procedures seem the only remedy. But must this condition occur? Research performed by the renowned Sir Edward Mellanby in 1934 demonstrated by experiments with laboratory animals that a lack of vitamin A can lead to diminished transmission of sounds.

At a symposium on metabolic functions of vitamin A at the Massachusetts Institute of Technology held in November of 1968, Dr. Oswald A. Roels of Columbia University reported findings that a lack of this vitamin causes cell membranes to break down. Vitamin A regulates the stability of the walls of tissue cells and he concluded that much hearing loss due to the aging process results from a vitamin A deficiency. All in all, it appears that plenty of vitamin A might keep many cases of otosclerosis from ever occurring.

# Vitamin A and Normal Vision

Vitamin A is essential for normal, healthy vision. About 1 percent of your daily intake of vitamin A is used by the retina, which receives and transmits the image formed by the lens. People who lack this vitamin often suffer from night blindness, the eyes' inability to adapt to the dark.

According to John E. Dowling, Ph.D., a professor of Biology at Harvard University, writing in *Scientific American* (October 1966), "Night blindness—insensitivity of the eye to dim light—is one of the oldest diseases known to man, and a cure for the disease has also been known since early times. Medical papyruses of ancient Egypt prescribed the eating of raw liver as a specific for restoring night vision." However, reported Dr. Dowling, it was not until the twentieth century that vitamin A was officially recognized as the key factor in better night vision.

Almost everyone experiences the common visual phenomenon of dark adaptation. The eye can adjust its sensitivity to nearly any level of light, be it dim or brilliant, and it functions more efficiently because of this ability. This mechanism goes to work when a person walks into a darkened movie theater from the brightly lit lobby. After being temporarily blinded, the eyes grow accustomed to the dark until they can finally define the location of the seats and aisles. Normal eyes become 90 percent adjusted to the dark in seven to ten minutes. However, this loss of sight lasts longer for the person suffering from night blindness.

The physiological cause of night blindness lies in the retinal pigment. The retina is composed of two kinds of cells; cones, which are sensitive to light and colors, and rods, which are sensitive to dim light and black and white. The cones are used primarily for daytime vision while the rods allow us to see at night. The rods contain rhodopsin (visual purple) which is composed of opsin, a protein molecule, and retinene (visual yellow), a form of vitamin A. When light reaches the retina, it breaks down the rhodopsin into these two components. This chemical reaction sends nerve impulses through the optic nerve to the brain. The nerve impulses form the image of whatever you are looking at. The breakdown rate of rhodopsin is a function of the amount of light entering the eye. High intensity light speeds the breakdown of visual purple, causing a brighter light sensation.

So that vision can be maintained constantly, rhodopsin is reformed from retinene and opsin as rapidly as it is broken down. This cycle of degeneration and regeneration continues all through life. However, in the splitting process some of the retinene is destroyed and, unless the body's vitamin A supply is constantly replenished, the eyes lose the ability to adapt to the dark efficiently. "The visual purple must be immediately regenerated by vitamin A if vision is to continue unimpaired. Should there be a deficiency of the vitamin, the regeneration is slow and the rods become less sensitive to light, which results in poor vision in dim illumination—night blindness," according to Glenn Kittler's *Richmond Times Dispatch* article (12 September 1965). George Wald, Ph.D., of Harvard University showed that a short supply of vitamin A also inhibits the sensitivity of cells necessary for vision in ordinary light because A is also important to their visual pigments.

Studies of subjects on vitamin A-deficient diets show that it takes longer for some people to develop night blindness. The reason for this, according to English researchers, is that humans vary in the amount of vitamin A they can store in their livers. As a result, a person who begins eating a diet poor in vitamin A, but has a large reserve of vitamin A, may not notice any change in his night vision for weeks or even months. Another on that diet, and with no store of vitamin A, might show signs of night blindness within a few days. Equally important, those who develop night blindness fall into two more categories: those who quickly regain their normal vision once vitamin A is restored to their diets, and those who recover more slowly (sometimes over a period of a few months).

In his experiments on night blindness in rats, who have a large number of cells responsible for vision in dim light, Dr. Dowling charted the animals' depletion of their vitamin A stores. As expected, when the animals did not receive the proper amount of vitamin A in their food, they drew on the store of vitamin A in their livers. In young rats the supply of vitamin A lasted three to four weeks. During this time the vitamin A level in the animals' blood and the rhodopsin in their eyes remained normal. When all the vitamin A in the liver was used up, the vitamin A level in the blood quickly fell, followed by a decline in the amount of A in the eyes. Two or three weeks later the opsin level began to drop.

Dr. Dowling and his colleagues were able to observe the actual effect of vitamin A deficiency on the animals' vision by measuring the rats' eye-sensitivity by the amount of light needed for a response. During the first few weeks of the experiment the rats' eyes responded normally. By the fifth week more and more light was needed to bring on even a slight reaction. By the eighth week the rats' rhodopsin levels had dropped to 15 or 20 percent of normal and it took almost a thousand times the normal light intensity to elicit any response. However, in spite of the difficulty the rats had in seeing, there was no permanent damage to their eyes. Large doses of vitamin A administered over a few days restored the rats' retinas to their normal performance.

At this point in the experiment Dr. Dowling ran into a problem. The rats didn't stay alive long enough for him to discover what was happening to their eyes. Vitamin A is essential for maintaining tissue health throughout the body. After eight or nine weeks on a vitamin A-deficient diet rats lose weight, experience trouble breathing, and become prone to infection. A rat who goes without vitamin A for 10 or 12 weeks usually dies. To combat this problem Dowling gave the rats vitamin A acid, which apparently is not converted into vitamin A in the rats' body tissues. The vitamin A acid kept the rats healthy and at the same time maintained their vitamin A-deficient condition. The investigators were able to keep the animals alive while observing the decline in vision brought on by a lack of actual vitamin A.

On this new diet the rats became severely night-blind. The visual cells in their retinas began to degenerate and were almost completely destroyed by the tenth month of the experiment. The animals were totally blind, unable to respond to light at any intensity. Even large doses of vitamin A failed to restore the rats' vision. Like all cells of the nervous system, vision cells cannot be regenerated once they are lost.

Of course, night blindness is little more than an inconvenience when one must walk through a darkened room, but this malady can lead to highly dangerous situations under some circumstances.

Night blindness was first recognized as a potential killer during World War II. Early in the war, fatal night accidents reached alarming numbers. Pilots lost sight of dim horizons and crashed; army truck drivers missed turns and drove into ditches when driving during blackouts; seamen couldn't see buoys; and soldiers missed enemy patrols which they should have spotted.

The Armed Forces Vision Committee was formed to investigate the problem. In their first study at Pensacola Naval Air Station, ophthalmologists tested men who had been on leave on the bright Florida beaches. All of the subjects failed the simplest night vision tests.

A second study was conducted in Rhode Island where Navy lookouts, who had been performing their duties with no difficulties, suddenly lost their night-seeing ability, yet each of the men had been picked for the job because of his superior vision. The researchers discovered that these men had been shoveling the snow which had blanketed the area two days earlier, and their loss of night vision was due to severe overexposure to the snow-reflected light.

When you drive at night, you encounter the same conditions which reduced night vision in the military men. Shining directly into your eyes, the glare from headlights of oncoming cars rapidly breaks down your visual purple. Research has shown that at 50 m.p.h. the average driver travels 73 feet totally blinded after meeting the headlights of other cars. For the person with low stores of vitamin A, the distance traveled is two to three times as great.

Since your night vision depends entirely on the vitamin A mechanism, even a mild deficiency affects it. If you are overly sensitive to headlight beams, if it takes a while to regain your vision after seeing headlights, and if you can't distinguish objects from their background, you need vitamin A.

# More Severe Deficiency Dangers

A more severe deficiency can bring on other problems such as tired and aching eyes after reading or close work. An acute deficiency causes burning and itching eyes, inflamed eyelids, headaches, and pain in the eyeballs. It can even lead to xerophthalmia, a major cause of blindness in malnourished children. In this condition the conjunctiva (inner lining of the eyelid) dries up and hardens. Tear secretions stop, the eyes become highly sensitive to light, the lids swell and become full of pus, and ulcers grow on the corners of the eye. If the dryness grows worse, the cornea can acquire a softness and become gray, dull, and cloudy. This condition is known as keratomalacia. At this stage irreversible blindness may occur.

A 1965 pamphlet published by the World Health Organization estimates that 25 percent of survivors from keratomalacia become totally blind, while about 60 percent suffer reduced vision in one or both eyes. The survey concluded, "Not only did a great many children show clinical manifestations of vitamin A deficiency, but low serum levels of vitamin A indicated the existence of a subclinical deficiency in an even larger number."

While the majority of us are not in danger of developing serious eye diseases such as xerophthalmia or keratomalacia, we could still be lacking a sufficient amount of vitamin A. Your need for vitamin A depends somewhat on your type of work or other activities. For example, office workers who read under bright lights need more vitamin A than those who work under moderate lighting conditions. On the other hand, people like miners and photographers who work in dim light, which requires good night vision, should also increase their consumption of vitamin A. And if you plan a vacation on the beach or at a ski resort, remember your vitamin A. The light reflected from the sand or snow affects your night vision.

# CHAPTER 20

# The Value of Vitamin A for
# Skin, Teeth, and Bones

Medical or nutrition books which discuss vitamins in detail usually mention vitamin A's important effect on the skin. Composed of epithelial tissue, the skin reacts early to a mild vitamin A deficiency. The cells on the surface (the stratum corneum) and on several lower layers shrivel up and die. This dead tissue plugs the oil sacs and pores, preventing oil from reaching the skin surface. The clogged pores, called whiteheads and blackheads, resemble goose pimples. In addition, the skin becomes dry and rough, especially on the elbows, knees, buttocks, and the back of the upper arm. Sometimes the entire body itches. Susceptibility to skin infections such as impetigo, boils, and carbuncles also increases.

Hermann Pinkus, M.D., and Rose Hunter demonstrated the vitamin's effectiveness in maintaining skin integrity by measuring and comparing the accumulation of hard, dry, dead cells with and without a vitamin A supplement. The researchers' method, described in the *Journal of Investigative Dermatology* (January 1964), involved repeatedly stripping dead skin cells from ten healthy adults by pulling cellophane tape off the subjects' backs. Dr. Pinkus and Ms. Hunter scraped the cells off the pieces of tape and counted the number of dry, roughened ones.

The volunteers then received a daily dose of 150,000 mgs. of vitamin A for a month. At the end of that time the number of horny cells stripped off a single area had decreased in all the subjects. The researchers concluded that vitamin A appeared to retard the development of the hardened cell. "Vitamin A has an 'antikeratinizing' effect," they said, "and . . . this is achieved by the cells remaining immature (young) longer."

## Teeth, Gums, and the Jawbone

Vitamin A, so important to the health of mucous membranes and skin, is just as important to the ameloblast cells which help to build the enamel of teeth. In fact, where there is insufficient vitamin A, calcified concretions (tumors) sometimes occur in the pulp of the teeth. Where there is vitamin A deficiency, bone growth is retarded. "These effects upon bone growth in vitamin A deficiency are of potential interest in the field of children's dentistry and orthodontics," reported James H. Shaw, Ph.D., of the Harvard School of Dental Medicine in *Modern Nutrition in Health and Disease* (Philadelphia, Pennsylvania: Lea and Febiger, 1964). "Since vitamin A deficiency causes such a profound influence on bone development, some of the inadequate growth patterns which result in orthodontic problems may have had their origin in prolonged periods of subclinical vitamin A deficiency during the developmental period of the child," Dr. Shaw observed.

Of course, healthy teeth require healthy gums. When the gums are afflicted with an inflammation called gingivitis, the gums tend to shrink away from the teeth inviting the formation of pockets where food debris can collect, leading to more infection and loosening of the tooth structure.

Dr. Karl Rinne reported in *Zahnarztl Rundschau*, a German dental journal (69: 15–18, 8 January 1960), that vitamin A is necessary to the health of the gums because it increases the resistance of the mucous membranes to infections. In four cases of severe gingivitis he used vitamin A together with vitamin E (vitamin E accelerates the blood circulation and "stabilizes" vitamin A, he noted). Three of his patients were in the menopause and were suffering from severe gingivitis and considerable loss of epithelial tissue. The dosage used was high: for six days— daily 500,000 I.U. vitamin A and 30 mg. vitamin E which he administered by intramuscular injection. For the next three weeks the schedule was as follows: three times daily—50,000 I.U. of vitamin A and twice daily one capsule (200 mg.) of vitamin E. His patients were completely cured. There were no relapses; one patient remained under observation for over two years, the other three from five to seven months.

## Important for Bone Growth

Vitamin A plays a major role in bone resorption. Although it is hard and inflexible, bone is as much a living tissue as the skin is. And, like the skin, old bone cells are constantly breaking down and falling away while new ones are created to take their place.

Asger M. Frandsen, D.M.D., reported in the journal *Oral Surgery* (April 1962) on what he referred to as the "profound influence of vitamin A on bone." When there was a deficiency of vitamin A, he observed, two things happened: first, there was a slight reduction in osteoblastic activity, or the process in which certain cells, the osteoblasts, create new bone material; and secondly, osteoclastic activity, whereby the osteoclasts, which are the cells responsible for dissolving old bone tissue, are either reduced or completely stopped.

If the skin on a certain part of your arm failed to slough off along with the rest of the skin on your body, yet underlying cells continued to replace it with new skin, the eventual results would be a large protrusion of dry, old skin. Exactly the same thing occurs with bone deficient in vitamin A. The osteoclasts no longer break down old bone tissue, yet the process of making new bone continues. The results can be serious. Dr. Frandsen described "degenerative changes in the brain and the cranial and peripheral nerves of vitamin A-deficient dogs." The continued overgrowth of skull bone eventually pressed into the brain.

Similar abnormal bone formations of the cranium were observed in laboratory animals deficient in vitamin A by Drs. B.

M. Kagan and R. S. Goodhart. Reporting on their extensive studies dealing with vitamin A deficiency and bone growth in test animals in a chapter entitled "The Vitamins" in *Modern Nutrition in Health and Disease,* third edition, (edited by Drs. Michael G. Wohl and Robert S. Goodhard, Philadelphia, Pennsylvania: Lea and Febiger Pub, 1964), the researchers observed malformations in the tunneling of cartilage and overly compacted bone areas, including a marked difficulty for laboratory rats to heal from bone fractures.

# CHAPTER 21

# The Genetic Code
# and Vitamin A

Biochemical research currently concentrates heavily on study of the genetic code. As it advances, scientists are documenting specific information about substances and mechanisms involved in the incredible ability of living things to maintain shapes, functions, and health.

If you break a bone, the bone cells around the break start reproducing themselves, rejoin the bone, and reinforce it at the break with a rim of extra bone called callus. What tells them to start reproducing, and what tells them to stop when the proper point has been reached? How does a cell know it is supposed to manufacture interferon when it is invaded by a virus? What tells the cells of the nose to reproduce in the particular pattern and at the particular rate that will give the nose the same shape the mother's nose has, and then to stop all this activity when that shape has been achieved?

These are fascinating and vital questions to which there were no known answers until the nucleic acids were isolated, examined, and tested. It was then found that one form of nucleic acid—messenger ribonucleic acid (RNA)—carries all the instructions that tell the individual cells how to perform so that life, health, and function may be maintained. Like all other living matter, however, RNA must also renew and reproduce itself to play its own key role. Otherwise, as it becomes old, its patterns blur and the body as a consequence develops more and more distortion such as "liver spots," lowered resistance to a particular disease, cancer, or other degenerative diseases.

Clearly, the ability of the body to synthesize fresh new RNA is absolutely fundamental to the ability to stay healthy or even to survive. Thus it would be impossible to exaggerate the significance of work at the University of Oklahoma School of Medicine and Medical Research Foundation which has established a close connection between our vitamin A nutrition and our daily ability to synthesize ribonucleic acid. Performed by three biochemists, Drs. B. Connor Johnson, Michelle Kennedy, and Naoki Chiba, the investigations were described in November, 1968, at a symposium sponsored by the Massachusetts Institute of Technology.

To form new ribonucleic acid containing the proper code of instructions, the body apparently must first obtain a blank matrix of nucleic acid containing few or no instructions. One of the best sources of such nucleic acid appears to be yeast, which yields a form that is called uridine. The University of Oklahoma biochemists set out to study the speed and efficiency of incorporation of uridine into the RNA of the livers of experimental animals. Why the livers? Because the liver, the most versatile organ of the body and one that performs the greatest variety of functions, contains greater concentrations of nucleic acids than any other organ.

Working with laboratory rats, Drs. Johnson, Kennedy, and Chiba set out to test a variety of conditions in which uridine was administered in the presence of vitamin A deficiency, normal amounts of vitamin A, and unusually large amounts of vitamin A.

"The data indicate a marked increase in incorporation of uridine into total liver RNA up to 30 hours after administration of 10 milligrams potassium retinoate (vitamin A)." It was found that while the liver deficient in vitamin A will continue to incorporate nucleic acid into its pool of RNA, "the extent of incorporation is much less . . . than in the case of the normal animals." The figures indicate that a normal vitamin A status will nearly double the rate of incorporation.

Having obtained this result, the researchers went on to experiment with administration of larger-than-normal amounts of vitamin A and found that this produced further increase in the rate of absorption, which is to say that it stimulated the synthesis of new RNA in the rat liver.

The results were then checked in various ways, through other studies involving malnourished rats as compared to normally fed ones, and also checking whether cortisone, an adrenal hormone whose production depends on vitamin A, had any influence on ribonucleic synthesis.

It was found that it was only vitamin A that changed the ability of the livers to manufacture new RNA. Even small quantities of vitamin A facilitated this process, but it was generally found that the more vitamin A there is in the liver, the faster the liver will manufacture RNA and the more it will manufacture.

The study was not limited to the liver. The same effect was discovered inside the nucleus of the individual cell. And in a tissue known to be particularly sensitive to vitamin A deficiency—in this case the mucous membrane lining of the intestine—"There was at least a three-fold difference in incorporation of labeled uridine into intestinal mucosal nuclear RNA between vitamin A-normal and vitamin A-deficient animals."

The researchers concluded that vitamin A "rapidly increases incorporation of uridine into intestinal mucosal and liver nuclear RNA."

They also said that "When normal and deficient (in vitamin A) animals are compared with regard to uridine incorporation into rapidly labeled RNA a three-fold difference was found. Also an increase rate of synthesis was indicated since peak incorporation was reached at or before 30 minutes for the normal as compared to one hour in the deficient." Thus we may well draw the additional conclusion that if your general condition is such that you have reason to suspect you are not synthesizing enough fresh, new RNA and are not producing it fast enough, you should check on your vitamin A status.

How is such a condition recognized? If exercise does not cause your muscles to toughen up and increase their endurance the way they used to; if the skin on your face, instead of regenerating itself fully, becomes dry and wrinkled; if you find yourself looking and feeling old; if your resistance to disease is not what it used to be. All these and the other signs that we ordinarily think of as "aging" are signs that we are becoming deficient in nucleic acid production.

# CHAPTER 22

# Vitamin A in Reproduction and Sexual Disorders

Vitamin A plays an integral role in the reproduction process and in the effectuation of a person's sexual identify. Probably none of your body's reproductive apparatus would work if vitamin A weren't there to participate in the synthesis of the sex hormones.

Experiments in animals and human beings over the past 20 years have provided researchers in this country and abroad with a steady stream of compelling data pointing to a direct link between vitamin A and sexual development and reproduction.

In the early 1950s Dr. A. Narpozzi studied the effects of various vitamins on men suffering varying levels of sperm deficiency, a deficiency which may often lead to sterility. In an article published in the Italian medical journal *Rivista Di Ostetricia e Ginecologia* (May 1954), Dr. Narpozzi reported that vitamin A—when administered with vitamin E—restored sperm levels to normal.

In 1966 Dr. Birthe Palludan of Copenhagan showed how an induced vitamin A deficiency in boars could stop or reduce sperm production. Describing the experiment in *Nature* (6 August 1966), Dr. Palludan noted an "administration of vitamin A to an A-avitaminoid (vitamin A-deficient) boar resulted in a complete normalization of the spermatogenesis (sperm production) within three months."

Dr. Thomas Moore of Dunn Nutritional Laboratory in Cambridge, England, noted in his chapter "Effects of Vitamin A Deficiency in Animals," in *The Vitamins* (ed. by W. H. Sebrell, Jr., and Robert S. Harris, 2nd edition, New York, and London: Academic Press, 1967), that mice, rats, and guinea pigs deficient in vitamin A had undersized, shrunken, and flabby testicles. And, as with Dr. Palludan's study of the effect on boars, Dr. Moore's experimental animals responded favorably to vitamin A treatment.

Dr. Moore concluded that the female experimental animal's reproductive organs also depend on a good supply of vitamin A, noting that a deficiency of vitamin A results in the female's failure to accept copulation or to conceive, or in the abortion of the fetus.

In experimental rats, even when the vitamin A-deficient females do conceive, they experience such difficulties as prolonged gestation, difficult births, or the death of the fetus. *Anophthalmos* (absence of eyes) and cleft palate and other congenital defects of the eyes and heart as well may also occur in the fetus.

The foregoing studies indicated that the correlation between vitamin A and reproductive disorders was due to a weakening of the epithelial lining of the sex organs through a deficiency called keratinization of the cells. Keratinization of the epithelial cells is the formation of hard, dry, scaly cells in the place of normal healthy cells which secrete mucus. The fiber buildup becomes a barrier, rather than a filter for the cell. The result is that the cell dies.

But research by Dr. Isobel Jennings, outlined in her book *Vitamins in the Endocrine Metabolism* (Springfield, Illinois: Charles C. Thomas, 1970) takes this area of vitamin A research further and suggests that the degeneration of the sex organs is due to an inadequate hormone supply stemming from the vitamin A deficiency. The body converts cholesterol into sex hormones (female estrogens and male androgens) and vitamin A is needed to activate two of the many chemical processes involved in the transformation.

Research involving male and female rats points to a direct relationship between the rats' vitamin A supply and sex hormones production. Studies showed that as vitamin A deficiency progressed, the rats' sex hormones diminished. Injection of vitamin A soon restored the needed hormones.

Male rats exhibited the same characteristics as animals in the previous studies by Drs. Palludan and Moore. Dr. Jennings reported that "advanced A-deficiency in the male rat is equivalent virtually to chemical castration and is associated with degenerative changes in the germinal epithelium of the testis (tissue covering the testis within the scrotum) and the production of abnormal spermatozoa."

Earlier studies had lead to the assumption that vitamin A deficiency directly caused the breakdown of the epithelium. However, rats who were equally vitamin A deficient, but received an injection of testosterone (the most powerful male hormone) suffered no degeneration of their testes and no decrease of sperm production. These results indicated that it was an absence of sex hormones (brought about by a vitamin A deficiency) which caused the breakdown.

Dr. Jennings also stresses the need for diabetics to take vitamin A as a preformed vitamin, i.e., a natural supplement of fish liver oil. For unknown reasons, diabetics are not able to convert carotene, found in abundance in carrots and green leafy vegetables, into fully formed vitamin A as found in fish liver oil.

## Impotency and Vitamin A

The diabetics' tendency to deficiency in vitamin A may explain one of the perils of the disease: impotence. According to an article by Dr. Alan Rubin (*M.D.*, March 1968) the incidence of impotence in diabetic men is two to five times greater than in nondiabetic patients. As Dr. Jennings indicated, vitamin A is essential for the synthesis of the sex hormones, so impotence in diabetics is probably related to the inability to convert carotene to vitamin A and consequent decrease in male hormone output.

# Vitamin A Deficiency and Birth Defects

Of course, vitamin A is not the whole story of sex and reproduction, but we have seen that a deficiency of the vitamin, especially during pregnancy, might drastically affect the process and degree of hormonal synthesis. And this could very well affect the degree of masculinity or femininity a child will carry in his or her chromosomes.

In a chapter entitled "Hormones and Vitamins in Prenatal Growth," Dr. Jennings remarks that "the whole wide range of defects in human morphogenesis (differentiation of cells and tissues during development) can be duplicated in most cases in experimental animals by dietary manipulation."

In other words, aside from those birth defects resulting from radiation, viruses, hormone therapy, harmful chemicals, drugs, and hereditary or genetic errors, the privation of nutrients essential to the fetus can cause equally serious results. Except for genetic defects, the type of abnormality—cleft palate, absence of limbs, heart anomalies, etc.—depends primarily "on the specific period of pregnancy during which the noxious stimulus acts," Dr. Jennings notes, rather than on what the teratogenic agent tending to cause the abnormality in the fetus happens to be. And, as animal experimentation has shown, nutritional deficiency must be counted on as one of those "noxious stimulants."

Studies on the effects of a vitamin A deficiency during pregnancy are, for the most part, confined to experiments with lower level animals because the effects of vitamin antagonists on humans during pregnancy are difficult to set up. One reason is that the most critical period from the standpoint of congenital malformations is the first three months of pregnancy and relatively few women visit maternity clinics this early. Further, the large number of pregnancies that would have to be followed to obtain statistically significant data is a serious problem. For example, to collect findings on 100 cases of cleft palate, experts estimate that about 100,000 pregnancies would have to be followed. However, when studies of human concerning vitamin antagonists during pregnancy have been made, the results have been consistent with those observed in lower animals.

# CHAPTER 23

# Vitamin A's Anticancer Role

When laboratory animals are made deficient in vitamin A, cancer-causing chemicals have more effect than they do in well-nourished animals—more tumors develop and they appear much sooner.

When certain cancer-causing agents (carcinogens) are added to cultures of prostate tissue from mice, their usual damage to the cells can be prevented by adding vitamin A at the same time. The vitamin can even reverse the damage when it is added to the culture after the carcinogen has begun its destruction.

In a number of cancers of ipithelial tissue (skin and various membranes that line the mouth, internal passages, and hollow organs), both human and mouse carcinomas can be made to regress under vitamin A treatment.

In an article in *Science* (27 December 1974) entitled "Vitamin A: Potential Protection From Carcinogens," Thomas H. Maugh II, Ph.D., cited these laboratory findings as examples of what has been discovered about vitamin A's anticancer role. Research presented at a workshop sponsored by the National Cancer Institute and Hoffmann-La Roche, Inc., suggests that cells may be protected after exposure to a carcinogen by the action of vitamin A, according to Dr. Maugh. It might be possible for the vitamin to "mediate a return to normalcy," after the intial damage has occurred, and thus prevent later full-blown "transformation" of the cell to malignancy.

Has science, then, really discovered the long-sought cure, or preventative of cancer and identified it as the familiar nutrient, vitamin A? Should we all load up on megadoses of vitamin A as our "anticancer insurance"?

Of course not. In the first place, vitamin A in megadoses can be toxic. As you probably know, large excess amounts of this oil-soluble vitamin are not harmlessly excreted, as in the case of vitamin C, but instead can build up in the body with harmful consequences. Secondly, no single nutrient will ever prove to be the one answer to cancer prevention. A healthy cell—one that can resist the attack of cancer-causing agents—requires not one but the full team of all essential nutrients, as the University of Texas' Dr. Roger Williams has repeatedly stressed in his book, *Nutrition Against Disease* (New York: Pitman, 1971). Dr. Williams documents the helpful role of quite a number of nutrients (including vitamin A) in preventing or retarding tumor growth in animals.

The evidence Dr. Maugh cites indicates that vitamin A plays an important nutritional role when it comes to keeping the body free of cancer. And, while megadoses of this nutrient are uncalled for, getting sufficient vitamin A in the daily diet is probably a very important anticancer measure.

## 'What's Wrong with the Brakes?'

When cancer develops, the malignant cell begins to multiply without restraint. One cell divides into two, the two into four, the four into eight, and so on, until large tumors are formed and malignant cells travel to many parts of the body. Healthy cells, on the other hand, don't "divide and multiply" except when more cells are needed—as in the case of the growing fetus, or in wound repair, or in the case of cells that require replacement, such as skin and blood cells.

# Why Nutrition Is Vital

Now, whatever the mechanisms that normally suppress the cell's tendency to proliferate, we can be sure of one thing: these mechanisms are dependent on nutrition. We can say this with absolute certainty because everything in the body—cell structures, enzymes, hormones, antibodies, everything the body possesses, synthesizes, and utilizes—is in the last analysis constructed out of what once was food and drink.

So where should we look to find out why cells turn malignant? The answer seems self-evident. If one or more nutrients are missing or insufficient among those required for the suppression mechanisms, it's obvious that the mechanisms won't work properly. The "brakes" will be off, so to speak. And a missing or deficient nutrient or nutrients will be the prime suspect as the factor permitting cell proliferation—in effect, deficiency may play a causative role in cancer.

# While the Cell 'Waits,' Vitamin A Acts

According to Dr. Maugh, vitamin A comes into the cancer-fighting picture at a stage in cancer development that has previously received very little research attention. The primary thrust of cancer therapy, he observed, has been to destroy malignant cells after they have been formed. A "somewhat smaller" effort has gone to reducing the incidence of exposure to cancer-causing agents. But almost no effort has been made "to discover what might be done during the period between exposure of a cell to a carcinogen and the cell's transformation to malignancy."

This waiting period, known as preneoplasia, is a lengthy one—often 20 years or more in the case of human cells. Initially, as Dr. Maugh explained, the carcinogen effects some relatively permanent change in one or more cells that may lead to cancer—such as a change in a gene. (Genes are hereditary units in the cell's nucleic acid, each containing an "instruction" for cell activity.) Many years after exposure, "transformation" takes place—"the cells rather abruptly show the properties characteristic of tumors and begin proliferating."

Just what has been happening inside the affected cells during the in-between years is still baffling the experts. "Almost nothing is known about cellular changes in preneoplasia," Dr. Maugh said.

Yet it is clear, he observed, that "in many cases, perhaps even a majority, the preneoplastic cells are repaired and 'spontaneously' revert to health." In other words, built-in body defenses (which, as we have seen, must be nutrition-dependent) are able to reverse the cell changes caused by the carcinogen and thus prevent the cell's eventual transformation to a cancer cell. Other changed cells, it is thought, may be destroyed by the body's defense system.

There is mounting evidence that vitamin A is a key player in this protective action. The most "crucial finding" and the most convincing to scientists, is the fact that "many carcinogens are much more potent in animals that have a long-term deficiency in vitamin A." Therefore, it is possible, according to Dr. Maugh and researchers who took part in the National Cancer Institute workshop, that vitamin A sometimes acts even prior to initial cell damage. In the case of some harmful substances, vitamin A is believed to inhibit the chemical's conversion in the body to an active carcinogen.

## Anticancer Action Probed

And sometimes, as was mentioned earlier, the vitamin can inhibit cancerous growth even after the cell has turned malignant. Vitamin A "can produce regressions in squamous cell and basal cell carcinomas (certain epithelial tumors) in mice and humans," Dr. Maugh wrote.

Just how vitamin A "works" in fighting cancer is still little understood. Research findings suggest that part of its anti-cancer action may be in weakening the attachment of a carcinogen to the cell's genetic material—the nucleic acid, DNA, which contains the genes. Since genetic disturbance is believed to be involved in the cell's loss of control over proliferation, such a weakening would help the cell "'spontaneously' revert to health," as Dr. Maugh put it. He cited a number of studies showing that "various carcinogens bind much more tightly to DNA" in cultures derived from animals made deficient in vitamin A.

There is also the possibility that vitamin A compounds "somehow stimulate the immune system to be more effective in countering malignancy." As scientists have learned in quite recent years, certain white cells or leukocytes of the immune system—those that have passed through and been treated by the thymus gland—recognize cancerous cells as a "foreign body" and seek to reject them. A number of drugs have an antitumor effect because they stimulate this immune response—and vitamin A has been shown to increase the antitumor action of such drugs 100-fold, according to Dr. Maugh.

It should be mentioned here, too, that vitamin A may boost the immune reaction against tumors by protecting the integrity and size of the thymus itself. In experimental animals, this small gland (situated in the chest) shrinks as tumors develop following the injection of a tumor-virus (Dr. Martin Zisblatt and colleagues, *American Journal of Clinical Nutrition*, August 1973, p. xxiv). When the animals are subsequently given large doses of vitamin A, the researchers report, both these happenings reverse—tumors diminish and the thymus reverts toward normal size. "Vitamin A," they speculate, "appears not to be working directly as a selectively antitumor compound, but rather, it appears to affect the process of rejection of the tumor." In other words, strong immune reaction to reject tumors depends on a healthy thymus, which in turn depends on adequate vitamin A.

Whatever future research uncovers about how vitamin A works against cancer, there seems little doubt that it contributes importantly to our natural defenses against malignant cells.

## Common Foods Rich in Vitamin A*

| | (International Units) |
|---|---|
| Spinach (1 cup, cooked) | 14,580 |
| Cabbage (1 cup, shredded, cooked) | 190 |
| Kale (1 cup, cooked) | 9,130 |
| Broccoli (1 cup, cooked) | 3,880 |
| Carrots (1, raw) | 7,930 |
| Corn (1 cup, cooked) | 660 |
| Eggs (1 large, raw) | 590 |
| Milk (1 cup, whole) | 350 |
| Liver (Beef, 3 oz., fried) | 45,390 |
| Kidney (Beef, 1 cup, cooked) | 1,610 |
| Apricots (3) | 2,890 |
| Cherries (1 cup, raw) | 1,550 |
| Cantaloupe (½ melon) | 9,240 |
| Peach (1) | 1,330 |
| Watermelon (1 piece) | 2,510 |

*Selected from tables in *Nutritive Value of American Foods in Common Units*, United States Department of Agriculture Handbook #456, November, 1975.

# THE B VITAMINS

## CHAPTER 24

# Thiamine, Vitamin B₁

Thiamine's primary importance to health stems from the part it plays in the oxidation process that goes on constantly in each individual body cell. The enzyme which carries on this process requires a collaborator (in this case thiamine) to do its work properly. Nervous tissue is especially dependent on carbohydrate oxidation for its functioning, so nervous tissue is one of the first to show the effects of vitamin B₁ deficiency.

Thiamine is also necessary for growth. Laboratory animals deprived of thiamine develop more slowly and do not attain the growth of their brothers and sisters who are on a diet containing ample amounts of this vitamin. Thiamine promotes good appetite and better functioning of the digestive tract. It improves the muscles of the stomach and intestines and has often been effectively used to cure stubborn cases of constipation.

The proper functioning of red blood cell transketolase, an enzyme that is active in blood metabolism, absolutely requires thiamine. In fact, doctors test for thiamine deficiency by checking the red cell transketolase activity. If this activity lags, the doctor knows his patient requires more thiamine for all normal bodily functions.

# The Beriberi Factor

Such sophisticated information about the vitamin's biochemical role is relatively recent. But people learned that thiamine is an essential element in the diet three-quarters of a century ago. They didn't call it thiamine, of course, and they had no idea what it consisted of. They only knew that it must exist.

It was in the 1890s in the Dutch East Indies, that Dr. Christian Eijkman found he could give chickens polyneuritis (beriberi in man) by restricting them to a diet of polished rice; he could reverse the process and cure them by feeding them the natural unprocessed brown rice.

Other scientists soon found that beriberi in humans, like the comparable disease in animals, could be cured, even prevented, if "primitive" rice were substituted for the "civilized" variety. These early researchers spoke of a "protective substance" in the rice polishings, and in 1911 a Polish chemist used the term "vitamin" to describe that substance—coining the word that has now become so common. It was not until 1926, however, that thiamine was chemically isolated in the same laboratory where Dr. Eijkman had made his original finding.

Today it is common knowledge that beriberi, which can cause paralysis, serious disorders of the heart, circulatory system, and liver, and eventually death, results from a severe thiamine deficiency. Such a deficiency can be brought on by a steady diet of polished rice, which has all of the thiamine refined out of it.

Fortunately, except in cases of extreme organic damage, simple thiamine therapy usually produces dramatic recoveries even in advanced cases of beriberi. In the *Canadian Medical Association Journal*, for instance, Drs. Weiss and Wilkins described how a man with advanced beriberi and heart failure showed a remarkably favorable reaction one and a half hours after the injection of 30 mg. of vitamin $B_1$, although at the time he was in a deep coma. Continued vitamin $B_1$ therapy saved his life.

## Thiamine Deficiency Today

While beriberi is rare in the United States, it is not unknown. According to *Food and Man* (New York: John Wiley and Sons, Inc., 1968), edited by Dr. Miriam E. Lowenberg, former head of the Department of Foods and Nutrition at Pennsylvania State University, "Beriberi has not been confined to the peoples of the world who eat rice. It has occurred in Labrador and Newfoundland and, in isolated cases, in institutions in the United States when white bread and white flour have been used as staples of the diet."

The authors of *Food and Man* go on to ask, "What about the people who get some thiamine but not enough? This can occur here or in any country; this condition is referred to as subclinical deficiency, meaning that the dietary lack is not so great as to cause definite illness, but the intake is not enough for good health. . . . Dietary studies where records are made of the kind and amounts of foods eaten by individuals or families and then the nutrient content of the diets calculated, indicate that many groups do not receive adequate amounts of thiamine (or of other nutrients) even though there are no obvious symptoms of disease."

## Why You Need More Thiamine

There are many reasons why we might not be receiving adequate amounts of thiamine. True, we are not in the dire position of the rice-dependent people stricken with beriberi, but the average American diet provides no insurance at all against thiamine deficiency.

"The cereal grains are good sources (of thiamine)," Dr. Lowenberg writes in *Food and Man*, "but the thiamine is in the germ and outer coatings so that refined cereals such as white rice and flour have lost their thiamine."

The chief crimes committed against rice in the name of civilization are those same ones committed against wheat when it is milled. The original brown rice, as it comes from the rice plant, contains protein, starch, fat, minerals, and vitamins, chiefly in its bran endosperm and germ. As brown rice is milled to make white or polished rice, these important nutrients are changed for the worse. Brown rice contains approximately 2.93 mg. of thiamine for every 100 grams, while white rice contains only .60 mg. of thiamine for every 100 grams. Wheat undergoes a similar loss. Even when white flour is "enriched," the thiamine content is about 20 percent less than that of whole wheat flour.

In addition to whole cereals, other rich natural sources of thiamine are yeast, liver, pork, and fresh green vegetables. But surveys such as the one the Department of Agriculture published in 1968 show that these foods are not staples of the average American family. Fresh vegetables, for example, have become a rarity in many homes.

Also, people today are eating a great deal more beef than they used to, and less pork. They are also eating less of the organ meats, such as heart and liver. This makes a tremendous difference in thiamine intake, because most cuts of pork have an average of ten times as much thiamine as beef does, beef heart has about eight times as much thiamine as muscle meat, while liver has about four or five times as much thiamine.

A bowl of hot oatmeal used to be a common breakfast, and oatmeal is a fine source of thiamine. (In fact, even two eggs will deliver only about one-third of the thiamine that is in a bowl of oatmeal.) When that bowl of oatmeal is replaced by "enriched" corn flakes, the thiamine content is reduced by more than half.

Potatoes and beans also used to be consumed in greater amounts than they are today, and both are excellent thiamine sources. So there is nothing very mysterious about the reason so many people today are not getting enough thiamine. It is the logical outcome of a shift in eating habits.

*Food and Man* gives additional reasons why a person's intake of thiamine is likely to be low: "Thiamine has the chemical qualities of being soluble in water and destroyed by high temperatures and by some chemicals including soda used in the treatment of foods. Since it is water-soluble, thiamine may be lost when large amounts of water are used in cooking vegetables or rice and the cooking water is thrown away. This water-solubility of thiamine explains why thiamine-containing foods should be eaten daily; this vitamin is not stored in the body—excess amounts are excreted."

## The Need for Thiamine Can Vary

A person's need for thiamine increases under various circumstances. Since thiamine is used in the oxidation of carbohydrates, consuming excess sugars and starches creates a need for more thiamine. Thus, eating polished rice or white unenriched bread or potatoes cooked in too much water, which in addition is discarded, makes for quite a vicious circle. Not only is the thiamine thrown out or destroyed in the preparation, but because these foods are all starches, the body requires more thiamine than it would if they hadn't been eaten.

Writing in *Newer Methods of Nutritional Biochemistry* (New York: Academic Press, 1967), Dr. Myron Brin says that extra supplies of thiamine are needed when antibiotics are being used over a long period, in cases of severe diarrhea, and "in any other situation that would affect adversely the absorption and/or utilization of the nutrient."

Pregnancy, lactation, fever, surgery, and other stressful conditions also call for an increase in thiamine intake. So does increased physical activity. The Committee on Foods and Nutrition of the National Research Council recommends 1.5 mg. of thiamine a day for a sedentary man and 2.3 mg. for one who is very active.

Older people seem to need a larger amount of thiamine. The New York Academy of Science's publication, *The Sciences* (vol. 1, no. 9) , reported significant research of Dr. Helen C. Olden: "In an experiment with one group of women aged 52 to 75 years, and another group aged 19 to 21 years, all subjects consumed the same quantity of thiamine, but the older women excreted less of the substance than did the younger (an indication that more was being used). Moreover, when both groups were deprived of sufficient thiamine, the older women showed adverse effects much more quickly.''

Probably the people most severely threatened by thiamine deficiency in the United States are alcoholics. A controlled study of twenty severe alcoholics, reported in the *American Journal of Clinical Nutrition* (November 1968), showed "a highly significant impairment of the thiamine absorption" in the alcoholics, compared to nonalcoholic controls.

Dr. P. A. Tomasulo and associates explained that severe liver disease leads to decreased conversion of thiamine into usable thiamine phosphate. The doctors pointed out that the impaired thiamine absorption is great enough to cause thiamine deficiency in alcoholic patients who have only marginally adequate intake. It is clear that those who drink large amounts of alcohol should get more than minimal thiamine intake.

## Insure Your Thiamine Intake

There are two ways to make certain you are getting all the thiamine you need. One is to eat generous amounts of thiamine-rich foods every single day. This means the daily inclusion in your diet of such foods as oatmeal or whole-grain rice and wheat, organ meats or pork, and potatoes, beans, peas, and asparagus. But many people simply don't and won't eat this kind of diet day in and day out. This is especially true with people who are watching their waistlines. Many health-conscious people today center their diets around lean beef, cottage cheese, salads, fruit juice, and similar low-calorie foods—all of which are also low in thiamine.

For such people thiamine is available in the concentrated food supplements of brewer's yeast, desiccated liver, and wheat germ, or in a variety of vitamin supplements. These sources will provide all the necessary thiamine (and other B vitamins) without the need to eat oatmeal and beans every day. It is best to take thiamine in supplements that contain the entire B complex, since it has been shown that the B vitamins work best when they work together. It is for this reason that "enriched" foods, where all the B vitamins are removed and only a few synthetic substitutes restored, are not reliable sources of complete nutrition.

There is no danger of getting too much thiamine, since excess amounts of this water-soluble vitamin are merely excreted. Megadoses of thiamine have been used successfully to treat myasthenia gravis and early multiple sclerosis, and in conjunction with other B vitamins, to treat a variety of nervous and mental disorders, and even alcoholism, all without side effects. Such large doses, however, should be taken only under the supervision of a doctor.

# CHAPTER 25

# Meeting the Needs
# of Your Nerves

A report in the *Journal of Applied Nutrition* (Spring 1975) stated that a deficiency in thiamine causes a dysfunction of the central nervous system, a degeneration of the peripheral nerves (nerves in the skin and near the surface of the body) and structural changes in intramuscular nerves. Thiamine is crucial to the enzymatic reactions that supply energy to the nerves and the brain and in the formation of *acetylcholine*, a compound involved in transmitting nerve impulses.

Beriberi, the disease of severe thiamine deficiency, is basically a disease of the nervous system. The medical term for beriberi is polyneuritis, which means "many types of nerve disease." There are two forms of the disease. In one form the muscle tissues waste away and paralysis, beginning in the legs, spreads through the whole body. In the other form swelling appears in the arms and legs and spreads to the trunk, while the heart, overworked from trying to pump blood throughout the swollen body, becomes enlarged and eventually fails.

Wernicke's syndrome is another disease attributed to severe thiamine deficiency. Its symptoms are confusion and complete disorientation. If the deficiency persists, the patient may lose coordination of voluntary muscle movements and the eye muscles may become paralyzed.

Both beriberi and Wernicke's syndrome can be reversed with large doses of thiamine, provided permanent neuromuscular damage has not occurred.

## Brain Damage Can Occur Before Severe Symptoms Are Apparent

A thiamine deficiency may start doing its damage where it hurts the most—in the brain—long before overt symptoms begin to appear. Early damage to certain cells in the brain stem has been found in laboratory rats fed a diet deficient in thiamine. A report on the frightening phenomenon appeared in the February, 1969, issue of *Nutrition Reviews*.

A significant point about these findings, as the editors explained it, is the appearance of lesions at a relatively early stage of the deficiency disease. Previously, using light microscopes, researchers had found pathological changes in the nerve cells of the brain (and elsewhere)—but only after the disease was far advanced.

However, in the series of experiments reported in *Nutrition Reviews*—experiments conducted in a number of laboratories over a period of years—electron microscopes revealed that some damage, though mild, occurs earlier, at just about the time that the laboratory rats show their first signs of abnormal posture and faulty equilibrium. These early lesions occur not in the nerve cells themselves but rather in the cells of the neuroglia (supporting elements of the nervous system).

At least in the case of rats, lesions within the brain have already formed by the time the animal shows any sign of deficiency beyond lack of appetite and loss of weight. *Nutrition Reviews* summarized: "Early lesions of acute thiamine deficiency . . . (are) coincident with the onset of neurological signs."

It has often been observed that long before the appearance of beriberi, signaling gross deficiency of $B_1$, an insufficiency of thiamine can produce vague and relatively mild mental symptoms which very few practitioners associate with dietary problems. Consider that "Recent studies have shown that a deficiency of thiamine, but not insufficient enough to provide beri-beri, would produce disturbances of the psyche. Even with to-day's enrichment of bread and flour, many people are probably subsisting on diets that are borderline in thiamine content" (article by Dr. M. R. Wilder, *Journal of the American Medical Association*, 162-17: 1956, abstracted in *Environmental Pollution and Mental Health*, Williams *et al.*, Washington, D.C.: Information Resources Press, Division Herner-Company, 1973).

Now, the possibility exists that irreparable brain damage may be caused by a deficiency in vitamin B, before a severe deficiency becomes apparent, so it makes good sense to insure an adequate thiamine intake with supplements.

## Early Symptoms of Thiamine Deficiency

The earliest symptoms of thiamine deficiency are deceptively commonplace. Writing in *Vitamins and Coenzymes* (New York: Interscience Publishers, Div. John Wiley, 1964), Drs. Arthur F. Wagner and Karl Folkers describe the first indications of illness as "fatigue, weight loss, and anorexia (loss of appetite)."

Typically, the person whose diet is poor in vitamin $B_1$ lacks energy and is constantly tired. The individual doesn't eat well or sleep well. Friends notice his irritability.

If thiamine deficiency worsens, more pronounced symptoms develop. Memory may become faulty, concentration poor. The person becomes unstable emotionally, overreacting to the normal stresses and strains. He is likely to be constipated and to have vague abdominal pains, and he may be bothered by pains in his chest as well.

As in the case of the laboratory rats, neurological disorders already present become apparent if the deficiency continues severe. The patient will feel a tingling and burning in the toes and soles of his feet, and his calves will become extremely tender.

# Improved Mentality

Happily, not all research on thiamine deals with deficiency. One of the most exciting areas of investigation concerns the possibility that supplemental thiamine can improve mental ability. In their book, *Diet and Disease,* (Emmaus, Pennsylvania: Rodale Books, 1968), Drs. E. Cheraskin, W. M. Ringsdorf, and J. W. Clark describe an experiment in this field conducted by Dr. Ruth F. Harrell of the Department of Educational Psychology at Columbia University.

Dr. Harrell selected two groups of children in an orphanage, ages nine to 19. The groups were closely matched in age, sex, weight, educational status, and mentality. One group was given a daily tablet containing two mg. of thiamine; the other group received a placebo. This procedure was continued for a year. It was a double-blind experiment—the children, of course, did not know which pills they were receiving, and neither did the investigators, who wanted to insure objectivity. Only after the results were all in did Dr. Harrell and her associates match up the testing scores to see how the vitamin group performed compared to the placebo group.

Both groups were tested at the beginning of the experiment and again at the end, and their percentage of improvement compared. Several categories of tests were used, each designed to measure an aspect of mental response. In all categories, the thiamine-supplemented group showed astonishing improvement when compared with the control group. "The percentage of improvement over controls," the authors of *Diet and Disease* commented, "ranged from approximately 25 to 3200. Thus it appears that mental achievement in children of presumably normal diet can be remarkably increased through employment of dietary supplements."

Mental alertness, then, is like emotional stability, serenity, and zest for life. All of these most valued intangibles have been shown to suffer when dietary intake of thiamine is low. With thiamine plentiful, they should thrive!

# CHAPTER 26

# Thiamine Plays
# an Important Role
# in Heart Function

Researchers have long known that thiamine is essential for a healthy heart. *The Avitaminoses* (Baltimore, Maryland: Williams and Wilkins Company, 1944), by Walter H. Eddy, Ph.D., and Gilbert Dalldorf, M.D., states, "Thiamine deficiency impairs the function of the heart, increases the tendency to extravascular fluid collections, and results in terminal cardiac standstill." The authors show how the famous English research physician, Sir Robert McCarrison, produced cardiac changes in pigeons by feeding them a diet deficient in vitamin $B_1$. Drs. Eddy and Dalldorf describe another experiment in which congestive heart failure was produced in pigeons and then cured by thiamine.

Many experiments with laboratory animals have supported the relationship between thiamine deficiency and heart disease. Dr. Earl E. Aldinger, of the Tulane School of Medicine, reported the stress observed in rats fed a thiamine-free diet for five weeks (*Circulation Research*, March 1965). During that time the tissues surrounding the heart showed a marked loss (69 percent) of tension and elasticity. The animals also developed an erratic heartbeat. Dr. Aldinger found that if the rats were given thiamine in the early stages of the deficiency, the heartbeat quickly returned to normal. However, if the deficiency lasted for five weeks or more, the heart became irreparably damaged and the rats died. Dr. Aldinger believed that thiamine is needed by the enzymes that provide the heart with energy. He concluded that the slowed heartbeat and decreased tension of the heart muscle could be attributed to a defect in energy production for the heart.

A more recent experiment involving rats confirms thiamine's role as a coenzyme in the production of energy for the heart. Dr. James B. Sutherland, of the Department of Pharmacology at the University of Ottawa's School of Medicine, and associates, used pair-fed rats to determine the effect of a lack of thiamine on *PDH* and *2-KGDH*, two enzymes that carry on energy metabolism for the heart. The rats on the thiamine-free diet developed slowed heartbeats, enlarged hearts, and eventually died of heart failure. According to a report of the experiment in the *Journal of Nutritional Science and Vitaminology* (vol. 20, 1974), "The appearance and severity of both bradycardia (abnormally slow heart rate) and cardiomegaly (enlarged heart) parallel the decrease in activities of pyruvate and 2-ketoglutarate dehydrogenases (PDH and 2-KGDH) in the heart. Thus, it appears that thiamine is an essential coenzyme for energy metabolism in the heart.

## Cardiac Victims Found Deficient in Thiamine

Not all research on the role of thiamine in heart failure has been confined to laboratory animals. A group of doctors, reporting in *Nutrition Reviews* (October 1955), measured the thiamine content of the heart muscle and of the liver and kidney tissues in 12 patients who died from heart failure with evidence of various kinds of severe organic heart disease.

These tissues were compared with similar tissues taken from 10 patients who had no heart disease and who died of other causes. The doctors found a consistent decrease in the average thiamine content of the heart muscle in the cardiac patients as compared with the control subjects.

The total thiamine in the "noncardiacs" was 1.37 mcg. per gram of tissue as compared to .60 mcg. for the cardiac subjects. *Nutrition Reviews* commented, "Because of the nature of the study it was presumably impossible for the author to obtain histories of food intake on either the cardiacs or control individuals prior to death so that these could be compared. The assumption would seem valid that the patients dying of severe cardiac disease had not been well nourished for a considerable period of time prior to death. Whether the deficiencies found were sufficient to impair the metabolism of the heart muscle was not known, although, as the authors indicate, these evidences of under-nutrition with respect to thiamine are certainly suggested."

## Less Thiamine, More Heart Trouble

E. Cheraskin, M.D., D.M.D., professor and chairman of the Department of Oral Medicine at the University of Alabama Medical Center, and associates, went one step further by testing the relationship between thiamine intake and heart trouble in living humans (*Journal of the American Geriatrics Society*, November 1967). Dr. Cheraskin recruited a group of dentists and their wives, 74 in all, to answer the questions in the standard Cornell Medical Index Health Questionnaire dealing with cardiovascular symptoms and signs: "Do you have pains in the heart or the chest?" "Are you often bothered by thumping of the heart?" "Does heart trouble run in your family?" "Do you get out of breath long before anyone else?" etc. Of the 74 subjects, 44.7 percent had at least one cardiovascular complaint, while 12.3 percent answered "yes" to three or more questions that might indicate cardiovascular problems.

To compare the cardiovascular complaints with thiamine consumption, the dentists and their wives were divided into two equal subgroups: of these 74 individuals, 37 consumed .13 to .91 mg. of thiamine a day; the remaining 37 consumed .92 to 2.95 mg. of thiamine a day. When the two groups were compared, it was found that the subjects consuming the lesser amount of thiamine had almost twice as many cardiovascular complaints as the subjects in the higher intake group.

## Carbohydrates, Thiamine, and Heart Trouble

The relationship between a high carbohydrate intake and a high rate of heart disease becomes increasingly obvious. The carbohydrates responsible for the increase in heart disease are the "empty" calories of refined sugar and refined starches. Thiamine, notably lacking in patients with heart trouble, is a known victim of excessive sugars in the body. It is possible that a diet high in refined carbohydrates and low in thiamine can lead to heart trouble.

Aware of this possibility, Dr. Cheraskin made a follow-up study of both thiamine and carbohydrate consumption in relation to cardiovascular complaints (*The International Journal for Vitamin Research,* vol. 37, no. 4, 1967). Using the same 74 individuals, Dr. Cheraskin again divided them into two equal subgroups according to the amount of thiamine intake. The subjects were then divided into groups according to the consumption of nonprocessed carbohydrates and processed carbohydrates.

When all of these groups were compared, the subjects with the highest number of cardiovascular complaints were also found to have a higher consumption of processed carbohydrates and a lower consumption of thiamine than the rest. Dr. Cheraskin commented, "It should be underlined that the relationships observed here do not, in themselves, prove cause-and-effect. However, it is noteworthy that the findings are consistent with other reports indicating the relationship of carbohydrate consumption to cardiovascular disease."

## Common Foods Rich in Thiamine*

|  | (milligrams) |
|---|---|
| Liver (Beef, 3 oz., fried) | .22 |
| Kidney (Beef, 1 cup, cooked) | .71 |
| Heart (Beef, 1 cup, cooked) | .36 |
| Ham (1 cup, cooked, chopped or diced) | .71 |
| Peas (Green, 1 cup, cooked) | .45 |
| Lima beans (1 cup, cooked) | .31 |
| Asparagus (4 spears, cooked) | .16 |
| Brown rice (Long grain, 1 cup, cooked) | .18 |
| Whole wheat flour (1 cup) | .66 |
| Brewers yeast (Debittered, 1 tbsp.) | 1.25 |
| Soybeans (1 cup, cooked) | .38 |
| Sunflower seeds (Hulled, 1 cup) | 2.84 |
| Rolled oats (Dry form, 1 cup) | .48 |
| Crabmeat (1 cup, flaked, cooked) | .20 |
| Raisins (1 cup, natural, seedless) | .16 |

*Selected from tables in *Nutritive Value of American Foods in Common Units*, United States Department of Agriculture Handbook #456, November, 1975.

# CHAPTER 27

# The Role of Riboflavin (Vitamin B₂) in Human Health

In 1879, long before its vitamin properties were discovered, riboflavin was recognized as a pigment in milk. It was sometimes referred to as the "old yellow enzyme." By 1933, riboflavin was identified and reported as isolated in pure form by Dr. Paul Gyorgy and others. Shortly thereafter, its significance as an essential growth factor was demonstrated by researchers.

Riboflavin is a fundamental constituent of living tissue and plays an important role in protein metabolism. New tissue cannot be formed nor can damaged tissue be repaired unless this vitamin is available.

Riboflavin's importance in nutrition stems from its reaction with protein to form flavoprotein enzymes that participate in a wide variety of reactions in metabolism. Once in the body, riboflavin is converted to two coenzymes, FMN (flavin mononucleotide) and FAD (flavin adenine dinucleotide). FMN and FAD are most active in the liver, the source of most of the body's enzymes. In the liver, these coenzymes are vital to the formation of oxidizing enzymes that control bodily processes.

Like thiamine, riboflavin is involved in the utilization of food. However, thiamine is used in the oxidation of carbohydrates, while riboflavin is concerned with the metabolism of lipids, such as fatty acids. Lipids, like protein and carbohydrates, are among

169

the principal structural components of the living cell. They are also involved in energy metabolism.

Riboflavin is needed for the metabolism of tryptophan, a naturally occurring amino acid that is essential for optimal growth in infants and for a proper nitrogen balance in adults. The body converts tryptophan to niacin when necessary, but riboflavin is needed for the conversion to take place.

Riboflavin is also a component of the retinal pigment of the eye where it participates in light adaptation. That riboflavin is "good for the eyes" has been known for some time, and is demonstrated by the fact that a deficiency of riboflavin can cause bloodshot eyes, conjunctivitis, and even cataracts.

## Deficiency Disorders of B₂

Deficiency of riboflavin most typically produced pathology of the lips, tongue, eyes, and skin. The lips are either unusually red or whitish. Ulceration and painful fissuring at the corners of the mouth are frequent. Scaly lesions may develop around the nose, cheeks, chin, and sometimes on the lobes of the ears. The scrotum or vulva may also be affected.

Among other things, riboflavin is needed by some tissue to utilize oxygen. In its absence, tiny blood vessels are formed in the body's effort to bring oxygenated blood into closer contact with the cornea. The result is bloodshot eyes.

Aside from these disorders, a riboflavin deficiency will cause serious impairment of the liver, the site of riboflavin's coenzyme activity. According to an article by Dr. Richard S. Rivlin in the *New England Journal of Medicine* (27 August 1970), tests with laboratory animals have shown the liver to increase in weight, fat content, and glycogen content during a B₂ deficiency. Structural changes within the cells of the liver also take place. Even more serious, the activity of flavoprotein enzymes that control vital bodily processes is depressed by a lack of B₂.

Anemia is usually associated with a lack of iron or folic acid, but a deficiency in riboflavin will also produce serious anemia. A report in *Blood* (April 1965) concluded that a lack of the riboflavin coenzymes prevents the production of red blood cells. According to Dr. Rivlin's article, anemia in riboflavin deficiency may be partly caused by reduced folic acid metabolism, since a lack of $B_2$ will reduce the amount of folic acid available to the liver.

## B₂ Deficiency Can Exist Undetected

While the overt physical symptoms of riboflavin deficiency can be recognized easily, damage to the liver can remain undetected for some time. It is also very difficult to pinpoint riboflavin deficiency as the cause of anemia. According to Dr. Rivlin, "Although the metabolic effects of riboflavin deficiency are widely expressed, few of these events can be detected clinically with ease."

A riboflavin deficiency may also cause personality disturbances without any apparent clinical signs of a deficiency. A study conducted at the United States Army Medical Research and Nutrition Laboratory, Denver, Colorado, placed six male volunteers on a riboflavin-deficient diet for 56 days. The men were given five standard personality tests from the Minnesota Multiphasic Personality Inventory (MMPI) as well as a hand-grip strength test both before and after the induced riboflavin deficiency. According to a report of the experiment in the *American Journal of Clinical Nutrition* (February 1973), "Significant changes were found in five personality subscales of the MMPI (hypochondriasis, depression, hysteria, psychopathic-deviate, and hypomania), as well as hand-grip strength. These effects were noted by the 39th and 52nd day of restriction, respectively, in the absence of any clinical symptomatology." The report concluded that the personality changes were due to stress brought on by a lack of $B_2$, and that the hand-grip strength was decreased by a reduction of flavoproteins in the muscles.

So now we know that, if a person doesn't get enough riboflavin, he or she will tire easily, have a poor appetite, be overly nervous, and perhaps suffer from digestive disturbances. If the deficiency is severe, it may become noticeable through signs of the deficiency state, such as pathology of the lips, tongue, eyes, and skin. However, the deficiency may cause a number of serious metabolic or personality disorders without any clinical signs of deficiency. Also, if the deficiency does not become severe, the person may go on feeling moody, tired, and nervous without realizing that a lack of $B_2$ is the cause.

# CHAPTER 28

# Are You Getting Enough Riboflavin?

Is it possible that significant number of Americans might be suffering from some degree of riboflavin deficiency today? The U.S. Recommended Daily Allowance for $B_2$ is 1.7 mg., but is everyone getting at least that much?

Harvard nutritionist Dr. Jean Mayer, who headed President Nixon's White House Conference on Food, Nutrition, and Health, told *Medical Tribune* (18 August 1969) that "realistically, not much has changed in this country since Steinbeck's *Grapes of Wrath* chronicled the extent of postdepression hunger and malnutrition."

Evidence of the poverty of the average American diet came to light in a survey of eating habits conducted by the Department of Agriculture, published in 1968. The survey compared eating habits in 1965 with those established in a similar survey ten years earlier.

Only half of the 7,500 households studied in 1965 (and selected as representative samples of the nation) consumed enough of one or more of the following essential nutrients: protein, calcium, iron, thiamine, ascorbic acid, vitamin A, and *riboflavin*.

How had the eating pattern changed, from the 1955 to 1965 survey? Much for the worse in terms of nutrition.

"Greater popularity of snacks is evident," the report stated.

"From 1955 to 1965 consumption increased for soft drinks, punches and "ades", potato chips, crackers, cookies, doughnuts, ice cream, candy, and peanut butter." Only peanut butter can be said to be nutritious—but the peanut butter, of course, was of the variety loaded with saturated fat found on most supermarket shelves.

While purchase of snacks increased during the 10-year period, purchase of fresh fruits and vegetables declined.

More than one third of the average family food budget in 1965 was spent on sugar, syrup, jelly, candy, bread, pies, and cakes. The baked goods, of course, were made from white flour with the vitamins and minerals of the wheat germ removed. While most refined grains are "enriched" today with riboflavin, the enrichment process restores only a fraction of what was removed, and replaces natural vitamins with synthetic compounds. As for sweets: refined white sugar is 99.5 percent carbohydrate; contains .1 mg. of iron and .2 mg. of copper per 100 grams; no calcium, no phosphorus, no vitamins at all.

It is small wonder, then, that some form of malnutrition exists at all levels of society. Nor is it remarkable that, of all the vitamin deficiencies, that of riboflavin is one of the most common. While riboflavin is found in a variety of foods (yeast, liver, wheat germ, eggs, cheese, green leafy vegetables, peas, lima beans, and organ and muscle meats), these very foods are the most neglected by the average housewife.

Unlike many of the B vitamins, there is no increased need for riboflavin when the carbohydrate intake increases. However, the need for riboflavin does increase as the protein intake increases. This is because riboflavin is essential for protein metabolism in the building of new tissue and in the production of flavoprotein enzymes.

## Riboflavin is Easily Destroyed

Riboflavin may be the most easily destroyed vitamin, because it is sensitive to light. Considerable amounts of the $B_2$ content of foods may be lost when exposed to ultraviolet rays, especially in the presence of alkali. This is particularly important in the case of milk, since milk is irradiated to give it vitamin D and is often packaged in glass or clear plastic containers. A report in the *Journal of the American Dietetic Association* (June 1975) confirmed that the riboflavin content of milk is lowered when the milk is exposed to light, and concluded by stating, "The milk industry and retail grocers should renew efforts to protect milk and reduce nutritional deterioration that occurs with light exposure."

Riboflavin is also destroyed by cooking and is vulnerable within the body to antibiotics and alcohol. Taking oral contraceptives will also destroy some riboflavin. Drs. N. Sanpitak and L. Chayutimonkul reported in the *Lancet* (4 May 1974) that women taking oral contraceptives had significantly lower levels of riboflavin than controls who took no contraceptives. Drs. Sanpitak and Chayutimonkul concluded that "prophylactic administration of riboflavin may be indicated for women taking oral contraceptives, especially in populations with poor vitamin nutrition. . . ."

## Where to Find Riboflavin

There is no danger of getting too much riboflavin; the body will simply excrete what it does not use. To assure an adequate intake of riboflavin, the best sources are natural foods that contain riboflavin along with other B vitamins. Whole grains, eggs, green leafy vegetables, peas, lima beans, and organ and muscle meats are good sources of riboflavin. Fish is a poor source, compared with beef and chicken. Beef liver is ten times as rich as beef muscle meats. In plants, riboflavin appears chiefly in the green leaves. Fruits, particularly of the citrus variety, contain only insignificant amounts of riboflavin.

# CHAPTER 29

# A Shortage of Riboflavin
# is a Familiar Cause
# of Birth Defects

There was a time—to quote the British scientist, Dr. D. H. Woollam of Cambridge—when the unborn baby appeared as "something alien and inhuman, a secure parasite immune from the stresses of the external world, born finally into that world, pristine and freshly minted" (*Journal of the College of General Practitioners*, November 1964). According to Dr. Woollam, the thalidomide tragedy changed our views. "We now feel as well as know that from the moment of implantation, if not indeed from fertilization, the embryo lies in an environment which possesses potentialities as dangerous to it as that which it will enter after birth."

We have learned that many environmental factors can cause congenital defects that once were considered solely the consequence of heredity. Of these environmental factors influencing the unborn baby, proper nutrition of the mother is an elementary, yet vital concern.

Riboflavin should be of particular concern in planning a pregnant woman's nutrition, for laboratory experiments have shown that a deficiency of riboflavin in pregnant mammals causes congenital malformations in their offspring. This discovery was first reported in the scientific journals over 35 years ago. Writing in *Science* in 1940 (92: 383), Drs. J. Warkany and R.

C. Nelson described malformations produced in rat fetuses whose mothers were deprived of adequate riboflavin in their diet. Since this pioneer work, much additional research has been conducted as investigators have tried to understand more clearly how riboflavin contributes to the normal development of the embryo and fetus.

Dr. Bruce Mackler and colleagues at the School of Medicine, University of Washington, Seattle, created riboflavin deficiency in varying degrees in four groups of pregnant rats (*Pediatrics,* June 1969). In all groups, a very large proportion of the fetuses— more than 95 percent—developed gross malformations.

Most of the defects, Dr. Mackler reported, were skeletal anomalies—abnormal development of the bones. Particularly common were incomplete development of the bones of the extremities—the baby rats' fore and hind paws—and abnormal smallness of the lower jaw. Dr. Mackler also mentioned cleft palate as an example of "a wide number of other anomalies" that have been produced in rat fetuses of mothers with a riboflavin deficiency.

## Effects of B₂ Deficiency in Pregnancy

The precise mechanism by which a pregnant mammal's riboflavin deficiency affects the fetus is incompletely understood, though studies such as Dr. Mackler's in *Pediatrics* shed light on the subject. In a biochemical analysis of the deformed fetuses, Dr. Mackler found a specific group of enzymes known to be dependent on riboflavin for their synthesis and concerned with the utilization of oxygen to produce energy, to be markedly reduced in activity compared to those of the normal control fetuses— those whose mothers received adequate amounts of riboflavin. One can see how deformities might easily develop if energy production is curtailed at a time when the cells—engaged in rapid multiplication and differentiation—have a high demand for energy.

A lack of B₂ can also increase the teratogenicity (fetal-damage potential) of certain drugs. As reported in *Research and*

*Technology* (26 April 1965), Dr. Lorene L. Rogers demonstrated that when teratogenic drugs were given to riboflavin-deficient pregnant rats, the incidence of birth defects was much higher than that caused by either the drug or the deficiency alone. In relating these findings to humans, Dr. Rogers stated that " . . . our results suggests that all physicians administering drugs of any kind during pregnancy should make every effort to see that the patient's nutrition is as nearly optimum as possible."

## Riboflavin Deficiency in Pregnancy

Dr. Mackler's report in *Pediatrics* showed that a lack of riboflavin may damage a fetus without any deficiency being apparent in the mother. In addition to examining the tissues of the deformed fetuses, Dr. Mackler studied the mothers' placentas and heart tissue. Here he found that enzyme activity was *not* significantly affected. "Fetal tissue," Dr. Mackler commented, "is apparently particularly susceptible to the effects of riboflavin deficiency." A level of deficiency that the mother can tolerate cannot be tolerated by the embryo at its crucial time of growth.

Can these laboratory findings on experimental animals be translated into human terms? How real is the danger that an expectant mother will have so low a supply of riboflavin that her baby may be deformed? Unfortunately, no studies have been made of malformed babies in relation to the mother's riboflavin nutrition. It is known, however, that riboflavin deficiency is considered one of the most common of vitamin deficiencies, and that malnutrition in this nutrient is widespread.

## Common Foods Rich in Riboflavin*

|  | (milligrams) |
|---|---|
| Liver (Beef, 3 oz., fried) | 3.56 |
| Kidney (Beef, 1 cup, cooked) | 6.75 |
| Heart (Beef, 1 cup, cooked) | 1.77 |
| Ham (1 cup, cooked, chopped or diced) | .32 |
| Beef (1 cup, cooked, chopped or diced) | .29 |
| Chicken (Dark meat, 1 cup, cooked) | .32 |
| Milk (1 cup, whole) | .41 |
| Eggs (1 large, raw) | .15 |
| Broccoli (1 cup, cooked) | .31 |
| Spinach (1 cup, cooked) | .25 |
| Kale (1 cup, cooked) | .20 |
| Peas (Green, 1 cup, cooked) | .18 |
| Lima beans (1 cup, cooked) | .17 |
| Brewers yeast (Debittered, 1 tbsp.) | .34 |
| Sunflower seeds (Hulled, 1 cup) | .33 |

*Selected from tables in *Nutritive Value of American Foods in Common Units,* United States Department of Agriculture Handbook #456, November, 1975.

# CHAPTER 30

# The Need for Niacin

Niacin is unique among the B vitamins because the body can produce small amounts of it. Tryptophan, an amino acid, can be converted to niacin through a number of biochemical steps. While the body does convert tryptophan for some of its niacin (babies get much of their niacin from the large amounts of tryptophan in milk), this is not a practical way to supply major niacin needs. It takes 60 mg. of tryptophan to make one mg. of niacin, and the conversion depends on ample supplies of other vitamins and protein.

Though the term "niacin" is commonly used, there are really two forms of the vitamin: *niacin,* (nicotinic acid) and *niacinamide,* (nicotinic acid amide, or nicotinamide). Both niacin and niacinamide perform the same vitamin functions within the body; both are equally effective in preventing a nutritional deficiency. Niacinamide is usually used when enriching foods.

The only differences between the two lie in the pharmacologic effects of nicotinic acid and nicotinamide. Nicotinic acid is a vasodilator (dilates blood vessels) and is sometimes used to increase peripheral circulation in the aging. Large doses of nicotinic acid are also prescribed to reduce cholesterol levels in the blood and to treat schizophrenics and alcoholics. (See index.) Niacinamide is used in treating a number of diseases involving the gastrointestinal tract, such as the sprue syndrome. It is also used to treat glossitis and stomatitis due to various causes. Recently the term "B₃" has become popular in referring to niacin, and is used mainly in relation to the pharmacologic effects of megadoses of the vitamin.

## Niacin Has Many Functions

While pellagra no longer rampages through the United States, the niacin-deficiency disease still seriously threatens several parts of the world today. According to Daphne A. Roe, M.D., nutritionist and dermatologist at Cornell University, "Pellagra remains a major health problem among the Bantu in South Africa, and it is still prevalent in Egypt and in the Deccan Plateau region of India. In these countries the disease continues to affect the rural poor, who, whether they subsist on maize or millet, cannot afford such pellagra-preventing foods as eggs and meat" *Natural History,* (October 1974).

Yet even in the United States, marginal deficiencies of niacin frequently lead to pellagra-like symptoms. A nationwide survey conducted by the U.S. Department of Health, Education, and Welfare in 1971-72 examined the nutritional status of a group that was designated as representative of the total United States population. Called the First Health and Nutrition Examination Survey (HANES), the study revealed that many Americans showed clinical signs of niacin deficiency. The elderly seemed to suffer the most—13.2 percent of all the people aged 60 years and over had fissures of the tongue—but other age groups were by no means exempt from such classic deficiency signs. Women between the ages of 18 and 44 showed a higher incidence of most deficiency signs than men in the same age group—9.2 percent of the women above the poverty level showed serrations and swelling of the tongue, compared with 8.6 percent of the men above the poverty level. It is important to note that only 6.8 percent of the women and 6.2 percent of the men *below* the poverty level showed the same clinical sign of deficiency. From this it is obvious that a higher income does not, of itself, insure better nutrition.

If so many Americans show clinical signs of niacin deficiency, there are probably many more who suffer from subclinical deficiencies of niacin. These shortages, not severe enough to bring on definite signs, may be responsible for weakness, irritability, mental fatigue, abdominal pains, sleeplessness, or even a red and furry tongue. Another common indication of niacin deficiency is a rash resembling prickly heat, which usually appears on the neck, forearms, and other uncovered parts of the body. The skin becomes dry and somewhat scaly, and usually has fine wrinkles and a coarse texture.

## Getting Enough Niacin

The HANES study shows that too few Americans get enough niacin from their diets. It also shows that poor nutrition in the United States is not tied to low income; in fact it is even worse in some higher income families.

Much of the problem is due to heavy reliance on foods that are highly refined or have a high carbohydrate content. Niacin, like most of the B vitamins, is used to metabolize carbohydrates, so the large amounts of sugar and starches in many processed foods rob the body of niacin that is needed for other functions.

Refining seriously diminishes the vitamin content of foods, and even though these foods might be enriched, the original quantities and combinations of vitamins are not restored. The complex of B vitamins must occur together to function properly. Niacin works with vitamins $B_1$, $B_2$, $B_6$, pantothenic acid, folic acid, and $B_{12}$ in alleviating deficiencies and in carbohydrate metabolism. Vitamins $B_1$, $B_2$, and $B_6$ are needed for converting tryptophan to niacin. The body also needs ample amounts of niacin to make proper use of thiamine and riboflavin.

Researchers have found that niacin sometimes occurs in "bound forms," meaning that the niacin is not released to the body from that food. According to a report in *Nutrition Reviews* (October 1975), "Additional evidence now indicates the presence in many foodstuffs, especially cereals, of niacin-containing compounds from which the niacin is not nutritionally available. . . . Later studies showed that the bound niacin was ineffective in curing niacin deficiency in the rat, chick, duck, or pig.'' It was the unavailability of the bound niacin in corn which caused pellagra among people subsisting on corn.

Niacin is also lost in cooking, and oral antibiotics interfere with its metabolism in the system. Many illnesses will decrease the absorption of niacin in the intestines, and as with all the B vitamins, alcohol is particularly destructive of niacin.

The U.S. Recommended Daily Allowance for niacin is 20 mg., but to protect yourself against factors that decrease niacin's availability, two to four times that amount would not be too much. Niacin is not toxic in large doses, but megadoses can produce uncomfortable side effects like burning, itching skin, flushing, and gastrointestinal upset. However, according to Dr. Roman J. Kutsky's *Handbook of Vitamins and Hormones,* (New York: Van Nostrand Reinhold Co., 1973), these effects begin with dosages of one gram or more.

# CHAPTER 31

# The Antipellagra Factor

Niacin first gained recognition as a cure for the dread pellagra, the disease which simultaneously attacks the skin, the gastrointestinal system, and the nervous system. Its effects, commonly referred to as the three Ds—dermatitis, diarrhea, and dementia—are potentially fatal.

Pellagra existed in Europe at least as early as the 1700s, but its cause was shrouded in mystery and ignorance. Because it was most common among rural people who ate lots of corn, authorities dismissed it as the "corn poison." Some argued that it was an infection, others believed it was caused by moldy maize or by sunlight.

From 1905 to 1915 there was an explosive outbreak of the disease in the southern United States. In 1914 Dr. Joseph Goldberger, a bacteriologist with the U.S. Public Health Service, was assigned the task of identifying the cause of pellagra once and for all.

As Herbert Bailey notes in his book, *The Vitamin Pioneers* (Emmaus, Pennsylvania: Rodale Books, Inc., 1968) "Here was a man who combined all the qualities of a pioneer in this field: imagination, powers of observation, and a deep compassion for sufferers. He was just the man who was needed at the time, for in 1915 more than 10,000 people died of pellagra in the United States. In addition, over 200,000 were suffering from it."

184

While orthodox medicine attributed the disease to poor hygiene, Dr. Goldberger was convinced that the poverty-level southern diet—limited almost exclusively to cornmeal and grits, cornstarch, white flour, corn syrup, pork fat, and sugar—was to blame. He could see that many of these people didn't raise any fruits or vegetables, and they couldn't afford meat. Their basic dependency on corn products eliminated sources of niacin and other essential nutrients not found in corn.

Checking state asylums in South Carolina, Georgia, and Mississippi, Dr. Goldberger found that the staff members—eating milk, meat, and eggs—were invariably free of the disease. The patients, on the other hand, were pellagra-psychotic. They ate mainly cereal.

Dr. Goldberger knew he was close to solving the puzzle that had stumped mankind for generations. However, a widely publicized report released by a private commission in 1916 threatened to wipe out his painstaking work. The Thompson-McFadden report officially concluded that pellagra was an infectious disease and was caused by the sting of the stable fly!

Dr. Goldberger had no choice. To prove once and for all that pellagra is not an infectious disease passed on by microbes, he bravely injected himself with excrement, mucus, and scaly skin droppings from pellagra victims. Bailey reports what happened. "Goldberger was given test after test and to everyone else's surprise (but not to his) nothing happened at all. No symptoms of pellagra appeared. None. At last, after more than a century, the old theory that pellagra was caused by an infection was swept away forever."

But the selfless doctor didn't stop there. Using healthy prisoner volunteers, he induced pellagra symptoms by feeding them a deficient diet and then cured them with a daily supplement of 30 grams of yeast, plus lean beef and milk. Dr. Goldberger knew he had found the "pellagra preventive," and that it was some unknown factor in the B vitamin complex, but he never succeeded in isolating the substance.

It was not until 1937 that Dr. Conrad Elvehjem of the University of Wisconsin identified the curative factor—nicotinic acid or niacin. He and his assistants injected 30 mg. of the substance into a dog with "black tongue," the canine equivalent of pellagra. "They didn't have long to wait," Bailey reports. "Within minutes, the dog began to show signs of improvement. There was suddenly no longer any doubt left. The item missing from corn had been found."

According to Bailey, when Dr. Tom Spies, a noted southern doctor, treated human pellagra victims with the vitamin, beneficial results were noted within 24 to 48 hours. Still other doctors discovered that in some cases niacin alone was not enough; other B vitamins such as thiamine and riboflavin were also needed. Apparently all of the B complex had to work together to insure health. The cure for pellagra was now a reality.

# CHAPTER 32

# Subclinical Pellagra
May Be Mistaken
for Mental Illness

It appears that pellagra, the niacin deficiency disease that is a common consequence of poverty, famine, and starvation diets, exists today in North America. Not in its most obvious form—with painful splotches on the skin, an inflamed tongue, raving madness, and serious digestive upsets that can end in death—but rather in a subclinical form whose symptoms are being mistaken for mental illness.

According to a noted Canadian psychiatrist reporting in the journal *Schizophrenia* (2nd quarter, 1971), both the hyperactive "problem" child who fails to do well in school and the schizophrenic confined to an asylum are victims of vitamin $B_3$ (niacin) deficiency. In effect, they are suffering from a form of pellagra; their illnesses are different in degree only. In his report, Abram Hoffer, M.D., of Saskatoon, Saskatchewan, who pioneered the highly successful megavitamin therapy for schizophrenics in the early 1950s, said, "Unfortunately, psychiatrists are no longer familiar with the clinical manifestations of pellagra. When the older literature is examined, it is clear that the best model of schizophrenia is pellagra. It is so good that for many years psychiatrists in mental hospitals could not distinguish between them."

The only certain diagnostic test was the therapeutic one, using crystalline vitamin B₃ once it became available. If the psychotic patient recovered in a matter of days on one gram per day or less he was labelled pellagrin. If not, he was termed schizophrenic. "What is not as well known," Dr. Hoffer continued, "is that long before pellagrins became psychotic they suffered from tension, depression, personality problems, fatigue. . . ." In other words, subclinical pellagra could easily be mistaken for mental illness.

Several years ago it was reported in *The Washington Post*, (2 April 1971), that pellagra had spread among the mentally ill and retarded in Maryland state hospitals. After personally inspecting Springfield State Hospital at Sykesville, Dr. Neil Solomon, then Secretary of Health and Mental Hygiene, said he found that "a tremendous number" of patients "had red, swollen tongues and lesions on exposed parts of their bodies"— a condition ignored by hospital personnel. When Dr. Solomon called for an investigation of the state's six facilities, probers discovered the institutional diets were deficient in niacin, protein, iron, and calcium. Ironically, one of pellagra's most common effects—mental derangement—is the very thing the state hospitals are trying to cure.

It appears that people most likely to exhibit the symptoms of subclinical pellagra are those who simply don't eat properly. It is an easy condition to develop, even amid an abundance of food, if it is nutritionally meager.

However, a poor diet may not always be the reason for an insufficient niacin supply. It is believed by such highly respected authorities as Dr. Linus Pauling and others, that victims of subclinical pellagra or mental illness may be suffering from a biochemical imbalance which creates a need for abnormally high doses of certain vitamins just to keep the mind functioning well. Noting that we have in our bodies a blood-brain barrier designed to keep undesirable molecules and contaminants out of the brain, Dr. Pauling suggested in *Schizophrenia* (2nd quarter, 1971), "This barrier may also sometimes operate to keep good molecules out of the brain. I have thought that it might well be that the value of megavitamin therapy for some patients is the result of their having a blood-brain barrier that is operating too efficiently, in such a way that even though in the peripheral tissues the concentration of vitamins may be essentially optimal, there could still be a local avitaminosis (vitamin deficiency) in the brain itself.''

## Symptoms of Subclinical Pellagra

While pellagra is rare, except under conditions of intense poverty and ignorance, symptoms of subclinical pellagra are not so rare, but may be mistaken for similar symptoms of other ailments. While dysperception is the clue to a correct diagnosis, its other symptoms, which include fatigue, depression, loss of appetite, headache, dizziness, weakness, and various aches and pains, are common to most any disease.

What are the chances that a family doctor would be able to diagnose subclinical pellagra in a patient suffering from it who came to be examined and treated? A lot depends on whether he knows the right questions.

R. Glen Green, M.D., in the publications *Schizophrenia* (2nd and 3rd quarters, 1970), recommended that physicians ask questions of such patients regarding, not physical, but perceptual changes involving the five senses. According to Dr. Green, the most pertinent questions are:

1. Does your face seem to change when you look in a mirror?
2. Do words move when you try to read?
3. Does the ground move when you walk?
4. Do you feel you walk on the ground or off the ground?
5. Do pictures move when you look at them?
6. Do you hear someone calling your name when you are alone?

If the patients say they have experienced some or all of these things—even sometimes—Dr. Green has them take the Hoffer-

Osmond Diagnostic (HOD) Test. The HOD Test is made up of 145 questions, to be answered true or false. Originally developed by Drs. Abram Hoffer and Humphrey Osmond to diagnose schizophrenic patients, it reveals perceptual difficulties in sight, hearing, taste, smell, and attitudes. The total score may vary between zero and 246. When used as a psychiatric method of diagnosis, a score of 40 or more may indicate that the patient is suffering from schizophrenia. Dr. Green, however, adapted the test to his medical practice, and discovered that a score of 40 or more also indicated subclinical pellagra.

## HOD Test Measures Progress of B₃ Therapy

Dr. Green presented a case history in his report to demonstrate his experience with subclinical pellagra. On 31 March 1969, a mother brought her nine-year-old girl to see Dr. Green, their family physician who had delivered the child almost ten years before. The girl, previously in the top third of her class, was now barely able to get passing grades in school. She spent much of her time in bed, and was constantly fighting with her brothers and sisters. Once active and happy, she was now utterly miserable. The reason her mother brought her to the doctor, however, was that the girl claimed to have daily abdominal pains, nausea, and leg pain, as well as spells of vomiting. Dr. Green examined the girl and found no physical explanation for these symptoms. Fortunately, he did not stop with a physical examination, but also asked her questions to determine her perception. That was what led to a successful diagnosis and treatment.

Dr. Green learned that his young patient suffered distorted vision. Upon looking in the mirror, she saw a blurred image of herself which got bigger as she gazed. In school, letters on the blackboard seemed to move in all directions, making them impossible to read. Even the ground she walked on appeared to move under her feet. She heard voices when nobody was around. When she picked up the blackboard eraser at school it felt fuzzy. Senses of taste and smell were disturbed. All these things brought on a state of depression, and the girl was afraid, although she could not say why.

The girl took the HOD Test on April 1 and scored 107, almost three times as high as the threshold figure. Dr. Green started her on one gram of nicotinamide three times a day. By April 16 the girl felt she was getting better, although the dysperceptions were still there.

Dr. Green reported that by 30 April 1969, "Her hallucinations were all gone, she could read without trouble, she could watch television, the ground stopped moving, she heard no voices, and so on. Her mood was happy, her fears evaporated. She had only two attacks of abdominal pain in the month and they were not bothersome. She looked and acted like a different girl."

When Dr. Green gave the girl another HOD Test on 2 July, she scored a safe 37. In checking two of her sisters, he found them suffering from the same thing, having scored 77 and 95 respectively on the HOD Test. After they each received the same amount of vitamin B₃ as their sister for three months, they took the test again and scored 10 and five respectively.

Should patients who score over 40 on the HOD Tests be referred to a psychiatrist to be treated for schizophrenia? Not necessarily, believes Dr. Green. He found that the response to vitamin B₃ treatment in his patients was enough to bring about a disappearance of their hallucinations and alleviation of the symptoms that would normally be considered reason for psychiatric treatment.

The significance of this discovery was put into words by Dr. Green himself when he said, "For the past 20 years I have been diagnosing (such patients) as neurotic, having flu, neurasthenia, sore throat, backache, etc., for want of something better. It is certainly true that patients have suffered perceptual changes in the past 20 years."

He added that, "In a seven-month period since November, 1968, I have diagnosed well over 100 cases of subclinical pellagra; 65 percent of the cases were under 16 years of age.

They all responded to vitamin B₃, which is niacin, or its amide, within a few days or weeks. The chief criterion for diagnosis of this disease is the presence or absence of perceptual changes.''

| **Common Foods Rich in Niacin*** | |
|---|---|
| | (milligrams) |
| Liver (Beef, 3 oz., fried) | 14.0 |
| Heart (Beef, 1 cup, cooked) | 11.0 |
| Kidney (Beef, 1 cup, cooked) | 15.0 |
| Beef (1 cup, cooked, chopped or diced) | 4.9 |
| Rabbit (White meat, 1 cup, cooked) | 15.8 |
| Turkey (White meat, 1 cup, cooked) | 15.5 |
| Chicken (White meat, 1 cup, cooked) | 16.2 |
| Ham (1 cup, cooked, chopped or diced) | 6.4 |
| Halibut (3 oz., cooked) | 6.9 |
| Tuna (1 cup) | 19.0 |
| Sunflower seeds (Hulled, 1 cup) | 7.8 |
| Whole wheat flour (1 cup) | 5.2 |
| Brewers yeast (Debittered, 1 tbsp.) | 3.0 |
| Peas (Green, 1 cup, cooked) | 3.7 |
| Peanuts (10 jumbo) | 3.1 |

*Selected from tables in *Nutritive Value of American Foods in Common Units*, United States Department of Agriculture Handbook #456, November, 1975.

# CHAPTER 33

# B₆, The Unsuspected Benefactor

Many nutrients, for better or worse, have a popular "label" attached to them in the eyes of the public. They may perform several vital functions in our bodies, but usually they come to be identified with one role, which may or may not be the most important one they play. Vitamin A, for example, is often thought of as the "night blindness" vitamin, because a deficiency can leave you groping and stumbling in semi-darkness. Mention vitamin C, and most people will instantly think of that nutrient's proven ability to fight colds. Vitamin D is the "sunshine" vitamin; thiamine is the "morale" vitamin, and so on.

But mention vitamin B₆, or pyridoxine, and most people are likely to come up with a complete blank!

Even John M. Ellis, M.D., a Texas physician who has used pyridoxine successfully in his practice for more than a dozen years, concedes that B₆ is like "an iceberg in foggy, uncharted Antarctic waters . . . a long time emerging from scientific obscurity." In his book, *Vitamin B₆: The Doctor's Report* (New York: Harper & Row, 1973), Dr. Ellis says that pyridoxine's image "is still blurred in medical circles, and even more so in the public mind. . . ."

Discovered in 1934 by Paul Gyorgy, M.D., Professor Emeritus of Pediatrics at the University of Pennsylvania School of

Medicine, pyridoxine was not recognized by the National Research Council in a recommended daily requirement until 1968. The nutritional significance of vitamin B6 has still not been fully explored. While giving a lecture at the University of Missouri in February, 1971, Dr. Gyorgy stated that, "At present we are facing an almost explosive interest in the metabolic role of B6 in man." He added that, "There are large numbers of findings of various types accumulating, but a clear, over-all picture of all connections and of their role is still missing."

## Activates Many Enzymes

Vitamin B6 is probably involved in more bodily processes than any other single nutrient. When B6 enters the body, it is transformed, with the aid of B2, into the coenzyme pyridoxal phosphate. This coenzyme is essential as an activator of a large number of enzymes, which in turn activate a wide array of health maintenance systems within our bodies. As the famous Soviet biochemist A. E. Braunstein wrote in *The Enzymes* (P.D. Boyer *et al,* ed., New York: Academic Press, 1960), "Pyridoxal phosphate holds an exceptional place among the coenzymes with regard to the unparalleled diversity of its catalytic function. . . ."

As pyridoxal phosphate, B6 is intricately involved in the metabolism of fats, carbohydrates, potassium, iron, and the formation of hormones such as adrenalin and insulin. Its most important role, however, is its function in protein metabolism. Amino acids, the building blocks of protein, can be absorbed and utilized by the body only if there is enough pyridoxal phosphate present. Thus, all the protein structures in our bodies, from glands to blood vessels and many more, are at the mercy of B6 sufficiency.

Pyridoxine is also necessary for the synthesis of DNA and RNA, the nucleic acids that contain the genetic instructions for proper growth, maintenance, and reproduction of all the cells in the body. Writing in *Today's Health* (March 1974), Dr. Philip L. White, director of the American Medical Association's Department of Food and Nutrition, pointed out that vitamin B6 "is needed for production of antibodies as part of the body's immune response and for synthesis of one of the components of hemoglobin." A $B_6$ deficiency can reduce immunity to attack by diphtheria or other organisms. Erwin DiCyan, Ph.D., in his book *Vitamins In Your Life* (New York: Simon and Schuster, 1974), speculated that pyridoxine's influence on the immunity system may be a result of the vitamin's importance to the production of DNA and RNA.

Pyridoxine performs these vital jobs with so little fanfare that most people never realize they have this unsuspected benefactor working for their good health. But $B_6$ has other important, more specialized abilities as well, and for certain people, its action can be dramatic indeed.

## Pyridoxine-Responsive Anemia

Anemia, a condition involving a reduced number of red blood cells, is usually believed to occur because of an iron deficiency. However, deficiencies of several other nutrients may also cause anemia. Vitamin E, folic acid, or $B_{12}$ are usually found to be lacking in cases where supplemental iron does not relieve the anemia, but in some cases doctors have found that a $B_6$ deficiency alone is responsible for the anemia.

One such case, involving a man who suffered from recurring anemia for several years, was reported by hemotologist Allen J. Erslev, M.D., in the *New England Journal of Medicine* (16 June 1960). Pyridoxine injections had helped the patient but never permanently. Dr. Erslev attributed the return of anemic symptoms to "intermittent pyridoxine deficiency." He suggested that "prolonged deficiency in pyridoxine may lead to irreversible changes in the synthesis of hemoglobin." Indeed, other researchers have noted that once this type of anemia appears, it rarely disappears; patients with pyridoxine-responsive anemia continue to require the vitamin in quantities much greater than the diet or even injections can provide.

A study by Eileen Harriss at the Postgraduate Medical School, London, helps to explain the interaction between iron and pyridoxine. It appears that while iron is necessary for hemoglobin synthesis, in the absence of sufficient pyridoxine, the mineral is not utilized properly and instead forms granular deposits within the blood cells.

Reprinted from a published symposium in *Hematology* (March 1962), the Harriss series of experiments revealed that mice fed a $B_6$-deficient diet and extra iron quickly developed anemia and died. Mice fed a pyridoxine-deficient diet without iron "survived somewhat longer before their hemoglobin concentration showed a marked fall."

The red cells of the pyridoxine-deficient mice were described as irregularly shaped and sized. Many were "markedly hypochromic" or pale. It was also noted that the iron content of the cells was excessively high. Yet when mice received pyridoxine in addition to iron in the diet, no anemia or iron overload appeared.

The researcher concluded, "The main fact of interest which emerges from these experiments is that a hypochromic anemia associated with tissue siderosis (iron infiltration) develops in pyridoxine-deficient mice despite normal or decreased absorption of iron. The presence of excess iron is not essential to the development of anemia, and in these animals the anemia can be attributed to pyridoxine deficiency alone."

## Helpful for Skin Problems

For the tearful teenage girl whose recurring premenstrual acne flare-up interferes with an active social life, vitamin $B_6$ can also be a very important nutrient. According to a report in *Obstetrical and Gynecological News* (1 May 1974), B. Leonard Snider, M.D., of Erie, Pa., gave daily $B_6$ supplements to 106 teenagers whose acne was under control, except for monthly flare-ups just prior to menstruation. The vitamin was taken for one week preceding and during the time of menstruation for an average of three menstrual periods. Seventy-six of the girls reported that $B_6$ reduced their acne flare anywhere from 50 to 75 percent.

Other doctors have reported success using pyridoxine ointment to treat another nagging skin problem, seborrhea. This chronic, inflammatory condition results when too much thick, greasy sebum is excreted by the body's sebaceous glands. Ugly scaling, redness, and crusted patches can appear on the face, ears, and scalp.

More than 20 years ago, Richard W. Vilter, M.D., one of the pioneers in early B₆ research, and three associates at the University of Cincinnati College of Medicine and Cincinnati General Hospital prepared an ointment by combining B₆ with a vanishing cream base, using 10 mg. of the vitamin per gram of base. This ointment was applied directly to seborrheic lesions on a number of patients. The researchers reported their success in the *Journal of Laboratory and Clinical Medicine* (vol. 40, 1952). "All twelve patients treated with local application of pyridoxine ointment had complete clearing of the areas treated in five to 21 days," they reported, "although two patients required concentrations of 50 mg. of pyridoxine per gram of vanibase to eliminate the last vestiges of the dermatitis. Itching disappeared first, then scaling, and finally the erythema (redness)."

## B₆ Related to Cancer Immunity and Atherosclerosis

Pyridoxine may also be involved in maintaining the body's immunity to cancer. When 10 baboons were fed a balanced diet intermittently lacking in just one nutrient—vitamin B₆—for two to six years, half developed premalignant nodules and other indications of liver cancer. These ominous changes occurred in animals that had received no carcinogenic substance—they were simply deprived of B₆.

Five other baboons *totally* deprived of pyridoxine failed to develop liver tumors, apparently because they didn't live long enough. All died of liver damage within six to eight months. Those results were reported by Henry Foy of the Wellcome Trust Research Laboratories in Nairobi, Kenya, and six other researchers in the *Journal of the National Cancer Institute* (November 1974).

Another animal finding which has been tremendously suggestive to practicing clinicians is that $B_6$-starved monkeys develop massive arteriosclerosis in virtually every part of their bodies. Discussing the relationship of $B_6$ to atherosclerosis and cholesterol-clogged arteries, Dr. Roger J. Williams in *Nutrition Against Disease* (New York: Pitman, 1971), says that Russian scientists have reported very low plasma levels of the coenzyme forms of vitamin $B_6$ in 31 of 48 atherosclerotic patients with high cholesterol counts. While the Russian scientists offered no explanation for this, Dr. Williams points out that $B_6$ is vital for production of lecithin, which is known to dissolve cholesterol.

Summarizing a number of other studies, Dr. Williams (an outstanding researcher who was the first to identify and isolate pantothenic acid, another B vitamin) declares: "From a consideration of the evidence we have reviewed, the surest guarantee against possible pernicious effects of various protein/fat/cholesterol combinations, in whatever proportions, is the daily intake of a sufficient amount of pyridoxine."

## $B_6$ May Help Prevent Tooth Decay

There is some evidence that pyridoxine plays a role in preventing tooth decay. The *New York State Dental Journal* (August-September 1956) reported on an experiment, led by Lyon P. Strean, Ph.D., D.D.S., which tested pyridoxine's effect on dental caries in hamsters. The results showed a dramatic six-fold difference in the number of dental caries between two groups of hamsters who differed only in the amount of pyridoxine they received in their diets. The first group, receiving barely enough $B_6$ to maintain life, averaged a 26.1 percent loss of tooth structure. The second group received 20 times as much $B_6$ as the first, and averaged a low 4.2 percent loss of tooth structure.

Several other animal studies over the years have shown that $B_6$ supplementation does indeed help to prevent tooth decay. Writing in *Vitamins and Hormones* (vol. 22, 1964), Lewis D. Greenberg, Ph.D., clearly demonstrated that young, developing monkeys deprived of adequate amounts of $B_6$ suffered from devastating tooth decay, while monkeys receiving sufficient B₆ did not. Studies with dogs showed similar results.

But what about tooth decay in people? A test, using supplemental B₆ lozenges, was conducted by Dr. Strean and reported in the *New York State Dental Journal* (March 1958). The study involved 28 children between the ages of 10 and 15 years. When the children who took pyridoxine lozenges for a period of one year were compared with a control group taking placebo lozenges, they showed a 40 percent reduction in tooth decay over the control group.

An article entitled "Effect of Vitamin B₆ on Dental Caries in Man," written by Robert W. Hillman, M.D., and appearing in *Vitamins and Hormones* (vol. 22, 1964), reviewed several studies that indicated pyridoxine lozenges reduced tooth decay in school children by as much as 50 percent. Dr. Hillman cited two studies which concluded that Cuban children who chewed sugar cane had fewer caries and higher blood concentrations of B₆ than did a peer group in New York City. Cane sugar has a relatively high concentration of B₆, while refined sugar has the B₆ (and virtually all other nutrients) processed out of it.

## B₆ Easily Destroyed in Processing

B₆ has also been shown to play an important role in the prevention or treatment of rheumatism, asthma, and kidney stones (see index), and is very beneficial in some cases of schizophrenia (see index). A deficiency of the vitamin can trigger a tic, a twitch, or a tremor. It can cause tension, irritability, insomnia, nervousness, an inability to concentrate, and severe halitosis. A severe deficiency can cause seborrheic dermatitis or eczema, appearing first in the scalp and the eyebrows, then around the nose, behind the ears, and around the genitalia. No other vitamin yet discovered by science seems to be involved in so many health functions as pyridoxine. Yet it is relatively easy to become deficient in pyridoxine.

Modern refining, processing, cooking, and storage all deplete the reserves of B₆ in the food we eat, according to an acknowledged authority on trace nutrients, Henry A. Schroeder, M.D. Summarizing laboratory analyses of hundreds of processed food products for their $B_6$ content, Dr. Schroeder reported in the *American Journal of Clinical Nutrition* (May 1971), that "Large losses occurred as a result of the canning of vegetables, ranging from 57 to 77 percent. Frozen vegetables showed losses of 37 to 56 percent in vitamin $B_6$." Average $B_6$ loss in frozen fruit juices was found to be 15.4 percent; in canned juices, 37.6 percent. Canned meats lost up to 42.6 percent of their pyridoxine content, while bologna, salami, and certain other processed meats lost an average of 68 percent. About 80 percent of the $B_6$ is removed from all-purpose flour. Precooked rice loses 93 percent of its original content of $B_6$.

A study conducted by the U.S. Army Medical Research and Nutrition Laboratory in Denver, Colorado, indicated that many people may be creating $B_6$ deficiencies in themselves by increased intake of protein. Reporting in the *Annals of the New York Academy of Sciences* (vol. 166, 1969), the army researchers demonstrated that a high-protein diet boosts the body's demand for $B_6$ and leads to a deficiency of that nutrient if the $B_6$ intake is not increased proportionately. People on a high-protein reducing diet should be particularly careful to increase their $B_6$ intake, perhaps with a supplement like desiccated liver.

## Many Don't Get Enough B6

It is easy to see that the wrong food choices might easily deprive a person of adequate amounts of this vitamin. Dr. Ellis believes this is now happening on a wide scale. "I have seen enough husbands and wives who ate from the same table and who suffered from the same symptomatology," he commented in his book, "to conclude positively that vitamin $B_6$ deficiency is the most prevalent deficiency in the United States today."

The Food and Nutrition Board of the National Academy of Sciences has set two mg. of $B_6$ daily as the Recommended Daily Allowance for healthy adult men and women. The RDA for women who are pregnant or nursing an infant is slightly higher, 2.5 mg. But when J.A. Driskell and two associates in Florida State University's Food and Nutrition Department analyzed the diets of 152 students, they found that three out of four were not consuming this much B6. The incidence of deficiency was independent of age, income, or the amount of money students budgeted for food, they told the annual meeting of the Federation of American Societies for Experimental Biology in Atlantic City, N.J., in April, 1974.

The problem is complicated by the fact that many people need much more of this nutrient than others to maintain health. Dr. Gyorgy stated in the *American Journal of Clinical Nutrition* (October 1971) that many individuals actually need *10 times the RDA* "as a precaution to prevent possible serious pathological conditions."

# CHAPTER 34

# Millions Need More B₆

"This I will not tolerate! This is the most foolish thing in the world!"

Such was the reaction of Dr. Paul Gyorgy, the codiscoverer of several B vitamins, to the Food and Drug Administrations's announced plan in 1974 to regulate the potency of vitamin supplements. The regulations proposed to limit vitamin D supplements to the FDA-sanctioned Recommended Daily Allowance (RDA), vitamin A supplements to twice the RDA, and all other vitamins to one and a half times their RDAs.

Dr. Gyorgy was particularly outraged at the proposed restrictions on vitamin B₆. The FDA based its recommendations on vitamin values rooted essentially in early research designed to discover how *little* of a vitamin is necessary to prevent outright deficiency disease. It does not reflect the recent sophisticated research at cellular and molecular levels, investigations showing the role of vitamins in enzymatic reactions and pinpointing subtle metabolic disorders in marginal deficiency states before there is any recognizable sign or symptom of overt deficiency disease. Dr. Gyorgy was dismayed over the proposed limits on B₆ potency because of evidence demonstrating that the "recommended daily allowance" for B₆ (two mg. for general use and

2.5 for pregnant and lactating women) must be not only doubled or tripled but increased 10-fold (and sometimes much more) in extremely large numbers of people to maintain normal metabolism.

Who are these individuals in need whose numbers mount into the millions?

The answer was spelled out at a 1970 international conference, held in Madison, Wisconsin, and sponsored by the University of Wisconsin Medical Center and the pharmaceutical house, Hoffmann-La Roche, Inc. The informative (though unwieldy) title of the gathering was: "The Biochemistry and Pathology of Tryptophan Metabolism and Its Regulation by Amino Acids, Vitamin B6, and Steroid Hormones."

Tryptophan is one of the essential amino acids incorporated in protein foods. Vitamin B6 is necessary for its proper metabolism in the body. In B6 deficiency, abnormal metabolism of tryptophan creates abnormal by-products or metabolites which can be harmful. As has been reported in the literature and was brought out strongly at the Madison conference, steroid hormones (including the adrenal corticosteroids such as cortisone and also the female hormone estrogen) have the effect of increasing the demand for B6 and therefore causing B6 deficiency if this vitamin is not supplied in large doses.

Raymond R. Brown, Ph.D., of the University of Wisconsin Medical Center, who was chairman of the conference, summarized the findings of the three-day scientific sessions in an article in the *American Journal of Clinical Nutrition* (February 1971). He listed the following categories of persons subject to B6 deficiency even though their diet is supposedly "adequate:" (1) women on the oral contraceptive, or OC (which contains estrogen); (2) pregnant women (who produce estrogen at elevated levels, one type of estrogen increasing to 1,000 times the normal level toward the end of term); (3) women at the peak of their estrogen output during the last two weeks of the menstrual cycle; (4) individuals—male and female, young and old—who are being treated with cortisone or other similar steroids.

# Millions At Risk

Let's stop right here and calculate what kind of numbers we're talking about.

There are about 54.2 million women (1970 census) in the age groups in which the female reproductive system is active.

This represents more than one-quarter (26 percent) of the entire U.S. population.

Of this large group, an estimated seven to eight million are current users of oral contraceptives.

Close to four million experience pregnancy in a year's time—a figure estimated from births plus miscarriages plus abortions.

So here we have 11 to 12 million persons with a greater-than-"normal" need for vitamin $B_6$ every day. The rest of this group—some 42 million teenage girls and mature young women—have a physiological demand for extra vitamin $B_6$ during a portion of each month.

Not counting the population on cortisone, then, more than one out of every four Americans would not be able to get the vitamin $B_6$ they require from the limited supplements the FDA favors. Furthermore, all of these people with their special $B_6$ demand are part of the "normal healthy population" which the FDA invariably refers to in justifying the amounts of vitamin supplements it claims are adequate for all "normal" needs.

In addition to these "normal healthy" persons, how many others have special $B_6$ needs because they are taking cortisone or one of the other steroids? No accurate figures are available here, but an estimate can be made. Consider arthritis and rheumatism, the most widespread disease conditions for which steroids are prescribed. The Arthritis Foundation estimates 17,000,000 Americans have arthritis severe enough to require medical care. At a 1968 symposium conducted by the Foundation, it was reported that steroid drugs are used in 23 percent of patients visits for arthritic/rheumatic disorders. One can conclude, therefore, that close to four million arthritics are getting steroid therapy.

The number of arthritics on steroids brings the total of

potentially B₆-deficient people to 58 million or 28 percent of the U.S. population. If you take into consideration *everyone* treated with cortisone, plus women of menopausal and post-menopausal age who receive estrogen replacement therapy, plus victims of certain diseases which research has found to be conducive to B₆ deficiency (Down's syndrome or mongolism, rheumatoid arthritis, diabetes), you can well assume that at least a third of the population, or one out of every three Americans, is, in effect, susceptible to a B₆ deficiency.

## Dangerous Metabolites in B₆ Deficiency

In his summary of the conference, Dr. Brown gave an account of what harm can result when someone with a special need for high levels of B₆ fails to get adequate quantities. Abnormal tryptophan metabolites are found in the urine of the B₆-deficient persons—xanthurenic acid being the best known of these substances and the one for which tests are usually made when checking an individual's B₆ status. These metabolites, Dr. Brown said, "retard oxidative phosphorylation," which means they interfere with carbohydrate metabolism. They also "form inactive complexes with insulin suggesting a diabetogenic action"—that is, they may induce diabetes. And they are "carcinogenic in the mouse-bladder assay"—that is, when implanted in mouse bladders these metabolites cause cancer. To date, no case histories of human cancer proven to be triggered by B₆ deficiency have been recorded. When it comes to diabetes, other causative factors have been investigated and stressed. However, at the joint meeting of the American Institute of Nutrition and the American Society for Clinical Nutrition, held at Cornell University in August, 1973, Dr. David Rose reported on controlled tests showing impaired glucose tolerance in OC users on a B₆-deficient diet—as opposed to non-OC users on the same diet. One of the OC users, Dr. Rose said, had such a severe impairment that her condition was regarded as "chemical diabetes mellitus," an effect "reversed by pyridoxine."

"The excretion of elevated levels of potentially hazardous

tryptophan metabolites may be reversed or prevented, or both, in almost all cases by the administration of vitamin B₆," Dr. Brown stated. As to quantity: "Specifically in the case of women on the oral contraceptive pill, tryptophan metabolism was normalized by levels of at least 20 mg. pyridoxine hydrochloride a day as contrasted with the Recommended Daily Allowances of two mg. a day for normal adult women in the United States.

Of course, not everyone on steroid therapy or with high levels of estrogen (self-produced or contained in the OC) has the characteristic metabolic disturbances indicative of B₆ deficiency—any more than everyone who smokes cigarettes automatically contracts lung cancer. Even where a metabolic disturbance does exist, the abnormal metabolites usually can be detected in the urine only after the individual has been given a tryptophan load—that is, a concentrated oral dose of this amino acid. Only then does it become apparent in laboratory tests that the body is manufacturing xanthurenic acid and many other abnormal tryptophan metabolites not manufactured by normal subjects handling the same tryptophan load.

## B₆ Levels Decline With Age

It may very well be that all people, as they get older, need extra vitamin B₆ to ward off the deteriorating effect of aging. After the age of 50, pyridoxine levels decline rapidly in almost everyone, according to Ronald Searcy, Ph.D., former Director of Diagnostic Research at Hoffmann-La Roche, Inc. In his book, *Diagnostic Biochemistry* (New York: McGraw-Hill, 1969), he points out that blood plasma levels of pyridoxal phosphate (B₆ coenzyme) average 11.3 millimicrograms per milliliter for ages 20 to 29. For ages 30 to 59, this level drops to only 7.1, and by age 60, the average level has fallen all the way to 3.4.

No one has as yet been able to clearly define, on a biochemical level, the process called aging, but certainly a failure of amino acids and the multitude of enzymes which contain amino acids is involved. B₆ is vital to these functions.

# Good Sources of Vitamin B6

How can you increase your intake of B6? Start by eating pyridoxine-rich foods such as liver, lean muscle meats (white meat of chicken is best), fish, whole grains, walnuts, filberts, peanuts, and sunflower seeds. Dark buckwheat flour, soybean flour, and sunflower seed flour are also rich in B6. If you bake your own bread, try adding any one of these to the mix.

Wheat germ is especially rich in B6. Ounce for ounce, it contains even more of this nutrient than liver. Bananas are another good source. "By chemical analysis, a banana has been found to be about five times richer in vitamin B6, gram for gram, than any other fruit," said Dr. Ellis. Bananas are doubly good because they are eaten raw. When one recalls what processing and cooking do to pyridoxine in many foods, it is easy to see the importance of eating as many fresh, raw vegetables and fruits as possible.

Even if you make a point of eating plenty of pyridoxine-rich foods at every meal, it is unlikely that you could take in much more than the RDA, if that. To obtain even half of what Dr. Gyorgy suggests, you would have to take additional B6 in supplement form.

If you are presently taking a B-complex supplement, look carefully at the label. It should be supplying at least two mg. of B6 every day at the suggested dosage.

# CHAPTER 35

# The Vitamin of Special Significance for Women in the Prime of Life

Pyridoxine has never been dubbed "the vitamin for women," but there are times in every woman's life when this fraction of the B complex can determine her physical and mental well-being.

It isn't that B₆ does not have great significance for men as well. Aside from playing an important role in a variety of metabolic functions, vitamin B₆ may well be a link in the prevention of such diseases as rheumatism, diabetes, arteriosclerosis, and associated heart attacks of the coronary occlusion type, all of which can lower the boom on men as well as women. However, B₆ has special significance for women. From the age of puberty right through menopause, hormone production has an enormous effect on a woman's life, and hormones and B₆ have a very special relationship. It is now known that at certain times in her life, a woman needs more B₆ to properly metabolize the increased supply of estrogens circulating in her body.

A woman's hormones, when they are channeled correctly, can be an exciting influence in her life—the kind that makes her glad she is a woman. But hormones, when they are not properly metabolized, can trouble a woman with a swarm of insidious symptoms—like depression, which is a frequent problem in women on the Pill, menopausal arthritis, edema, and weight gain every month just before menstruation, and a host of problems associated with pregnancy.

Dr. John Ellis, a general practitioner in Mt. Pleasant, Texas, has done pioneer work in this field. Long before the facts were established in controlled studies at university research centers, he had discovered the helpfulness of B6 therapy during pregnancy, the premenstrual period, and during oral contraceptive use. In his book, *Vitamin B6, The Doctor's Report* (New York: Harper & Row, 1973), Dr. Ellis recounts how high-level B6 supplements eliminated many symptoms characteristic of women with the high estrogen levels typical of these three conditions.

## Pregnancy Increases Need For B6

"All pregnant women," according to Dr. Ellis, "have an increased need for vitamin B6. It is a factor in the prevention and treatment of toxemia of pregnancy and the convulsions of eclampsia." Other signs and symptoms that appear during pregnancy that are responsive to B6 are swelling in the hands and feet, cramps in the legs, hands and arms that "go to sleep," and painful neuropathies (functional disturbances) in the fingers and hands.

Edema is so common that at least one-third of all pregnant women in the United States and England suffer with it. It is particularly worrisome because it may presage toxemia of pregnancy, a form of poisoning that frequently threatens the life of the mother or fetus or both. Toxemia in turn may lead to eclampsia or convulsions, both extremely serious situations.

There is a theory in obstetrical circles that water retention is caused by excessive salt in the diet. Therefore many obstetricians restrict salt intake and prescribe diuretics to pregnant women who show signs of edema. This procedure has been discredited.

The need for salt during pregnancy was recognized by the 1969 White House Conference on Food, Nutrition, and Health, which issued this statement: "Sodium retention is, in fact, a normal physiological adjustment during pregnancy, and is directly related to normal blood volume expansion and tissue growth. If dietary sodium is limited, there is increased·stimulation of the normal sodium conservation mechanisms. The resulting increase in aldosterone secretion increases the quantity of sodium reabsorbed from the kidney filtrate. Sodium restriction observed in laboratory animals produces extreme enlargement and even exhaustion of the aldosterone-secreting cells of the adrenal cortex. Examination of the fine structure of these cells indicates extreme pathology when animals are subjected to the double stress of sodium restriction and pregnancy." The statement condemned "promiscuous use of diuretics" during pregnancy as "antagonistic" to the physiological adjustment and a stress on the salt-conserving mechanism.

In his treatment of 225 pregnant women, Dr. Ellis made no effort to restrict salt intake and gave no diuretics. He found that vitamin $B_6$ controlled edema so effectively—and safely—that these steps were not necessary. A ten-mg. daily dose seemed to be sufficient for many patients, but it soon became evident that it was not enough to relieve a number of symptoms, especially swelling of the hands and feet. Some patients suffered from pain in the joints of the fingers until he administered 50 to 450 mg. of pyridoxine daily.

## Cramping Isn't Always Caused by Calcium Deficiency

The leg cramps so frequently suffered by pregnant women (and occasionally women experiencing menopause or menstruation) are often interpreted as a calcium deficiency. Dr. Ellis found some of the worst leg cramps in women who were taking high quantities of calcium. Their leg cramps were not relieved until they began taking $B_6$. When in some instances the pyridoxine alone did not relieve foot and leg muscle spasms during pregnancy, the addition of potassium as a daily oral supplement usually eliminated muscle spasms completely. He has also had a high degree of success by adding magnesium supplements to the therapy during the prenatal period.

One patient who was given prenatal vitamin-mineral capsules that included 10 mg. of pyridoxine complained a month later that her feet and legs were more swollen and she now suffered severe nocturnal muscle spasms in her legs. Dr. Ellis prescribed 50 mg. of pyridoxine daily in addition to her prenatal capsule. By the third night, muscle spasms in her legs had subsided and within 14 days she had lost 11 pounds.

Dr. Ellis sees B6 as a possible link in the prevention of diabetes, for he has found that his pregnant diabetic patients do much better on large, almost massive doses of B6 without insulin. The eclamptic patient, he has found, is hypersensitive to insulin, which in some patients may trigger a convulsion.

The need for B6 apparently increases as pregnancy advances. Even 50 mg. daily was inadequate to control edema in nine out of 16 cases. Five of these nine were then controlled by increasing the pyridoxine to 100 mg. daily. The remaining four required injections of 150 mg. daily. Two of the four who required 150 mg. by injection delivered twins, a logical explanation of their heightened need for the vitamin, Dr. Ellis pointed out.

Based on his experience, Dr. Ellis concluded that a pregnant woman may need from 50 to 450 mg. of pyridoxine daily, and up to 1,000 mg. daily for short intervals in a few cases. If she is threatened with eclampsia, she needs more B6. She also may need more magnesium, which is a cofactor of B6. These deficits are made worse if she drinks great quantities of milk. The oversupply of calcium in the milk adds to the imbalance because milk is a poor source for both magnesium and B6. A magnesium deficit is associated with nausea and vomiting.

B6 itself has been used as a measure against nausea in pregnant women for many years. William H. Sebrell, Jr., M.D., discussed its effectiveness in *Vitamins and Hormones* (vol. 22, 1964): "Vitamin B6 has long been used clinically on an empirical basis in the treatment of nausea and vomiting during the first trimester of pregnancy . . . it would appear that pregnancy either alters vitamin B6 metabolism or increases the demand so that the requirement during pregnancy is higher than usual, creating a need that is not being met by dietary intake of some pregnant women."

## Depression on the Pill Linked to Lack of B6

Vitamin B6 can also bring dramatic relief to women who suffer from depression as a result of taking oral contraceptives, according to a report in the *Lancet* (28 April 1973). Dr. P. W. Adams and associates as St. Mary's Hospital Medical School in London reported that mood changes are quite common in those taking the Pill, as is B6 deficiency. When the researchers examined 22 women thus affected, they found that 11 were seriously deficient in B6. The women were pessimistic, dissatisfied, and irritable. They complained of tiredness and a loss of sex drive.

The altered excretion of tryptophan metabolites observed in women on the Pill is similar to that found in nutritional B6 deficiency. (The tryptophan load test is used to assess the extent of a B6 deficiency.) When large amounts of xanthurenic acid, one of the breakdown products of tryptophan, appear in the urine, this is regarded as an indirect sign of B6 deficiency. About 80 percent of women on the Pill have abnormal tryptophan metabolism, indicating a relative B6 deficiency, said the London physicians. Some have an absolute deficiency. One of the consequences of this deficiency is a derangement of the metabolites in the cerebrospinal fluid, a condition which leads to depression.

Dr. Adams found that 20 mg. tablets of pyridoxine hydrochloride taken twice a day for two months relieved the symptoms of depression—but only for those women who were severely B6- deficient at the beginning of the study. A larger study, involving 39 oral-contraceptive users, produced similar results and was reported by Dr. Adams and his colleagues in the *Lancet* (31 August 1974).

## Puffiness and Soreness of Menstruation Can be Prevented

There is hardly a woman who does not experience some discomfort a week to ten days before her menstrual cycle begins. Perhaps her clothes feel too tight, or her hands and face get puffy. Sometimes her hands are so painful she thinks she has arthritis. Gynecologists have for years been prescribing diuretics and hormones in attempts to control this premenstrual edema and the so-called arthritis so often associated with it.

Since vitamin B₆ seems to regulate the water balance in the body, Dr. Ellis wondered if it might relieve these premenstrual torments.

Over the years, Dr. Ellis reports, he has used B₆ to treat many patients with edema of the hands during the menstrual period linked with abdominal distension, involuntary muscle spasms of the legs and feet, and swelling of the eyelids and face. In one group of eleven treated for these disorders, four had previously taken diuretics for control of edema, with little success. When they took 50 to 100 mg. of pyridoxine daily, all their signs and symptoms were relieved after the first menstruation cycle. Yet, Dr. Ellis never mentioned the word salt (which retains water in body tissues) nor did he use diuretics at any time. Vitamin B₆ was the only agent.

## Why Some Women Can't Cope With Menopause

If you have a long-term vitamin deficiency, your body may be inadequately prepared for the stress of menopause, and you could leave yourself wide open to some well-known tortures. One of them is a kind of rheumatism that has been labeled "menopausal arthritis," which brings in its wake the particular distress of Heberden's nodes, painful little burrs, or knots, that appear on the sides of the finger joints. Dr. Ellis found that these nodes are responsive to pyridoxine if they are not of long-standing duration. Two patients who were nearing menopause and had been troubled for several months by these bright red, distinctly circumscribed nodes on the finger joints, reported that the pain subsided and the redness disappeared within five weeks on pyridoxine therapy.

"Menopausal arthritis" isn't always menopausal. One of Dr. Ellis's patients suffered from numbness and tingling of the fingers and hands and could not bring her right index finger to reach her thumb with enough strength to hold a pencil. At night she

suffered cramps in her leg muscles and would have to get out of
bed to massage away the painful spasms. She had what Dr. Ellis
termed the "reddest Heberden's nodes that I have ever seen."
After she started taking 50 mg. of pyridoxine daily, her improvement was almost miraculous—she had no pain. After a year on
the B₆ the nodes disappeared. She continued to menstruate pain-
lessly and without edema for seven years before the onset of
menopause.

Everyone has a critical need for this vitamin, but women in
the prime of their lives seem to need it most of all.

## Common Foods Rich in Pyridoxine*

| Portions of 3½ oz. | (milligrams) |
|---|---|
| Brewers yeast (debittered) | 2.50 |
| Sunflower seeds (hulled) | 1.25 |
| Wheat germ (toasted) | 1.15 |
| Brown rice (raw) | .55 |
| Soybeans (raw) | .81 |
| Beans (White, raw) | .56 |
| Liver (Beef, raw) | .84 |
| Liver (Chicken, raw) | .75 |
| Chicken (White meat) | .68 |
| Mackerel (Atlantic, raw) | .66 |
| Salmon (canned) | .30 |
| Tuna (canned) | .43 |
| Bananas | .51 |
| Walnuts | .73 |
| Peanuts (roasted) | .40 |

*Selected from tables in *Pantothenic Acid, Vitamin B₆ and Vitamin B₁₂ in Foods*, United
States Department of Agriculture Home Economics Research Report #36, August,
1969.

# CHAPTER 36

# B$_{12}$: The Miracle Factor in Liver

Not long ago, a diagnosis of pernicious anemia was virtually a death sentence; before 1926, six thousand Americans died of the disease each year. Doctors watched helplessly as the debilitating disease took hold of its victims.

The first signs of the anemia are usually a sore tongue and tingling or burning sensations in the hands or feet. Patients tend to be pale and white-lipped, and develop a variety of abdominal difficulties: gas, constipation or diarrhea, nausea, vomiting, pain, and poor appetite. Ringing in the ears, spots before the eyes, chronic fatigue, drowsiness, and irritability plague the victim as vital organs starve for oxygen because not enough red blood cells are being formed. The liver and spleen often become enlarged, and neurological damage increases as the disease progresses. When the anemia becomes severe, the heart may fail.

In 1922, however, Dr. George Hoyt Whipple, a University of Rochester pathologist, discovered that dogs suffering from a condition similar to pernicious anemia could be cured by eating large amounts of raw beef liver. This discovery led two Harvard physicians, Drs. George R. Minot and William P. Murphy to test the benefits of liver on human patients, and in 1926 they reported that eating large amounts of raw liver did indeed cure victims of pernicious anemia. The three doctors, who were awarded a Nobel Prize for their work in 1934, launched a twenty-year search for the therapeutically active substance in raw liver.

Over the years, the liver therapy was refined. At first, patients had to eat nauseating amounts of uncooked liver—half a pound or more a day. Later, patients no longer had to force down chunks of raw liver; they could be given liver extract injections. Unfortunately, these injections were expensive, uncomfortable, and inconvenient, and many patients couldn't tolerate them for very long. People were still dying of pernicious anemia.

Finally, in December, 1947, 21 years after the initial work of Drs. Murphy and Minot, a team of scientists at the Merck Institute in Rahway, New Jersey, extracted a small amount of red crystals from liver. For testing they needed a pernicious anemia victim who was not receiving other treatment. It took two months to find such a patient. In February, 1948, a critically ill 66-year-old woman was brought to Brooklyn Hospital. She was given a single, minute injection of the crystalline red substance. Five days later she was making healthy new red blood cells at an enormous rate. A few weeks after that she had completely recovered. The antipernicious anemia factor had been isolated. It was named vitamin $B_{12}$.

## $B_{12}$ Deficiency Damages Both the Blood and the Nerves

With the discovery of $B_{12}$ came knowledge of both the cause and the cure of pernicious anemia. The anemia develops because a lack of $B_{12}$ causes damage to both the blood-forming process and the nervous system. The bone marrow produces abnormally large red blood cells, called megalocytes or macrocytes, whose life span is only half that of normal blood cells. The bone marrow turns red and jelly-like, and both red and white blood cell counts drop. The red blood count may go below 1,000,000 compared to a normal count of 5,000,000. White blood counts fall to 3–5,000 compared to normal levels of 5–10,000. Blood cells show both arrested maturation and unusually rapid destruction—many probably never reach the bloodstream—and both these events account for the anemia.

Damage to the nervous system may range from tingling sensations in the fingers to profound and irreversible damage to the nerves; 40 to 95 percent of pernicious anemia victims suffer some degree of neurological damage. When symptoms of nerve damage appear before signs of anemia, accurate diagnosis and treatment are much more difficult. Severe $B_{12}$ deprivation, even without pernicious anemia, may cause progressive degeneration of the protective myelin sheath surrounding the nerves of the spinal cord and brain.

While pernicious anemia is still a serious condition, treatment today is a relatively simple matter. The object of the treatment is to replace depleted $B_{12}$ stores rapidly and to maintain them at normal levels. Actual dosage varies with different patients, but a typical regimen may consist of 15 mcg. of $B_{12}$ injected intramuscularly every two or three hours for three or four doses, followed by 30 mcg. weekly for two months; doubled doses are sometimes recommended when complications exist. Oral therapy is not recommended at the start of treatment but daily doses ranging from 250 to 400 mcg. by mouth will often keep a patient in remission.

## Intrinsic Factor

A $B_{12}$ deficiency can develop for several reasons, but pernicious anemia is usually the result of not being able to absorb the vitamin. Due to $B_{12}$'s particularly complex structure, it cannot be simply absorbed like most nutrients. Among its many juices, the stomach secretes a substance called the "intrinsic factor," which binds to $B_{12}$ so that it can be absorbed through the intestinal walls. There are, however, a number of people who are missing or are underproducing the intrinsic factor, and cannot absorb the vitamin, no matter how much of it they eat.

Why some people are unable to produce the intrinsic factor is not entirely clear. Stomach surgery accounts for some cases of

$B_{12}$ deficiency by removing the portion of stomach that produces the intrinsic factor. According to James H. Jandl, M.D., in the *Cecil-Loeb Textbook of Medicine* (Paul B. Beefson, M.D., and Walsh McDermott, M.D., ed., Philadelphia: W. B. Saunders Co., 1971), a prolonged iron deficiency may cause the intrinsic factor-producing tissues in the stomach to atrophy. The actual amount of the intrinsic factor produced varies from person to person, and it is probably that stomach surgery, iron deficiency, or other factors such as pregnancy or aging could cause a failure in the secretion of the intrinsic factor in people who have an inborn tendency to produce low amounts.

Dr. Jandl also suggests that a large portion of the people lacking the intrinsic factor may be suffering from a defect in their immune system. The immune system normally protects the body from disease organisms by producing antibodies that fight foreign matter. Sometimes, however, the immune system goes haywire and produces antibodies against the body's own tissues; this defect is called an autoimmune disease. According to Dr. Jandl, 90 percent of patients with pernicious anemia were found to have antibodies against the stomach cells that produce the intrinsic factor, and roughly half of the patients had antibodies specifically against the intrinsic factor.

If a person suffering from a $B_{12}$ deficiency lacks the intrinsic factor, oral supplementation will do little or no good. For this reason, $B_{12}$ injections have become the accepted means of restoring depleted $B_{12}$ levels. The injections put the $B_{12}$ right into the bloodstream, bypassing the need for absorption. While oral $B_{12}$ supplements have sometimes been combined with intrinsic factor taken from animal stomachs, $B_{12}$ shots work faster and are more economical.

# CHAPTER 37

# B₁₂ for the Blood, Nerves, Growth, and . . .

The vital role of vitamin $B_{12}$ in maintaining normal red blood cell formation and the integrity of the nervous system is quite clear. The vitamin is also recognized as essential for normal growth in man and in many animal species. It has been named by both the Food and Drug Administration and the National Research Council as a necessary nutrient. But a report in *Nutrition Today* (January/February 1973) best summed up the scientific sentiment concerning $B_{12}$'s significance when it stated, "Recent discoveries suggest that the principal role of vitamin $B_{12}$ may not be its effect on the hematopoietic system but in its role as a master substance that affects all kinds of biological functions in ways which, for the most part, remain unknown." In spite of its importance, the set requirements for $B_{12}$ in man are the smallest of any known active nutritional substance—vitamin, mineral, or hormone. The Recommended Daily Allowance of the vitamin has been set at six micrograms (mcg.)—only six thousandths of a milligram.

Even in such small quantities evidence shows that the vitamin plays a primary role in nucleic acid synthesis. In animals fed $B_{12}$-deficient diets, the total amount of RNA and DNA in critical body organs—liver, spinal cord, cervical ganglia—was reduced, and the bone marrow of pernicious anemia patients showed similar results. Other studies have shown that $B_{12}$ is indirectly involved in converting folic to folinic acid; in carbohydrate metabolism, especially the conversion of carbohydrates to fat; and as an aid in the utilization of fats, carbohydrates, and proteins. It is also deeply involved with neural functions and the maintenance of nerve cells.

$B_{12}$ also seems to be an integral factor in maintaining fertility, as evidenced by a letter to the editor of the *Lancet* (6 January 1968). Drs. John H. Blair, Harlan E. Stearns, and George M. Simpson of the Rockland State Hospital Research Center, Orangeburg, New York, reported that cases of infertility they had investigated "improved greatly during a seven-month course of weekly injections of 30 mg. of vitamin $B_{12}$." This led them to suggest that "Vitamin $B_{12}$ might be beneficial in the treatment of low fertility in other cases"—other, that is, than in anemia.

## Deficiency Can Be Subtle But Devastating

Many people seem to think that if they haven't developed a good case of diagnosable pernicious anemia, they're getting enough vitamin $B_{12}$ in their diets. In fact, unless they have developed anemia, many people don't even think about $B_{12}$. It's not one of the vitamins one hears about every day.

But the results of a $B_{12}$ deficiency may not show themselves for quite some time before anemia develops, according to a study conducted by Oded Abramsky, M.D., a member of the Neurology Department of Hadassah University Hospital and Hebrew University Hadassah Medical School in Jerusalem, Israel. Dr. Abramsky concluded that the results can be devastating—and irreversible.

Writing in the *Journal of the American Geriatrics Society* (February 1972), Dr. Abramsky described the cases of three $B_{12}$-deficient patients. From his case studies, he concluded that "mental or psychiatric manifestations such as mental apathy, fluctuations in mood, memory disturbance, paranoia, or frank psychosis may more often precede the blood changes (of anemia) by a number of years." In addition, there may be adverse changes in the nervous system. These changes may include such problems as soreness and weakness of the limbs, diminished reflexes and sensory perception, changes in temperature in parts of the body, difficulties in walking, stammering, and jerking of limbs.

Even worse, a $B_{12}$ deficiency is something even a doctor might not think of looking for, or not find if he did look. He could easily check a patient's blood, find the blood levels of $B_{12}$ relatively normal and no sign of anemia, and misdiagnose the problem. This lack of parallelism between the condition of the blood and the symptoms the patient may be suffering, said Dr. Abramsky, is "the chief reason for the failure to make an early diagnosis." He warned, however, that "the early recognition of vitamin $B_{12}$ deficiency is important, for it enables prompt treatment. Otherwise, the end result of untreated cerebral or spinal lesions may be severe dementia and paraplegia, which may be completely irreversible when treatment is delayed by failure in diagnosis." In simpler terms, if a $B_{12}$ deficiency is not spotted in its early stages, it may result in permanent mental deterioration and paralysis.

The surest way of detecting a hidden $B_{12}$ deficiency is to administer a Schilling test, which measures the actual absorption of the vitamin. This test consists of giving the patient a measured amount of radioactive vitamin $B_{12}$ by mouth, then following it with an intravenous dose of regular $B_{12}$ to help flush the first. The doctor then measures the amount of radioactivity in the urine over a 24-hour period. He then repeats the test, adding the intrinsic factor, an amino acid and enzyme mucoprotein compound necessary for the assimilation of vitamin $B_{12}$. If the level of $B_{12}$ is low and then becomes normal when the intrinsic factor is given, the doctor has pinpointed a $B_{12}$ deficiency and oncoming anemia.

What makes this vitamin so important is its effect on myelin, the protective sheath that covers the spinal cord and other elements of the nervous system. Although the need for vitamin $B_{12}$ is generally minute, if that small amount is missing from the diet or is absorbed improperly, the result may be disastrous. The myelin will begin to disintegrate, opening the door to damage to the nervous system and possible psychosis.

## B₁₂ Is a Growth Factor

If you've ever noticed how grass shoots up after a rain as it never does after a watering with the garden sprinkler, you know there is something different about rainwater. Bruce Parker, Ph.D., a botanist at Washington University in St. Louis, told the *New York Times* (15 August 1968) that B$_{12}$ may be responsible for the spurt of growth noted after a heavy rainfall. According to Dr. Parker, the B$_{12}$ is synthesized by microbes in the air and then deposited in the ground by the rain. The mechanism by which the vitamin stimulates growth is still unknown.

Evidence that this vitamin can stimulate growth in humans is not new. The results of a school nutrition study, reported in the *Journal of Clinical Nutrition* (September/October 1953) support the conclusion that vitamin B$_{12}$ exerts a "growth-promoting effect" when given as a dietary supplement to children suffering from growth failure. With the increase in growth came other manifestations of improved health. Teachers in the classrooms became aware that some of the pupils were improving in behavior, attitude, and scholastic work, while others were showing less strain and fatigue, greater interest and attention, and hence better all-around progress. Parents, too, concurred in these findings.

A group of Ohio scientists, headed by Norman C. Wetzel, M.D., conducted an experiment at the Children's Fresh Air Camp and Hospital in Cleveland. Eleven children between five and 12 years of age were given vitamin B$_{12}$ by mouth over a two-month period. "Dramatic" responses by five of the 11 children were reported by the Cleveland scientists in the journal *Science* (December 16, 1949).

Every morning B$_{12}$ was fed to the children who were under care at the institution for varying degrees of malnutrition and growth failure. In addition to the vitamin doses, all the children were continued on whatever programs of rest, exercise, and diet they had been following in efforts to improve their growth and physique.

After getting the $B_{12}$, the children not only showed a change in growth rate but also had more physical vigor. They were more alert, better behaved, and there was a significant improvement in their appetites.

## Improved Growth, Greater Resistance To Germs

Later studies have confirmed the earlier findings linking $B_{12}$ to improved growth. One study, conducted by two researchers at the Department of Nutrition and Food Science at the Massachusetts Institute of Technology, demonstrated that the vitamin influences not only growth, but also enhances resistance to infection, and is of great importance both before birth and later in life. Reporting in *Nature* (March 23, 1973), Paul M. Newberne, Ph.D., and Vernon R. Young, Ph.D., also underscored the importance of vitamin $B_{12}$ in amounts considerably larger than the minimum doses required to prevent deficiency disorders.

Drs. Newberne and Young mated rats, then gave some of the females a standard $B_{12}$ diet (50 mcg. per kilogram of diet), an amount which exceeds the estimated requirement for the pregnant, lactating, and growing rat. Another group of rats were given an amount of $B_{12}$ in considerable excess of this intake—50,000 mcg. per kilogram of diet, or 1,000 times as much $B_{12}$ as the control group. Both groups received the same food during pregnancy. After giving birth, all the rats were put on the standard $B_{12}$ diet. After weaning, their progeny, too, were given a standard $B_{12}$ diet. This way the researchers were able to measure the effects on the offspring of a higher maternal intake of $B_{12}$ during pregnancy, as those effects carry over into the first months of life.

The results showed that $B_{12}$ benefited the baby rats in more ways than growth. Rats born to mothers who had received more $B_{12}$ weighed more than the other animals, and this greater weight continued during the first year of life. Those babies whose mothers had more vitamin $B_{12}$ also had more protein per body weight and less fat than did the others. Offspring of supplemented mothers also showed more active liver enzymes, suggesting they might be better protected against infection.

In fact, further studies revealed that those babies whose mothers had received more $B_{12}$ experienced lower mortality and more resistance to infection during the first month of life than did those whose mothers had received only "normal" amounts of $B_{12}$.

Improved resistance to infection was proven experimentally by Drs. Newberne and Young. When the baby rats were three months old, they were injected with *salmonella typhimurium* (a deadly parasite). Eighteen hours after infection, positive cultures were found in blood samples in about equal numbers for both groups. But, bacteria were cleared more efficiently from circulation—within 48 hours—in those rats born to the mothers who received the high doses of vitamin $B_{12}$. After 10 days, mortality was much lower in the offspring of the high $B_{12}$ group, indicating a greater resistance to the experimental infection. Twenty-one of the low $B_{12}$ group succumbed to the infection after 10 days; only nine of the high $B_{12}$ group succumbed. This experiment, according to Drs. Newberne and Young, suggests "a long-term beneficial clinical effect on the offspring of the higher $B_{12}$ intake group during intrauterine development." They responded much more favorably to the stressful stimulus of a systemic infection.

## Pregnancy Makes Big Demands on $B_{12}$

$B_{12}$ is unusual in that it is a water-soluble vitamin that can be stored by the body. Every expectant mother would do well to provide her liver with good reserve stores of this essential factor, since pregnancy makes unusual demands on those stores.

Twenty-six women in the last trimester of pregnancy were studied by Louis Wertalik, M.D., and colleagues of the Ohio State University College of Medicine. They were all in good health and eating normally. Most of them were receiving iron and vitamin supplements which contained 0.1 mg. of folic acid and two mcg. of B$_{12}$. However, according to a report of the study in the *Journal of the American Medical Association* (September 27, 1972), B$_{12}$ values continued to decrease in pregnancy despite daily oral administration of this amount of the vitamin.

If a woman has been on the Pill she has two strikes against her as far as B$_{12}$ stores are concerned. Dr. Wertalik's research team found that healthy young women who were taking oral contraceptives experienced a rapid fall in serum B$_{12}$ values. They were found to have a mean serum B$_{12}$ level of 221, which was 40 percent lower than the control group mean of 372.

The stress of pregnancy on top of the depletion caused by the Pill can put both mother and baby in jeopardy as far as B$_{12}$ stores are concerned, unless the mother takes more of this vitamin than many prenatal vitamin supplements provide.

## Vegetarians Easily Become Deficient

Vitamin B$_{12}$ is different from all the other members of the B family in another respect. Most of the B vitamins are found largely in yeast, wheat germ, rice polishings, and liver. B$_{12}$, however, is made by bacteria in the sea and deep lakes, and in the intestinal tracts of mammals. The human body can make B$_{12}$ in the colon, but little is absorbed. The only dietary source is food of animal origin, such as milk, eggs, meat, cheese, and liver. Liver, however, is by far the richest source.

Vegetarians are particularly susceptible to a B$_{12}$ deficiency, since the avoidance of meat excludes the main sources of the vitamin from their diet. Vegetarians who eat eggs and milk in generous amounts are not as vulnerable as are vegans, who avoid all animal products and by-products. To be nutritionally safe, it would be wise for all vegetarians, especially vegans, to take a daily supplement of the B complex that is rich in B$_{12}$. The B$_{12}$ found in vitamin supplements is derived from bacteria, and is neither synthetic nor of animal origin.

A B$_{12}$ deficiency can also be caused by liver disease, since the vitamin is stored in the liver. For this reason alcohol, with its detrimental effect on the liver, may contribute to a lack of the vitamin.

## Does Vitamin C Destroy $B_{12}$?

In 1974, Victor Herbert, M.D., and Elizabeth Jacob, M.D., published a report in the *Journal of the American Medical Association* (14 October 1974) which claimed that "High doses of vitamin C, popularly used as a home remedy against the common cold, destroy substantial amounts of vitamin $B_{12}$ when ingested with food." Such a statement quite naturally caused concern among the many thousands of people taking large doses of vitamin C for its many beneficial effects.

In truth, Drs. Herbert and Jacob did not demonstrate that vitamin C would destroy $B_{12}$ in people taking large doses of vitamin C. Their experiment was conducted totally *in vitro*, that is, in the test tube. It is easy to demonstrate *in vitro* that high concentrations of vitamin C alter DNA and RNA—the vital carriers of heredity; but in the blood of a living human being, it simply doesn't happen.

An actual examination of patients receiving large doses of vitamin C showed that what happened in the test tubes of Drs. Herbert and Jacob does not necessarily happen in the human body. In a letter to the editor of the *Journal of the American Medical Association* (April 21, 1975), Mehr Afroz, M.D., and associates at the Veterans Administration Hospital in St. Louis explained that spinal cord-injury patients in their care routinely received doses of ascorbic acid of four grams or more a day to enhance urinary acidity. Concerned by the claim that vitamin C destroys $B_{12}$, Dr. Afroz and his associates decided to examine their patients for themselves. They measured serum $B_{12}$ levels by the technique of radioisotope displacement in ten male patients aged 17 to 69 years. According to the letter, each of these patients had received ascorbic acid in this dose for more than 11 months. All had been on unrestricted diets and all took their medication in four divided doses each day. The vitamin $B_{12}$ levels were all well above the low normal value (300 mg/ml) and three were above the high normal (1,000 mg/ml).

## Common Foods Rich in Vitamin $B_{12}$*

| Portions of 3½ oz. | (milligrams) |
|---|---|
| Liver (Beef, raw) | .080 |
| Liver (Chicken, raw) | .025 |
| Kidney (Beef, raw) | .031 |
| Heart (Beef, raw) | .011 |
| Beef (Raw) | .001 |
| Clams (Soft, raw) | .098 |
| Oysters (Eastern, raw) | .018 |
| Sardines (Raw) | .011 |
| Crab (Cooked or canned) | .010 |
| Crayfish (Raw) | .002 |
| Mackerel (Salted and smoked) | .012 |
| Trout (Raw) | .003 |
| Herring (Raw) | .010 |
| Eggs (Raw) | .002 |
| Cheeses (Blue, Brick, Cottage, Limburger, Mozzarella or Swiss) | .001 |

*Selected from tables in *Pantothenic Acid, Vitamin $B_6$ and Vitamin $B_{12}$ in Foods*, United States Department of Agriculture Home Economics Research Report #36, August, 1969.

# CHAPTER 38

# Folic Acid, the Other Antianemia Vitamin

Folic acid, also known as folacin and folate, was so named because it was first discovered in green leafy vegetables, or foliage. It was first isolated from spinach leaves in 1941 as a factor necessary for the growth of certain microorganisms.

At about the same time, medical researchers were reporting cases of anemia in animals and humans that were similar to pernicious anemia, but did not respond to the usual treatment. The anemia was definitely a nutritional macrocytic (giant cell) type, but liver extracts had no effect on its progress. Further work resolved the mystery. It was discovered that liver contains two distinct antianemia substances: $B_{12}$, effective against pernicious anemia; and a second substance, folic acid, which was being removed in the process of refining liver extracts for the treatment of pernicious anemia. Folic acid, effective only against certain other macrocytic anemias, was later isolated from both liver and yeast, and was recognized as the same growth factor isolated from spinach a short time earlier.

Both vitamins are vital to the blood-forming processes, and while each vitamin is needed to treat its particular type of anemia, folic acid deficiency anemia is similar to $B_{12}$ deficiency anemia. The red blood cells become extremely large, abnormally shaped, and have a very short life span. The symptoms are not sudden and obvious, but creep up on the victim and make themselves apparent very gradually. Eventually the victims become weak and easily fatigued, they behave irritably, and may even suffer from sleeplessness or forgetfulness.

Today, anemia caused by a lack of folic acid is much more common than $B_{12}$ deficiency anemia, and it is alarming to note that folic acid deficiency is much more prevalent and easier to develop than was once thought. According to a report in the *British Medical Journal* (19 October 1975) from the Department of Hematology, London Hospital, doctors were surprised to find megaloblastic anemia developing in two men under intensive care for surgery. Apparently, the doctors did not realize to what extent severe injury or surgery could deplete folic acid stores. The report stated, "Our experience suggests that it is unwise to rely on the folic acid stores of severely traumatized patients even for short periods."

Of course, severely injured people aren't the only ones in danger of developing a folic acid deficiency. Increased tissue demand which occurs while a person is under intensive medical care may seem more dramatic and serious, because the person is in a life-endangering situation from the start. But at least there are doctors around to see the deficiency taking its toll. People whose bodies develop folic acid deficiencies in response to the slow, steady stress of everyday life may never be so lucky as to have their problems identified.

## Folic Acid Has Many Important Functions

Like $B_{12}$, folic acid is vital to the proper growth of cells, and is directly related to the synthesis of DNA and other nucleic acids. Megaloblastic anemia is commonly thought of as the most prevalent symptom of a deficiency, but that is because megaloblastic anemia, although similar to other anemias in obvious symptoms, is relatively easy to confirm as a folic acid deficiency. Other symptoms aren't so easy to pinpoint as a folic acid deficiency; sore tongue, mouth sores, impaired wound healing, gastrointestinal inflammation, mental illness, and reduced resistance to infection. These varied symptoms point out the many facets of good health that folic acid is involved with. In fact, wherever there is a rapid turnover of cells, wherever the body builds or repairs itself, folic acid is vital.

If a pregnant woman doesn't get enough folic acid, irreversible damage to the developing fetus can result. A "nutritional time bomb" is what MIT Professor of Nutrition and Food Science, Paul M. Newberne, Ph.D., calls one possible result of a deficiency of dietary lipotropes—folic acid, vitamin $B_{12}$, choline and methionine. Writing in *Technology Review* (December 1974), Dr. Newberne explained that an early deficiency of these chemical substances can severely hinder the body's ability to fight off disease just when it's needed most, later in life. The body's immune system, which is regulated by the thymus gland, needs folic acid and other lipotropes to develop properly. In laboratory tests, offspring of mother animals fed diets with marginal amounts of folic acid and methionine were significantly less able to fight off common food poisoning bacteria.

Getting marginal amounts of folic acid during pregnancy can result in having a child more susceptible to illness, but severe folic acid deficiency can render a child mentally retarded. In a South African study detailed in *Nutrition Reports International* (November 1974), 57 percent of the children born to mothers who got little folic acid during pregnancy showed abnormal or delayed development.

## All Mothers-To-Be Need Supplements

While British mothers-to-be, as a rule, receive folic acid supplements, their American counterparts do not. American medicine's prenatal care has not advanced to the point where all pregnant women receive adequate vitamin supplementation. When Victor Herbert, M.D., and associates examined 110 pregnant women at a New York City municipal clinic, they found that 16 percent of the women had a definite folic acid deficiency and another 14 percent had borderline deficiencies. Also,

64 percent of the women had serum levels that were at the lower limit of the normal range.

"It is estimated that half the pregnant women in the world may be folacin (folic acid) deficient," according to Erwin Di-Cyan, Ph.D., in *Vitamins in Your Life and the Micronutrients* (New York: Simon and Schuster, 1974). "The fetus drains the pregnant mother of much of her folacin stores, so she needs supplementation daily." Megaloblastic anemia is one of the well-recognized complications of pregnancy, and, says Dr. DiCyan, "Birth defects are among the grave results of (folic acid) deficiency in pregnant women."

Folic acid deficiency has also been linked with many complications of pregnancy such as toxemia, *abruptio placentae*, premature birth, and afterbirth hemorrhaging. Toxemia is a complication, brought on by infection, which is characterized by high blood pressure, edema, the presence of albumin in the urine, and, if unchecked, headache, spots before the eyes, dizziness, and convulsions. Such a condition may be dangerous to both the mother and the unborn baby.

*Abruptio placentae* is the premature separation of the placenta from the wall of the uterus before the baby is born. Since it is through the placenta that the unborn baby receives its nourishment and oxygen, this constitutes a severe threat to the infant and will be fatal if the separation is complete. It is also a danger to the mother because the separation may be accompanied by bleeding and shock.

## Folic Acid Linked to Mental Illness

Pregnancy is not the only situation in which folic acid supplementation is needed. In a Massachusetts General Hospital study published in the *New England Journal of Medicine* (16 October 1975), the author reported that several mentally disturbed or retarded individuals were helped with folic acid. One mildly retarded teenage girl suffered from schizophrenic delusions, withdrawal, and catatonia. All her psychotic symptoms disappeared, however, when she was treated with oral folic acid and vitamin B6. When the treatment stopped, the symptoms returned within five to seven months. When the vitamins were resupplied, the symptoms again disappeared.

Schizophrenic patients have responded to folic acid in other studies. At Northwick Park Hospital, Middlesex, England, mentally ill patients treated with folic acid were released from the hospital from 23 to 36 percent sooner than those not given folic acid (*Lancet,* 9 August 1975). As yet, no confirming trials have been carried out. But the clinical improvement necessary to warrant release from a mental hospital is generally regarded as a relatively stable bias-free criterion.

## Disease Susceptibility

Controlled studies have been performed, however, investigating the relationship between folic acid deficiency and increased susceptibility to infection. An African study, reported in the *Lancet* (14 December 1974), found that patients with bacterial infections could not absorb dietary folic acid as efficiently as healthy persons. An American study appearing in the *American Journal of Clinical Nutrition* (March 1975) has shown that the cells' ability to defend themselves against infection is impaired during severe folic acid deficiency. These two studies, taken together, suggest a vicious cycle, wherein the folic acid-deficient person becomes particularly susceptible to viral, fungal, parasitic, and certain bacterial infections, which in turn may interfere with absorption of the vitamin.

A folic acid deficiency may also compound itself by creating still another disorder. One of the major causes of folic acid deficiency is impaired absorption of the vitamin in the small intestine. Yet, Charles Halsted, M.D., of the University of California School of Medicine, reported in *Nutrition Reviews* (February 1975) that folic acid deficiency can ravage the mucosal lining and impair the nutrient-absorbing function of the small intestine. Consequently, a person who is not getting enough folic acid is in danger of not using all he does get.

# Deficiency Common

All this information is more than academic, because folic acid deficiency is not nearly so rare as was once believed. Between 1974 and 1976, the number of patients with disorders resulting from congenital defects in the uptake or utilization of the vitamin has nearly doubled, according to Richard W. Erbe, M.D., of the Genetic Unit at Massachusetts General Hospital (*New England Journal of Medicine,* 9 October 1975). A study of black school children in Mississippi, reported in the *Journal of the American Dietetic Association* (November 1974), revealed that the average daily intake of folic acid was about one-fifth of the recommended amount. Over 99 percent of the children consumed less than half the daily recommended amount.

Besides pregnant women and their babies, the estimated eight million American women on oral contraceptives run a special risk of folic acid deficiency, as scientific journals have been reporting since the beginning of the 1970s. In an article in the *Journal of the American Medical Association* (17 December 1973), a team of researchers referred to the "increased incidence of megaloblastic anemia and other abnormalities of folate metabolism in users of oral contraceptives."

The elderly also appear to face an increased risk of folic acid deficiency. During routine investigations at an English hospital, authorities discovered that more than a third of an unselected group of 72 patients, over age 70, had low levels of folic acid in their blood. Two of the patients had such serious folic acid deficiency that megaloblastic anemia resulted from it. The article in the *British Medical Journal* (23 July 1966) also remarked that 67 percent of the patients unable to care for themselves because of mental disorders were folic-acid deficient. Doctors were inclined to believe the shortage was largely due to simple malnutrition.

As with other nutrients, deficiencies of folic acid can result from more than just not getting the Recommended Daily Allowance (RDA) which is set at .4 mg., or 400 mcg. Since vitamin C is necessary for the reduction of folic acid to the active form the body can use, a deficiency of that vitamin can further aggravate the ill effects of a marginal supply of folic acid. And not only can body tissues need more folic acid because of trauma, infection, or growth, but certain factors in the diet can compete for dominance in the system—and win. Alcohol is primary among these factors.

Most individuals can control their intake of alcohol. Controlling one's intake of folic acid—trying to get enough—is not quite so easy. Although folic acid is plentiful in liver, wheat bran, asparagus, and the greens of beets, kale, endive, spinach, and turnips, the vitamin is easily destroyed in cooking and by simple exposure to air and light. Any water that vegetables are cooked in should be saved for soups or stews, since much of the vitamin dissolves in the water when heated.

## Government Restrictions

The Food and Drug Administration sets a limit on the amount of folic acid that can be included in a supplement. The limit equals the RDA of 400 mcg., yet many supplements don't even supply that much, if any at all. The government might be worried about epileptics getting too much folic acid, since large amounts may cause anticonvulsant drugs to lose their effectiveness. But the real reason for the restriction is that folic acid seems to mask some of the effects of vitamin $B_{12}$ deficiency anemia. Folic acid was once used to treat this anemia—until it was discovered that while removing most of the symptoms, folic acid allowed the neurological deterioration to continue. The government's reasoning, then, is that to protect those who do not get enough $B_{12}$, we must restrict the availability of another, equally important nutrient.

Of course, as in most instances, the problem is more complex than government reasoning would seem to indicate. Actually, according to a study appearing in the *Lancet* (24 May 1975) a deficiency of $B_{12}$ can impair the cell's utilization of folic acid. Today, folic acid deficiency is far more common than $B_{12}$ deficiency.

## Common Foods Rich in Folic Acid

No standard food composition tables are available as yet from the United States Department of Agriculture for this vitamin, but the following foods are generally recognized as the richest sources.

| | |
|---|---|
| Spinach | Turnips |
| Liver | Potatoes |
| Kidney | Broccoli |
| Wheat bran | Orange juice |
| Asparagus | Swiss chard |
| Beet greens | Black-eyed peas |
| Kale | Lima beans |
| Endive | |

# CHAPTER 39

# Pantothenic Acid, the Missing Vitamin

Methyl bromide is the perfect insecticidal fumigant. It kills every insect under the sun—domestic or foreign, common or exotic. Sprayed into a sealed warehouse—which is the way it is almost always used—it will even kill mice. Any squirrels, chipmunks, lizards, bats, or birds which happen to be in the food storage area at the time of spraying will also be killed. So will human beings. In fact, there is no living thing which could come out of a silo or warehouse or ship's hold which has been fumigated with methyl bromide in any other condition except dead.

But once fresh air is permitted to enter the fumigated area, the methyl bromide quickly evaporates, leaving scarcely any trace of its murderous presence. Repeated applications can be made without exceeding the residue tolerance of 50 parts per million. Furthermore, no matter how heavily applied, it leaves no telltale taste or odor which might be detectable to the person eating the grain, dried milk, meat, or any other product fumigated with methyl bromide.

In short, it seems to be an ideal insecticide and rodenticide for stored foodstuffs, and is therefore very extensively used by food wholesalers in the United States and other countries.

Unfortunately for people who eat the food which has been fumigated with methyl bromide, doctors in Japan are now convinced that it has caused 10,000 or more people in that country to fall victim to a disease known as subacute myelo-optic neuropathy, which produces, among many other symptoms, gastrointestinal tract disturbances, impaired vision, decreased resistance against infection and stress, and degeneration of the spinal cord.

Oddly enough, the Japanese researchers believe that this horrendous disease is caused by eating food which contains not the slightest trace—perhaps not even a single molecule—of methyl bromide or any related chemical.

## Disease Linked to Lack of Vitamin

Actually, the Japanese doctors at first had no reason to suspect that methyl bromide or any other insecticide might be involved in the genesis of subacute myelo-optic neuropathy, they told the Ninth International Congress of Nutrition in Mexico City. Dr. Yoshikazu Yomura and his colleagues of the Department of Neurology at Kanto Rosai Hospital in Kawasaki did notice, however, that there was a striking similarity between the symptoms displayed by their patients and the symptoms produced both in animals and in human beings who are deficient in the B-complex vitamin pantothenic acid.

Gastrointestinal disturbances, strange itching and burning sensations, and weakened resistance to every kind of stress, including infection, all of which are seen in the neuropathy patients, are all classic symptoms of pantothenic acid deficiency.

Drawing blood samples from the neuropathy patients, the Japanese team discovered that they did, in fact, tend to have low levels of pantothenic acid.

The next step was to see if large doses of pantothenic acid would help these patients. Their suspicion was dramatically confirmed: of 77 neuropathy patients treated with injections of pantothenic acid, 52 experienced what the Japanese called either "excellent" or "extremely marked" relief. Results in 16 others were described as "fair."

The doctors were still at a loss to explain how these patients became deficient in pantothenic acid, because it is not usually considered a vitamin which is difficult to get.

While puzzling over this question, the Japanese neurologists happened to treat a patient suffering from acute methyl bromide intoxication. His job was to fumigate food with methyl bromide, and somehow, perhaps because his mask was not on properly, he had been felled by fumes. The doctors were able to pull him through this crisis satisfactorily, but after his acute symptoms subsided, they noticed that he now suffered from a new set of symptoms which were very similar to pantothenic acid deficiency. Was it possible that there was some kind of obscure link between methyl bromide and pantothenic acid deficiency?

Eager to thoroughly investigate any clue that presented itself, the investigators decided to see what would happen to rats whose entire food ration had been fumigated with methyl bromide in much the same manner as food for humans is fumigated in warehouses. In contrast to a group of control rats, those eating the fumigated food did not gain weight normally, and displayed such symptoms as tiredness, diarrhea, excitation, and discolored hair, skin, and eyes. Although most of the symptoms subsided as the rats grew older, the autopsy showed that many of the animals had suffered serious damage to their nervous systems.

The doctors were still puzzled, because analysis of the fumigated ration fed to these animals showed no residue whatsoever of methyl bromide. However, when the investigators analyzed food before and after fumigation, with a technique known as infrared spectrophotometry, they made a startling discovery: fumigation changed pantothenic acid into another, unknown compound!

This was the link that they were looking for. True, the methyl bromide was gone from the fumigated food, but it had taken with it all the pantothenic acid, a nutrient vital to health. In the case of the worker who had been felled by methyl bromide fumes, the vitamin destruction apparently had taken place within his body. The other patients, apparently, had suffered because the vitamin had been destroyed in the food they ate. The victims probably ate very large amounts of polished rice which had been sprayed.

The idea that the nervous disorder known as subacute myelo-optic neuropathy can be caused by eating food fumigated with methyl bromide is a theory. A good theory, but still, only a theory. On the other hand, that fumigating food with methyl bromide destroys the vital pantothenic acid content is a fact. It is also a fact that this B vitamin is essential to good health. Symptoms of pantothenic acid deficiency, which range from balky bowels to lowered resistance to infection can be present to a relatively mild extent when deficiency is relatively mild. In other words, absence of gross nervous disorders is not proof that a person is not suffering to some degree from a deficiency of pantothenic acid.

## Reproduction is Damaged

The Japanese experiments are not the only evidence of the nutritive destruction wrought by methyl bromide. In 1960, a group of researchers at the Texas Agricultural Experimental Station at College Station, Texas, published a bulletin entitled, "Effects of Fumigation For Insect Control on Seed Germination." Fumigation with methyl bromide, their tests revealed, interfered with the germination of every kind of seed tested. Two fumigations, which is not in the least uncommon in practice, "always caused severe injury." When temperature and moisture were relatively low, little immediate damage was seen. However, after the seed was stored for 12 months, which again is not at all unusual, "drastic reductions in germinations appeared." This latter fact is significant because it suggests that even after methyl bromide has disappeared from food via evaporation, the nutritive damage which it has initiated grows progressively worse.

Another important revelation from these tests is that seed which does sprout after fumigation with methyl bromide shows signs of abnormality. As the researchers put it: "Seed injured by some fumigants produced seedlings with certain structures which failed to grow. The primary root and tubule often become necrotic (dead) in corn and sorghum seed, largely due to overgrowth of molds on these weakened structures. The failure of certain seedling parts to develop often resulted in excessive growth of other parts of the same seedling. . . . Fumigated seed of all crops produced seedlings that were less vigorous than non-fumigated seed even when germination percentages revealed little or no differences."

When these tests were made at the Texas Agricultural Experimental Station it was not known why methyl bromide caused such destruction of the integrity of the seeds. All the researchers knew was that the seeds contained no residue, just as the fumigated food in Japan contained no traces of methyl bromide. They were aware, of course, that pantothenic acid occurs nearly universally in all growing things and is regarded as a growth stimulant. But they had no reason to connect the sprouting failure of fumigated seeds with this nutrient.

However, in light of the Japanese discovery, it can be assumed that the reason for the failure of the fumigated seed to sprout and grow normally was that its pantothenic acid had been destroyed in whole or part.

Reproductive damage caused by a lack of pantothenic acid is not limited to grains. According to *Executive Health* (January 1976), animal studies have shown pantothenic acid to be vital to normal reproduction. Depending on the severity of the vitamin deficiency, fetuses of pregnant rats were either resorbed or born deformed. The more pantothenic acid that was made available to the mother rats, the less damage there was to the fetuses.

Roger J. Williams, Ph.D., wrote in *Nutrition Against Disease* (New York: Pitman Publishing Corp., 1971) that, "There are reasons for thinking that a substantial number of human reproductive failures—stillbirths, premature births, malformed babies, and mentally retarded babies—are due to the lack, during pregnancy, of enough of the very same vitamin, pantothenic acid, that . . . investigators showed was so crucially important for rats."

# CHAPTER 40

# The Antistress Vitamin

Although pantothenic acid was discovered in 1933 by Roger J. Williams, Ph.D., little attention has been paid to what it does and what a lack of it can do. In *Nutrition Against Disease* (New York: Pitman Publishing Corp., 1971), Dr. Williams wrote that pantothenic acid "has received almost no attention. Most physicians have been taught its name, but they have never been introduced to the idea that the quantity present in the diet may be crucial. While it can safely be asserted that no one in any country of the world ever ate a meal or snack without getting some pantothenic acid in it, it is wishful thinking to suppose that people always get enough."

Pantothenic acid's name is derived from *pantos,* the Greek word for everywhere, because it occurs in all living cells. Since it is present to some extent in all foods, there has been a common assumption that a deficiency in this vitamin is very rare. But in today's chemical environment with its many processed foods, it may be difficult with some diets to obtain even the Recommended Daily Allowance (RDA) of 10 mg. Many people may have individual requirements for pantothenic acid (and other vitamins) that exceed the RDA, making supplementation necessary. Dr. Williams believes that everyone would benefit from getting more pantothenic acid. In *Nutrition Against*

*Disease* he wrote, " . . . it is probably an inherent characteristic of the human system to require relatively large amounts of this vitamin. . . . Human muscle, the most abundant tissue in our bodies, contains about twice as much pantothenic acid as the muscle of other animals, and it must all be acquired through nutrition. Human milk, which nature provides for human babies, is relatively rich in the vitamin."

What happens when the human body is deprived of pantothenic acid? To find out, physicians at Iowa State University College of Medicine gave volunteers from the Iowa State Prison a diet adequate except for pantothenic acid. The results were reported in the *Proceedings of the Society of Biology* (vol. 86, 1954). The young men complained of fatigue and a desire to sleep during the day after only two weeks of deprivation. Loss of appetite and constipation plagued them by the third week. They became quarrelsome, discontented, and totally out of sorts by the fourth week. Urine analysis showed a decrease in adrenal hormones, which fell progressively lower as the experiment continued. The subjects also developed low blood pressure, extreme fatigue, stomach distress, constipation, and continuous respiratory infections. The digestive enzymes and stomach acid were markedly reduced. By the fifth week of the experiment, these men were extremely miserable, and burning feet added to their suffering.

These results are extraordinary for several reasons. First, it is very unusual to produce such severe symptoms by removing a single nutrient for only a few weeks. Healthy young people deprived of vitamin C, for example, may not show any obvious symptoms for months. This is ironic, because the human body is absolutely unable to synthesize vitamin C, while intestinal bacteria are able to provide us with a certain amount of pantothenic acid which they themselves synthesize out of other nutrients. Obviously, the need for pantothenic acid from dietary sources on a regular basis is much more critical than most people imagine. Without it, we soon develop a whole catalog of ills that few would ordinarily associate with inadequacy of a single fraction of the B-complex family.

# Vitamin Needed to Handle Stress

Pantothenic acid is involved in several vital functions of the body, and is often referred to as the antistress vitamin because it is needed by the adrenal glands and by the body's immune system.

In mice, deficiency of pantothenic acid produces a devastating effect upon the adrenal glands. The glands literally die, often hemorrhaging as they do so. Production of the many vital steroids, including cortisone, normally produced by the adrenal glands, ceases. Because these steroids regulate literally dozens of metabolic functions, the pantothenic acid-deficient mouse suffers from a host of severe symptoms, including ulcers.

The adrenal glands are known to protect man from all kinds of stress, both physical and mental, and oral doses of calcium pantothenate help man to get through periods of stress with less wear and tear. This was shown in a dramatic series of experiments by Elaine P. Ralli, M.D., with the cooperation of some very brave volunteers. As explained in the *Nutrition Symposium*, (National Vitamin Foundation Ser. 5, 78, 1952), Dr. Ralli subjected the male adult volunteers to stress by immersing them in freezing cold water for long periods of time. Various tests were made immediately following this ordeal to chart the effects on body chemistry.

Following six weeks of oral doses of calcium pantothenate, the volunteers were once again subjected to the freezing cold water treatment. This time, Dr. Ralli noted that the various blood tests showed far fewer signs of stress than the first series. One change was that after taking the pantothenic acid, the volunteers were not depleted of ascorbic acid, as they tended to be the first time. Dr. Ralli concluded that pantothenic acid apparently increases the capacity of our tissues to withstand stress. Another form of stress which pantothenic acid helps to protect against is allergic reactions (see chapter 104).

Pantothenic acid is an essential element of coenzyme A, which is very involved in the utilization of nutrients and the production of energy. Thus, the vitamin is important to the integrity of all the cells in the body, and is concentrated in the organs.

Pantothenic acid is also one of the B vitamins which have been identified as absolutely essential to the production of antibodies which help fight off infection. Experimental studies carried out on mice by Abraham E. Axelrod, Ph.D., of Pittsburgh University Medical School show clearly why the volunteers from the Iowa State Prison who were denied pantothenic acid suffered from continuous respiratory infection.

Dr. Axelrod told a seminar on Nutrition and the Future of Man, conducted by the Vitamin Information Bureau in December of 1971, that the B vitamins necessary for the creation of antibodies against infection "are pyridoxine, folic acid, and pantothenic acid." If any one of these three is missing, he explained, test animals simply cannot produce circulating antibodies. Any regimen which one might choose to help resist infection, including vitamin C, vitamin A, antibiotics, or any other agents, obviously cannot be depended upon to do much good if your system is deficient in any of these three B-complex vitamins.

## Deficiency Linked to Arthritis

Hormones produced by the adrenal glands, including cortisone, control a tendency towards inflammation, which may be caused by still other hormones. A team of English researchers, reporting in the *Lancet* (26 October 1963), looked into the relationship of pantothenic acid and arthritis and observed that rheumatoid arthritics had lower blood pantothenic acid levels. The lower the level, the greater was the severity of their arthritis symptoms. Daily injections of pantothenic acid and ingesting royal jelly (a secretion of the honey bee which is rich in pantothenate) led to a gradual rise in blood pantothenic acid levels and an improvement in the general condition, mobility of joints, and a fall in the sedimentation rate. When treatment was reduced, blood pantothenic acid levels fell and clinical relapse occurred.

According to *Executive Health* (January 1976), two English scientists—E.C. Barton-Wright, D.Sc., a biochemist, and W.A. Elliot, M.D., Physician-in-charge of the Rheumatic Clinic of St. Alfege's Hospital, London—have worked with arthritics for many years, and are convinced of a definite relationship between low blood pantothenic acid levels and arthritic symptoms. Dr. Barton-Wright believes that insufficient intake of pantothenic acid is a factor in arthritis, and he blames today's increase of rheumatoid and osteoarthritis on an increasing use of processed foods which have most of their vitamin content removed.

One of the most profound and least-understood forms of stress to which the human body can be subjected is radiation injury. Is it possible that these same properties of pantothenic acid which help both animals and humans resist infection, allergy, and severe stress might also protect against the lethal effects of radiation?

The answer—resoundingly affirmative—comes from Dr. I. Szorady of Hungary, in his study of pantothenic acid reported in *Acta Paediatricia* (6:1, 1963). The Hungarian physician found that mice which were given pantothenic acid for a week and then irradiated a week later, had a survival rate fully 200 percent better than those which were given the same radiation dose but no pantothenic acid.

Dr. Szorady commented: "Due to its metabolic key position, pantothenic acid thus seems to induce slow biochemical processes which ensure enhanced protection against radiation injury. The capacity of pantothenic acid to protect the epithelium, to promote tissue regeneration, protein synthesis, antibody production, and corticoid synthesis . . . as also its antiallergic properties, may all be involved in those biochemical processes."

Citing a German study published in 1961, Dr. Szorady mentioned another therapeutic use of pantothenic acid: "As proved by experimental results and clinical observations, pantothenic acid mitigates the side effects and toxicity of several antibiotics produced from streptomyces, such as streptomycin, dehydrostreptomycin, neomycin, kanamycin, and viomycin."

# Vitamin Stimulates Intestinal Motility, Relieves Gas

Pantothenic acid is also needed for the normal functioning of the gastrointestinal tract. When dogs were fed a diet deficient in pantothenic acid, they suffered the discomfort of abdominal distention which usually results from an inhibition of bowel motility (capability of movement) a condition known medically as ileus (Vitamin Information Bureau, Inc., New York). Experiments also showed that when pantothenic acid was given after surgery, there was a much shorter period of discomfort.

Ileus usually occurs after intestinal surgery. In its mildest and perhaps most common form, ileus causes postoperative distention with accompanying wind pains and abdominal discomfort which may follow the simplest operation, possibly not even involving the abdomen, stated an editorial in the *British Medical Journal* (14 September 1963). In its severe form, fortunately rare, the intestines become completely paralyzed and all function ceases so that the patient's life is in grave danger.

The finding that pantothenic acid lessened the period of ileus in dogs encouraged surgeons to evaluate the possibility of similar treatment in postoperative human patients.

Several investigators observed 100 patients suffering paralytic ileus and found that pantothenic acid produced good results with an early passage of flatus (gas, wind, or air in the gastrointestinal tract). Their report, appearing in the *American Journal of Surgery* (97:75, 1959), revealed that there was also much less postoperative nausea and distention.

When a double-blind study of hospital patients was conducted, researchers found a significant difference between the controls and the trial group. According to the report in *Surgery, Gynecology and Obstetrics* (112:526, 1961), those who got pantothenic acid were able to expel trapped gas in an average of 10 hours, while those who did not get pantothenic acid suffered gas pains for 77 hours. Also, the length of the hospital stay was shortened from 14 days for those who got no pantothenic acid to two days for those who received the vitamin. No adverse effects were observed.

Why is it that pantothenic acid has such an influence on intestinal motility? Without pantothenic acid, a very important substance called acetylcholine cannot be produced. Acetylcholine is a chemical which transmits messages at the nerve endings. Without it, the nerves cannot control motor and secretory intestinal activity. It has, in fact, been found in experimental animals, that after a period of stress, the acetylcholine reservoir in the body is diminished (*British Medical Journal*, 14 September 1963). However, if pantothenic acid is given, the acetylcholine level may be increased by as much as 50 percent. This was determined by researchers reporting in the *Journal of Applied Nutrition* (11:177, 1958).

It is possible that people who have never had surgery but constantly suffer from gas may be helped by getting more pantothenic acid. Carlton Fredericks, Ph.D., reported in his *Newsletter of Nutrition* (1 October 1972) that "250 mg. daily has not only been reported to relieve postoperative gas pains, but to prevent them. My recent observations," he wrote, "suggest that those who are troubled by intestinal gas and distention for which no physical cause has been found sometimes respond to pantothenic acid—so much so that I am persuaded that these people have an elevated requirement for the vitamin, difficult to fulfill even with a reasonable choice of foods."

## Part of the B Complex

The role of pantothenic acid as an individual nutrient can hardly be overestimated, but it does its work best in combination with other related B vitamins. All these vitamins occur naturally and plentifully in brewer's yeast and desiccated liver.

The best table food sources of pantothenic acid are the organ meats—heart, liver, kidney, and brain. Soy flour, sunflower seeds, dark buckwheat, and sesame seeds are all top-notch providers of pantothenic acid. Most vegetables and nearly all fruits contain very little pantothenic acid.

# CHAPTER 41

# Do You Grind Your Teeth?
# You Might Need
# Pantothenic Acid
# and Calcium

There are millions of people who wake every morning with aching jaws after a night of grinding their teeth while they sleep. Spouses have been led to threaten divorce and on occasion to seek one, in response to too many noisy and sleepless nights. In some, the habit is so out of control that the grinding goes on intermittently during the day.

Bruxism—tooth grinding—is more than an unpleasant habit. It is a prominent cause of tooth loss and of gum recession, both resulting from the loosening of the tooth in its socket that frequent grinding induces.

People who gnash their teeth have tried everything from dentistry to psychiatry, and have even tried stuffing their mouths with a wet towel in despair. However, there is evidence that bruxism is related to nutrition, and that the grinder doesn't need the dentist or psychiatrist as much as he needs more calcium and pantothenic acid.

While many parents tend to consider bruxism a temporary phase—something the child will grow out of—it is not a practice which should be ignored. A Swiss dental scientist, Peter

Schaerer of Bern, has reported in the *Journal of the American Dental Association* (January 1971) that persons who clench their teeth during sleep or during a "confrontation" can cause damage to the teeth, gingiva (gums), jaw joint, and muscles.

While the practice is usually associated with children, adults also contribute to the nocturnal cacophony and their own gum problems and malocclusion. In fact, the percentage of adults who grind their teeth, five percent, is the same as the percentage of children who grind their teeth.

These statistics were revealed by George R. Reding, Ph.D., assistant professor of psychiatry at the University of Chicago, and John E. Robinson, Jr., M.D., associate professor in the Walter T. Zoller Dental Memorial Clinic of the same university. These two men investigated bruxism by means of dental examination, interviews, and sleep-laboratory techniques, and reported their findings in a University of Chicago News Release (13 February 1968).

While psychiatrists, psychologists, and dentists who have considered the problem of nocturnal teeth grinders often assumed it was associated with mental illness or emotional disturbance, according to Dr. Reding, there is no demonstrable evidence of such an association. Psychological tests of matched groups of grinders and nongrinders recruited among University of Chicago students gave no indication the grinders were more emotionally disturbed than the nongrinders.

## Antistress Vitamin Helps

According to a report in the *Dental Survey* (December 1970) by Emanuel Cheraskin, M.D., D.M.D., and W. Marshall Ringsdorf, Jr., D.M.D., M.S., bruxism is a nutritional problem that can be greatly ameliorated with increased dosages of calcium and pantothenic acid, the antistress vitamin.

In order to explore the relationship between diet and nocturnal teeth gnashing, Drs. Cheraskin and Ringsdorf set up a multiple testing program using a group of dentists and their wives. Each one was asked to fill out an Oral Health Index

Questionnaire in which one of the questions was, "Do you clench or grind your teeth or are you conscious of the way your teeth fit together, awake or asleep?" Each one was also asked to complete a questionnaire designed to reveal the nutrient content of his diet. Then the group listened to lectures on diet.

One year later, each participant again completed both questionnaires. By this technique it was possible to relate dietary habits to the practice of tooth grinding.

Of the 94 people studied, 58 (group one) reported no bruxism at the first visit. On the second visit they reported a higher intake of protein, calcium, vitamin A, $B_1$, $B_2$, niacin, C, $B_6$, pantothenic acid, iodine, and vitamin E. They again reported no tooth grinding at all on the second visit a year later.

There were five people established as group two who had not improved their nutrition at all and developed the habit of grinding their teeth during the course of the experimental period.

Sixteen people placed in group three were tooth grinders at the beginning of the study. These 16 increased their intake of calcium, vitamins A, C, pantothenic acid, iodine, and vitamin E. Without any other change in life situations—without any deliberate effort—by the end of the year they were quiet sleepers no longer disturbing their families' slumber with the sound of a nocturnal cement mixer. More important, they were not loosening their teeth in their sockets or tearing them away from their gums. The 15 people in group four, who were tooth grinders before and remained tooth grinders, increased their intake of vitamins A, C, iodine, and vitamin E.

What nutrients did group three get that group four did not get? Calcium and pantothenic acid. But why should these two nutrients be involved in a phenomenon that disturbs the slumbers of millions of people every night of the year?

## Muscles Need Calcium

It is well known that calcium is vital to the strength of the bones. But nerves, muscles, and various organs of the body also depend for their health on a regular supply of calcium. Calcium is used by the nerves and indeed has been found by 1970 Nobel Laureate Sir Bernard Katz to be the key requirement for transporting impulses along the nerves from one part of the body to another. It is urgently needed by muscles; lack of calcium will cause cramps or convulsions. What is a convulsion? A violent involuntary series of contractions of the voluntary muscles. What is bruxism? An involuntary movement of the muscles of the mouth bringing the teeth together in a grinding movement.

What about pantothenic acid? When a deficiency of this B vitamin was induced in volunteers, the symptoms included headache, fatigue, gastrointestinal disturbances, numbness in extremities, and both *muscle cramps and impaired motor coordination.*

"Thus," Drs. Cheraskin and Ringsdorf pointed out, "it would appear to be of some note that in the subjects who stopped bruxing there was an increase in pantothenic acid intake."

Pantothenic acid is known as the antistress vitamin, essential to the proper functioning of the adrenal glands. When pantothenic acid is undersupplied, the adrenals do not function properly and may not produce cortisone and other important hormones. A lack of these hormones will leave anyone vulnerable to situations that cause stress.

Situations of stress use up the body's stores of pantothenic acid which is part of the complex molecule of coenzyme A, the substance essential for the production of acetylcholine. Acetylcholine is the chemical transmitter at the autonomic nerve endings controlling motor activity.

While, by psychiatric standards, tooth grinders are considered normal, Peter Schaerer noted in his report that "the primary causes of bruxism seem to be changes in central nervous activity—as in sleep, in states of nervous tension, or in conflict situations. Psychological studies have shown that persons suffering from bruxism frequently display emotional disorders such as excessive fright or aggression, irritability, and tenseness."

Tooth grinders, then, are not candidates for the psychiatrist's couch—it's just that their stresses are showing. A good supply of pantothenic acid may be just what they need in order to cope with their stresses.

## Common Foods Rich in Pantothenic Acid*

| Portions of 3½ oz. | (milligrams) |
|---|---|
| Liver (Beef, raw) | 7.70 |
| Liver (Chicken, raw) | 6.00 |
| Kidney (Beef, raw) | 3.85 |
| Heart (Chicken, raw) | 2.56 |
| Heart (Beef, raw) | 2.50 |
| Buckwheat flour (Dark) | 1.45 |
| Wheat bran (100%) | 2.90 |
| Sesame-seed flour | 2.76 |
| Brewer's yeast (Debittered) | 12.00 |
| Sunflower seeds | 1.40 |
| Soybeans (Dry, raw) | 1.70 |
| Peas (Dry) | 2.00 |
| Peanuts (Raw) | 2.80 |
| Eggs (Raw) | 1.60 |
| Lobster (Raw) | 1.50 |

*Selected from tables in *Pantothenic Acid, Vitamin B6 and Vitamin B12 in Foods,* United States Department of Agriculture Home Economics Research Report # 36, August, 1969.

# CHAPTER 42

# Biotin—A Necessary Coenzyme

Biotin, one of the lesser-known vitamins in the B complex, was stumbled upon in a rather unusual manner. A researcher at the Lister Institute of Preventive Medicine in London was using raw egg white as a source of protein in the diet of rats. After a few weeks the animals developed dermatitis and hemorrhages of the skin. Their hair fell out, their limbs became paralyzed, they lost considerable weight and eventually died.

Only raw or cold dried egg white produced these symptoms. Cooking made the egg whites harmless. Subsequent investigations showed that the effects of raw egg white could be alleviated or prevented by any one of a variety of food stuffs. This protection occurred, it was thought, because of some substance common to all these foods. This then unknown factor was labeled "Protective Factor X."

Through experimentation, Paul Gyorgy, Ph.D., learned that liver is a good source of the protective factor. In 1940, he identified the factor and called it vitamin H. However, before too long, scientists confirmed that the substance was actually a member of the B complex, and today biotin is recognized as being widely distributed throughout the body. In fact, it is an essential constituent of almost all living cells, both plant and animal. Yet, its potency is so great that no cell contains more than a slight trace of it. It is normally measured in micrograms, with the Recommended Daily Allowance set at 300 mcg.

Biotin is now recognized as a coenzyme necessary for a variety of important bodily functions. It is involved in the metabolism of carbohydrates, proteins, and fats, especially the unsaturated fatty acids. Active throughout the entire body, the vitamin is needed for normal growth, and its physiological functions include maintenance of the skin, hair, sebaceous glands, nerves, bone marrow, and the sex glands.

## Deficiency Symptoms

Biotin occurs in a wide variety of food substances, and can, to some extent, be manufactured in the intestines of both animals and man. Consequently, a full-fledged deficiency is rare. But deficiencies do occur, and they present real medical problems.

Several years ago, a 62-year-old woman suffering from a bewildering set of symptoms was admitted to a hospital in Birmingham, Alabama. Her appetite was poor; her mouth and lips were sore; she had a severe case of dermatitis. Besides that, she was suffering from nausea and vomiting, mental depression, pallor, muscle pains, and pains around her heart. Her hands and feet suffered from a tickling sensation.

After undergoing a battery of tests, according to a report which appeared in the *American Journal of Clinical Nutrition* (February 1968), the woman was found to be anemic, she had abnormal heart action, unusually high cholesterol levels, and strange liver symptoms.

Upon questioning the woman, hospital staff doctors learned that she suffered from a liver ailment which her own family doctor said could be cleared up by eating a high protein diet. Accordingly, her doctor put her on a diet that included six raw eggs and two quarts of milk daily along with her regular meals; a regimen she followed for 18 months.

Little did she—or apparently her doctor—know that the dietary program she was following had led to her condition by short-changing her system of biotin. The symptoms were actually caused by eating the large numbers of raw eggs over a long period of time. Raw egg whites have a special protein in them called avidin which combines with biotin in the intestinal tract. This complex mixture cannot be broken down and digested. As a result, biotin is passed through the intestinal tract and excreted. If this condition is allowed to continue for four weeks or more, a disease known as "egg-white injury" occurs which can only be overcome by feeding the patient a biotin-rich diet and including plenty of egg yolk, liver, or yeast.

A deficiency of biotin can be induced in dogs, chicks, and other fowl merely by leaving the biotin out of an experimental diet. In rats, mice, and monkeys, a deficiency can be induced by giving the animals antibiotics or sulfa drugs which lower the number of intestinal microorganisms, thereby preventing biotin from being produced in the intestines by bacteria. Animals that are made deficient in this nutrient for experimental purposes first exhibit signs of skin disease and a loss of fur and later develop swollen joints. Eventually, they develop paralysis of the hindquarters and multiple disorders of the genital tract.

Two skin diseases in infants, seborrheic dermatitis and desquamative erythroderma, are apparently connected with a biotin deficiency and respond to biotin therapy, according to John Marks in *The Vitamins In Health and Disease* (Boston: Little, Brown and Co., 1969).

Writing in *Pediatrics* (December 1969), Aaron Nisenson, M.D., of the Department of Pediatrics at the UCLA Center for the Health Sciences, reported that several cases of seborrheic dermatitis in infants were cleared up by administering biotin by injection and feeding liver to the nursing mother. Dr. Nisenson noted that biotin in food is bound to protein. To be effective, the biotin must be broken down by acid hydrolysis and gastric enzymes to the unbound, or "free" form. During the first three months of life, the mechanism for hydrolysis and gastric enzyme digestion in some infants may be defective and "free" biotin may not be available in adequate amounts. A nursing mother, he noted, is able to convert bound to unbound biotin which is excreted in her milk.

To clear up the skin problem, Dr. Nisenson recommended feeding the child a biotin-rich diet (egg yolk, yeast, liver), but he also said, "However, improvement in the infant is much more dramatic when the nursing mother is given large amounts of liver orally for 10 days."

## Biotin's Availability

Although biotin is found in many different foods, there are several factors that can affect its availability. As with practically all the B vitamins, cooking losses do occur. The presence of avidin in certain foods will decrease the amount of biotin absorbed. But the biggest threat to biotin availability comes from the use of antibiotics and sulfa drugs. These drugs destroy the intestinal bacteria that produce the vitamin. Over the years, the use of antibiotics in cattle has increased, raising the possibility that food from these animals contains less biotin than it once did.

Biotin, along with the rest of the B complex, is most plentiful in yeast, liver, eggs, and a variety of grains, nuts, and fish. Until recently, biotin was not manufactured and so it was missing from many commercial vitamin formulas. Manufacturers considered biotin too expensive to add to their products, and many still do not add it today. Check the label of the supplement you buy to be sure it contains biotin, if you are relying on the product as a source for that nutrient.

---

### Common Foods Rich in Biotin

No standard food composition tables are available as yet from the United States Department of Agriculture for this vitamin, but the following foods are generally recognized as the richest sources.

| | | |
|---|---|---|
| Brown rice | Lamb | Kidney |
| Bulgar wheat | Beef | Eggs |
| Rolled oats | Veal | Milk |
| Brewer's yeast | Fish | Cheese |
| Chicken | Liver | Nuts |
| Pork | | |

---

# CHAPTER 43

# Inositol: A Vitamin
You "Don't Need"
that is Vital
to Your Health

The label on a jar of vitamin B-complex tablets lists some strange-sounding names, many of them followed by asterisks. At the bottom of the label there's another asterisk and after it the words: "Need in human nutrition has not been established."

No need? Then why take them? Why put the stuff in tablets, anyway? Why write about them?

Why? Because scientists may not yet understand the need for these vitamins but our bodies are not so ignorant. Deep in the vitals of every key organ in the human body there exist vitamin or other food factors whose reason for being—and for being in that particular place—can barely be guessed at by the most learned scientists. Does this mean that the vitamins are triflers, physiologic loiterers? Or does it mean that we cannot yet understand why they are there, a reflection on the state of science rather than the importance of the vitamin?

In some cases, there has been considerable investigation into the role of these little-known food factors and the results are extremely suggestive. Inositol, a member of the B complex, is a good example. Inositol is one of those "asterisk vitamins" whose presence in a supplemental food such as yeast must be accompanied by the notation that the need for it in human nutrition has not been proven.

A peculiar thing about inositol is that it occurs in extraordinarily high concentrations in the human brain. High amounts are also found in the stomach, kidney, spleen, and liver, as well as the heart. And although inositol occurs naturally in a number of foods, the human body apparently possesses the ability to synthesize it through the action of intestinal bacteria, perhaps even in tissue.

It is apparent from this that inositol is playing an important role—an extremely important role—in health. That may be so, but if intestinal bacteria can make inositol, why do we need more from our food? Would it serve any real purpose?

## Controls Cholesterol

Two of the first researchers to answer this question with enthusiastic affirmation were Drs. Gross and Kesten, who in 1940 reported the astonishing effectiveness of inositol in treating psoriasis patients whose blood levels of cholesterol were above normal. They announced in the *New York State Journal of Medicine* that no less than 55 out of 64 patients had a significant reduction in blood cholesterol after taking an inositol preparation made from soybeans.

In 1949, Drs. Felch and Dotti reported the same kind of results when this B vitamin factor was administered to another group of patients: 30 diabetics suffering the familiar raised blood level of cholesterol. The researchers said in the *Proceedings of the Society for Experimental Biological Medicine* that their tests showed inositol to be of real value in lowering serum cholesterol, at least in diabetics.

The same year, Drs. Leinwand and Moore reported in the *American Heart Journal* that they, too, had encouraging results using inositol to control abnormal lipids, or fats such as cholesterol. They gave three grams daily to patients with atherosclerotic symptoms and reported that after an initial rise, there was a substantial fall in blood cholesterol after treatment continued. The initial increase could well have been caused by the flushing out of cholesterol deposits from arteries into the bloodstream, and the subsequent drop a reflection of the liberated cholesterol having been excreted or broken down.

The ability of inositol to break up abnormal deposits of fat has also been demonstrated by its use in connection with the treatment of fatty infiltration or cirrhosis of the liver. A study reported in the *Proceedings of the Society for Experimental Biological Medicine* (vol. 54, 1943) demonstrated that administration of inositol reduced liver fat to nearly normal levels in only 24 hours in patients whose livers were heavily infiltrated with fat as a result of gastrointestinal fat.

Apparently, cholesterol control is not the only function of inositol. No one knows how or why it should be so, but this B factor has also been demonstrated to have a mild inhibitory effect on cancer. *Science* (vol. 97, 1943) reported that intravenous shots of inositol slowed down the growth of transplanted tumors. Researchers wrote in the *Journal of Urology* (vol. 59, 1948) that when inositol was given to six patients suffering from bladder cancer, their tumors grew smaller and blood stopped appearing in their urine.

A study appearing in *Federation Proceedings* (vol. 6, 1947) reported that inositol has also been used with some success in treating nerve damage in certain forms of muscular dystrophy, but only when used in conjunction with vitamin E. Alone, neither vitamin has any effect. Similarly, inositol has been reported by some researchers to have greater power to break up fat when it is given along with another B factor, choline, to which it is related (*The Biochemistry of Inositol*, Pittsburgh, Pennsylvania: Mellon Institute, 1951). Still another related factor, biotin, has been shown to have a complex relationship with inositol, both in their effect on pathological fat in the liver, and the well-being of bacterial flora.

If all this sounds rather complicated, that's because it is, fantastically so. And science has barely scratched the surface. The metabolic complexities of inositol are such that experimenters have frequently clashed with each other over findings. Results achieved by one scientist are often not achieved by another. This would seem to indicate that there are more factors involved than scientists can control in their laboratories. It is indicative of where we stand that although the existence of inositol was discovered in Europe in 1850, its true status as a vitamin was not established until 1956. There are many questions begging for answers.

Is the ability of inositol to mobilize and reduce cholesterol related to the nearly identical action of vitamin C (see index)? Are the two vitamins perhaps synergistic, as are inositol and vitamin E in treating nerve damage? And by what possible mode of action did it reduce tumor size and stop urinary bleeding in every one of six cancer patients?

No answers exist yet for these questions, but two things are fairly certain: inositol has important protective functions in human health, and some people are not getting enough of it. If they were, why would they get healthier upon receiving extra amounts?

Taking inositol as an isolated vitamin is not recommended. Too little is known about how it works, especially in terms of its effects on other vitamins and enzymes, to take substantial amounts of it with any kind of real security. On the other hand, getting enough inositol—either in carefully compounded supplements or in whole foods, where it occurs along with the rest of the B complex in a balanced form, makes good nutritional sense.

## Heart vs. Steak

The question of inositol's occurrence in foods is rather interesting. The best sources are beef brain, beef heart, and wheat germ, but few Americans eat any of these foods. Yet primitive man, when he killed an animal, ate the heart, liver, brain, and other organs first, and let his dogs gnaw on the muscle meat, or steaks. And when he ate grain, he also ate the germ, because his grain was not refined. Today, all that is changed. Not only does man eat white bread bereft of its germ and bran, but he concentrates on steak, which is the poorest of all animal sources of inositol, and gives his dogs the nutrient-packed organ meats.

There is little question, then, that most of us are getting significantly less of this B vitamin than our ancestors did during the millenia that our physiology and metabolism evolved. It's possible, of course, that we might compensate for this if our intestinal bacteria churned more of it out, but there is no reason to believe this is so. If anything, what with antibiotics killing off beneficial intestinal bacteria by the billions, and a host of other chemicals from plastics to synthetic hormones insinuating their way into our metabolic systems, there would be less absorption of the needed vitamin.

---

### Common Foods Rich in Inositol

No standard food composition tables are available as yet from the United States Department of Agriculture for this vitamin, but the following foods are generally recognized as the richest sources.

| | | |
|---|---|---|
| Beef brain | Bulgar wheat | Molasses |
| Beef heart | Brown rice | Nuts |
| Wheat germ | Brewer's yeast | Citrus fruits |

---

# CHAPTER 44

# Choline, a Vital Link
# in the Nervous System

Choline is rarely recognized by the public as a vitamin, and is excluded from most popular multivitamin supplements. Although choline is sometimes added to animal feeds to insure good nutrition, there has been no Minimum Daily Requirement or Recommended Daily Allowance established for humans. Yet this member of the B complex is not only concerned with the body's general health, it is needed for the proper functioning of the all-important nervous system. In fact, because it is needed by the nervous system, it is tied in with every bodily function: without it, even the heart would stop beating.

Choline is an essential ingredient of the nerve fluid acetylcholine, which is needed to jump the gap between nerve cells so that impulses can be transmitted. This phenomenon is particularly apparent at the point where a nerve cell all but joins the muscle cell which it controls. In order for the muscle to carry out the instruction coming from the brain, it must first receive the message. However, a small gap or "synapse" separates the nerve cell from the muscle. Acetylcholine bridges the gap and gets the message across.

Acetylcholine is stored in the "synaptic vesicles" of every

nerve cell where it waits passively to relay the message it will receive. The inactive acetylcholine, when jolted by a nerve impulse rippling through that cell, rushes into the synaptic gap to allow the message to cross over to the next nerve or muscle cell. When it does, the acetylcholine reaching the next cell comes into contact with receptor sites, where another chemical, cholinesterase, breaks acetylcholine down into its components, allowing the cells once again to come to rest after the message has passed.

The ability of acetylcholine to relay an impulse is essential to healthy nerve functioning, and choline is an essential component of acetylcholine. If there is a shortage of the substance, the muscles cannot be properly stimulated and will become damaged. If that happens, the whole body will become weak and listless. A severe deficiency can result in paralysis, cardiac arrest, and death.

## The Liver Also Needs Choline

In order to stay healthy, the liver also needs choline. Otherwise, fatty deposits build up inside that vital organ, blocking its hundreds of functions, and throwing the whole body into a state of ill health. This fact was brought out at an Atlantic City symposium of the American Institute of Nutrition, the results of which were reported in *Federation Proceedings* (January-February 1971).

"It is known from histological and biochemical evidence that withdrawal of choline from the diet in one single meal causes accumulation of lipid in the liver," wrote Sailen Mookerjea, of the medical research department of Charles H. Best Institute, University of Toronto. He stated that experiments conducted by him and his colleagues, as well as those reported in the *Journal of Lipid Research* (7: 10, 1966) show that "the increase of liver lipids within one or two days of choline deprivation, uncomplicated by unnecessary manipulations, has always been an irreproachable fact."

Richard H. Follis, Jr., M.D., explained why in his book, *Deficiency Diseases* (Springfield, Illinois: Charles C. Thomas, 1958). He noted that fats must leave the liver in the form of phospholipids. When choline is deficient in the diet, this phospholipid turnover is reduced. Choline, he added, also enables the liver to burn up fatty acids. "By these two mechanisms," wrote Dr. Follis, "the liver cells are normally able to clear themselves of fatty acids which are brought to them by the bloodstream, whether from ingested lipids or from the breakdown of fats elsewhere, particularly in the deposits of subcutaneous tissues and other areas."

But if choline is not available, fat droplets settle within the liver cells, where they may form cyst-like structures. This fatty infiltration inhibits the liver's ability to detoxify substances that enter the bloodstream, to metabolize proteins and carbohydrates, or to regulate the electrolyte balance in the body's tissues. In time, the whole body may eventually become diseased by poisons that the liver has been unable to eliminate.

Such a situation is less likely to occur if the diet contains a maximum of choline and a minimum of fats. A study demonstrating the combined effect of choline deficiency and excessive fat upon the liver was conducted by N.W. King, D.V.M., an assistant pathologist at the United States Army Medical Research and Nutrition Laboratory in Denver, Colorado. The *American Journal of Clinical Nutrition* (January 1965) gave an account of the significant experiment.

Dr. King observed that rats fed a choline-deficient diet developed "severe" damage—30 to 40 percent of the cells composing the liver lobules became infiltrated with fat. Half the rats in this group also received fat injections which caused 75 to 80 percent of these cells to fill with fat droplets. When choline was added to the diet, the changes were not as severe. The livers of rats fed a diet rich in choline throughout the duration of the experiment appeared normal in every way.

In humans, also, choline supplements have been found to diminish a fatty condition called liver steatosis. The *American*

*Medical Association Journal* (24 February 1951) reported that two groups of infants suffering from this ailment were put on a high protein, low fat diet. One group also received choline supplements, and was reported to have "had less fatty infiltration after a given length of time."

## Deficiency Can Raise Blood Pressure or Lower Resistance

A choline deficiency may also cause a rise in blood pressure, which can be reduced by adding choline to the diet, as shown by a report in the *Journal of Vitaminology* (vol. 3, 106, 1957). When 158 patients suffering from hypertension were given choline, those who suffered from headaches, dizziness, palpitations, and constipation got partial or complete relief within ten days. Blood pressure in all the patients dropped by the third week, at which time it was down to normal in one third of the patients. Had those patients been getting enough choline throughout their lives, they might well have avoided hypertension and its accompanying discomforts altogether.

The *American Journal of Public Health* (March 1966) published a paper by W. Stanley Hartroft, M.D., Ph.D., professor of physiology at the University of Toronto, which was first presented at the ninety-third annual meeting of the American Public Health Association in Chicago in October, 1965. In it, Dr. Hartroft reported that lack of choline was found to set young rats on the path to high blood pressure. More important, such a deficiency probably does the same thing to human infants.

Choline is also one of the three B-complex factors identified by a team of researchers at the Massachusetts Institute of Technology as being of enormous importance in building lifelong resistance to disease. Reporting in *Science News* (17 August 1974), Paul Newberne, M.D., and his associates named choline, folic acid, and vitamin B₁₂, along with the amino acid methionine as key nutrients in the development of the immune system.

Dr. Newberne's studies have shown that it only takes a slight deficiency of these nutrients in pregnant animals to shortchange the immune system of their offspring. Although they appear perfectly normal at birth, in later life they turn out to be more susceptible to infections than the offspring of plentifully nourished mothers. Also, there is reason to believe that they are also more likely to succumb to cancer.

What is true of these laboratory animals, is very probably true of humans, too. "Even a subtle impairment in the immune system may open a child to disease later in life," said Dr. Newberne. "The many unexplained illnesses in children, and the wide variation among children in their susceptibility to illness may very possibly be explained by what their mothers ate during pregnancy."

From a biochemical standpoint, all four nutrients are classified as lipotropes, and are involved in a very basic metabolic process known as the transfer of methyl groups. Perhaps more to the point, all four substances are also needed for the synthesis of nucleic acids in the formation of new cells. That means that even a slight shortage of these nutrients could—theoretically—interfere with the extremely rapid growth of the fetus.

In fact, Dr. Newberne and his research team found just such retarded growth in the thymus glands and other organs of the lymph system in their test animals. The lymph system, and especially the thymus, is crucial to the body's immune response in fighting infection.

Although the animals born to mothers marginally deficient in these nutrients appeared to be normal, later autopsy revealed that their thymus glands were only three-fifths the size of the glands in animals born to properly nourished mothers.

This reduction in thymus size was linked to an even more dramatic difference in resistance. When the control (well-nourished) animals were infected with salmonella bacteria, three out of 20 died. Among the animals whose mothers were just slightly deficient, 14 out of 20 died—almost five times as many.

# Choline Plentiful in Lecithin

Choline is a basic constituent of lecithin, the emulsified phospholipid (combination of fatty acids and phosphorus). Its most common source in the average diet is egg yolk, although abundant supplies of lecithin are also contained in soybeans.

It is very important to note that human breast milk also contains lecithin, while cow's milk is lacking in it. Apparently, the infant whose mother does not nurse him, but raises him on a cow's formula, has a vastly increased chance of developing a deficiency in choline, which is in short supply at birth. In light of the studies just discussed—Dr. Hartroft's study linking an early choline deficiency with high blood pressure, and Dr. Newberne's study demonstrating choline's importance in the early development of the immune system—breast feeding would appear to be an important step in insuring a child against a host of possible ills.

Breast feeding is just the beginning of a lifetime of good nutrition. As far as choline is concerned, eggs and soybeans should become important in one's diet. Liver and brewer's yeast are also good sources. Each gram of desiccated liver contains about 10 mg. of choline, while brewer's yeast contains 2.4 to 3.6 mg. per gram. While no official intake of choline has been set, estimates of the amount contained in a good diet vary from 500 to 900 mg. a day.

Choline should be taken as part of the B complex, because of its interaction with other B vitamins. It is closely related to inositol, another constituent of lecithin, and its relationship with folic acid and $B_{12}$ has been pointed out.

What should not be in a diet is just as important as what should be in it. According to Adelle Davis, too many calories, particularly from alcohol and refined sugar, greatly increase the need for choline. Alcohol inhibits normal blood flow and keeps fat from being absorbed the way it normally would, while it dumps extra calories into the body and uses up vital supplies of several nutrients, including choline.

## Common Foods Rich in Choline

No standard food composition tables are available as yet from the United States Department of Agriculture for this vitamin, but the following foods are generally recognized as the richest sources.

| | |
|---|---|
| Brewer's yeast | Beef liver |
| Fish | Eggs |
| Soybeans | Wheat germ |
| Peanuts | Lecithin |

# CHAPTER 45

# PABA, the Vitamin within a Vitamin

Para-aminobenzoic acid (PABA) is one of the lesser-known constituents of the B complex. It is unique among vitamins in that it is actually a vitamin within another vitamin. Within the body, PABA forms one of the basic constituents of folic acid. PABA also stimulates intestinal bacteria to produce folic acid, and is involved in the utilization of pantothenic acid.

The need for PABA has not yet been established, and some authorities question its status as a true vitamin. Yet PABA is an important part of the B complex. Not only is it needed by folic acid and pantothenic acid; it also functions as a coenzyme in the metabolism of proteins and the production of blood cells. PABA is found with other B vitamins in such rich sources as liver, yeast, wheat germ, molasses, and eggs. The vitamin can also be synthesized by intestinal bacteria.

What we know about PABA we know mostly because it is, in chemists' terms, antagonistic to the sulfa drugs. In the body, substances are linked together in chains of molecules. The substances that make up the sulfa drugs are almost the same as those that make up PABA. When the sulfa drugs are taken into the body they combine with other protein substances in the digestive tract. Because they are so much like PABA chemically, they will naturally combine with the same substances PABA should combine with. If the sulfa drugs get there first, and if they are there in greater quantity than PABA, they will crowd out the vitamin. On the other hand, if PABA is present in greater quantities and manages to combine first, the sulfa drugs will become ineffective.

Thus, it is possible that taking sulfa drugs may induce a deficiency not only of PABA, but of folic acid and pantothenic acid as well. Curiously, the possible side effects of sulfa drugs—digestive disorders, nervousness, and depression—are also symptoms of deficiencies in these B vitamins.

Although no need in human nutrition has been established for PABA, it has been found to have great therapeutic value as a sunscreen and a possible preventive for skin cancer (see index). The vitamin has also been successfully used as a treatment for another skin disorder, vitiligo (see index).

---

### Common Foods Rich in Para-aminobenzoic Acid

No standard food composition tables are available as yet from the United States Department of Agriculture for this vitamin, but the following foods are generally recognized as the richest sources.

| | |
|---|---|
| Liver | Brewer's yeast |
| Eggs | Wheat germ |
| Molasses | |

---

# VITAMIN C AND
# THE BIOFLAVONOIDS

# CHAPTER 46

# The Universal Antitoxin

Throughout the medical profession there is widespread disbelief that there can be such a thing as a general detoxicant, and one that is a vitamin at that. Doctors tend to hold, with good reason, that a chemical (and ascorbic acid, like every other substance, has its own specific chemistry) reacts with other particular chemicals. No chemical reacts with everything.

How, then, can vitamin C help to detoxify all kinds of toxic substances? Obviously, it can only do so indirectly by reinforcing the hundreds of defenses the body naturally possesses. And why vitamin C should have this remarkable effect has finally been explained convincingly for the first time.

Irwin Stone, the man to whom Linus Pauling dedicated his book, *Vitamin C and the Common Cold* (San Francisco: W.H. Freeman, 1970), doesn't believe that vitamin C is a vitamin at all. And he doesn't believe that the vitamin C deficiency disease, scurvy, should be so classified or regarded as a nutritional disorder. In fact, he argues, the prevailing concept of ascorbic acid as "vitamin C" (which cures scurvy when given in trace amounts) is the single biggest reason why medical research has failed to test the therapeutic value of ascorbic acid given in massive doses—doses which are logically called for under a quite different concept of what ascorbic acid is all about.

Stone, who is a biochemist and author of *The Healing Factor* (New York: Grosset and Dunlap, 1972), explains that man's dietary need for ascorbic acid is a biological accident. And a human being's chronic shortage of ascorbic acid—a shortage which becomes extreme in the case of scurvy—is the consequence of a genetic disease, which he calls hypoascorbemia. We inherit hypoascorbemia from a remote primate ancestor who suffered the "biochemical catastrophe" of a mutation (damage to a gene) which destroyed a liver enzyme necessary for ascorbic acid synthesis. Almost all mammals possess this enzyme (L-gulonolactone oxidase) and manufacture their own ascorbic acid—and so did man's ancestor before the mutation took place.

Although the species became totally dependent on food for its ascorbic acid needs, Stone says, it is nevertheless incorrect, biologically speaking, to define ascorbic acid as a nutrient or vitamin; rather it is a "missing endogenous product"—that is, a substance "normally" synthesized within the body.

In judging how much ascorbic acid is required for optimum human health, we should be guided by how much is synthesized by "normal" mammals. Stone points out that mammals produce ascorbic acid plentifully, saturating blood and tissue, and—most important—stepping up production under conditions of stress when the body draws most heavily on its ascorbic acid stores.

Stone suggests "correction" of man's genetic disease, hypoascorbemia, by ascorbic acid intake in an amount comparable to that produced by other mammals—in other words, in the amount humans would be synthesizing for themselves had the genetic defect never occurred. These amounts are measured in grams—not the milligrams of the Food and Nutrition Board's Recommended Daily Allowances.

Infectious diseases, cardiovascular disorders, collagen diseases, cancer, and the aging process—these are some of the human ills, Stone says, that scanty evidence suggests might be unequivocally moderated by ascorbic acid given at the dosage level called for by the genetic concept. For conclusive evidence, he calls on the medical community to test his theory with widespread clinical studies.

# A Lone Investigator

In the mid-1930s, Stone developed for his laboratory the use of ascorbic acid as an antioxidant for food preservation—receiving a patent for the process that is now widely in use. But it was the medical rather than the industrial use of ascorbic acid that fascinated him, sending him to haunt New York's medical libraries, comb and analyze research as reported in the medical literature, and eventually come to his conclusion that the vitamin C concept, with its presumptions about "trace" amounts, is all wrong.

Acting on his own convictions, Stone (and the rest of his family) began taking daily doses of ascorbic acid in large amounts, working up to between three and five grams daily as compared with 60 mg. in the Recommended Daily Allowances. The size of the dose Stone calculated from the amount of ascorbic acid synthesized by the rat—equivalent to 4.9 grams a day for man and 15 grams under conditions of stress.

In 1960, when Stone was the victim of a near-fatal automobile accident, he upped his dosage to the even higher stress levels of 30 to 40 grams a day and succeeded in leaving the hospital in three months instead of the full year predicted by his physician. Except for the accident, Stone comments, he has enjoyed vibrant health under his ascorbic acid regime and has suffered no illness, not even the common cold.

As to any possible "toxicity" of ascorbic acid in large doses, Stone points to ascorbic's acid's long-documented record as "the least toxic of any known substance of comparable physiological activity." Furthermore, he elaborates, while human investigators have not tested the safety of large amounts of ascorbic acid taken over long periods of time, nature has.

"There is good evolutionary reason," he writes, "for (ascorbic acid's) complete lack of toxicity. Living organisms have been exposed to fairly high levels of ascorbic acid throughout eons of time, if this can be judged from its widespread occurrence in all forms of present-day life from the simplest to the most complex. If ascorbic acid had any toxicity that would have been detrimental to survival, it would have been eliminated long ago by the evolutionary process."

# A Genetic Accident

Only a very few species throughout the entire animal and plant world have lost their ability to synthesize ascorbic acid. Among animals, only man and other higher primates, the guinea pig, an Indian fruit-eating bat, and a bird (the red-vented bulbul) are known to be dependent on food for their ascorbic acid needs and can contract and die of scurvy.

Now, there is little disagreement that a past mutation is responsible in each case for this deviant physiology. Stone is certainly not the first to suggest it. Where he offers a new insight is in seeing man as continuing to be disabled, handicapped, in fact, "diseased" by his ancestor's genetic accident.

We must presume that, originally, the mutation presented no problems to the species because of ample food stores of ascorbic acid in year-round vegetation. (A gorilla living in a comparable habitat is estimated to consume about 4.5 grams of ascorbic acid in his daily enormous intake of vegetation.) In the case of man's ancestor, we must even presume that the mutated individuals had an actual survival advantage over their brothers whose liver enzyme, L-gulonolactone oxidase, remained intact—otherwise the latter group would have been the one to have survived to the twentieth century. Discussing this matter in his book, Linus Pauling points to geneticists' finding that there is biological "economy" with survival value in losing a physiological function, providing the species can adjust to the change without disadvantage.

But what happens when an advantageous situation changes?

"As soon as man or his primitive ancestors left their original tropical or semitropical environment and moved to the temperate climes where fresh vegetation was no longer available the year round, they were in trouble," Stone writes. And the dietary habits they developed only compounded their distress. "With the discovery of fire and the development of cooking, the fresh raw meat and fish of man's early diet which were fairly rich sources of exogenous ascorbic acid lost much of this vital substance because of its sensitivity to heat-enhanced oxidation. . . . Primitive agriculture with its emphasis on the easily storable cereal crops provided foodstuffs essentially devoid of any ascorbic acid.''

Stone theorizes: "It is mute testimony to the ruggedness and adaptability of the human organism that man was able to survive on such low levels of ascorbic acid compared with the amounts produced by other mammals. Survive he did, but the toll in disease, misery, and death must have been great.''

Scurvy has caused more deaths, Stone speculates, and created more human misery and has altered the course of human history more than any other single cause. For centuries, scurvy has been associated with dietary needs. For the past half century, as the nutritional sciences and the vitamin theory developed, the accepted explanation of scurvy is that it is a nutritional disorder due to the lack of the trace nutrient, vitamin C, in foodstuffs.

But the *true* cause of scurvy (as well as of less obvious forms of ascorbic acid deprivation) is the missing enzyme, according to Stone. Hypoascorbemia fits perfectly into the genetic disease classification: "A disease caused by an inherited defect in the gene which controls the synthesis of the particular enzyme whose absence or lack of activity causes the specific pathologic metabolic syndrome.''

As Stone observes, there is more to his contention than a fascinating concept or a mere matter of semantics: "The genetic concept provides a new rationale for the therapeutic use of high levels of ascorbic acid either alone or in combination with other medicaments, and opens vistas of clinical testing in many areas that have lain fallow in the decades since the discovery of ascorbic acid (1932).''

# CHAPTER 47

# This Physician Names
# Megadoses As the Norm

A very frightened man burst into the office of Fred R. Klenner, M.D., of Reidsville, North Carolina, complaining of severe chest pains and shortness of breath. The man thought he was dying. After hearing that the man had been stung or bitten by a bug about ten minutes earlier, Dr. Klenner gave him an injection of calcium gluconate, thinking that the man had been attacked by a black widow spider. But that didn't work, and the man remained in agony.

Seeing that the man had an adverse reaction to the injection, Dr. Klenner immediately pulled 12 grams of vitamin C into a 50 cc. syringe and gave the man an injection. Even before the injection was completed, the man began to experience relief from the symptoms. He was sent home and returned later with an object that looked like a mouse. It was an inch-and-a-half long with long brown hair. There was a dark ridge running down the entire back. It had several pairs of legs and a tail much like a mouse. The next day, Dr. Klenner had "the thing" identified as a Puss caterpillar. This unusual caterpillar left 44 red raised marks on the back of its victim. In Dr. Klenner's words, "Except for vitamin C, this individual would have died from shock and asphyxiation."

For the past generation, this iconoclastic southern doctor has been waging virtually a one-man war against the Washington establishment with his "radical" views on vitamin C. He is convinced massive doses of vitamin C are an absolute necessity in the body's 24-hour-per-day struggle against the ravages of illnesses ranging from pneumonia to burns to diabetes and even overdoses of barbiturates.

And when Dr. Klenner uses the word "massive," he means just that. He has been known to give a woman suffering from pneumonia 140 grams—almost five ounces—of vitamin C and had her recover within 72 hours! That's 140,000 mg. But the patient was well in three days.

According to a report in the *Journal of Applied Nutrition* (Winter 1971), Dr. Klenner presented a survey of available literature on vitamin C and cited a number of cases he treated himself. In addition the doctor criticized the minimum daily requirements, calling them an "illegitimate child" co-fathered by the National Academy of Sciences and the National Research Council and representing "a tragic error in judgment. There are many factors which increase the demand by the body for ascorbic acid (such as stress), and unless these are appreciated, at least by physicians, there can be no real progress."

Based on what science has learned, according to Dr. Klenner, it is no longer possible to set a numerical unit in terms of minimal daily requirements—if indeed it ever was. The simple fact is, as he notes, people are different. The same people experience different situations at various times. With vitamin C, what may be adequate today means little or nothing in terms of tomorrow's needs.

## Combats Carbon Monoxide

Dr. Klenner has found that vitamin C is of value in dealing with the environmental pollutant carbon monoxide, thrown off by automobiles. He said clinical experience suggests that if sufficient ascorbic acid is suddenly placed into the bloodstream—12 to 50 grams—that through "flash oxidation" a concentration is made high enough to pull carbon monoxide from hemoglobin to form carbon dioxide. This reaction is similar to the one a patient gets when given pure oxygen from a tank.

Not many of us, of course, are foolish enough to run our engines in closed garages and get critically poisoned by carbon monoxide. But wherever there is heavy traffic, the accumulations of this poison gas are great enough, in the opinions of some experts, to make us all suffer from mild chronic carbon monoxide poisoning. Those of us, that is, who do not have enough vitamin C in our systems to counteract the odorless, tasteless, invisible, but deadly gas.

Pregnant women can benefit from large doses of vitamin C too. For example, Dr. Klenner observed over 300 consecutive obstetrical cases using supplemental vitamin C by mouth. The lowest amount of ascorbic acid he used was four grams and the highest amount 15 grams each day. He estimates requirements are roughly four grams during the first trimester of pregnancy, six grams during the second and 10 during the third. As a result of supplemental ascorbic acid by mouth, hemoglobin levels were much easier to maintain. Leg cramps were less than three percent and were always associated with the patient's running out of vitamin C tablets.

In addition, the capacity of the skin to resist pressure of an expanding uterus was improved. Labor was shorter and less painful. There were no postpartum hemorrhages. No patient required catheterization, evidence of the diuretic effect of vitamin C. Also, there were no toxic manifestations over the 300 pregnancies.

## Vitamin C for Other Trauma

Dr. Klenner also found that vitamin C is an absolute must in the treatment of burns, both internally and externally. He uses a three percent ascorbic acid solution as a spray over the entire area of the burn. This is used every two to four hours for a period of five days. The external use of vitamin C is combined with massive doses of ascorbic acid by injection and mouth. For example, Dr. Klenner would give a 220-pound burn victim at least 50 grams of vitamin C burn solution every eight hours for the first several days, then continue the treatment at 12-hour intervals as indicated.

Dr. Klenner is even more emphatic about massive vitamin C dosages in patients having diabetes mellitus. He found that 60 percent of all diabetics could be controlled with diet and 10 grams of ascorbic acid daily. The other 40 percent will still need insulin—but considerably less than would be expected—and less medication overall. He observed "every diabetic not taking supplemental vitamin C could be classified as having subclinical scurvy. For this reason they find it difficult to heal wounds. The diabetic patient will use the supplemental vitamin C for better utilization of his insulin. It will assist the liver in the metabolism of carbohydrates and reinstate his body to heal wounds like normal individuals."

Dr. Klenner also believes that vitamin C is necessary for patients undergoing surgery. He found that samples of blood taken six hours after surgery showed drops of approximately one-quarter the starting amount. At 12 hours, the levels were down to one-half. Samples taken 24 hours later, without ascorbic acid added to the fluids, showed levels three-quarters lower than the original samples.

A researcher named Schunacher (*Ohio State Medical Journal*, 42: 1248, 1946) is cited by Dr. Klenner as having reported that the preoperative use of as little as 500 mg. of vitamin C given orally "was remarkably successful in preventing shock and weakness" following dental extractions. Other investigators, according to Dr. Klenner, have shown in both laboratory and clinical studies that optimal primary wound healing is dependent to a large extent upon the vitamin C content of the tissues.

In experimental work, guinea pigs fed a diet free of ascorbic acid showed a 600 percent acceleration in cholesterol formation in the adrenal glands. Dr. Klenner found cholesterol levels could be controlled when daily intakes of ascorbic acid were high. By taking ten grams or more of vitamin C each day you can eat all the eggs you want, according to Dr. Klenner.

It has been suggested that ascorbic acid metabolism may be an index of total metabolism and a diagnostic guide. His recommendations are, therefore, that adults "taking at least 10 grams of ascorbic acid daily and children under 10 at least one gram for each year of life, will find that the brain will be clearer, the mind more active, the body less wearied, and the memory more retentive."

# Emergency Procedure

Dr. Klenner summed up his philosophy towards vitamin C at the October, 1972 meeting of the International Academy of Preventive Medicine: "I have seen children dead in less than two hours after hospital admission, having received no treatment simply because the attending physicians were not impressed with their illness. A few grams of ascorbic acid given by needle while they waited for laboratory procedures or examinations to fit their schedule would have saved their lives. I know this to be a fact because I have been in similar situations, and by routinely applying massive doses of ascorbic acid, I have seen death take a holiday."

Dr. Klenner believes that it should be a rule of medicine for large doses of vitamin C to be given in all pathological conditions, while the physician ponders a diagnosis. The reason for this treatment has been backed by hundreds of cases under his supervision, he said. "Victims of house fires, especially children, succumb more often to monoxide poison which is overlooked in this course of treating the burn. A dose of 500 mg. per kilogram of body weight of vitamin C given intravenously will immediately neutralize the monoxide poisoning and there will be a major factor in stopping the development of third degree burns."

Nobel prize winner Dr. Linus Pauling, at the same meeting, commented, "I must say I found it astonishing that at this late date, 40 years after ascorbic acid was recognized as vitamin C, we still do not really know reliably what the optimum intake of ascorbic acid is. There are great differences of opinion."

The Food and Nutrition Board of the National Academy of Sciences Research Council has advocated 60 mg. for an adult male per day, Dr. Pauling pointed out. "I have been taking 6,000 mg. a day and I may well increase my intake because I have faith in Dr. Klenner, who takes 20,000 mg. a day. I think he may well be right. There is very good evidence about this."

The question of how much vitamin C should be taken remains an enigma. Only two animals have been studied to determine exactly how much they manufacture in their bodies, the rat and the housefly. The rat manufactures vitamin C at a rate ranging from two grams a day to as high as 15 grams a day under stress calculated in relation to a person who weighs 154 pounds. If you had a 154-pound housefly, it would manufacture 10 grams of vitamin C a day, Dr. Pauling said.

"These theoretical considerations lead us to the conclusion that the animals would not manufacture more vitamin C than is needed for good health, and in fact that they would manufacture less than would correspond to the optimum health. Accordingly," Dr. Pauling continued, "this rather large figure, 100 times the Recommended Daily Allowance, can be considered as the lower limit."

# CHAPTER 48

# How the Blood
# Uses Vitamin C

This moment, as you sit reading, you are surrounded by millions upon millions of tiny, unseen microorganisms, many of which can cause disease. They cannot be eliminated, even by the sterilization procedures of a hospital. Attempts at wholesale elimination have always been disastrous, upsetting the natural balance through which various species of bacteria control each other. Since bacteria can't be wiped out, our health and in many cases our very survival hinges upon the ability to coexist with these ever-present, potentially dangerous germs without letting them take charge in our bodies.

Yet the body, for many reasons, cannot depend completely on natural balance for protection against hostile organisms. One strain can get out of hand for a while, causing serious infective disease. Some types of bacteria are such deadly outlaws that our bodies have to take a "shoot on sight" attitude.

For such situations, it is the white cells of the blood that are our chief defense. The blood goes everywhere. Let any organism or material be recognized as hostile, and the white cells attack it, literally digesting it to put it out of commission. Without this protection we could not exist.

Studies have shown that for the height of activity and effectiveness, the white cells of the blood require a rich supply of vitamin C.

## Direct Stimulator of White Cell Activity

Lawrence R. DeChatelet, Ph.D., Charles E. McCall, M.D., and M. Robert Cooper, M.D., of the departments of biochemistry and medicine at the Bowman-Gray School of Medicine in Winston-Salem, N.C., reported to the sixty-second meeting of the American Society of Biological Chemists at San Francisco in June of 1970 that initial results of experiments indicated that ascorbic acid has a direct role in the killing of bacteria by white blood cells. Not only that, they said, but ascorbic acid added to isolated white cells also stimulated greater defensive activity than that observed in normal, healthy cells, and triggered a similar reaction in diseased cells previously known to be incapable of killing bacteria.

Their report came practically on the heels of Dr. Linus Pauling's book, *Vitamin C and the Common Cold* (San Francisco: W. H. Freeman and Company, 1970), in which the world-renowned chemist and twice Nobel Prize winner advocated taking large doses of vitamin C daily to protect against colds and improve health generally by aiding body resistance to germs and reducing susceptibility to infections.

For more than 30 years medical researchers have known that the white blood cells which respond to bacterial invasion in the bloodstream accumulate ascorbic acid, the pure form of vitamin C. And it's no secret to anybody who can read a newspaper that vitamin C has been called the best protection against colds and other infections. But nobody has been able to show that the ascorbic acid in white blood cells is directly involved in the fight against bacterial infection—until now.

Not all bacteria are harmful. For example, we must have certain types of bacteria in our intestines at all times if our food is to be completely digested and assimilated. Outside our bodies bacteria are used in fermentation, they improve the soil by fixing atmospheric nitrogen into the ground, and they break down dead matter into soluble food for plants as well. However, if you eat food that has been decayed and contaminated by bacteria, the result is often fatal food poisoning. Other types of bacteria, if they catch hold in the body, may result in a whole range of diseases that include pneumonia, tonsillitis, tuberculosis, and diphtheria. It is these latter kinds of bacteria that must be destroyed as soon as they enter the body. Otherwise, an infection sets in.

When bacteria enter the bloodstream, certain white blood cells called phagocytes attack, engulf, and kill them, the process being known as phagocytosis. However, the bacteria can also get the upper hand when the body's defensive network is not up to par. If you have ever suffered a raw, sore throat, then you've acquired first-hand experience in what happens when the body is unable to throw off a bacterial infection right away.

Dr. DeChatelet and associates studied the process of phagocytosis by testing the reactions of phagocytes before and after ascorbic acid was added to the blood cell samples. They knew that three types of metabolic activity take place during phagocytosis: oxygen is used up, hydrogen peroxide is produced, and a series of biochemical reactions known collectively as the hexose monophosphate shunt (HMS), by which the body uses glucose, also steps up its normal pace. But why these activities occur, or how they are related to the bactericidal aspect of phagocytosis, remained a mystery.

So the three researchers isolated human and animal phagocytes, adding foreign particles to these samples to test the rate of response to invaders. They noted that human white cells increased HMS activity six-fold as they engulfed the intruders. Rabbit cells, when foreign particles were added, doubled their shunt activity.

Then they took a comparable sampling of human and rabbit cells, but this time added ascorbic acid to the resting phagocytes instead. When they did, the HMS activity when measured was found to be even greater than the response usually noted when the cells are involved in defending the body. In other words, ascorbic acid increased the biochemical activity which is directly associated with killing bacteria.

Further investigation showed that when an oxidated form of ascorbic acid, called dehydroascorbic acid, was added to these resting cells, the HMS stimulation which indicates a fighting response to invaders increased even more than when plain ascorbic acid was added.

The research team proposed that when ascorbic acid is added to the phagocytes it is first changed into dehydroascorbic acid, which explains the increased oxygen consumption associated with phagocytosis, while hydrogen peroxide is formed and the hexose monophosphate shunt activity is increased.

It stands to reason that since white blood cells use ascorbic acid under normal circumstances, and since ascorbic acid has been postulated to be responsible for the killing mechanism of phagocytosis, that when the body is besieged by a wave of infectious bacteria, such as the kind that cause tonsillitis, the need for ascorbic acid rises and can only be filled if the body is getting enough vitamin C with which to wage the battle.

## Diseased Cells May Be Returned to Normal

The most gratifying discovery made by the Bowman-Gray researchers came when they studied leukocytes, or white cells, that were taken from a patient suffering from a rare disease of childhood known as chronic granulomatous disease, a condition in which the white blood cells are unable to kill bacteria. Instead, the phagocytes respond to infection by engulfing the bacteria, but then nothing else happens. The bacteria, although surrounded, travel the bloodstream throughout the body and may establish an infection anywhere, while impotent white cells are helpless to do anything about it.

Significantly, the researchers noted that these diseased white cells, when particles were added to them, showed no increase in hydrogen peroxide or HMS activity, both of which are associated with the killing of bacteria under normal conditions. However, when a little ascorbic acid was added to samples of the isolated, diseased white cells, increased HMS activity was initiated to 400 percent of that which occurred when foreign particles were added. "This observation suggests a therapeutic potential for this vitamin. . . ." the trio reported, and they are now studying whether the killing power of chronic granulomatous disease leukocytes can be improved with vitamin C.

This most recent study helps to explain countless, previous, successful administrations of vitamin C as an antibiotic. For example, Fred R. Klenner, M.D., told the Tri-State Medical Association of the Carolinas and Virginia in February of 1951 that as infection gets worse, the body's need for vitamin C mounts, and body tissues are depleted. What vitamin C there is in food, he said, is rapidly used up fighting infection.

Dr. Klenner, in his book, *The Key to Good Health: Vitamin C,* with F. H. Bartz (Chicago: Graphic Arts Research Foundation, 1969) tells about his experiences in treating patients—who had both viral and bacterial infections—with from one to 20 grams of ascorbic acid per day. Long before that, he reported in the *Journal of Applied Nutrition* (vol. 6, 1953), in an article entitled, "The Use of Vitamin C as an Antibiotic," that he had successfully treated cases of measles, virus pneumonia, encephalitis, and poliomyelitis with massive doses of vitamin C.

Another early report showed ascorbic acid to be a more potent germ fighter than bactericidal drugs such as hydrogen peroxide. In the *Annals of the Pasteur Institute* (102, No. 3, 278–291, 1962) four of the Institute's research workers reported experiments with *Escherichia coli,* one of the most common of the food poisoning bacteria, which often shows up in precooked frozen foods that have been thawed and then refrozen. Comparing the effect on *E. coli* of hydrogen peroxide, ferrous sulphate, and ascorbic acid, the Pasteur Institute researchers found that ascorbic acid would not only destroy as many bacteria as the other two known germicides, but would also destroy the poisonous bacteria considerably faster than the other two.

In most cases, the beneficial effects of nutrients are noticed long before the biochemical explanations for these effects are uncovered. But that doesn't mean we should wait for a chemist or biologist to come up with a precise reason why eating a particular food or supplementing our diet with additional nutrients in tablet form does us good. The scientist who told us 10 years ago that we needed only 50 or 60 mg. of vitamin C a day, and that there was no evidence of additional benefits from added amounts, is today conceding that several thousand mg. a day may well be valuable.

Scientific studies into the biochemical effects of nutrients in our bodies are certainly welcome. If additional experiments support the initial findings of the Bowman-Gray researchers, perhaps their work will spark a new round of investigations into more reasons why vitamin C is so important in maintaining good health.

# CHAPTER 49

# Does It Really Prevent Colds?

Should you take vitamin C to prevent colds this winter? Yes, indeed. Should you take it in extraordinary quantities, far beyond the recommendations of the Food and Drug Administration and the National Academy of Science? You certainly should if you want the vitamin to give you real protection against colds. And will it really keep you from getting colds all winter long? Maybe. And maybe not.

No, it is not a contradiction, any more than it is a contradiction to say that dogs and cats have far better natural resistance to colds than we do, while recognizing that dogs and cats do sometimes get colds. It has frequently been pointed out by such authorities as Linus Pauling and Irwin Stone that dogs and cats, like practically all other mammals except man, synthesize their own vitamin C at a rate that, pound for pound, would translate into something like 11 or 12 grams a day (11,000 to 12,000 mg.) for an average man. And there is little doubt remaining that this ability to synthesize vitamin C and increase the amount synthesized when necessary, affords most animals superb protection against viral infections of the upper respiratory tract, otherwise known as the common cold.

By such simple observable facts we can easily see that vitamin C does not afford complete protection against colds, but that those who are well fortified with the vitamin are far less likely to spend their winters nursing stuffed and runny noses, sinus headaches, coughs, sore throats, and general discomfort.

The reason is nearly as obvious as the fact, if we go into a standard medical textbook, *The Cecil-Loeb Textbook of Medicine* (Philadelphia: W.B. Saunders Company, 1971). The section on the common cold by George Gee Jackson, M.D., states that "many viruses and some nonviral filter-passing agents can cause the common cold. No single strain of virus accounts for more than a small proportion of the illnesses." Dr. Jackson estimates that there are well over 100 viruses that can cause infections of the respiratory tract in man, as well as some nonviral agents. And that, of course, is the reason that controversy exists. If we suppose that vitamin C, in very large doses, is effective against 90 cold-causing viruses, or even 100, that would still leave a few viruses against which it is not effective. And if it is effective against all the cold-causing viruses, there are still the nonviral agents. We can be quite sure that vitamin C will never prevent all colds from all sources, and we can be quite sure that there will always be some doctors who will try it on one patient, find it ineffective, and conclude that vitamin C has no value against colds.

## Recognition of Cold-Prevention Factor in Vitamin C

Researchers and some practicing physicians have long been aware of the role that vitamin C plays in the prevention of the common cold. A letter in the prestigious *British Medical Journal* (21 April 1951), from Drs. John M. Fletcher and Isobel C. Fletcher expressed surprise that there was not more material appearing in medical journals on the potency of vitamin C in protecting against cold germs. The two physicians wrote that in their own practice they found vitamin C excellent for that purpose. The profession's indifference to using the vitamin as a cold preventive, the doctors suggested, might be due to the difficulty among the experts in reaching agreement on the actual daily requirement of vitamin C.

It fell to a world-renowned Nobel Laureate, Linus Pauling, to provide an acceptable solution to the problem of dosage. In his book, *Vitamin C and the Common Cold* (San Francisco: W. H. Freeman, 1970) Dr. Pauling's statement, buttressed by reasonable, readable, and fascinating information about our need for the nutrient, is very simple: as a regular ongoing practice, take one to three grams of ascorbic acid a day (Dr. Pauling himself takes two grams a day according to the 15 February, 1976 issue of *Modern Medicine*) or approximately 17 to 50 times as much as the traditional Recommended Daily Allowance; at the first sign of a cold symptom, step up your intake of the vitamin by 500 to 1,000 mg. every hour for several hours up to 10 grams a day. The common cold might be eradicated from this country within a few years, Dr. Pauling contends, if the practice he recommends should become general.

Up and down and across the United States, hundreds of thousands of people responded. Vitamin C sales skyrocketed. Druggists and supermarkets were caught with empty shelves. Wholesalers ran short of stock. "The demand for ascorbic acid has now reached the point where it is taxing production capacity," a spokesman for the Merck Chemical Division told the *New York Times* (5 December 1970).

Obviously, to the American public, Dr. Pauling's prescription of vitamin C to control the common cold came as "news." Apparently none of the people who raided the vitamin shelves had ever before thought of protecting themselves against the sniffles and sneezes and coughings and serious aftermaths of a cold through such a simple and harmless method—no drugs, no nose drops, no atomizers, nothing but an essential nutrient that belongs in the human body.

## Massive Doses the Key

The massive doses which Dr. Pauling recommends are the key to his "case" for vitamin C. It is his contention that much past research on the effectiveness of vitamin C in fighting the common cold has been inconclusive—or, rather, not strikingly conclusive—because the vitamin C supplements given to experimental subjects have been too small. Usually in the neighborhood of 200 mg.

Only five to 15 mg. of ascorbic acid are necessary to prevent scurvy (the vitamin C-deficiency disease), Dr. Pauling points out; therefore, doctors oriented to this small amount consider 200 mg. a "large dose" and assume that experiments based on a supplement this size are a fair test. But there's a great difference, the author adds, between the amount needed to prevent death from scurvy and the optimum amount for the best of health. He cites evidence that the optimum amount (varying because of varying individual needs) lies in the range between 250 mg. and 10,000 mg. (10 grams) a day.

## Individual Requirements Vary

Dr. Pauling suggests that each person may test his own individual requirement: if, on one or two grams a day, the individual still comes down with colds, the indication is to step up the preventive dose. Dr. Pauling cites scientific evidence for "a more than 20-fold variation in the need for ascorbic acid," giving particular attention to the studies of Roger Williams, Ph.D., of the University of Texas, who is a specialist in the field of biochemical individuality and the first scientist to identify and synthesize pantothenic acid, one of the important B vitamins.

Dr. Williams pointed out at a meeting of the National Academy of Sciences, on 27 April 1967, that vitamin C requirements vary too much among individuals to rely on blanket recommendations. "By avoidance of individuality in human needs, possibly in an attempt to keep their science pure, medical scientists are overlooking and failing to develop a set of major weapons against disease." The vitamin specialist from the University of Texas also criticized the attitude of the Food and Drug Administration for suggesting that food supplements are valueless for the average person. In Dr. Williams' view this agency is "yielding to an unscientific taboo."

The strong opinions expressed by the Texas scientist were

based on experiments concerning the vitamin C requirements of laboratory-bred guinea pigs. The tests showed a surprising 20-fold range in the vitamin C needs of individual guinea pigs. This difference was apparent even in small groups of animals. Of course, Dr. Williams reasoned, since human beings are the least uniform of all species, "on nonemotional scientific grounds it would appear that interindividual variation in human vitamin C needs is probably just as great."

Examining the evidence, it becomes clear that there is no universal answer to the question: How much vitamin C should I take? For most people, 1,000 mg. a day should be enough to forestall most colds. If it doesn't do the trick, try more. At the first sign of a cold, without delay, start increasing intake. You needn't take more than 100 to 200 mg. at a time, but take it frequently—every hour, or even every half hour. You'll have to discover for yourself the right frequency and the right amount to eliminate colds.

In his book, Dr. Pauling tells us that when our ancestors lived on a diet of green plants, it was possible for them to lose (through mutation) the ability to synthesize their own vitamin C (an ability possessed by almost all animals except the guinea pig and primates) because of the richness of vitamin C in their food. Dr. Pauling checked the amount of vitamin C (per 2,500 kilo-calories of energy, i.e. in one day's food for an adult) in 110 raw natural plant foods and also in 14 plant foods richest in this vitamin. In the two cases, he found respectively a vitamin C content of 2.3 grams and 9.4 grams. These calculations he presents as part of his evidence that man's natural daily need for vitamin C is many, many times greater than the daily allowance recommended by the Food and Nutrition Board.

## Vitamin C Safest Cold Remedy

Dr. Pauling's warnings about the dangers of drug "remedies" for the common cold (as opposed to the non-toxic vitamin C) may alarm many people. However, those people looking for an alternative to many of the over-the-counter remedies and prescription drugs will be the first to salute Dr. Pauling's inspired proposal for labeling cold remedies. Instead of the usual warning *(Keep out of reach of children)*, the Nobel Laureate suggests that cold medicines should be labeled: *Keep this medicine out of reach of everybody. Use ascorbic acid instead!*

Doctors prescribe aspirin and antibiotics for winter illness despite evidence that neither one does much good. Worse than being ineffective, aspirin and antibiotics can actually hurt you. And aspirin, the all-time favorite for cold and fever symptoms, is not the safe, effective, wonder-in-white the TV commercials suggest.

## The Truth About Aspirin

Edith D. Stanley, M.D., of the Infectious Disease Section of the Abraham Lincoln School of Medicine, University of Illinois College of Medicine, Chicago, published a report in the *Journal of the American Medical Association* (24 March 1975) which demonstrated some interesting facts about aspirin.

Volunteers infected with cold viruses, and treated with aspirin, experienced only moderate reduction in severity of symptoms. To be statistically significant, the reductions would have to have been great enough to be obviously accountable to the treatment rather than chance or error. None of the reductions was statistically significant.

What was significant was that volunteers treated with aspirin shed from 17 to 36 percent more viruses than placebo-treated groups. This means that the amount of viruses contained in the nasal discharge of the aspirin-treated volunteers was considerably greater. So persons taking aspirin for relief of their winter illness are increasing the threat of spreading their illness to husbands, wives, children, or co-workers.

Aspirin has also been shown to inhibit the infection-fighting leukocytes from traveling to inflammatory tissue. By suppressing the body's natural response to the infection, aspirin may "relieve" symptoms which are a result of the leukocytes doing battle with the invading viruses. But the reproduction of the virus is left unchecked. At the very least, the person treating his cold with aspirin becomes more likely to spread his cold to someone else. And viruses unchecked by the body's infection response system can spread within the body and prolong or complicate the illness.

## Antibiotics Worse Than Useless

The antibiotics-for-winter-illness picture is no less upsetting. These drugs are no more effective than aspirin, and far more dangerous. Yet in a survey cited by Lester F. Soyka, M.D., in his article on "The Misuse of Antibiotics for Treatment of Upper Respiratory Tract Infections in Children" in the April 1975 issue of *Pediatrics,* 95 percent of physicians surveyed gave patients one or more prescription drugs for the common cold and more than half of those drugs were antibiotics.

Dr. Soyka's paper cites half a dozen controlled studies, all of which demonstrate that antibiotics do not shorten the duration of upper respiratory infections, do not prevent complications or secondary infections, and do not reduce the amount of disease-producing organisms in the nose and throat.

Antibiotics are effective in producing side effects. Vomiting, diarrhea, and skin rash are common. Drug reactions, in which antibiotics often play a prominent role, account for 3 to 5 percent of all hospital admissions. But more sinister is the possibility that use of an antibiotic will sensitize the patient to the drug, thereby preventing future use for a real life-threatening illness.

## Canadian Studies Bolster Vitamin C's Reputation

Terrence W. Anderson, M.A., B.M. (equivalent to M.D.), B. Ch., Ph.D., a noted epidemiologist at the University of Toronto, reported in the *Canadian Medical Association Journal* (5 April 1975), the results of the third of his tests of vitamin C's effectiveness against winter illness. The results showed that vitamin C significantly lessened the severity of illness and reduced by 25 percent the number of days spent indoors because of illness.

Dr. Anderson first set out in 1971 to *disprove* Dr. Linus Pauling's contentions that vitamin C could dramatically reduce the suffering of the common cold. He gave vitamin C to half of the 1,000 subjects, and an inert placebo to the other half in his double-blind study. Dosage was one gram (1,000 mg.) daily increased to four grams during the first three days of any illness.

The results surprised Dr. Anderson. Of the 818 people who stayed with the experiment to the end, those taking vitamin C had 30 percent fewer days in which the illness kept them indoors. And 40 percent more of the vitamin C group were entirely free of illness.

For his most recent study, Dr. Anderson used smaller doses of vitamin C: one 500 mg. tablet each week, increased to three tablets on the first day of an illness, and two tablets on days two through five. Half of the people taking vitamin C received sustained release capsules, half received regular tablets.

Dr. Anderson took great care to insure that the double-blind format of his study was not broken by volunteers who might guess whether they were taking vitamin C or a placebo. Similar tasting tablets were used. And instructions were deliberately phrased to sidetrack suspicious volunteers. Apparently these measures were successful. More than half of both groups, 68 percent, said they didn't know which they were taking. And of those that did profess to know, half were right and half were wrong.

## Reduces All Illness, Not Just Colds

In evaluating the results, Dr. Anderson did not attempt to differentiate between "colds" and a wide range of respiratory maladies. Such symptoms as confinement indoors, days off from work, throat soreness, chest soreness or tightness, feverish feeling, chills, aching limbs, and depression were recorded.

And when the results were in, vitamin C significantly reduced severity of typical winter illness symptoms—especially days confined indoors, chest soreness, feverish feeling, chills, and aching limbs.

Dr. Anderson reported: "There is now little doubt that the intake of additional vitamin C can lead to a reduced burden of 'winter illness'. . . . Furthermore, the effect does not seem to be restricted to 'colds,' for the effect observed was as great or even greater on illness not involving the nose. . . ."

So why hasn't the medical profession scrapped the futile, dangerous use of antibiotics and aspirin? Resistance to the adoption of vitamin C as a treatment for winter illness might be accounted for in several ways. First of all, vitamin C is not promoted by drug companies, because it cannot be exclusively patented. Therefore, competition among vitamin C manufacturers keeps profit margins low relative to patented medicines. High-profit drugs, like antibiotics, are vigorously promoted to doctors in the form of elaborate advertising brochures and free samples. And since doctors obtain most of their information about drugs from drug companies, they are at a disadvantage when it comes to knowing what is really available for what purpose.

Also, there seems to be a real prejudice against vitamin C, perhaps because many of its champions are outside the medical-drug establishment. Many of the early studies which set out to disprove vitamin C's effectiveness failed to report or evaluate beneficial results adequately. For whatever reason, many medical writers go to great lengths to downgrade vitamin C.

In the *Journal of the American Medical Association* of 10 March 1975, Thomas R. Karlowski, M.D., reports the results of a trial at the National Institute of Health in Bethesda, Maryland. No attempt was made to measure the real effect of vitamin C on the whole range of bothersome symptoms associated with winter illness. Unlike Dr. Anderson's study, only an "all or nothing" effect was regarded as worthwhile.

Writes Dr. Karlowski: "It was assumed that there was no need to try to detect a reduction of less than 30 percent because in the possible application of the study results to the general population, less than a 30 percent reduction would not be worth the trouble involved in taking two capsules three times a day."

Dr. Karlowski would do well to let individuals decide for themselves if under 30 percent less sickness is "worthwhile."

## Better Nutrition Could Save Billions of Dollars

If that 25 percent reduction in days of confinement measured in Dr. Anderson's study were duplicated nationwide, the savings would be enormous. No one in the United States has current records of how many work days are lost to winter illness, and the resulting cost. But Canada's annual bill for lost work time because of respiratory illness exceeds $270 million, according to an article in *Nutrition Reviews* (October 1973). The United States, which has a population 10 times that of Canada, might be expected to have a much larger loss. A conservative estimate of the United States' cost based on Canada's figures would be in the neighborhood of two billion dollars.

And that figure does not include the millions of dollars lost because of decreased efficiency on the part of workers who are ill, but who come to work anyway. Nor does it include the cost of doctor bills, the cost of all that useless, dangerous medication, the loss of time and money because of adverse drug reactions, or the inestimable loss of "good times" to days of stay-at-home blahs.

Despite all this, it appears that reducing your "down time" from winter illness is only one small part of the benefits to be gained from vitamin C. Research and clinical experience have established a role for vitamin C in the prevention of a host of common diseases. These benefits range from those which are well proven, such as protecting against the toxicity of certain drugs, to those which are still experimental, such as protecting against cancer.

# CHAPTER 50

# The Perfect Pair
# for Powerhouse Protection
# Against Colds

To bring out the total protective quality of vitamin C, wheat germ should be added to the daily diet, according to Dr. Albert Szent-Gyorgyi, the Nobel Laureate who first isolated vitamin C. In his book, *The Living State* (New York: Academic Press, 1972), Dr. Szent-Gyorgyi describes how, about a year after this great discovery, he became aware that whatever permits ascorbic acid to function in human respiration as it does in plants seemed to be missing in the pure vitamin. Some years later, a friend told Dr. Szent-Gyorgyi that he credited a mixture of yeast and wheat germ eaten for breakfast every day as the reason he had been without colds for several years. Being a chronic sufferer from colds himself, Dr. Szent-Gyorgyi adopted the same breakfast custom and found that he, too, had no more colds.

Dr. Szent-Gyorgyi made an intensive biochemical investigation and found that the only function of the yeast in the mixture was to split the glucosides in the wheat germ. Since the body is able to accomplish this without help, he decided to eliminate the yeast from his breakfast and found that the wheat germ alone is just as successful. In a footnote Dr. Szent-Gyorgyi states that his daily breakfast consists of a sliced banana, over which he pours about two ounces of wheat germ, adding milk. He also drinks tea to which he adds about a gram (1,000 mg.) of ascorbic acid (vitamin C) instead of lemon. In the afternoon he has another cup of tea, once again containing a gram of ascorbic acid.

## Two Ounces or More Daily

Through further investigation Dr. Szent-Gyorgyi was able to establish a complex series of reactions between ascorbic acid and quinones produced by the splitting of the glucosides of wheat germ. These reactions were triggered by the manganese content of the wheat germ. Materials that are present in most plant foods to a very limited extent are present most richly in wheat germ. Thus, it is the belief of Dr. Szent-Gyorgyi that almost any plant food we eat will potentiate our vitamin C intake to some extent, and the vitamin C will have its beneficial effect. But to fully potentiate the large amounts of vitamin C recommended by him and many other renowned scientists, he believes that two ounces or more of wheat germ every day is necessary for the full utilization of vitamin C. "My finding wheat germ useful against colds is not at variance with Dr. Linus Pauling's statements," says Dr. Szent-Gyorgyi. "If one is deficient in two factors, administration of one of them may help to some extent, while full benefit may be derived only by taking the two in combination."

When the scientist speaks of "full benefit," of course, he is talking about far more than merely preventing colds, important as that single activity may be. Dr. Szent-Gyorgyi believes the length, continued good health, and activity of his life are attributable to the combination, and that is certainly more than a matter of just staying free of colds.

Vitamin C, as is explained biochemically in *The Living State*, functions as an antioxidant in relation to a wide variety of materials that we call "toxic" because, if they are permitted to oxidize within our systems, they initiate chain reactions that disrupt the normal orderly processes of life. There are hundreds—perhaps even thousands—of such toxic materials. There are poisonous metals like cadmium and lead. There are toxins produced by harmful bacteria. There are the venoms of insect stings and snake bites. There are numerous viruses like the hundred or so of the common cold.

All the above toxic hazards attack us in essentially the same way. They disrupt the normal activities of the body when they are oxidized. Vitamin C prevents the oxidation. What the wheat germ does is to furnish the vitamin C with otherwise missing chemical elements that permit the vitamin actually to regenerate itself so that it is not used up the first time it functions as an antioxidant, but is able to perform the same protective role many times.

# CHAPTER 51

# Who Are the People
# with Special Needs
# for More Vitamin C?

Most people taking vitamin C want more than just protection against colds. They are seeking all-around optimum health. If this is your desire, you will probably need even more vitamin C if you fall into one of several special categories. There is evidence that smokers, heavy drinkers, diabetics, and those who use aspirin regularly need additional vitamin C.

Consider those categories one by one. If you smoke a pack of cigarettes a day, you can expect to have 25 percent less vitamin C in your blood than a nonsmoker. If you smoke more than one pack a day, the deficiency is close to 40 percent. Those figures apply to men and women alike, and were reported by Omer Pelletier, Ph.D., director of Canada's Bureau of Nutritional Sciences of the Canadian Food Directorate. Dr. Pelletier's findings are based upon a nationwide Canadian survey involving more than 2,000 subjects. According to an article in the *Medical Tribune* (13 November 1974), he found that smokers did not necessarily get any less vitamin C in their diet than non-smokers, but their bodies apparently aren't able to absorb as much.

Anyone drinking a lot of beer, wine, or whiskey is also going to need extra vitamin C. A report by four Scottish doctors in the

*Lancet* (21 September 1974), noted that the liver depends on vitamin C to produce an enzyme—alcohol dehydrogenase—that helps usher alcohol out of the bloodstream. The less vitamin C there is, the longer the body stays polluted.

Researchers at the Coatesville, Pennsylvania Veterans Administration Hospital have reported that vitamin C in conjunction with thiamine and the amino acid cysteine may offer "a means of protection against chronic body insult" caused by drinking and smoking. Dr. Herbert Sprince, who directed the study, says vitamin C helped laboratory rats detoxify otherwise *lethal* doses of acetaldehyde, an alcohol breakdown product also found in tobacco smoke (*Medical Tribune*, 15 May 1974).

## Diabetics, Many Arthritics, Could Do Better with More 'C'

If you are diabetic, your vitamin C requirements are likely to be in excess of other individuals, in the opinion of Dr. George V. Mann, associate professor of biochemistry and medicine at Vanderbilt University. Writing in *Perspectives in Biology and Medicine* (Winter 1974), Dr. Mann theorized that diabetics lack the ability to transport all the vitamin C they ingest across cell membranes to places where it is needed. This results in the serious blood vessel disorders frequently associated with lifelong diabetes. If this theory is correct, extra vitamin C could help prevent many of the complications that diabetes brings with the passing years.

Arthritics and others who must take aspirin regularly because of pain are also depleting their bodies of vitamin C. After discovering that aspirin, in commonly used dosages (equivalent to about two tablets), immediately blocks the absorption of vitamin C by human blood cells, Dr. H. S. Loh and two other researchers in the University of Dublin's Pharmacology Department in Ireland warned that "supplementary ascorbic acid should be administered to individuals receiving aspirin therapy" (*Journal of Clinical Pharmacology*, November–December 1973). Other medical researchers have found that prednisolone, a steroid drug used by arthritics, can cause skeletal damage in children, unless large doses of vitamin C are administered (D. Liakakos *et al., Archives of Diseases in Childhood,* 1974, 49).

The more you are exposed to chemicals and drugs, the more you need vitamin C to minimize their harmful effects on your health. How *much* more vitamin C? Let common sense be your guide, because at present, there is no other. A reasonable estimate of increased need might be from 100 to 500 mg. of additional vitamin C for each problem area, depending on severity. Remember that whether you are looking to vitamin C as a preventive of the common cold, or as protection from toxins in the environment, there is no one dosage that will be right for you and everyone else. You are an individual with very special and unique needs, so adjust your vitamin C intake accordingly.

# CHAPTER 52

# The Teenage Tendency
# Toward Deficiency

A double surprise in nutritional research as related to adolescents was reported in 1972 by a team of pharmacists and doctors at the University of Dublin, Trinity College, in Ireland. They found that vitamin C can help make the youngsters healthier and provide them with a higher degree of resistance to disease.

One of the surprises is that it takes more than eight times the so-called Recommended Daily Allowance of vitamin C to give growing boys optimal levels of systemic vitamin C, or ascorbic acid.

Writing in the *International Journal of Vitamin and Nutrition Research* (4, 1971) Drs. H. S. Loh and C. W. M. Wilson described the results of a 14-week study done with 191 Irish boys and girls from Dublin schools, ranging in age from 11 to 19.

The doctors divided the students into several groups, giving some vitamin C supplements and some placebos. Their most important finding was that when a supplement of 200 mg. of vitamin C daily was given to the boys, the ascorbic acid concentration in their blood (leucocyte ascorbic acid concentration) increased significantly. But when the supplement was boosted to 500 mg. daily, there was still more improvement of vitamin C levels.

Why is this important? Leucocyte ascorbic acid measurement is a vitally important sign. It's a reliable indication of just how much vitamin C is actually in the body and ready to go to work. From this measurement, it can be determined just how well the body will be able to mobilize vitamin C to counteract infection and disease, and repair injury and burns. A high leucocyte ascorbic acid concentration means better over-all health, while a low leucocyte ascorbic acid concentration is often the first clinical sign of scurvy.

## Large Doses Found Very Effective

The surprise is that the large dose of 500 mg. of vitamin C resulted in the measurably higher stores of vitamin C in cells. It is sometimes said that when large amounts of vitamin C are taken by people who do not have scurvy, the excess is merely excreted from the body within five hours. But here is firm evidence that these high doses actually build up more useful concentrations of vitamin C than smaller amounts.

And this same phenomenon was observed with increases of hemoglobin. It has been known for some time that when vitamin C is taken, hemoglobin levels tend to rise even though no iron is taken with it. This is because the ascorbic acid mobilizes iron out of other tissues and puts them to work in the vital red blood cells, which carry oxygen to every part of the body. But in this experiment, it was shown that when 500 mg. of vitamin C were taken, the increase in hemoglobin was greater than with 200 mg., again showing that far from being "wasted," large supplements of vitamin C perform very useful work.

The second major surprise in this Irish study is that this increase in hemoglobin when large doses of vitamin C were taken only occurred in the boys. In the girls, there was actually a slight reduction in formation of red blood cells when a supplement of 200 mg. of vitamin C was given daily. Drs. Loh and Wilson pointed out that this is apparently the result of low iron stores in the girls. Because of menstruation, girls lose iron on a regular basis. And with inadequate stores of iron, the researchers reported supplements of vitamin C actually interfere with the normal creation of red blood cells.

Many nutritionists insist that any woman, young or old, should take supplemental iron every day. Iron taken without vitamin C will not be utilized very well. In fact, if vitamin C levels are very low, the iron may not be utilized at all. On the other hand, it doesn't make sense for a woman to take vitamin C without taking supplemental iron as well. This is a classic example of partnership between two or more nutrients.

Drs. Loh and Wilson emphasized, however, that boys are by no means exempt from the problem of low iron or hemoglobin levels. Although the boys in the experiment showed an increase in these levels, they still did not achieve the "optimal levels found in adult males." So it wouldn't have been a bad idea for these youngsters to have taken iron, too, along with their vitamin C.

## Need for C Grossly Underestimated

Another study focusing on the need of youngsters for more vitamin C was presented by Dr. Man-Li S. Yew of the University of Texas at Austin at the October 1972 meeting of the National Academy of Sciences held in Washington, D.C.

The implication of Dr. Yew's work is that growing children might have need of 40 times more vitamin C than the amount now officially recommended. Dr. Yew said that "although 44 years have elapsed since the isolation of vitamin C, the amounts required for human health are far from established. Dr. Pauling's suggestion that human needs for this vitamin have probably been underestimated by a factor of 10 or more, has frequently been ignored or refuted by rhetoric rather than sound experimentation."

In describing the experiments, Dr. Yew said he fed young, healthy guinea pigs a diet which was supplemented with ascorbic acid at four widely different levels ranging from .05 mg. to 50 mg. for every 100 grams of body weight. "Growth rates both before and after surgical stress, recovery time after anesthesia, scab formation, wound healing . . . all support the conclusion that young guinea pigs ordinarily need about 5.0 mg. per 100 grams of body weight," Dr. Yew said.

"This is far beyond what is needed to prevent scurvy . . . and . . . under stress the needs are even higher. On a body weight basis, this is equivalent to the need on the part of a developing 65-pound youngster for 1,500 mg. of ascorbic acid daily, rather than the Food and Nutrition Board's recommendation of 40 mg.," the scientist declared.

# CHAPTER 53

# Advancing Years Demand
# Extra Vitamin C

The average levels of vitamin C in the blood decrease in old age. It's not a question of whether people consume less vitamin C when they get older; rather, their low levels appear to reflect an inability to utilize vitamin C in the same manner as younger people do. Dr. Michael L. Burr and colleagues of the Medical Research Council of Cardiff, Wales, reported in the *American Journal of Clinical Nutrition* (February 1974) that older persons who included more vitamin C in their diet *still* had less of the nutrient circulating in their systems than younger people in the study who still maintained a comparable diet.

The significance of these findings is still open to conjecture. It could mean that older people don't need as much vitamin C as younger people do. But it could also mean that they need *more,* either because they're using more of it, or because they use what they do obtain *less* efficiently. There is good cause to believe that old people should be taking extra vitamin C and that building up sagging vitamin C levels can go a long way toward maintaining youthful vigor in later years.

# Studies on Aging and Vitamin C Deficiency

Dr. H. LeCompte, a well-known Belgian doctor, theorizes that whereas aging is a process of slow oxidation of body tissue, vitamin C is the *antioxidant* needed to retard or reverse the process. In his article "Vitamin C and the Prevention of Aging," published in *ACTA Gerontologica et Geriatrica Belgica* (1971, vol. IX, no. 4), Dr. LeCompte reports the case of his own father-in-law. At the age of 67, before beginning the doctor's "geriatric cure," he was "totally old and worn out." After the "cure," which consisted of several grams of vitamin C every day for a year, Dr. LeCompte's father-in-law began a new career as a journalist. At the age of 82, still a working journalist, he was picking up spare cash writing translations and studying Russian just to keep busy.

Dr. LeCompte is not the only researcher to associate vitamin C deficiency with many of the diseases accompanying old age. George V. Mann, Sc.D., M.D., writing in *Perspectives in Biology and Medicine,* Winter 1974), reported that some diseases which accompany diabetes also accompany old age. Diabetics need extra insulin to enable their bodies to metabolize carbohydrates and sugars. But carbohydrate intolerance also strikes 40 percent of the people past the age of 50, Dr. Mann noted. While diabetics have a tendency to develop cataracts, Dr. Mann says that changes in the lens of the eye occur in 65 percent of *all* people 50 to 60 years old and in 95 percent of people over 65! Diabetics are also especially prone to develop circulatory problems, another disability that troubles older non-diabetics.

The connection between these facts and the need for vitamin C is that "Human beings, and perhaps other species requiring vitamin C, need insulin for the transport of the vitamin into the cells of certain tissues. Impairment of insulin function, whether by its absence, as in juvenile diabetes, or by its inhibition, as in adult-onset diabetes, will lead to impaired transport of vitamin C," Dr. Mann explained.

He also pointed out that there are certain "insulin-sensitive" tissues which tend to develop what he calls "a kind of 'local scurvy' with faulty collagen formation." In the circulatory system, this can lead to abnormalities in blood vessels. "In the eye, lenticular opacities (cataracts) are another result," Dr. Mann said.

Dr. Mann, who is associated with the biochemistry department of Vanderbilt University in Nashville, Tennessee, and is a career investigator of the National Institutes of Health, stated boldly that, "A combination of a large intake of AA (ascorbic acid) and adequate insulin will prevent these lesions."

In separate lab tests cited by Dr. Mann, researchers injected animals with diabetes-producing substances. Animals who produced their own vitamin C, or who were fed supplemental vitamin C, developed none of the devastating complications associated with diabetes. Guinea pigs, who cannot manufacture their own ascorbic acid, developed cataracts only when fed a vitamin C-deficient diet.

" . . . Human cataracts," suggests Dr. Mann, "may be a late consequence of marginal intake of AA, the diabetic being especially prone to cataracts because he also lacks insulin to facilitate its transport. . . ."

# Vitamin Fights the Ravages of Aging

"A nutritionally optimum amount of vitamin C would be important in any attempts to slow the aging processes," reported Dr. A. L. Tappel, biochemist of the University of California at Davis, in a provocative paper titled "Will Antioxidant Nutrients Slow Aging Processes?" in *Geriatrics* (October 1968).

Dr. Tappel dealt at some length with the nutritional destruction caused by free radicals. These free radicals result from peroxidation of essential fatty acids, and their ability to affect the tissue cell in countless ways, from destroying its membranous structure to subtly altering cell organization. In many aspects aging is the cumulative result of damage done by free radicals, and vitamin E is considered the great prophylactic that prevents free radicals from forming by preventing peroxidation of lipids.

As Dr. Tappel observed, however, even if you have a good intake of vitamin E, there are times when the consumption of fats out-balances the amount of the vitamin available, and then free radicals will be formed. It is at this point that vitamin C enters into the picture and is found to be another major nutrient that fights to keep you young. It does this in two ways, according to Dr. Tappel. This particular vitamin is a scavenger of free radicals, breaking down and cleaning up any of these destroyers that have been formed because of an insufficiency of vitamin E. Also, "Through antioxidant synergism it (vitamin C) can increase the effectiveness of vitamin E. . . ."

Two such heroic roles might seem enough, but as has often been pointed out, vitamin C is the most versatile of vitamins with functions and effects so far-reaching that it can actually replace any other vitamin for a limited period of time and keep the body functioning and healthy.

With regard to aging, there is one important aspect that is unrelated to the damage done by free radicals and cannot be countered by antioxidants. That is the aging of *collagen,* described in the *Journal of the American Geriatrics Society* (December 1968) by Donald G. Carpenter, Ph.D., and James A. Loynd, M.S. in their article "An Integrated Theory of Aging." Drs. Carpenter and Loynd reported that "The collagen fibers . . . shrink with age and 'choke off' the surrounding tissue; thus the surrounding tissue becomes increasedly anoxic (lacking oxygen) and wrinkled." These two researchers are among many holding that the deterioration of collagen is integral to the process of aging. And here again, vitamin C plays a vital role in holding back the process.

If you are past 40, and a cut heals slowly, your physician will probably tell you that you can't expect to heal as fast at your age as you healed in your teens. If you have pains in the small of your back, you may be put into traction to relieve them, and you may be advised to try to put up with this "normal" symptom of aging. Rheumatoid arthritis and rheumatism of the muscles, thickening of the skin with formation of inexplicable stains, ulcerative colitis, gout, hardening of the arteries, and even heart disease and cancer have all been interpreted as "normal" results of the aging process.

Yet there is ever-increasing reason to believe that vitamin C can either fully prevent or play a significant role in preventing all of these afflictions. So if these are the symptoms of aging, why not look to vitamin C to keep you young?

## The Role of Collagen

The resistance which vitamin C helps to provide comes by way of a stabilizing fiber called collagen. Actually vitamin C is indispensable to the formation of collagen. Even an early edition of the *Merck Service Bulletin, Vitamin C* (West Point, Pennsylvania: Merck & Co., Inc., 1956), stated that collagen formation is one of the "most important roles of ascorbic acid." Collagen, a protective substance constituting about 40 percent of the body's protein, can be pictured as a cement whose "glue-like" ability holds our cells in a healthy and natural formation of firmly walled tissue.

As long as our tissues have the strength provided by collagen, they are far better able to resist penetration by any invading infections. But, if collagen is not manufactured properly (due to an ascorbic acid deficiency), our cells can no longer stand firm. Instead of acting as the main supportive protein of skin, tendon, bone, cartilage, and connective tissue, defective collagen assumes a watery appearance and leaks uselessly into the bloodstream.

Naturally, if collagen is not performing its binding job, cellular chaos results. And at this stage—when tissues begin to deteriorate—our health is placed in a position of real danger. If tissues lack the strength they once had, how can they ward off the diseases continually trying to invade the body?

Unfortunately, the answer we must accept is both frightening and obvious. Fragile and unstable tissues are certainly capable of little, if any, resistance. When collagen is liquefied or broken down and therefore not doing its job, the cells are easily permeated and diseases can run rampant. The following conditions (collectively referred to as "collagen diseases," "group diseases," or "connective tissue diseases") are all related to the abnormal functioning of collagen: aging; defective wound healing; inflammation of muscle tissues (aches and pains); gout; rheumatic fever; low back pain; rheumatoid arthritis; muscular rheumatism; receding and bleeding gums; scleroderma—thickened, hard, rigid, and pigmented patches of the skin; ulcerative colitis; vasculitis—inflammation of a blood vessel; and inflammation of the coats of the small and medium sized arteries of the body with inflammatory changes around the vessels.

Our ability to resist these diseases depends largely on the ability of collagen (connective tissue) to regenerate itself fast enough. And the best (and only) way to prevent its slowing down is with increased vitamin C in the diet.

In the *Archives of Pediatrics* (October 1954), Dr. William J. McCormick wrote that "the degree of malignancy of an illness is determined inversely by the degree of connective tissue resistance. And this, in turn, is dependent on the adequacy of vitamin C intake." (The less resistant the connective tissue is, the more serious the trouble is likely to be. And lack of ascorbic acid is the basic cause of lack of resistance.)

It is prolonged insufficiency of this vitamin that makes it increasingly hard for collagen to offer proper resistance to disease. The deficiency usually is not apparent till middle age. That is why it has been possible to confuse it with "normal aging."

Although it has been established that vitamin C is fundamental to the proper manufacturing of collagen, scientists do not know exactly how an insufficient intake of ascorbic acid is related to defective collagen metabolism. In the *New York State Journal of Medicine* (15 May 1965), Gerald M. Rivers, Ph.D., said that derangements in connective tissue should "ultimately be referable to the biochemical and physiologic function of ascorbic acid at the molecular level." Dr. Rivers goes on to say that though the precise mechanism has not yet been learned, "Collagen synthesis is significantly depressed in ascorbic acid deficiency."

# CHAPTER 54

# Atherosclerosis—A Disease of Vitamin C Deficiency

One of the most common and deadly diseases of the older years is atherosclerosis—or the narrowing and hardening of the interior of the arteries—as solidified cholesterol and other substances are deposited to form plaques on arterial walls. Premature senility is often traceable to atherosclerotic lesions in arteries leading to the brain, because the narrowed vessels restrict the blood flow and hence the supply of oxygen and nutrients to the brain cells. And, of course, lethal heart attacks are commonly the result of narrowed arteries in which blood clots get lodged, completely cutting off the flow of blood to the vital organ. Strokes are known to result from hemorrhages caused by the increased pressure.

According to Dr. M. L. Riccitelli, of the Yale School of Medicine, there has been evidence since 1949 stating that atherosclerosis could be related to a vitamin C deficiency. In an article entitled "Vitamin C Therapy in Geriatric Practice," which appeared in the *Journal of the American Geriatric Society* (January 1972), Dr. Riccitelli reported that Dr. J. B. Duguid, writing in the *Lancet* (2: 925, 1949), showed that guinea pigs deprived of vitamin C developed lesions similar to those of human atherosclerosis patients. Subsequent investigators, according to

Dr. Riccitelli, discovered that atherosclerotic lesions in vitamin C-deprived animals could be completely cured by prolonged corrective vitamin C therapy. And, he added, animal studies conducted 20 years ago by A. L. Myasnikov demonstrated that ascorbic acid has "a partial anticholesterolemic and antiatherogenic effect." In other words, vitamin C reduces serum cholesterol levels and inhibits cholesterol build-up on artery walls. However, Dr. Riccitelli noted, "very little has been reported in the literature regarding the effects of vitamin C in the etiology of atherosclerosis."

There are those researchers who look upon atherosclerosis as a deficiency disease—like scurvy, beriberi, rickets, and pellagra—induced by malnutrition and treatable by nutritional corrections. One of those holding this belief is an English pathologist, Dr. Constance Leslie, who noticed that she could vary the amount of cholesterol in her own blood serum simply by varying the amount of vitamin C she included in her diet. She brought her cholesterol count down from 230 to 140 simply by increasing her vitamin C intake and she reversed the process when she restricted her vitamin C intake.

Dr. Leslie, formerly Dr. Constance Spittle, of Pinderfields Hospital in Wakefield, Yorkshire, England, has come to the conclusion that atherosclerosis, or hardening of the arteries, "is a long-term deficiency (or negative balance) of vitamin C, which permits cholesterol to build up in the arterial system, and results in changes in other fractions of the fats." This is admittedly an hypothesis, though consistent with other published findings about vitamin C and atherosclerosis. In actual findings, Dr. Leslie has shown that in young persons with healthy arteries, blood levels of the fatty substance cholesterol go down significantly on a daily supplement of one gram of vitamin C, whereas the same supplement causes increased serum cholesterol in patients who have been diagnosed as atherosclerotic. In her view, the extra cholesterol in the blood of these patients comes from formerly hardened cholesterol deposits which the vitamin has mobilized or reamed out from arterial walls. Thus, according to Dr. Leslie, the high readings signify decreased, not increased pathology—vitamin C is acting to move cholesterol away from the arteries.

Dr. Leslie's discovery of the effects of vitamin C on serum cholesterol was accidental. According to Dr. Leslie, several years ago she became curious about the claims of a pharmaceutical company that one of their products derived from pineapple had clot-dissolving properties. Testing the pills, she found no supportive evidence and dismissed the claim as unfounded. Later, though, when more refined techniques had been developed for testing, Dr. Leslie pursued the testing of the product once again. "If it was something in the pineapple, I thought, why not try eating the pineapple itself? In fact, why just the pineapple? Why not other fruits, too?"

Dr. Leslie then proceeded to live on an all-fruit diet, to which she found she had to add salad vegetables for their salt content. Each day thereafter she extracted a blood sample, tested it for clot-dissolving properties (she found no change), and dated the samples. She continued this regimen for several months when serendipity stepped in. It was a Saturday afternoon and a patient had just been admitted to the hospital with a bleeding problem. Familiar with the problem of trying to find a donor on such short notice on a weekend, Dr. Leslie—as she had often done before—climbed up on the table to have her own blood taken. But this time she went into partial shock after giving blood. Her restricted diet, short especially on protein, had ill equipped her for this generous gesture.

Now, as a patient in treatment for shock herself, Dr. Leslie routinely had her blood checked for something besides clotting properties. What startled her in the report from the hospital was the cholesterol reading—it seemed unusually low. Once on her feet again, Dr. Leslie dug out the frozen samples of her blood and checked for cholesterol. Sure enough, during a one-month period of her diet her serum cholesterol had gone down from 230 (mg. per 100 ml. blood) to 160. As she continued to eat largely of fruits and vegetables, her cholesterol later dropped to 140, despite the fact that she was now on a varied diet that included plenty of cholesterol-rich foods such as cheese and eggs.

"That convinced me," she explains, "that there was an active principle at work. It wasn't the absence of other foods but the presence of fruits and vegetables that did the trick. Mostly I had eaten raw fruits and greens, so I wondered what would happen if I cooked them. I found out: after three weeks with everything cooked, my cholesterol started going up again. Of course, that directed my attention to vitamin C because of its well-known destruction under heat treatment."

## A Pattern of Protection Emerges

At this point, Dr. Leslie stopped being her own solitary guinea pig and enlisted the participation of others in the hospital. Again, she was in for a surprise. Only the younger volunteer subjects consistently reduced their serum cholesterol by taking vitamin C, while the supplement had the reverse effect on atherosclerosis patients. A third group, older volunteers presumably in normal health, showed no consistent pattern: by taking daily vitamin C tablets, some lowered their cholesterol level, others raised it.

In Dr. Leslie's view, the older "normal" volunteers who showed elevated cholesterol following vitamin C therapy had, in fact, undiagnosed atherosclerosis—their artery walls under the influence of vitamin C were releasing unsuspected atherosclerotic cholesterol deposits. For them, and for recognized patients with this disease, the important thing about cholesterol is not how much is in the serum, Dr. Leslie says, but "Where is it going?" Dr. Leslie mentioned a study by researchers Zaitsev, Myasnikov, and Sheikman (*Kardiologyia* 4:30, 1964) in which radioactive cholesterol was fed to animals. In animals receiving vitamin C, the cholesterol went to the liver (which converts cholesterol into bile acids) and to the adrenal glands (which use cholesterol in the synthesis of steroid hormones); but in animals not given vitamin C, the cholesterol was deposited in the aorta, a principal artery.

For help in steering cholesterol away from arteries into more appropriate sites, Dr. Leslie recommends one gram (1,000 mg.)

of vitamin C a day for people with suspected or confirmed atherosclerosis. For other adults who may have "lagged behind" in their vitamin C consumption, she advises around 250 mg. in a daily supplement. (Going on an all-fruit diet, as Dr. Leslie herself demonstrated, is not a wise approach.)

Dr. Leslie suggests that her findings could also be used as a diagnostic test for arterial health. In an interview in *Emergency Medicine* (June 1975), she advised doctors to check a patient's serum cholesterol (an average of several readings), prescribe vitamin C for a period, then check cholesterol again. "If the cholesterol goes down and stays down, your patient's arteries are pretty good," she is quoted. "If it goes up and stays up, then they are pretty poor."

Except in advanced cases, the presence or absence of atherosclerotic damage to arteries is extremely difficult to determine (unless, of course, Dr. Leslie's proposed test proves valid and becomes accepted). In research on atherosclerosis, therefore, it's not easy to compare atherosclerotic patients with normal persons of comparable age, since the "normals," too, may have the disease, though undiagnosed.

## Attention Turned to Veins

"I wanted to get on unarguable grounds with my vitamin C research," Dr. Leslie claimed. "That's why I decided to leave the problem of arteries for a while and go into the somewhat comparable problem of clots, or thrombi, in the veins."

In both arteries and veins, damaged or weakened spots on vessel walls are believed to contribute to thrombi formation, and vitamin C might be expected to strengthen these structures because of its well-known role in the synthesis of collagen or intercellular "cement." The vitamin's influence on blood lipids, or fats, might also affect the clotting behavior of both arterial and venous blood. But, of the two vascular systems, the veins offer the most clear-cut experimental model. In the case of deep-vein thrombosis, patients at risk are readily identified, and a highly sensitive, convenient method is available for studying clot development.

With research support from a pharmaceutical firm and the cooperation of doctors at Pinderfields General Hospital, Dr. Leslie set up her double-blind experiment, giving either one gram of vitamin C or a dummy placebo tablet to patients, ages 35 to 85, all at high risk for clot development. Of these, about half were surgical cases (prostate, hip, and cancer), and the rest had various serious disorders related to cardiovascular disease, including 17 who had had heart attacks.

In double blind trials, according to the *Lancet,* (11 December 1971), the researchers tested legs for deep-vein thrombosis, looking for even minute thrombus formation unaccompanied by any discernable clinical signs (such as swelling and tenderness of the calf). The results: "The incidence of deep-vein thrombosis in the placebo group was 60 percent, compared to 33 percent in the vitamin C group," Dr. Leslie reported. But even more striking than this two-to-one difference in the incidence of clots, Dr. Leslie believes, was the dramatic difference in degree of severity.

The patients' legs were scanned to detect a rise in radioactivity, indicating a clustering of radioactive-tagged fibrinogen which has been given to them. (Fibrinogen is a blood protein associated with the clotting process.) A radioactive rise of 15 percent is accepted as "positive"—that is, indicative that thrombus formation is taking place. Of the 10 vitamin C patients who tested positive, six had rises of 25 percent or less, i.e., barely over the normal range. None had a rise exceeding 80 percent, whereas in the placebo group quite a few had rises of over 100 percent and a number went over 200 percent.

Reflecting these ratings, only one vitamin C patient showed actual physical signs of thrombus, whereas such signs were evident in 12 instances in patients given only placebos. Though not considered statistically significant, three pulmonary emboli developed in placebo patients, none in patients receiving vitamin C.

# 'Oh, We Don't Get Thrombosis Here'

Even as she was setting up this clinical experiment, Dr. Leslie discovered heartening support for her thesis. In the hospital's Regional Burns Unit, she was told: "Oh, we don't get thrombosis here." Since badly burned patients must sometimes be immobilized for weeks, the incidence of thrombosis is generally expected to be high—but not at Pinderfields. How come? Dr. Leslie discovered that, since its founding in the mid-sixties, this unit had routinely treated burn patients with one gram daily of vitamin C to promote tissue healing. Protection against deep-vein thrombosis was apparently an incidental benefit.

As word of Dr. Leslie's study circulated in the hospital, a number of surgical services began routine vitamin C administration to protect their patients. In the six months following completion of the experiment, Dr. Leslie wrote to the *Lancet,* (28 July 1973), that Pinderfields' surgeons on six wards, giving 500 mg. of vitamin C daily to their patients, had only three cases of deep-vein thrombosis and three cases of pulmonary embolism (two of which were slight). Even this small number, she added, might be eliminated if the daily supplement were increased to a full gram.

Today, unfortunately, only the burns unit at Pinderfields continues the practice of vitamin C protection. Dr. Leslie is not sure why. Research published in England by others, she says, has emphasized the failure of vitamin C to eliminate thrombotic episodes, though the amounts used in these trials have been well below the one-gram supplement her own experiment proved effective. The situation appears similar to what happened a few years ago in the controversy on vitamin C as a preventive against the common cold. It was "proved" over and over again that vitamin C therapy had no effect in forestalling or reducing the severity of colds—until Linus Pauling's writings forced researchers to repeat experiments, using massive, not token, doses of the nutrient.

Dr. Leslie wishes someone would repeat her clinical study on deep-vein thrombosis and verify her findings. She wishes she had funds for further research so she could continue her experimental work in conjunction with her regular job in the hospital's clinical laboratory. She wishes surgeons at Pinderfields hadn't gradually dropped their vitamin C programs for reasons she can't understand. Perhaps, she speculates, it's too simple for ready acceptance—the notion that a vitamin can make so much difference.

But, though temporarily frustrated, Dr. Leslie has no doubt that the future will bear out her major thesis: that inadequate intake of vitamin C—a "negative balance" as she calls it—is largely responsible for major diseases of the blood vessels. She's convinced that protection against these threatening disorders lies in adequate vitamin C supplements plus a diet plentiful in vitamin C-rich foods.

## Another Theory on the Importance of Vitamin C and Atherosclerosis

Anthony Verlangieri, Ph.D., a young biochemist at Rutgers University in New Brunswick, New Jersey, is another researcher investigating the possibility that a deficiency in vitamin C may be one of the major underlying causes of atherosclerosis. After more than six years of animal research, Dr. Verlangieri is convinced that there is such a relationship.

Dr. Verlangieri is well aware of earlier work, both with animals and human beings, which indicates a protective role for ascorbic acid, or vitamin C, in the entire circulatory system. But the importance of his work, according to Dr. Verlangieri, is that he has found what he believes to be the mechanism by which the vitamin wards off atherosclerosis. And this new understanding, he feels, places the earlier indications of vitamin C's effectiveness on a much sounder and more scientific basis.

According to an official spokesperson for Rutgers University, "What is new in Dr. Verlangieri's findings is that he has identified the loss of certain chemical compounds that are the building blocks of the artery lining; this loss occurs when atherosclerosis is induced in laboratory animals. . . . When vitamin C is added to the disease-producing diet, however, these same compounds do not disappear but are actually increased above normal levels, his results show. And along with this change, the extent of the disease is greatly reduced, as compared to the artery damage in rabbits receiving no vitamin C."

## What Causes Artery Disease to Take Hold?

One of the intriguing aspects of Dr. Verlangieri's work is that it points to a possible new understanding of how atherosclerosis actually begins. Many people believe that the trigger is an excess of cholesterol or other fats in the bloodstream. But while cholesterol doubtless plays some role, most medical evidence, according to Dr. Verlangieri, suggests that cholesterol will only attach itself to blood vessels if there is something wrong with them—if they are rough or irregular or otherwise abnormal. What happens to the blood vessel lining in the first place to permit the cholesterol to grab hold and form plaques is not known.

Dr. Verlangieri's findings suggest two possible explanations: "Apparently, vitamin C is needed for the body to produce these particular compounds in the lining of the arteries. If these compounds begin to disappear, the lining may become more permeable—it is something like a sieve, held together by these materials. Without them, cholesterol and other fatty substances may be squeezed through the lining and begin to form plaques," according to Dr. Verlangieri.

"The other possibility is that these compounds in the arteries help metabolize, or break down, cholesterol or other fats in the bloodstream. If these compounds aren't there, fats may build up on the vessel wall simply because the normal mechanism for removing them isn't working."

It seems, however, that vitamin C is not the only factor involved in protecting arteries—which should come as no surprise to anyone who appreciates the total interrelatedness of human metabolism. In the case of Dr. Verlangieri's experiments it seems that vitamin C is working hand in hand with sulfur-containing compounds in such a way as to transfer the sulfates to other compounds inside arterial cells.

The particular compound which has come under Dr. Verlangieri's scrutiny—and led to an unexpected bonus in his research—is known as chondroitin-4-sulfate. The biochemist explains that he singled it out because, although there were changes in a whole group of compounds he was studying, this one showed the most dramatic increase when vitamin C was added to the rabbits' diet—it jumped 150 percent.

## Heart Disease Deaths Cut Dramatically

Only after making his own observations did Dr. Verlangieri learn that chondroitin-4-sulfate has been used—with astonishing success—as an experimental treatment for coronary atherosclerosis by a team of medical researchers headed by Dr. Lester Morrison in Culver City, California. Although the number of patients treated there with chondroitin-4-sulfate (also known as CSA) has been small, Dr. Morrison has published results indicating that the death rate among heart patients given CSA has been a remarkable 80 percent less than among the control group with the same disease history, according to Dr. Verlangieri.

"What is exciting is the way our research fits together," Dr. Verlangieri reported. "They have used this compound therapeutically, as a replacement for what has been lost—while my findings show that vitamin C stimulates the production of the same compound within the body."

## 'Maybe It's Not So Strange That We Need More Vitamin C'

The role of cholesterol itself, which has long been regarded as a major risk factor in atherosclerosis, may be clarified by these new findings on vitamin C. Studies by a Czechoslovakian scientist, Dr. Emil Ginter, have shown an inverse relation between cholesterol and vitamin C levels—when one increases, the other declines. According to Dr. Verlangieri, "This may be where cholesterol is playing a role as a trigger. It may lower the vitamin C level in the body, and as the chondroitin-4-sulfate in the artery decreases, we now have the foundation laid for the beginning of the disease."

Other risk factors follow a similar pattern, the Rutgers biochemist adds. Smoking and psychological stress, both associated with atherosclerosis, also reduce vitamin C levels; female hormones increase the levels of vitamin C, and women, until they reach menopause, are less prone to the disease than men,

"The vitamin C level of the body is very changeable, and can be modified by many things," according to Dr. Verlangieri. "You can have tissue saturation of the vitamin at breakfast, and be down to half that by dinner time. . . . The Recommended Daily Allowance of vitamin C, after all, was established on the basis of the amount that would prevent scurvy. But it may be that you can prevent scurvy with a relatively low level, while it simply takes a higher one to prevent atherosclerosis."

Dr. Verlangieri also reported that a colleague has independently achieved the same results with vitamin C. And these findings indicate that the vitamin has a dual effect, reducing blood vessel abnormalities which can be seen with a microscope, while also reducing cholesterol and plaque formation. So far, let us emphasize, the protection vitamin C affords our arteries is—strictly speaking—theoretical. Dr. Verlangieri puts it this way: "I can say absolutely this is what happens in rabbits. I can't yet say absolutely in humans, though I'm 99 percent convinced."

# CHAPTER 55

# Vitamin C Protects Against High Blood Cholesterol

*by Dr. Emil Ginter*

*Dr. Emil Ginter of the Institute of Nutrition in Bratislava, Czechoslovakia, is internationally recognized as one of the leading researchers in the field of vitamin C metabolism and health. His scientific articles have appeared in the medical journals of continental Europe, England, and the United States.*

Here in the Research Institute of Human Nutrition, many years of experimentation with animals and human beings have recently culminated in some findings that we believe can help protect against both heart attacks and cerebrovascular disorders.

Why did we undertake this research in the first place? The underlying reason is that one of the more recent developments of our rapidly changing civilization is a profound change in the major causes of death, both in Europe and the United States. Even though we cannot claim that the problem of fighting infectious diseases has been completely solved, it is nevertheless true that today, these infections threaten mankind in a far less menacing way than in past years.

On the other hand, it is clear that mankind's number one enemy today is atherosclerosis—the clogging and hardening of the arteries with fatty deposits—which cause abnormalities in the functioning of our vital organs, particularly the heart and brain, and is involved in the death of nearly half of all people. Physicians the world over are today searching for a more effective way of fighting against this mass killer.

The great majority of scientists involved in atherosclerosis research share the opinion that more than one factor is responsible for the continuously rising number of heart attacks. Along with whatever inherent predisposition one may have for falling victim to this disease, one of the chief contributing causes is insufficient physical activity. Other factors which probably play a role are excessive smoking and pollution of the environment by industrial contaminants and automobile exhausts. Stress situations doubtless also play a role here. As far as the role of nutrition goes, it is well known that the uncontrolled consumption of calories, particularly those produced by animal fats and sucrose, may also have a damaging effect.

## Work Began a Decade Ago

More than a decade ago, a work team of the Biochemical Department of the Research Institute of Human Nutrition in Bratislava, Czechoslovakia, started a research program with the aim of finding out to what extent vitamin C can affect cholesterol levels in the blood, and blood vessel disease as such.

This team is not the first to try to solve this problem. Pioneering work had been done by Russian, American, and Indian scientists who published reports claiming that vitamin C has the ability to decrease the cholesterol level of the blood and thus protect the human organism against atherosclerosis. Unfortunately, soon after the publication of their research, contradictory papers were published which shed doubt on the protective effect of vitamin C in fighting high blood cholesterol levels.

We tried to find out what might have caused these discrepancies, and we finally came to the conclusion that more sophisticated investigation methods were necessary to pinpoint the exact role of vitamin C in the metabolism of cholesterol and atherosclerosis.

From the beginning, we attempted to carry out all our experimentation under conditions approaching very closely those which actually occur in human nourishment. Compared with other vitamins, the importance of vitamin C is very special, because only man, monkeys, guinea pigs, and a few other species of animals need to receive vitamin C through food consumption. All other animals produce vitamin C themselves—in the liver from sugars—and these animals, as well as plants, are therefore never deficient in this vitamin. Animals in this category are obviously able to control in a very economic way their vitamin C supplies, which is confirmed by the experience that feeding them with large quantities of vitamin C has no effect on the level of the vitamin in their tissues.

On the other hand, the human organism and guinea pigs respond to vitamin C supplementation quite directly: with decreasing doses of vitamin C, the concentration of this vitamin in their blood, liver, and other vital organs decreases.

Considering this fact, it is useless to apply to human beings any results obtained in experiments with commonly used laboratory animals such as mice, rats, or rabbits, as these animals are richly endowed with vitamin C regardless of whether or not the vitamin is present as such in the food they eat. In contrast, lack of this vitamin in the diet of human beings may result after approximately 100 days in symptoms of a very dangerous and ultimately fatal disease—scurvy.

## Experiments Carefully Structured

We decided, therefore, to use guinea pigs in our experiments, as these animals, like us, are highly dependent on receiving vitamin C in their food. We would like to point out, however, that we did not use a model simulating a total deficiency of vitamin C. If a guinea pig is completely deprived of vitamin C, it dies with typical scorbutic symptoms within four to five weeks. Such a total deficiency of vitamin C occurs today only rarely. While the explorers of yesterday died in great numbers during their long sea crossings for lack of fresh vegetables and fruits, today vitamin C deficiency is more often found in what we call the latent form, or marginal deficiency.

Despite the fact that scurvy occurs only rarely, it is very probable that today a large number of people suffer from this latent vitamin C deficiency. This has been confirmed in past years by many scientists in Great Britain, Australia, and in the German Federal Republic. However, as to what biochemical changes take place in the human organism as a result of this latent deficiency, not very much has been known until recently.

With these considerations in mind, we developed a model of latent vitamin C deficiency for application to guinea pigs which has enabled us to observe biochemical changes which take place over a long period of time, sometimes in experiments lasting as long as one year. During these experiments, no external signs indicating vitamin C deficiency were observed. The guinea pigs grew normally and also had a normal appetite and behavior.

## Animals Looked Healthy But Had High Cholesterol

Despite their apparent health, we observed that after several months on this marginally deficient diet, there was a significant rise in the cholesterol level in their livers and blood. This unexpected finding raised all sorts of questions in our minds, as it would in anyone who was involved in trying to fight the modern plague of atherosclerosis. We then set out to discover *why* a relative deficiency of the vitamin C produces an increase in cholesterol.

Cholesterol metabolism in human beings is a very complicated process. We get part of our cholesterol in the form of food (exogenous cholesterol) but our organism produces more cholesterol by itself in the liver and in the gastrointestinal tract (endogenous cholesterol). Cholesterol is synthesized from bicarbonaceous fragments produced from oxidation of sugars, fats, and even proteins. As cholesterol is a lipoid or fatty substance nearly insoluble in water, it circulates in our blood complexed with proteins, the so-called lipoproteins.

Cholesterol present in the blood penetrates all the tissues of the organism, the speed of its displacement to various tissues varying widely. For example, it enters the brain only very slowly, but can move in and out of the liver almost instantly. Because of this dynamic nature, problems concerning the absorption, synthesis, and distribution of cholesterol in the living organism can be solved only by using radioisotope methods, which involve marking cholesterol in various parts of the molecule by a radioactive atom whose progress through the body can be traced with special measuring devices.

In the early years of our experiments aimed at finding the underlying cause of the rise in cholesterol levels in guinea pigs with less than optimal vitamin C, the results we obtained were rather discouraging. Using various radioactive compounds, we found only that the rise of the blood cholesterol level in the deficient guinea pigs was *not* caused by changes in cholesterol absorption from food. Nor was it a result of an increase in cholesterol being internally synthesized. We could not even observe any change in distribution of cholesterol between the blood and the various tissues. There seemed to be only one logical explanation left, and we then decided to study intensively the processes of cholesterol *elimination* from the organism.

Cholesterol is eliminated from both human and animal bodies in two ways. One way is that cholesterol is released in an unchanged state by the gallbladder and through the intestinal wall into the bowels, from which it is eliminated by the stools, often chemically changed by bacterial activity in the intestines.

The second manner of cholesterol elimination is more complicated, but for most animals, more important. By enzymatic action, which today is not yet well understood, cholesterol converts in the liver to bile acids, and these are eliminated by the gallbladder into the intestinal tract and out of the organism.

We zeroed in on this latter process by "tagging" cholesterol on the molecular side chain with a radioactive carbon atom. During the cholesterol conversion to bile acids, a part of the side chain splits off and the radioactive carbon then appears in the carbon dioxide breathed out by the organism.

Through use of this method, we were able to obtain evidence that in guinea pigs suffering from latent vitamin C deficiency, the speed of cholesterol conversion to bile acids is rather slow, causing an accumulation of cholesterol in the liver and blood of the animals.

# Vitamin C Deficiency Hinders Cholesterol Elimination

The liver of a normal guinea pig, we found, converts on a daily basis about 40 percent more cholesterol to bile acids than the liver of a vitamin C-deficient guinea pig.

We also observed that high doses of vitamin C applied to vitamin C-deficient guinea pigs markedly speeds up the degradation of cholesterol. In addition, a very close relationship between the amount of vitamin C in the liver and the ability of the liver to oxidize cholesterol has also been observed; an increasing amount of vitamin C producing an increased ability of the liver to degrade cholesterol through oxidation.

The question now is: What importance have these findings in connection with atherosclerosis? In the diagram, we show the process of cholesterol conversion to bile acids in the liver, and the effect of the reduced speed of this process when vitamin C is deficient. A retarded process of cholesterol oxidation finally results in a larger cholesterol accumulation in the liver and blood. The blood flowing through the coronary arteries and nourishing the cardiac muscle contains, in the case of a vitamin C deficiency, an increased number of cholesterol molecules. Consequently, more cholesterol accumulates in the walls of the vital blood vessels.

This explanation is confirmed by the fact that signs of atherosclerotic changes were observed in the blood vessels of some guinea pigs that suffered for a long time from vitamin C deficiency.

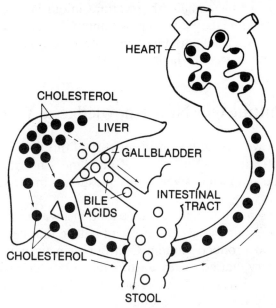

*The role of vitamin C deficiency in atherogenesis is seen in this schematic illustration by Dr. Ginter. In the normal organism, most of the liver cholesterol (black circles) is transformed to bile acids (empty circles). Cholesterol in this form is eliminated through the gallbladder and intestinal tract. In latent vitamin C deficiency, the transformation of cholesterol to bile acids is impaired, as indicated by the broken arrow, and cholesterol accumulates in the liver. Increased amounts of cholesterol are transported by the blood to the heart, and cholesterol deposits in the coronary arteries are formed.*

What about human beings? Professor Knox from the University of Birmingham in Great Britain recently carried out a correlation analysis which statistically compared the mortality ratios for heart disease and cerebrovascular disease in different regions of England and Wales to the dietary intake of a number of nutrients. Vitamin C intakes showed a strong negative correlation with these diseases: in the regions with high vitamin C intake, the mortality for ischemic heart disease and cerebrovascular disease was low, while in areas where vitamin C intake was low, the occurrence of these diseases was higher.

Recently, we have made observations in our laboratories that the blood of animals with latent vitamin C deficiency contains not only an increased amount of cholesterol, but also of triglycerides, an excess of which are known to be involved in atherosclerosis.

## Putting Our New Knowledge to Work

How can we best utilize the discovery of this new biochemical function of vitamin C in terms of mankind's nutrition? In my opinion, the simplest answer to this question is in the area of *prevention*.

It is necessary for us to consume food in a way that allows our systems to repair the genetic error of nature that deprives us of the ability to produce vitamin C in our own tissues. Our food must be very varied, with a sufficient daily supply of fresh vegetables and fruits. If this is not always possible, the use of supplemental vitamin C is recommended.

According to our experiences, a daily dosage of 200 mg. of ascorbic acid, given to men and women 40 to 60 years old during the winter months, decreased in a statistically significant way the blood cholesterol level.

It is possible that high dosages of ascorbic acid will have some curative effects for people suffering from atherosclerosis. Undoubtedly, however, the far more simple and more effective way is prevention of atherosclerosis by means of well-balanced nutrition and a healthy life regimen.

# CHAPTER 56

# More Vitamin C, Less Chance of Gallstones

The studies of Dr. Constance Leslie and Dr. Emil Ginter lead to one conclusion: with vitamin C as its companion, there is no need to fear cholesterol. It can be a friend. It is converted into bile which is an important digestant. Lack of bile leads to problems with the gallbladder, which means a lack of vitamin C can lead to gallbladder problems or an inability to digest fats including cholesterol—a whole round-robin of problems which many people currently on low cholesterol programs are beginning to experience.

With plenty of vitamin C in the diet a person doesn't have to be a Jack Spratt. He can eat the fats his body needs. And they can be metabolized so that they cause neither atherosclerosis nor gallstones—which are too frequently the result of a shortage of bile acids in the gallbladder. When gallstones are removed from patients, they are 60 to 100 percent cholesterol, Dr. Donald Small, associate professor of medicine and chief of biophysics at Boston University told the Society of University Surgeons in New Orleans in 1973 (*Medical World News,* 30 March 1973).

Normal gallstone bile carries completely dissolved cholesterol along with bile salts and lecithin. Therefore, gallstones must reflect the insolubility of the cholesterol in a bile that is abnormal. What is it that renders bile an inadequate solvent for cholesterol in the first place? Dr. Small suggested an innate metabolic defect in the organ secreting the gallbladder bile—the liver. Cholesterol builds up in the bile, until, at some critical point, the excess is precipitated as microcrystals which grow and stick together to form gallstones.

Instead of resorting to surgery to remove the gallbladder, Dr. Small urged a less radical course, such as changing the metabolism to increase the solvent capability of gallbladder bile. The drugs that are used medically to achieve this end, Dr. Small commented, "may cure gallstones but cause atherosclerosis."

Dr. Ginter in Czechoslovakia may well have the answer to the problem of increasing the solvent capability of gallbladder bile without causing any side effects like atherosclerosis. Dr. Ginter suggests, on the basis of his experiments, that the amount of vitamin C in the liver is the factor which determines the rate of cholesterol transformation to bile acids. Increasing your vitamin C, according to Dr. Ginter's study, means more bile acid. And more bile acids mean that cholesterol remains in solution and does not precipitate out as gallstones—or arterial plaques.

But, how much vitamin C is enough? A person who is getting the U.S. Recommended Daily Allowance (U.S. RDA) may not show any outward signs of vitamin C deficiency, yet may have a hidden deficiency that can significantly reduce the rate of cholesterol transformation to bile acids. Dr. Ginter observed that animals marginally deficient in vitamin C consumed food normally and had a normal outward appearance, but the vitamin C concentrations in their livers and spleens were significantly lower than those in the control group and the total cholesterol concentration in their blood and livers was significantly higher.

One of the answers may indeed be to increase intake of vitamin C greatly. Our early ancestors who never worried about cholesterol consumed a diet of raw natural plant foods which provided between 2.3 grams and nine grams of vitamin C per day for a 150-pound man, according to Linus Pauling, professor of chemistry, Stanford University.

Those who have been subsisting on the RDA of 60 mg. of vitamin C daily may be astounded at the suggestion of taking C by the gram (1,000 mg.). But Dr. Boris Sokoloff brought about "improvement ranging from moderate to impressive" in 50 out of 60 atherosclerotic patients whom he treated with one to three grams of vitamin C daily, according to a report in the *Journal of the American Geriatric Society* (1966, 14, 1239).

# CHAPTER 57

# A Key to Better Brain Power

Dr. Linus Pauling, twice winner of the Nobel Prize and perhaps America's most acclaimed scientist, asked the following question at the Second International Conference of Social Psychiatry in London in 1969: "What would be the consequence for the world if the national leaders and the people as a whole were to think just 10 percent more clearly?" Dr. Pauling was really asking, "What would be the net effect on society if everyone consumed the optimum amount of vitamin C?" for he is convinced that 10 percent improvement in both physical and mental health is the result of such nutrition. While most of us are familiar with the physiological benefits that vitamin C can confer, not so many of us realize that it also benefits our mentality. Psychiatrists have made tremendous strides in recent years treating their patients with megavitamin therapy. The basis of this therapy is massive amounts of niacin (vitamin $B_3$), usually given along with other members of the B complex. But very large doses of vitamin C are an integral part of this therapy, and there is considerable evidence that schizophrenics have a very special need for this vitamin.

A simple deficiency of vitamin C is enough to produce confusion and listlessness in a person who is not afflicted with any specific psychiatric disorder. Persons with very poor eating habits or chronically ill persons eating very little food are the most susceptible to extreme vitamin C deficiency, which will produce both physical and mental symptoms of scurvy.

Whether or not an active person who has a good appetite would be able to play a better game of chess or better direct the affairs of a nation if he took a vitamin C supplement remains to be seen. Nevertheless, Dr. Pauling's question underlines the indisputable fact that insufficient vitamin C can cause impaired mentality—in anyone.

## Vitamins the Brain Needs

Why should vitamin C be important to clear thinking? In one sense, the answer is quite simple. As Dr. Pauling explained in an article in *Science* (19 April 1968), " . . . the proper functioning of the mind is known to require the presence in the brain of the molecules of many different substances. For example, mental disease, usually associated with physical disease, results from a low concentration in the brain of any one of the following vitamins: thiamine ($B_1$), nicotinic acid or nicotinamide ($B_3$), pyridoxine ($B_6$), cyanocobalamin ($B_{12}$), biotin, ascorbic acid (C), and folic acid. There is evidence that mental function and behavior are also affected by changes in the concentration in the brain of any of a number of other substances that are normally present. . . ."

An impressive demonstration of the relationship of vitamins to mental function, specifically in the elderly, was reported by M. L. Mitra, working with geriatric patients in a British hospital. In a report entitled "Confusional States in Relation to Vitamin Deficiencies in the Elderly" (*Journal of the American Geriatrics Society,* June 1971), Mitra described seven cases of confusional states caused solely or largely by vitamin C deficiency.

A 70-year-old woman, on admission to the hospital, was feverish, lethargic, and confused. Antibiotic treatment cleared up a serious infection, but the patient still complained of lethargy, depression, painful legs, and bruises all over her body, the latter two being known symptoms of vitamin C deficiency. Tests confirmed the deficiency, which was corrected with one gram of ascorbic acid daily for three weeks. At that time, her physical and mental symptoms disappeared, and she felt so well that she was discharged and required no further medical attention. Mitra cited other similar cases which demonstrate the link between mental states (which may be incorrectly diagnosed as "senility") and a deficiency of ascorbic acid.

## Brain Cells Require Large Amounts of Vitamin C

The brain, in fact, has a greater concentration of vitamin C in it than most of the other tissues of the body, according to *The Vitamins* (W. H. Sebrell, Jr., and Robert Harris, editors, New York: Academic Press, 1967). Guinea pigs suffering from scurvy, the vitamin C deficiency disease, develop significant biochemical changes in their brain tissues, according to the famous European researcher Dr. Emil Ginter, *Biologia* (17, 771: 1962). In view of these two facts, it is not surprising that a deficiency of vitamin C in human beings can produce mental symptoms, which include listlessness, confusion, and depression.

Vitamin C plays a very special role in the mental status of the schizophrenic. According to Dr. Allan Cott, psychiatrist, vitamin C assists in the conversion of a body substance called adrenochrome to one called leucoadrenochrome, a non-toxic substance. In persons suffering from schizophrenia, he points out, the adrenochrome is instead converted into a toxic substance called adrenolutin. Dr. Cott writes that " . . . vitamin C was added to the (megavitamin) treatment when it was found that ascorbic acid retarded the oxidation of adrenalin and in this way reduced the production of adrenochrome. . . . Adrenochrome combines with vitamin C and uses it up more quickly, leaving a C-deficiency in schizophrenics. Vanderkamp's test shows requirements of 10 to 30 grams or more in schizophrenic patients before free ascorbic acid is found in the urine."

The precise significance of the fact that vitamin C spills into the urine of schizophrenics only after a huge intake has not been ascertained. Some doctors, including Dr. Cott, believe that it may involve the destruction of vitamin C by hormonal by-products of the almost constant state of stress in which the schizophrenic lives. Stress, it is known, rapidly uses up vitamin C.

Dr. Roger J. Williams, in his book *Nutrition Against Disease* (New York: Pitman Publishing Corp., 1971), writes, "We cannot be absolutely certain yet that all mentally diseased individuals have ascorbic acid deficiency and are improved by massive doses. But the evidence points strongly toward the conclusion that ascorbic acid is a link in the chain and giving the brain cells an ample supply is one way to help insure healthy brain functioning."

What about the great majority of people—those who are not schizophrenic? Is it possible that some of us have unusually high requirements for vitamin C? Dr. Williams, one of America's leading nutrition researchers, thinks that many people do indeed have extraordinary requirements for vitamin C. In his research Dr. Williams discovered that guinea pigs, like human beings, require dietary vitamin C because they cannot manufacture it, and vary in their need for this vitamin tremendously. His study "Individuality In Vitamin C Needs," which he wrote with G. Deason, appearing in the *Proceedings of the National Academy of Sciences* (57, 6, 1967), showed that some guinea pigs require 32 times more vitamin C than others in order to maintain health. Tests by other scientists have confirmed these findings, and some researchers claim that the difference in requirements for vitamin C among individual guinea pigs can be as high as a factor of 250.

There is, then, at least a good probability that many people consuming no more than the minimum daily allowance of vitamin C are not getting all that they require for top physical and mental well-being. Irwin Stone, author of *The Healing Factor* (New York: Grosset and Dunlap, 1972), and Dr. Linus Pauling both recommend an average daily intake of at least several grams.

Perhaps this much is required by some people. A more conservative goal might be one-half gram (500 mg.) to one gram (1,000 mg.) every day. During periods of stress or illness this should, of course, be increased.

# CHAPTER 58

# Protection Against Poisoning from Toxic Substances in the Environment

Children who live in highly congested urban areas, whether or not they eat flakes of lead paint, have shown dangerously high levels of this toxic metal in their systems. The major source of this poison is automobiles. According to the National Air Pollution Control Administration, cars emit no less than 500 million pounds of lead into the atmosphere each year. Other sources of lead are some of the glazed earthenware eating and serving dishes, some toothpaste tubes, and sealants such as those used in the preservation of canned evaporated milk. Much of the commercial food that is sold today also contains excessive amounts of lead.

It's authoritatively estimated that some 200,000 American children are the victims of chronic lead poisoning, whether diagnosed or not, while 400,000 others are very close to developing symptoms. In fact, the average American already harbors more than a quarter of the amount of lead necessary to meet the medical definition of lead poisoning in adults. The systems of those living in urban areas are even closer to the critical level.

As the level of lead rises in you, the ability of your body to rid itself of this poison is crippled. As lead accumulates, the progressive results are irritability, fatigue, insomnia, constipation, confusion, kidney damage, convulsions, paralysis, and finally death. Many children with lead poisoning suffer from hyperactivity and irreversible retardation, besides the purely physical symptoms.

In several studies attempting to determine the rate of toxicity of lead ingestion, it has been noted that vitamin C often appears as an antidote to the devastating effects of lead poisoning. A study published in the Yugoslavian journal, *Acta. Pharm. Jugosl.* (December 1962) named vitamin C as a useful antidote in cases of lead poisoning.

In the United States, Dr. E. D. Hobart and associates at Rush Medical College in Chicago found that muscle damage from lead poisoning is much more severe when vitamin C levels are low. The vitamin C-deficient test guinea pigs, which were fed lead, developed widespread damage of muscle fiber and calcium deposits around the damaged cells. Vitamin C, the researchers noted, is essential in producing connective tissue which surrounds and protects muscle fibers. Experiment results reported in Japan's *Tohoku Journal of Experimental Medicine* (46: 295-322, 1944) said that vitamin C administered to test animals on high lead diets actually prolonged their lives.

## Mercury Poisoning Also Inhibited by Vitamin C

Mercury is still another heavy metal which poses at least a potential threat to the health of all of us. In Japan, catastrophic crippling and death have resulted from eating seafood contaminated with mercury. Here again, vitamin C can be a literal lifesaver. This was demonstrated in a dramatic series of experiments reported in 1964 by Momcilo Mokranjac and Ceda Petrovic in the *Comptes Rendus Hebdomadaires des Seances de l'Academie des Sciences* (Paris).

The scientists first established the dose of mercury chloride that is fatal to guinea pigs. Then they gave each one of a fresh group of guinea pigs 200 mg. of vitamin C a day for six days (the human equivalent of almost 14 grams a day). On the sixth day all the C-fortified guinea pigs were given lethal doses of mercury—and not one of them died. Maintained on 0.2 grams of vitamin C each day after poisoning, all the animals were alive and well.

Variations of this experiment showed that while vitamin C is useful as an antidote to mercury poisoning, it is much more effective when the system is already saturated with it at the moment the poisoning occurs. In other words, vitamin C should be taken every day as a preventive measure.

## Also Protects Against other Environmental Poisons

This vital nutrient also offers protection against cadmium poisoning, an increasing danger. Although the element is relatively scarce, comprising only 0.00002 percent of the earth's organic crust, recent findings indicate that, due to industrial pollution, there are ever-greater concentrations of cadmium in our food, water, and air. Excessive levels of cadmium are known to be detrimental to human health, "causing high blood pressure in low concentrations and testicular atrophy and brittleness of the bones in high concentrations" *Ecologist* (November 1975).

It's almost impossible to escape cadmium if you live in the United States. If you eat white bread, it is depositing significant quantities of cadmium into your stomach and they are ultimately getting into your bloodstream. If you drink coffee or tea, your system is accumulating still more cadmium. If you live any place where automobiles drive along the road then both the automobile exhausts and the tires wearing down in use are putting cadmium into your lungs when you breathe. If you smoke, or even if you sit in a room where someone else is smoking, your lungs are accumulating still more cadmium from the tobacco smoke. If you eat food that has been fertilized with phosphates, that food contains cadmium from the fertilizer. So how are you going to avoid this particular mineral, and more important, how are you going to avoid the harm it does you?

That harm is something to avoid. Cadmium is named as a major cause of high blood pressure and stroke by Henry Schroeder, M.D., former director of the famed Dartmouth Trace Elements Laboratory, who has himself conducted exhaustive experiments with rats to uncover the relationship between cadmium and blood pressure.

"When the rats were given traces of cadmium in drinking water from the time of weaning, hypertension (high blood pressure) began to appear about a year of age, increasing the incidence with age. Once hypertensive, they remained so until death."

Could the finding be applied to human beings? That was where the study had actually begun, when autopsy examinations of victims of strokes, made by Dr. Isabel H. Tipton at the University of Tennessee, revealed that victims of stroke and hypertensive heart disease had high levels of cadmium in their bodies. Dr. Schroeder's study established that it was more than coincidence, and the cadmium was actually causing the disease. "Hearts were also enlarged," said Dr. Schroeder, "renal arteriolar sclerosis was found frequently and some of the systolic blood pressures were over 260. . . ." He also found typical atherosclerotic plaques in the coronary arteries of the mice exposed to cadmium. He concluded that if the mice had not been sacrificed for examination, they would have developed full scale atherosclerosis.

## Wide-ranging Damage from a Little Cadmium

Hypertension and heart disease are far from being the sum of the damage done by cadmium, however. Some scientists are beginning to consider this mineral pollutant the chief reason that tobacco smoke causes lung cancer. One of the most widespread harmful effects of cadmium is to displace zinc and deplete the body of that valuable element that is intimately connected with sexual health, wound healing, and even, some think, mental function.

Cadmium also depletes the body of iron, thus inducing

anemia. It was in the course of investigating this particular toxicity of cadmium that two FDA nutritionists established that vitamin C is an excellent detoxifier of the poisonous metal. Reporting in *Science* (4 September 1970), M. R. Spivey-Fox and Bert E. Fry, Jr., described a study of the ability of vitamin C to protect Japanese quail against cadmium. They used this particular bird because it is one of the most sensitive creatures on earth to environmental pollution, and anything that will protect the quail against a pollutant will surely protect human beings even better.

Their very well controlled study demonstrated that this is exactly what vitamin C will do in relation to cadmium. In four weeks' time young birds fed an adequate diet to which cadmium had been added grew slower than their controls and gained less weight. Seven of the 51 birds exposed to cadmium died while none of the controls did. But when cadmium plus vitamin C were added to the diets of a third group, it was found that the birds were given a strong measure of protection against the toxic mineral. The vitamin C improved the ability of the birds to utilize iron and zinc and not only did they stay alive but they showed far better growth and health.

And thus, while the administrative heads of the FDA were urging the public to reduce its intake of vitamin C, that agency's own Nutrition Division was establishing that we desperately need the vitamin to detoxify one of the most vicious and omnipresent of all pollutants.

## Nitrite Danger Lessened by Vitamin C

One of the most controversial subjects in scientific circles today concerns the legal use of nitrates and nitrites as preservatives and flavoring agents in such foods as hot dogs, bacon, canned ham, most luncheon meats, and smoked fish. Under laboratory conditions, it has been shown that once in the stomach nitrites can combine with substances known as secondary amines to create new compounds known as nitrosamines, which are powerful cancer-causing chemicals.

The battle rages with physicians and scientists who insist that both nitrates and nitrites should be forbidden as additives on one side, and, on the other side, the food processors and the Food and Drug Administration, who claim that the possibility of developing cancer is less important than the ready availability of these foods.

But what is the sensible course to take while the battle continues? One answer is to increase your vitamin C intake whenever you eat food which you suspect may contain nitrates or nitrites.

The special protection afforded by vitamin C was demonstrated at the Eppley Institute for Research in Cancer, a branch of the University of Nebraska Medical Center. An elaborate series of tests showed that when vitamin C is present in sufficient quantity, the transformation of nitrite into potentially deadly nitrosamines is blocked almost completely (97 to 99 percent). Dr. Sidney S. Mirvish and his colleagues were so impressed that they recommended vitamin C as a routine precautionary measure whenever any one of a large number of nitrite-treated foods or drugs are ingested.

# CHAPTER 59

# Minimize Drug Toxicity

A good reason to take vitamin C along when one goes to the hospital, or the doctor, or anywhere, is vitamin C's power to detoxify many common drugs. Corticosteroids are prescribed for a wide range of common illnesses, including acne, rheumatic fever, eczema, allergies, bronchial asthma, inflammatory bowel diseases, and myasthenia gravis. Many arthritis patients have been given these drugs. These "wonder drugs" are also accompanied by an impressive list of toxic side effects including: increased susceptibility to infection, edema, hypertension, hyperglycemia, acne, mental disturbances, congestive heart failure, thin fragile skin with impaired wound healing, menstrual irregularities, and glaucoma to name just a few. But in taking vitamin C along with the drug, chances of avoiding these complications are greatly improved. A study led by Jane Henkel Chretien, M.D., clinical instructor of medicine at Georgetown University Hospital and published in the *Journal of the Reticuloendothelial Society* (vol. 14, 1973), used vitamin C to correct defects caused by corticosteroids in patients' immunologic defense systems. Two grams of vitamin C administered orally over a 12-hour period fully reduced the steroid-induced block in the patients' infection-defense systems. Dr. Chretien concluded: "Correction of intracellular metabolic defects induced by steroids suggests the use of ascorbic acid in patients treated with steroids for long periods.''

Another study, by Drs. Vincent G. Zannoni and Paul H. Sato of New York University School of Medicine, which was reported in *Medical World News* (19 July 1974) showed that vitamin C can prevent toxicity of drugs by speeding up their metabolism, so they don't build up to excessive levels in the blood.

Vitamin C was said to lessen the side effects of levodopa treatment of Parkinson's disease by Dr. William Sacks, Research Center, Rockland State Hospital, Orangeburg, New York, in a letter to the *Lancet* (1 March 1975). So dramatic was the elimination of side effects that a 62-year-old man, who had discontinued his treatment because of intolerable nausea and salivation, was able to resume levodopa therapy with a reduced dosage.

"Within four weeks of starting ascorbic acid (vitamin C) the ability to move his head had increased. Salivation also decreased and his speech and handwriting improved considerably. He began to play the organ again, something he had not been able to do for several years,'' reported Dr. Sacks. To double-check the results, Dr. Sacks alternated ascorbic acid with a placebo under double-blind conditions. Side effects returned with the placebo and disappeared once again with vitamin C.

# CHAPTER 60

# The Answer
# to Internal Bleeding
# in Aspirin Users

One of the least publicized side effects of aspirin is its tendency to cause internal bleeding when misused or taken unwisely. It's difficult for many of us to accept the notion that a medication that can relieve headaches so well can just as easily damage the stomach lining when taken in excess or over a long period of time. The deleterious effects of aspirin were demonstrated by researchers D. J. Parry and P.H.N. Wood who reported in the British medical journal *Gut* (8:1967) that hospital patients suffering from intestinal bleeding are twice as likely to be regular aspirin users as patients hospitalized for some other reason.

Experienced physicians see a number of aspirin-induced problems. And they are aware that the aspirin habit is difficult to stop for many of the longtime users; hence, what is needed is a way to counteract the internal problems which confront aspirin users.

Such, at least, is the conclusion of a group of Scottish physicians under the direction of Dr. R. I. Russell of the University of Glasgow Department of Medicine. In two thorough studies published simultaneously in the *Lancet* (14 September 1968), Dr. Russell and associates describe research that led to their conclusion that vitamin C plays a definite role in counteracting the tendency of aspirin to cause bleeding of the gastrointestinal tract.

"It has long been known that repeated aspirin ingestion may cause chronic blood-loss in the gastrointestinal tract," reported Dr. Russell and associates.

## Vitamin C Deficit Linked to Hemorrhage

Dr. Russell reported on a case which suggested that ascorbic acid deficiency was a factor in causing internal hemorrhaging. The case was that of a woman of 43 who had been taking aspirin regularly for one month and had taken two 300 mg. tablets a few hours before admission to the Western Infirmary in Glasgow in 1965. She had multiple bruising of both legs and internal examination revealed multiple punctures of the mucous membranes of the gastric mucosa. Further diagnostic examination revealed that the patient had mild scurvy which suggested itself as a possible factor in her gastric hemorrhage. Challenged by this case, Dr. Russell and his group of Glasgow investigators worked out a further investigation to try to relate the vitamin C status of all patients admitted to the hospital with acute gastrointestinal hemorrhage, and further to relate the condition of these patients to their ingestion of aspirin and alcohol.

"Forty of the 60 patients with gastrointestinal hemorrhage (67 percent) had taken aspirin, alcohol, or both in the week before admission to hospital. But it was further found that despite these precipitating factors, a significantly higher proportion of those who had developed hemorrhage were low in ascorbic acid as compared with those who had taken the same precipitants but had not developed hemorrhage."

A further question now presented itself to the doctors. Was it perhaps the aspirin or alcohol or the bleeding that induced the vitamin C deficiency rather than being caused or permitted by it?

"To examine the effect of aspirin on L.A.A. (leucocyte ascorbic acid) levels, we asked four healthy volunteers to take 300 mg. aspirin twice daily for a week. The L.A.A. levels were measured twice in the week before ingestion, twice during the period of ingestion, and twice during the following week. L.A.A. levels were not significantly different," according to Dr. Russell.

It was established that the association of low vitamin C levels with gastric hemorrhage was that of a cause rather than an effect.

## Slight Deficiency Leads to Bleeding

This of course raised a further question. If vitamin C deficiency permitted toxic substances, notably aspirin, to irritate the gastric mucosa to the point of causing hemorrhage, how severe a deficiency is necessary to permit that extremely dangerous effect? "Although L.A.A. levels are low in patients with gastrointestinal hemorrhage, only six of them had any clinical evidence of scurvy. Many, therefore, suffer a subclinical form of the disease," reported Dr. Russell.

So it is not very much of a deficiency that is needed. You don't have to get so little vitamin C in your diet that you will develop hemorrhages of the skin capillaries and mouth, the first clinical signs of scurvy. There may be no obvious sign whatsoever. But if there is even a slight deficiency, the chances are enormously increased that taking aspirin or an alcoholic drink will cause bleeding in the stomach. Furthermore, the Scottish doctors discovered that "patients with low tissue levels of ascorbic acid, in which bleeding from a gastric erosion may have been precipitated by aspirin or alcohol, may . . . continue to bleed or restart bleeding due to faulty wound healing." The ultimate result is often a perforated ulcer, which certainly requires major surgery for its repair.

The Scottish research group further pursued the question of why there were low levels of vitamin C in the bleeding patients since they had found that the low levels were not caused by the aspirin or alcohol. Diet histories revealed that there was the simplest possible reason—the patients just didn't get enough vitamin C in their diets.

And finally Drs. Russell and A. Goldberg experimented on guinea pigs themselves to determine whether they could change the effects of aspirin by changing the level of vitamin C.

"Bleeding points were found significantly more often in the animals on the scorbutogenic diet than those on normal diet, and when aspirin had been administered the difference was even more striking," the team reported.

Thus checking in every imaginable way, these Scottish physicians emerged with a study showing that the amount of vitamin C in the diet can make all the difference, to a user of aspirin or alcoholic beverages, between mortally serious illness and a relatively mild illness that can be eliminated simply by eliminating use of the provoking factor.

# CHAPTER 61

# A Barrier
# to Bladder Cancer

In 1972, the federal government launched a multimillion-dollar program aimed at preventing, diagnosing, and treating bladder cancer. Obviously the government was reacting to the mounting incidence of the disease, which is already responsible for 10,000 deaths annually in the United States. Bladder cancer strikes most frequently between the ages of 50 and 70, and three out of four times it strikes a man. What makes it such a dread disease is the lack of success in treating it. According to statistics compiled by the American Cancer Institute, 42 percent of the people who develop bladder cancer die within five years.

As early as 1968, Tulane's Dr. J. U. Schlegel reported that vitamin C can prevent recurrences of tumor formation in the bladder. The key to prevention, Dr. Schlegel noted, is to provide this water-soluble vitamin in such ample amounts of the vitamin that an excess of it spills over into the urine and is carried to the bladder. Dr. Schlegel found that for most of his patients, 500 mg. of vitamin C taken three times a day kept bladder cancer from recurring (*Medical World News*, 21 June 1968).

Vitamin C in the bladder, which Dr. Schlegel called "a cesspool of active ingredients," apparently prevents the formation of cancer-causing compounds. Dr. Schlegel and three colleagues in the Department of Surgery at Tulane University School of

Medicine found that when vitamin C was added to the drinking water of laboratory mice, the animals resisted bladder tumor formation even when implanted with 3-hydroxyanthranilic acid (3-HOA), a proven bladder carcinogen. They theorized that the antioxidant effect of vitamin C prevented 3-HOA from being oxidized into toxic breakdown products.

As a result of their experimental studies, the researchers recommended a daily dose of 1,500 mg. of vitamin C "as a possible preventive measure of spontaneous bladder tumor formation and recurrence in man." They noted that, "the administration of 500 mg. ascorbate (vitamin C) three times a day should have no harmful consequences" (*Journal of Urology,* vol. 103, February 1970).

## Other Suspected Causes of Bladder Cancer

Alcoholic beverages, soft drinks, and coffee have all been implicated as causes of bladder cancer in test animals. People who drink alcohol are more likely to develop bladder cancer than those who don't, according to Dr. Meera Jain of the University of Toronto's Department of Preventive Medicine. Relating her findings in an interview, she noted that, along with her colleague, Dr. Robert W. Morgan, she had studied 233 bladder-cancer patients and a like number of healthy control subjects before she discovered that risk factor.

Even more startling, according to Dr. Jain, was the uncovering of a similar bladder-cancer risk factor among people who consume cola drinks. "We are not sure what causes this," she noted. "It may be aflatoxin mold that has contaminated the cola nuts, a prime ingredient in cola drinks. Or perhaps it is related to the caffeine content of these drinks." Dr. Jain's research was published in the *Journal of the Canadian Medical Association* (16 November 1974).

Dr. Jain also noted that people who consume large amounts of alcohol or cola increase the risk of bladder cancer if they smoke. This confirms earlier reports, by National Cancer Institute researchers and others, that there is a strong association between bladder cancer and smoking—a habit that rapidly depletes stores of vitamin C.

Still another clue to the puzzle of bladder cancer was turned up by Dr. Philip Cole of the Harvard School of Public Health in Boston. After interviewing 468 bladder-cancer patients in eastern Massachusetts, Dr. Cole reported "an unanticipated finding is association of the disease with coffee-drinking. . . . for both sexes, drinkers of less than one cup of coffee per day have lower bladder-cancer risk than any other 'exposure' category." Dr. Cole concluded in the *Lancet* (26 June 1971) that about a fourth of all bladder cancer in men and half of such cases among women might be caused by coffee drinking. Caffeine (a known mutagen) or artificial sweeteners such as saccharin might be responsible, he theorized.

With these facts in mind, it appears to be no mere coincidence then that while coffee is still the number one drink in terms of overall popularity, the consumption of several of the beverages linked to bladder cancer has also gone up. According to a report in the *New York Times* (28 July 1973), the average American consumed 30.3 gallons of soft drinks in 1972, up from 16.8 in 1962. And cola sales make up 63 percent of all soda sales. During that same 10-year period, beer sales increased almost 50 percent, whiskey sales 33 percent, and wine sales almost doubled. It's known, for example, that bladder-cancer death rates are higher in those states where per capita beer consumption is greatest (*Journal of the National Cancer Institute,* September 1974).

# More Evidence of Vitamin C's Protective Role in Bladder Cancer

One man who can vouch for the value of vitamin C in protection against bladder cancer is Dr. Lyle A. Baker, a veterinarian at Cornell University. "My father came down with bladder cancer about two and a half years ago," Dr. Baker recalled, "and the urologist who did the operation pointed out to me that in doing hundreds of these he had never seen bladder cancer himself in a non-smoker. In other words, it was always a smoker and my father was a two- or three-pack a day smoker. About that time I read a report from Tulane University which indicated that megavitamin doses of vitamin C would prevent the recurrence of bladder cancer, so I merely put my father on a couple of thousand milligrams per day and he has done very nicely for two and a half years with no recurrence. I cannot say that is what did it but here again, you see, what about people who smoke and what about their vitamin requirements? I would say that anybody who smokes should definitely be taking vitamin C" (*New Dynamics of Preventive Medicine,* New York: Intercontinental Medical Book Corp., 1974).

One way that vitamin C protects against the harmful effects of alcohol was reported recently by four researchers at Stobhill General Hospital in Glasgow, Scotland. N. Krasner and associates measured the time it took for alcohol to disappear from the blood of healthy volunteers before and after receiving a gram of vitamin C daily for two weeks. They found that the more vitamin C in the body, the quicker the alcohol was whisked away and destroyed by alcohol dehydrogenase, a liver enzyme (*Lancet,* 21 September 1974).

## 'Public Should Be Informed'

Vitamins C, $B_1$, and cysteine (a sulfur-containing amino acid) protected rats against the toxic effects of acetaldehyde, produced as a first step when the body metabolizes alcohol, reported Dr. Herbert Sprince of Philadelphia's Jefferson Medical College (*Medical World News,* 27 May 1974). Acetaldehyde is also found in tobacco smoke.

"I don't want to go on record . . . saying that once you've taken some vitamin C and $B_1$, to drink and smoke all you want and it isn't going to hurt you. I can't do that for one second," cautioned Dr. Sprince. "But I generally think the public should be informed of this, even though the work was done with rats. There's some strong feeling that this may be helpful for human therapy."

Obviously, scientists don't have all the answers yet about how the toxins we ingest may be triggering bladder cancer and other ailments. But as long as alcohol, soft drinks, coffee, and cigarette smoke remain a fact of daily life for millions of Americans, the advice of Drs. Sprince, Schlegel, and others to boost our intake of vitamin C makes good sense.

# CHAPTER 62

# Frostbite Preventive

According to some interesting studies undertaken in Canada, a country where the thermometer dips to frostbite levels, a person can actually regulate his internal thermostatic mechanism to produce more body heat—if he gets plenty of vitamin C. "Low temperatures increase the need for vitamin C and beneficial effects of ascorbic acid have been observed in people exposed to extremely low temperatures," reported Dr. Marie-Louise Desbarets-Schonbaum, assistant professor of pharmacology at the University of Toronto (*Toronto Star,* 7 February 1973). She studied the role of vitamin C in maintaining adequate body temperature in cold environments.

"People exposed to chilly temperatures and whose food supply was limited have been found to develop disturbances in the circulation of their feet," Dr. Schonbaum said. "Such problems could be relieved or avoided, if these people were given extra ascorbic acid."

Some people get acclimated to cold weather as the seasons change. Others, though they insulate themselves with warm clothing, just seem to shiver in their snuggies all winter long and just can't wait until the first robin makes his appearance in the garden. To these people, winter is a cold misery. According to the Canadian study, people who just can't stand the cold, would get more joy out of the beauty of the season if they also got more vitamin C. Apparently, vitamin C can be to your body what antifreeze is to your car.

# Vitamin C Improves Circulation

How it works is still a mystery, but Dr. Schonbaum believes that when ascorbic acid is in short supply, a certain enzyme which, through an intricate pattern of activity, encourages full circulation of the blood, may not be able to do its job. Lacking vitamin C, the enzyme is unable to do its work properly and, according to Dr. Schonbaum, this could account for some of the circulation disturbances people suffer in a cold climate.

According to an earlier study also done in Canada, by Dr. Louis-Paul Dugal of the department of biology, University of Ottawa, and reported in the *Annals New York Academy of Science* (21 April 1961), it is possible that the beneficial effects of vitamin C may be due, at least in part, to its action on the precursors of particular heat-raising hormones. "We recently observed in our laboratory," reported Dr. Dugal, "that both exposure to cold and vitamin C administration accelerate the metabolism of tyrosine and phenylalanine, precursors of thyroid and medullary hormones."

In a series of experiments, Dr. Dugal was able to show, convincingly, that vitamin C, in large doses, helps to keep the body temperature up when exposed to a cold environment. With both guinea pigs and rats, the percentage of survival was always enhanced by vitamin C. With guinea pigs, moreover, Dr. Dugal found that more and more vitamin C was needed as the temperature of exposure was lowered. The guinea pig, like man, does not synthesize vitamin C within its body. Most animals do. It may be as important as fur in helping them endure the rigors of winter.

# Resistance to Freezing

In both man and monkey, it appears, vitamin C can help prevent frostbite as well as keep the body temperature up without raising the room thermostat. A group of monkeys given a fairly large dose of ascorbic acid daily for six months, Dr. Dugal found, were able to endure a freezing climate with far fewer consequences than another group of monkeys getting only 25 mg. of ascorbic acid daily. In the monkey study, a control group of 11 monkeys was kept constantly at room temperature and fed regular dog food plus an oral supplement of 25 mg. of ascorbic acid daily for six months. Another group consisting of eight monkeys was given the identical diet and the same amount of ascorbic acid, but was kept in a mildly cold environment of 10° C. for six months. Finally, five monkeys, kept at the same mildly cold temperature for six months and on the same diet as the other two groups, received 325 mg. of ascorbic acid daily. Then, all the monkeys were exposed to an intensely cold environment of minus 20° C. for a period of two hours.

The results? In the first group, the fall in rectal temperature was three degrees Centigrade. (This group had not been pre-exposed to the cold before exposure to the minus 20° C. temperature.) Group two, which had been preexposed at 10° C., had grown a much thicker fur than group one but experienced the same fall in rectal temperature. But group three, preexposed to the same cold temperature and receiving 325 mg. of ascorbic acid daily, experienced a fall in rectal temperature of only 2.1 degrees Centigrade, a difference of .9 degrees. This, says the research team, is statistically very significant.

Did vitamin C protect the monkeys from frostbite? Yes. As many as 35.4 percent of the monkeys who were getting 25 mg. a day of ascorbic acid experienced frostbite of the tail. But only 3.6 percent of those who were getting 325 mg. a day experienced frostbite. In other words, there was 10 times as much frostbite among the animals on low vitamin C.

The thermal effect of vitamin C is, according to another research study, just as beneficial for man as it is for monkeys. A team of researchers headed by Dr. J. M. Leblanc has shown that large doses (425 mg. a day) of vitamin C were beneficial in cold climates according to an article appearing in the *Canadian Journal of Biochemical Physiology* (32: 407, 1954). Skin temperature was better maintained, Dr. Leblanc reported, foot trouble was greatly decreased as compared with the low vitamin group (25 mg. a day), and sensation of discomfort was decreased.

How much vitamin C should you give your children to help keep their fingers from numbing on their way to school? Forty times the amount recommended by the Food and Nutrition Board of the National Academy of Science is what is needed by the growing child even when he is not exposed to cold, reported Dr. Man-Li S. Yew of the University of Texas at Austin (*Associated Press Dispatch,* 17 October 1972).

Dr. Yew told the conference of the National Academy of Science that when young, healthy guinea pigs were fed a diet supplemented with ascorbic acid at four different levels, there was a decided difference in their growth rate, their recovery time after surgical stress, and in wound healing. Young guinea pigs, Dr. Yew said, ordinarily need about five mg. per 100 grams of body weight daily. "This is far beyond what is needed to prevent scurvy . . . and . . . under stress the needs are even higher," reported Dr. Yew. "On a body-weight basis, this is equivalent to the need on the part of a developing 30 kilogram (65 pounds) youngster of 1,500 mg. of ascorbic acid daily, rather than the Food and Nutrition Board's recommendation of 40 mg."

Remember that stress creates the need for more vitamin C. And cold is a stress on the system. It took 325 mg. of vitamin C daily to help prevent frostbite of the tail in the experimental monkeys. Now do your own calculations, based on your own weight and the stress conditions under which you live. One thing is certain. Vitamin C in large quantities can help you avoid the shivers this winter.

## Common Foods Rich in Ascorbic Acid*

| | (milligrams) |
|---|---|
| Honeydew (½ melon) | 172 |
| Cantaloupe (½ melon) | 90 |
| Oranges (1) | 66 |
| Strawberries (1 cup) | 88 |
| Blueberries (1 cup) | 20 |
| Papaya (1 cup, cubed) | 78 |
| Kale (1 cup, cooked) | 102 |
| Brussels sprouts (1 cup, cooked) | 135 |
| Peppers (green, 1) | 210 |
| Broccoli (1 cup, cooked) | 140 |
| Cauliflower (1 cup, cooked) | 69 |
| Spinach (1 cup, cooked) | 50 |
| Lima beans (1 cup, cooked) | 29 |
| Cabbage (1 cup, cooked) | 48 |
| Tomatoes (1) | 28 |

*Selected from tables in *Nutritive Value of American Foods in Common Units,* United States Department of Agriculture Handbook #456, November, 1975.

# CHAPTER 63

# Bioflavonoids: The "Useless" Vitamin We Need

It was back in the thirties that the Hungarian scientist, Dr. Albert Szent-Gyorgyi—then at work isolating vitamin C, or ascorbic acid—stumbled on the bioflavonoids.

What are the bioflavonoids? They are brightly colored substances that appear in fruits, along with vitamin C. They have also been called vitamin $C_2$, vitamin P, flavones, flavonols, flavonones, and so forth. Vitamin P, whose organic structure as a vitamin is disputed by some physicians, is a substance that occurs along with vitamin C in foods. So when you take vitamin C made in a laboratory you don't get any vitamin P, of course. But when you eat foods rich in vitamin C, such as citrus fruits or green peppers, the vitamin P comes right along with the vitamin C. And researchers have discovered that in many situations where vitamin C alone is not effective, the combination of the two will work wonders. Biologically active, they are widespread in nature but found most abundantly in the white pulp of citrus fruit. Dr. Szent-Gyorgyi found in his earliest studies that the bioflavonoids (which he named vitamin P) play a role in strengthening the body's smallest blood vessels, the capillaries.

For his work in crystalizing and isolating vitamin C, Dr. Szent-Gyorgyi won the Nobel prize in medicine in 1937. And in the years that followed, both vitamin C and vitamin P figured in thousands of animal and human studies conducted all over the world. Physicians prescribed the bioflavonoids (usually in company with vitamin C) for literally dozens of disorders believed to be related to faulty capillary function—habitual and threatened abortion, postpartum bleeding, nosebleed, skin disorders, diabetes retinitis, bleeding gums, heavy menstrual bleeding, hemorrhoids, and many others. Papers appeared in the journals testifying to clinical success.

Nevertheless, American scientists came to doubt that the bioflavonoids could classify as vitamins. Were they really essential to human health—that is, a substance normally involved in human metabolism? Or did they merely have some helpful pharmacological properties? The very name, bioflavonoids, came into common usage because of unwillingness to use the term vitamin P.

But this downgrading of an important nutrient was just the beginning. By the late 1960s, the United States Food and Drug Administration (FDA) had decided not only were the bioflavonoids not a vitamin; they had no nutritional value at all.

## Plentiful in American Diet

There's a ready explanation, Dr. Szent-Gyorgyi says, why the American scientific community has failed to accept the bioflavonoids as vitamins. Writing in his book, *The Living State* (New York: Academic Press, 1972), the scientist points out that most fruits and vegetables are rich in these substances, and the citrus fruits extremely so. Almost all Americans get enough of these foods to prevent gross vitamin P deficiency and obvious unmistakable signs of deficiency disease. It's not that vitamin P is unnecessary—but that it's already there.

But such superior nutritional conditions were not true of Hungary after the war, where citrus fruits were a rarity and vegetables in very poor supply. And physicians in that unhappy country found that there were indeed deficiency disorders that yielded specifically and only to administration of bioflavonoids.

Edema, or the accumulation of fluid in the tissue, and bleeding into the tissue (noticeable as red spots and splotches when it occurs close under the skin) both can be the result of fragile faulty capillaries. Vitamin C has a recognized role in maintaining capillary health. Capillary breakage is characteristic of the vitamin C deficiency disease, scurvy. But vitamin P, which in nature is found in close association with vitamin C, has an essential role also.

Just what is the function of the capillaries? It is not too much to say that the entire cardiovascular system—heart, arteries, and veins—exists for the whole purpose of serving the capillaries. For these narrowest of blood vessels, just wide enough to let blood cells go through in single file, are the business end of the circulatory system.

It is here and here only that the cells receive from the bloodstream the oxygen, nutrients, hormones, antibodies— everything the bloodstream delivers. And it's here the wastes are taken up. All the rest of the circulatory vessels—arteries that carry fresh oxygenated blood from the heart to all parts of the body and the veins that carry the used blood back to the heart for reoxygenation in the lungs—these vessels are impermeable, watertight. It's only at the capillary level—the network of capillaries that form links joining the tiniest arteries (arterioles) to the tiniest veins (venules)—that fluid from the bloodstream seeps out of this otherwise closed system and mingles with the fluid that constantly surrounds all the body's cells. And then seeps back again.

For this seepage to take place, the walls of the capillaries must be permeable. But not *too* permeable. The blood cells and blood proteins normally stay within the capillaries. It's the presence there of the blood proteins that provides the osmotic pressure which accounts for the fluid's eventual return to the bloodstream at the venule end of the capillary. The proteins, as Dr. Roger James expresses it in his book, *Understanding Medicine* (Baltimore: Penguin Books, 1970), "give to the blood an osmotic pressure which acts so as to draw fluid into the capillary from the outside like a kind of magnet."

When capillaries are too fragile and break, or too permeable.

the blood itself passes out into the intercellular fluid. Bruises are a concrete sign of capillary breakage near the surface of the skin—and a skin that bruises easily is a signal that capillaries are not as strong as they should be. Edema develops when the osmotic pressure is insufficient to draw accumulated intercellular fluid back into the flowing bloodstream, and this condition, too, can be caused by capillaries that are too permeable; they allow the escape of blood proteins that are needed inside for the maintenance of proper osmotic pressure. Fluid accumulates around an infected or wounded area because, in defensive action, the nearby capillaries become extremely permeable; the cells that form the capillary wall pull apart leaving spaces in between, thus allowing the white blood cells to leave the circulating blood and pour into the affected area to fight invading microorganisms. Blood proteins also flow into the intercellular fluid through the enlarged spaces, and the osmotic pressure that normally pulls back the fluid is temporarily lost.

## Abundant Evidence in Scientific Reports

With this brief description of capillary function it is clear that any nutrient that is involved here has indeed a vital role to play in human health. When we learn that vitamin P helps decrease capillary fragility and helps prevent abnormal permeability, we can recognize that this is a characteristic of prime importance to the well-being of every cell in the body. For all the cells depend totally on the capillaries to bring them everything they need and to take away every waste that would poison them.

The literature describing the benefits of bioflavonoids in treating ailments stemming from capillary disorders is lengthy and convincing. Even the conservative *Medical Letter* (9 February 1968), which approved of the FDA action in banning bioflavonoid medications as ineffective, had to agree that the many studies demonstrating effective therapy with the bioflavonoids were done by competent investigators whose "studies were of about the same quality as many of the studies now being reported." The publication went on to quote from articles which had appeared in half a dozen respected journals from 1955 to 1963, including this report from the *Annals of the New York Academy of Sciences:* "Taking everything together, there can be little doubt that flavonoids are not only useful therapeutic agents in conditions of capillary fragility, but have many diverse actions in the animal body."

Fresh fruits and vegetables in general provide both vitamin C and vitamin P. And the citrus fruits are especially rich in both. When eating an orange or grapefruit or cutting up a lemon for seasoning or juice or dessert, don't throw away the pulp. Especially the little white core that runs down the middle—that's a treasure trove of bioflavonoids.

The citrus fruits have a mixture of flavonoids, and a good commercial product of bioflavonoids from lemon (the citrus fruit from which vitamin P is usually extracted) contains the entire lemon bioflavonoid complex—not a select few. At the present time bioflavonoids are not sold separately but in combination with vitamin C.

When making salads, think of vitamin P and be generous with the green pepper strips and include the white pulpy portion where bioflavonoids are concentrated.

## Bioflavonoids and Menstrual Problems

Bioflavonoids are of special importance to women suffering from any of a wide variety of ailments usually summed up by the phrase, "female problems." But men as well as women are likely candidates for some surprising benefits from the bioflavonoids.

A series of reports comes from Strasbourg, France, where Dr. T. Muller and his associates at the Hospices Civils announced the results of a study in which flavone (another name for bioflavonoid) compounds were used on a large number of women coming to their hospital with gynecological problems, according to an article in *Family Practice News* (15 March 1974).

The French team of doctors said the major finding was that "flavone compounds are highly effective substitutes for hormone therapy in most cases of functional uterine bleeding." In 18 of 20 women who were treated for irregular or painful menstrual flow (which was not caused by anatomical damage), results were rated as good to excellent. Improvement was progressive, with most improvement achieved by the third menstrual cycle. Few, if any, side effects were noted. In addition, the doctors reported, these same flavone or bioflavonoid compounds are also useful in preventing the bleeding that often follows the insertion of an intrauterine contraceptive device. Of 40 women who took bioflavonoids after insertion of an IUD, only one failed to return to a normal menstrual flow by the third cycle.

What is it about bioflavonoids that exerts this protective effect against abnormal bleeding? The published report of this work mentions that the flavone compounds "have been shown to improve venous (vein) tone and increase capillary wall resistance." In other words, when generous amounts of bioflavonoids are added to the diet, they have been observed to help prevent pressure problems and leaks in the vast internal pumping system which distributes and returns blood to the heart.

If bioflavonoids are so good for the veins and capillaries, you might expect that there would be other uses to which doctors could put them besides irregular uterine bleeding. And it turns out that Dr. Muller and his associates did just this.

## Varicose Veins and Hemorrhoids Reported to Improve

When bioflavonoids were given to 60 women complaining of varicose veins, they reported pain, discomfort, and swelling of the legs were significantly relieved. Hemorrhoids, another common problem of pregnancy, were also relieved by bioflavonoid treatment, the doctors reported.

Women who were helped the most were those whose problems were relatively mild. Women who had given birth to several children and had more serious problems with their legs had somewhat less improvement. Nevertheless, in this latter group of women, fully two-thirds obtained relief from painful throbbing and swelling.

Pregnant women who were suffering the most with leg problems, some of whom had varicose ulcers, did not show very much improvement in the appearance of their veins that could be physically measured. Despite this, most of the women "reported a prompt disappearance of pain and swelling sensations" after taking bioflavonoids.

The fact that bioflavonoids can give great help with cases of hemorrhoids and varicose veins—not necessarily accompanying pregnancy—had been demonstrated earlier by Dr. Bernard A. D. Wissmer of the Medical Policlinic of the University of Geneva, reporting in *Current Therapeutic Research* (August 1963). Dr. Wissmer said that he had cured many patients suffering various types of hemorrhoids with a bioflavonoid compound. In most cases, he said, pain and hemorrhaging stopped after two to five days. He also noted that varicose veins often improved strikingly during treatment with his bioflavonoid compound.

## Saving the Babies with Bioflavonoids

Fragility and poor tone of veins and capillaries can cause a woman pain and distress, but they can prove fatal to a developing fetus, which depends on the integrity of its mother's small blood vessels to keep it growing. Back in 1955, an Atlanta, Georgia, physician discovered that women who had a history of habitual abortion frequently developed large discolored spots from the smallest bruises. This led Dr. Robert B. Greenblatt, of the Medical College of Georgia, to test them for abnormal capillary fragility. At a conference on bioflavonoids and the capillary sponsored by the New York Academy of Sciences on 11 February 1965, Dr. Greenblatt reported that "positive tests were obtained in over 80 percent, a much higher incidence than that found in a control group."

Working on the then new theory that bioflavonoids could reduce capillary fragility, Dr. Greenblatt gave them along with vitamin C (the two are almost always found together in nature) to a total of 21 expectant mothers. Of 13 patients who had two previous spontaneous abortions, 11 delivered live infants after the nutritional treatment. Available statistics, Dr. Greenblatt said, indicate that the expected number of live babies from this group would be only eight. In a group of seven patients who had anywhere from three to eight previous successive abortions, four were delivered of live infants, whereas statistics indicated that only one live baby should be expected.

One would expect that this study made medical history, but that wasn't to be the case, because it was not "controlled." (That is, one group of women would get bioflavonoids while another group would be given something else—or nothing—to demonstrate a difference in response.) In addition, Dr. Greenblatt, anxious to take every possible precaution, gave all the women vitamins, minerals, hormone therapy and bed rest as part of their preventive care. So it is impossible to say exactly how much of the unexpected success was due exclusively to the bioflavonoids. But Dr. Greenblatt suggested that at the very least, it does seem to be a good idea to give bioflavonoids to all women with a history of habitual abortion who are also found to have capillary fragility. And he added that whatever its statistical significance, the use of bioflavonoids in his own practice resulted in a considerable improvement in the "salvage rate" of babies carried by habitually aborting mothers.

According to an article in *Science News Letter* (17 January 1959) Dr. Thomas F. Dowd, attending physician to the Philadelphia Eagles, reported on his experience giving bioflavonoids to professional football players. He told a symposium on stress and circulation held in Detroit that ordinarily, about 40 percent of football players show large bruises after a game, and all but five percent of the remaining players have smaller bruised areas.

After going on a regimen of three citrus bioflavonoid capsules a day, only five percent of the players were discovered to have large bruises after a game. Physiologically, this makes perfect sense since bruises are nothing but a mass of broken or damaged capillaries.

# A Natural Antithrombosis Factor

The work of Dr. R. C. Robbins of the University of Florida has vastly extended the frontiers of our knowledge about bioflavonoids and pointed the way toward health benefits that might far outweigh those already known.

The essence of Dr. Robbins' discovery is that the bioflavonoids, particularly certain citrus bioflavonoids, are natural and potent antithrombosis agents. He found this to be true in test-tube experiments, animal experiments, and blood studies of human beings.

These new findings would not make the bioflavonoids the first natural antithrombosis factor, however. Another such agent is heparin, manufactured and secreted by the liver, and which is often injected by physicians into patients who seem to be at a very high risk of developing a thrombosis (a pathological blood clot which may form in the veins of the leg, tear loose, and wind up blocking a major blood vessel). This can lead to severe injury to the lungs and heart, all too often causing the swift death of cardiac tissue which is deprived of its oxygen-rich supply of blood.

In an article in the medical journal *Atherosclerosis* (18, 1973, 73–82), Dr. Robbins described an experiment in which he tested the antithrombogenic potency of heparin against that of nobiletin, one of the most physiologically active of the bioflavonoids. Of course, he didn't decide to conduct this complicated test purely on a hunch. Over the past six or seven years, he explained, little-known but fascinating research has shown that the flavonoids "have antiadhesive effects on blood cells." By this, he means that they tend to prevent blood cells, and to a lesser extent, blood platelets, from clumping together in clots that can seriously interfere with the normal flow of the circulating blood. He further explained that "flavonoids such as hesperidin and rutin" have been shown to increase the life span of rats which were fed diets calculated to induce thrombosis.

With this in mind, he set out to observe the effects of the bioflavonoid compound nobiletin on laboratory rats which had been injected with adenosine diphosphate (ADP), a chemical which is known to induce blood clumping, widespread lung thrombosis, and death in animals. At the same time, another group of animals which were given ADP were also given heparin, so that the protective effect of heparin could be compared to that of the bioflavonoid substance, nobiletin.

The tests showed that the nobiletin was, in fact, far more effective in preventing death from thrombosis than was heparin. In one group of 11 animals which were infused with ADP, all those given the bioflavonoid complex survived, while in the group given heparin, four died. In the second group, which was given a larger dose of ADP, all those given the bioflavonoid complex survived again, and again four in the heparin group died. When the dose of ADP was increased drastically, six of 11 animals in the bioflavonoid group lived, but only three of 11 in the heparin group lived.

In another series of tests, Dr. Robbins measured the blood of animals to see what effect nobiletin had on blood-clotting time. He found that it had almost no effect at all—which is considered a safety factor, because any substance which significantly raises the clotting time of blood poses a threat of excessive bleeding.

He cautioned, however, that bioflavonoid compounds "should be approached with guarded enthusiasm as a sole treatment against thrombosis." Thrombosis triggered by ADP, he warned, is not necessarily the same kind of thrombosis which most often arises in human arteries. Usually, thrombosis in the body involves an excess of a substance known as fibrin, which seems to act like a net in the bloodstream, catching various particles and causing them to stick together in a clot. And while heparin is effective against fibrin, bioflavonoids are not.

## Not the Sole Answer, But Helpful

Nevertheless, Dr. Robbins feels that because of the proven antiadhesive potencies of the bioflavonoids, their presence in the bloodstream would probably serve to slow down the growth of a pathological clot considerably, and notes that heparin and the bioflavonoid nobiletin are compatible in use. He further suggests that "antiadhesive compounds are not only indicated in impending thrombosis and embolism of large blood vessels but may be useful in disease and traumas where aggregated blood cells interfere with the microcirculation." He added that another plus in favor of the bioflavonoids is that they are safe, and do not interfere with the ability of the blood to clot when clotting is required to close an injury.

Dr. Robbins also published another study of bioflavonoids in *International Journal of Vitamin and Nutrition Research* (43, 1973, 494–503) in which he described in detail the ability of various bioflavonoid compounds to reduce abnormal blood clumping. He concluded: "A dietary role for flavonoids is suggested by evidence of a widespread low-level blood cell aggregation in apparently healthy subjects, which is inhibited by flavonoids that are normal components of certain foods." And he added: "The significance of blood cell aggregation is that it interferes with the microcirculation, causing a variety of adverse effects, and promotes thrombosis and embolism of large vessels."

Later in the article, discussing the protective effect of nobiletin against experimentally induced thrombosis, Dr. Robbins suggested that "this (inhibition of thrombosis) may be a relevant observation in view of the high incidence of cardiovascular diseases in Western countries that terminate in thrombotic episodes."

Dr. Robbins' work indicates that the bioflavonoids, besides easing the discomfort of varicose veins, probably also reduce the risk of a thrombosis arising in these inflamed veins. It also shows that, although the bioflavonoids seem to restore normal resistance to capillary walls, they don't do this by causing any "thickening" of the blood. In fact, since they act to prevent abnormal blood clumping, it is fair to say that the bioflavonoids act as normalizers of blood flow in the capillaries and veins. And this, of course, is in contrast to the effect of drugs, which invariably have only one-dimensional effects, and because of this, always pose a risk.

## Citrus Bioflavonoids Most Potent

It is worth noting that Dr. Robbins, after testing a number of the bioflavonoid compounds, reported that the greatest biological activity is shown by certain compounds from the rind and pulpy portions of citrus fruits. Among the most active are tangeretin, nobiletin, and sinensetin. Oranges and lemons are particularly excellent sources of these bioflavonoids, so eat as much of the inner rind as possible. Tangerine juice happens to be exceptionally rich in tangeretin and nobiletin, so although the tangerine doesn't have any edible rind to speak of, the juice itself is loaded with bioflavonoids.

Orange juice that you buy frozen is a relatively poor source of bioflavonoids, for the simple reason that the bioflavonoids give an off-taste to the juice, so the amount of pulp that is squeezed is carefully controlled by processors.

Fortunately, citrus bioflavonoids are available in concentrated form, and in much greater potencies than you could get by eating whole fruit. The easy availability of these substances results from the fact that when oranges are squeezed to make juice, there is a tremendous amount of pulp left over, which can be inexpensively processed to extract the bioflavonoids.

Most researchers who have worked with the bioflavonoids agree that they have the greatest beneficial effect when taken together with vitamin C. This makes sense, because in nature, the bioflavonoids and vitamin C almost invariably occur together—oranges being the classic example. As Dr. Linus Pauling has pointed out, it is quite certain that our distant ancestors ate a much greater quantity of fruits and berries, rich both in vitamin C and bioflavonoids, than we do today.

## Common Foods Rich in Bioflavonoids

No standard food composition tables are available as yet from the United States Department of Agriculture for this vitamin, but the following foods are generally recognized as the richest sources.

| | | |
|---|---|---|
| Citrus fruits (skins and pulps) | Grapes | Papaya |
| Apricots | Green peppers | Broccoli |
| Cherries | Tomatoes | Cantaloupe |

# VITAMIN D

## CHAPTER 64

## Vitamin D
## —The Sunshine Vitamin

Vitamin D is not just a single nutrient; it is a family of various chemically related sterols, some of which have to be produced synthetically and some of which occur in provitamin form in plants and animals. Vitamin D is best known for its integral role in maintaining the health and growth of bones, but it is also vital to metabolic functions that directly affect the heart, nervous system, and the eyes.

The need for vitamin D is obvious, but obtaining ample and safe amounts of the nutrient is not always simple. It is commonly referred to as the "sunshine vitamin" because natural vitamin D (also known as $D_3$) is formed when the ultraviolet rays of the sun, hitting the skin, change a form of cholesterol which is a precursor of vitamin D in the skin into cholecalciferol ($D_3$)—the same substance that we get as natural vitamin D in fish liver oils. Chemical laboratories have managed to synthesize $D_3$, as well as a number of stronger members of the vitamin D group—including vitamin $D_2$, $D_4$, $D_5$, and $D_6$.

The best supplementary source of vitamin D is the natural product from fish liver oil. Fish are somehow able to manufacture this substance without the benefit of ultraviolet rays, and it is stored in their livers in relative abundance. The important thing is that, unlike the artificially synthesized forms of vitamin

D, fish liver vitamin D₃ is the identical substance that our own bodies manufacture. Because of this compatibility, it is unlikely to have the toxic effects that can result from large doses of the man-made vitamin.

A flurry of cases of vitamin D-hypervitaminosis occurring in the United States and Great Britain in the 1940s has been directly related to the widespread introduction of synthetic vitamin D. "In the years 1942 to 1952," reported Dr. Daphne A. Roe in the *New York State Journal of Medicine* (1 April 1966), "when calciferol (D₂) had recently been introduced for the treatment of lupus vulgaris (a skin disease) as well as such benign conditions as chilblains and psoriasis, signs of overdosage with vitamin D were not so uncommon."

Vitamin D, like vitamin A, is a fat-soluble vitamin. Unlike the water-soluble vitamins whose excess can be eliminated easily by the body, excess vitamin D is stored in the liver. Since vitamin D plays an integral regulatory role in the metabolism of calcium, an oversupply of this important nutrient can cause serious problems. Vitamin D is needed for the absorption of calcium through the intestinal wall, increasing the level of calcium in the blood serum, and it is partially responsible for depositing calcium into the bones. Theoretically, an over-accumulation of vitamin D could lead to excess calcification of the bones, to hardening of the arteries, and possibly, to retarded mentality in children.

But is vitamin D responsible for infantile hypercalcemia? The FDA seems to think so. In their own words: "Daily ingestion by infants of doses between 1,000 and 2,000 I.U. has produced hypervitaminosis D, usually manifested as the infantile hypercalcemia syndrome." *Federal Register,* (14 December 1972, p. 26619).

The FDA's concern about hypercalcemia has its roots in the United Kingdom of 20 years ago. Officials there, concerned about the rising toll of rickets in the nation's children and embarrassed over the ease of cure, began to fortify milk powders, infant cereals, and other foods with synthetic vitamin D. It is estimated that the average infant in England subsequently consumed about 2,000 I.U. of vitamin D daily. But as the rate of rickets began to fall, hypercalcemia began to appear with unusual frequency. So, in 1957, reductions were made in the vitamin D content of various infant's foods and supplements. Soon the rate of hypercalcemia began to fall.

It was shown that vitamin D did cause hypercalcemia in infants. But the FDA ignores a crucial fact: Dr. Ogden Johnson of the FDA, in an interview on 16 February 1973, said that in every single report used by the FDA to document vitamin D's harmful effects, only vitamin $D_2$, the synthetic form, was used. The British experience likewise involved only synthetic D.

And there is a difference between synthetic and natural vitamins. Dr. Isobel Jennings of the University of Cambridge, England, has written a book, *Vitamins in Endocrine Metabolism* (Springfield, Illinois: Charles C. Thomas, 1970) which discusses in length the subtle but crucial differences between the two.

Dr. Jennings reports, "In many cases synthetic vitamins are now available which may be identical with the naturally occurring substance or only closely related. The close relations, although useful in many ways, pose some problems in that they may have only a fraction, whether large or small, of the biological activity of the natural product. They may substitute for several, but not all, of the functions of their natural counterparts, so that *it is essential to use extreme care in their use.*"

And the difference between synthetic vitamin $D_2$ and natural vitamin D? According to Dr. Jennings, "$D_2$ is structurally different from $D_3$ in having an unsaturated side-chain. It is prepared by irradiation of ergosterol, a vegetable sterol present in ergot and yeasts. $D_2$ varies in its antirachitic (antirickets) potency in various animal species, *and is rather more toxic than the naturally occurring animal vitamin.*"

## Where Do We Get Vitamin D?

Vitamin D does not exist in great quantities in nature nor is it found in many foods. Those that do contain it are the oils of some fish, most notably cod and halibut. Egg yolks also contain some, and milk is "vitamin D-enriched" through ultraviolet irradiation. As a result of the paucity of natural vitamin D in food-stuffs, humans need to get it from the principal source: the sun. And if they don't, diseases overcome the natural systems of the body.

As the sun is the earth's source of life, so is it the source of much vitamin D that we need. When ultraviolet sunlight strikes the skin, it sparks the synthesis reaction of the provitamin 7-dehydrocholesterol, a form of cholesterol, into vitamin D under the skin and easily satisfies the vitamin D requirement.

The skin has a remarkable capacity for manufacturing vitamin D. In an abstract which appeared in the *Medical Journal of Australia* (24 August 1968), it was estimated that one square centimeter of white human skin could synthesize 18 I.U. of vitamin D in three hours. The quantity of vitamin which is synthesized depends on the amount of sunshine which penetrates the skin's outermost horny layer.

Vitamin D is either manufactured under the skin or ingested in foods. After the body receives it, most vitamin D is transported to the liver for storage. "Other deposits are found in the skin, brain, spleen, and bones. The body can store sizeable reserves of vitamin D, just as is the case with other fat-soluble vitamins. These reserves probably account for the infrequency of vitamin D deficiency in adults; the most common deficiency is in the rapidly growing infant who has little opportunity to accumulate adequate body stores," according to *The Heinz Handbook of Nutrition* (New York: McGraw Hill Book Company, 1965). This, of course, is the orthodox opinion, which is not without substance though it overlooks the extent of rickets, osteomalacia, and osteoporosis. Even among those who cannot be said to suffer from such a frank vitamin D deficiency, however, lack of the vitamin does commonly take its toll each year as winter drags along.

## Pollution Makes Winter Even Worse

One important reason why wintry skies just can't deliver the sunshine vitamin in amounts we need is the staggering concentration of dirt and grime that modern man has added to the atmosphere. Soot and other particles do a very effective job of filtering out the sun's vital ultraviolet rays. In fact, the first widespread epidemics of rickets occurred in Europe in the seventeenth century, when the air had become fouled with a pall of smoke, from the increasing use of soft coal.

Three hundred years later, people who live in industrialized, urban areas are still succumbing to what Professor W. Farnsworth Loomis of Brandeis University called "the earliest air-pollution disease." The number of elderly people dying after bone-breaking falls in Britain over a 35-year period was closely related to the amount of coal smoke in the air, Dr. T. P. Eddy of the London School of Hygiene and Tropical Medicine reported in *Nature* (13 September 1974). Bone fragility caused by lack of sunshine is the suspected cause.

"When smoke pollution was at its height in 1937–39," Dr. Eddy noted, "it was estimated that in Leicester (latitude 53 degrees north) at least 30 percent more ultraviolet daylight would have reached the center of the city in winter if all the smoke in the atmosphere had been eliminated, and occasionally the loss was more than half." He concluded, "The steep rise in femoral (thighbone) fractures with advancing age in Britain may be attributable to an absolute or relative deficiency of vitamin D."

There is every reason to expect that the air quality over our cities and even much of our rural area will get worse, much worse, screening out still more sunshine. According to a report in *Science News* (17 June 1972), airline crews and passengers note a growing pall of dirty, murky air stretching from horizon to horizon over much of the United States. Weather bureaus have reported that occasions of low visibility (six miles or less) are occurring 54 percent more often than they did just three years before (*Environment*, April 1972).

But even if air pollution could be eliminated tomorrow, suddenly making our skies crystalline, winter would still play havoc with our bones. From November through March, the sun rises so late and sets so early that those of us who work in offices or factories often go from weekend to weekend without spending any time in bright sunshine. And what little time we do manage to spend out-of-doors is virtually useless for vitamin D accumulation, because we are heavily wrapped in coats, scarves, and gloves.

## Sunlight: Vital, but Elusive

For the housebound or bedridden individual, the situation is even more grave, as a study by Dr. Robert M. Neer of Harvard Medical School demonstrated. Dr. Neer studied 33 soldiers' home residents, aged 52 to 93, for four-week periods during two consecutive winters. All were in reasonably good health at the start of the experiment, but they were advised to stay indoors and away from windows.

One group was exposed to ultraviolet light from fluorescent tubes that duplicated the full spectrum of natural sunlight. The second group was exposed to ordinary fluorescent lighting only. Intestinal absorption of bone-strengthening calcium *increased* in the first group from 38 to 41 percent the first year, and from 41 to 47 percent the second year. But calcium absorption *fell* in the group deprived of ultraviolet light from 39 to 30 percent the first year, from 43 to 32 percent the next. Dr. Neer concluded that adult vitamin D requirements should be reexamined in light of the evidence that many otherwise healthy people apparently suffer winter deficits (*Medical World News,* 8 January 1971).

The farther north you live, the more difficult it is to obtain your vitamin D from sunshine. Above 40 degrees north latitude, the winter sun never rises as much as 20 degrees above the horizon, leaving many city streets in shadow from dawn to dusk. The sunlight never penetrates. Many large cities in North America lie north of that line, including Philadelphia (which straddles it), New York, Cleveland, Chicago, Pittsburgh, and Seattle.

It would be great to just jet away for a week to the sunny Caribbean in February when mid-winter cold and the vague aches and pains of vitamin D-deficient bones are at their peak. There you could soak up enough sunshine to recharge your vitamin D batteries, perhaps enough to carry you through the remainder of winter.

But if the Islands aren't on your itinerary, you can still be certain of getting all the vitamin D your bones will need for the long winter months by supplementing with natural vitamin D derived from fish liver oil.

# CHAPTER 65

# Some Consequences of Severe Vitamin D Deficiency

Although knowledge of vitamin D requirements has been with us for more than 50 years, many people still suffer the effects of deficiency. It's easy to understand how the cold season compounds our problems when it comes to the need for vitamin D. In winter, when people can bring themselves to go outside, they carefully bundle up and in shielding their flesh from the biting cold, they also shield the body from the vitamin D-inducing ultraviolet rays of the sun.

In reality, the lack of sunshine need not be worrisome in the 1970s since all people can—and should—literally swallow their sunshine in the form of vitamin D supplements, thereby protecting themselves from a rash of problems brought on by a shortage of that important vitamin.

Vitamin D protects individuals from suffering from a number of diseases such as rickets in infants and children, osteomalacia in adults, and osteoporosis in the elderly.

## Rickets

Essentially, rickets affects the very young. It throws their bone-growth metabolism off, resulting in malformation. Bone formation during childhood and infancy is very important because the skeleton is still in the process of active growth and development. Obviously, this early growth sets the pattern for a child's frame as he grows into an adult. Manifestations of rickets include fragile and easily broken bones, and soft teeth, extremely susceptible to decay. The outward signs of rickets include bowed legs and bent backs.

In adults, vitamin D deficiency can bring on osteomalacia, or adult rickets, a condition marked by the softening of the bones along with accompanying pain, tenderness, muscular weakness, anorexia (loss of appetite), and loss of weight.

The elderly also suffer from a lack of vitamin D. In their case, the disease is called osteoporosis, a condition marked by a mineral depletion of the bones, leaving their normally solid structure pitted with holes like a sponge. Consequently, the bones become weak and brittle. The elderly, as a result of this problem, live in fear of simple falls which could—and often do—lay them up for months unless their systems have an adequate supply of vitamin D.

## Vitamin D Deficiencies Are Overlooked

Vitamin D-deficiency diseases today are rarely recognized by doctors as such, and so are rarely reported. Physicians are conditioned to the idea that there is no longer a vitamin D deficiency in this country, so they look for other causes. But rickets does exist, and evidence of this was reported in the *American Journal of Clinical Nutrition* (November 1967) by Sister Mary Theodora Weick of the Nutrition Department of Mercy Hospital, Buffalo, New York. She found, in studying official records from 1910 through 1961 that 13,807 deaths were caused by rickets, and that from 1956 to 1960, 843 cases of rickets were reported. She doubts that all cases of rickets are reported, and states that rickets "is still noticeably prevalent, and only constant, continual efforts will bring about its complete elimination."

The *Journal of the American Medical Association* (31 August 1964) stated that " . . . cases of common nutritional-deficiency disease are being missed because it is assumed they no longer occur and because the diagnostic features have been forgotten. Two examples are outstanding—scurvy (a vitamin C deficiency) and rickets (a disease created by deficiencies in calcium and vitamin D)." The article went on to point out that these diseases are occurring "with disturbing and increasing frequency even under apparently good circumstances and unrelated to other diseases."

The blame must be put at the doorstep of nutritionists who were so certain that rickets would be eradicated by the addition to bottled milk of 400 I.U. of vitamin D$_2$ (ergocalciferol) per quart, that they never bothered to check on whether it actually was.

## Fish Replace Unavailable Sunlight

Dr. W. Farnsworth Loomis, professor of biochemistry at Brandeis University, called rickets "the earliest air pollution disease." What relation does rickets have to air pollution? Writing in the *Scientific American* (December 1970) Dr. Loomis said that it took years for researchers to realize that people who suffered from rickets were simply not manufacturing vitamin D in their bodies, because pollution blocked the healthy effect of the sun, preventing the ultraviolet rays from reaching the skin, thus preventing vitamin D from being made.

Researchers, Dr. Loomis continued, were thrown off the track for a while by the fact that rickets was not rampant in the Northern European countries where sunlight was scarce, but where the population ate a lot of fish. Only later did they discover that fish are able to manufacture calciferol, one form of vitamin D, without the aid of ultraviolet rays from the sun, and that the people who ate the fish acquired the vitamin in their diets. Later studies showed that certain fish liver oils were rich in the antirachitic ingredient and that cod liver oil, for example, taken over the sunless winter months, offered effective protection from rickets.

# Vitamin D's Role in Evolution

Dr. Loomis, writing in *Science* (4 August 1967) said the imprint of vitamin D goes back in history a million years or more. He theorized that it was because of the human body's need to take in a certain amount of vitamin D, but not too much, that the human species has developed into three principal racial groups distinguished by skin color and loosely called black, yellow, and white.

The control of skin color over vitamin D synthesis, he said, explains the distribution of the races of man in prehistoric and early historic times. As far as anthropologists can tell, human beings originated in Africa near the equator. Almost certainly, they had black skins. Many anthropologists have argued that dark skin evolved as a protection against sunburn and skin cancer. Dr. Loomis, however, says dark skin came first and light skin evolved as a protection against a deficiency of vitamin D.

Black skin allows only 3 to 36 percent of ultraviolet rays to pass while white skin passes 53 to 72 percent. As early man moved north from the equatorial region, beyond the fortieth parallel—roughly the latitude of Madrid and Naples—Loomis says he got into a zone where black skin filtered out too much ultraviolet, resulting in rickets. Even today, black children are more susceptible to rickets than are white children, especially in the northern states.

When ultraviolet rays strike the skin, the pigment-producing cells produce melanin—and a suntan. The black races (Negro, Bushman-Hottentot, and Australoid) with a more abundant supply of melanin, are, in effect, permanently tanned. Members of the white race are transparent-skinned in winter, when they must make the most of the limited ultraviolet available to synthesize vitamin D, but they take a tan in summer, when they might suffer from an excess.

But even with the knowledge of what vitamin D is and how it works, there is mounting evidence to show that man is simply not getting enough of the vitamin, especially in winter.

# Vitamin D and Osteomalacia

For those people who can truly feel the cold and gloom of winter in their aching bones, the wait for spring seems doubly long. However, medical researchers have now discovered that without protection with ample amounts of the "sunshine" vitamin D, the aches, pains, and possible fractures that weakened bones are heir to can rage well into the warm months.

Our bodies need vitamin D to help assimilate the calcium in food and carry it to skeletal sites where it is deposited to form new bone. Contrary to what many people assume, the adult human skeleton is *not* a static structure. Our frames are constantly being broken down and "remodeled" as calcium and other minerals flow from the bones to the bloodstream and back again to bone. When not enough vitamin D is available, newly-formed bone becomes soft, pliable, and even misshapen. If calcium privation continues long enough, osteomalacia develops. This bone disease, the adult equivalent of childhood rickets, brings pain, tenderness, and muscular weakness. If the bones are allowed to demineralize severely, they may fracture very easily.

"Osteomalacia should be considered in any patient who has vague generalized aches and pains and who is known to be on an unusual diet," stated a *Medical Digest* (September 1970) summary of a study by Drs. C. E. Dent and R. Smith. The pair came to that conclusion after examining a number of osteomalacia patients at London's University College Hospital. One "unusual diet" they referred to—low-fat—is hardly unusual at all in our calorie-conscious society. But it could lead to osteomalacia, because vitamin D is usually only absorbed with fats and oils.

# Cold Weather Bad for the Bones

Over a five-year period three doctors, J. E. Aaron and colleagues in Leeds, England examined small biopsy samples of hip bone taken from 134 patients who had suffered suspicious fractures of the femur, or thighbone. In the *Lancet* (13 July 1974) they reported that signs of osteomalacia were found in 37 percent of the cases. Most interesting, however, was their discovery that disease symptoms were heavily clustered in those patients whose fractures occurred in February through June.

"As would be expected if this seasonal variation was attributable to variation in the supply of vitamin D dependent on sunlight," the doctors reported, "the proportion of cases with osteomalacia is highest in the spring and lowest in the autumn."

The two- to six-month lag between the days of absolute least sunlight (the third week of December) and the highest incidence of osteomalacia is explained when we remember that vitamin D is fat-soluble, and thus easily stored in the body. All summer while the sun shines brightly you are stockpiling this vitamin for the cold dark days ahead. Reserves are most likely to run out at the very tail end of winter or even early spring.

Vitamin D content of the blood can dip much earlier in the year, however. In normal individuals, blood levels of 25-hydroxycholecalciferol, the circulating form of vitamin D, were found to be at their lowest in December, a full two months or more before the aches and pains of osteomalacia are at their worst. The subjects were all hospital workers whose exposure to sunlight may parallel your own. They were only able to go outdoors on weekends and during their summer vacations. (Serum levels of vitamin D were at their highest in September.) These findings were reported in the *Lancet* (30 March 1974) by Dr. Marilyn McLaughlin and five other researchers at Westminster Hospital and Royal Free Hospital, London, England.

## Why Mature People Are Most Vulnerable to Winter Woes

Unless you are getting supplementary vitamin D in your diet, each winter brings a new and serious challenge to your bones. And as you grow older, that challenge becomes more severe with each passing year. After the age of 30 to 35, the total amount of bone in an individual actually shrinks "about 10 percent per decade in women and five percent per decade in men," explained mineral metabolism expert Dr. Louise Avioli in an interview recorded in *Medical World News* (19 October 1973). That's probably why seasonal bone loss may cause no pain in a woman of 25, but real suffering in a woman of 55.

As bone structure weakens with age, osteomalacia and osteoporosis (a related disease in which the bone becomes pitted and loses critical mass) are more likely to develop. According to Dr. Avioli, "The usual symptoms of adult osteomalacia are weakness and generalized bone aches; of osteoporosis, localized back pain on arising or bending over, or pain in areas where the spinal vertebrae may actually have collapsed. The ordinary x ray picks up only 30 percent bone loss or more. By this time the horse is already out of the barn, so to speak."

## Rheumatism—Or Hungry Bones?

Some people, at this point, mistakenly blame their aching bones and joints on rheumatism. But the most frequently voiced complaint—pain in the mid- to lower-back region—is actually a symptom of osteoporosis. Dr. William Brady, a well-known physician and syndicated columnist was on the right track when on 20 May 1965, he suggested to his readers that they start each morning as he did: by taking six capsules of calcium, and vitamin D to help absorb it. "To this," he wrote, "I attribute the fact that I have no 'rheumatiz', no nondescript ache or pain, no headache, no backache, and no other manifestation of calcium deficiency."

All the bone-building calcium in the world won't do you any good if there is insufficient vitamin D to help the body to absorb and use it. And time after time, studies have shown that in the absence of sunshine or supplementation, dietary intakes of the vitamin often fall far short of the recommended 400 I.U. daily. A British study published in the *Lancet* (28 April 1973) involved 103 hospitalized geriatric patients, whose confinement dictated that they obtain all their vitamin D from dietary sources rather than sunshine, and the results were appalling. The average daily intake of vitamin D was just 64 I.U. One 72-year-old woman, who had been housebound for 14 years, was found to be ingesting only 40 I.U. daily! Needless to say, she suffered from severe osteomalacia. Deficiency on such a wide scale is not so surprising when we consider that vitamin D occurs naturally in only a handful of foods.

Whether or not you can ignore diet and depend on sunlight for your vitamin D depends on where—and how—you live. "In many populations exposed to adequate sunshine, the dietary intake of vitamin D is probably irrelevant," said Dr. J. Chalmers, a physician at Princess Margaret Rose Orthopedic Hospital in Edinburgh, Scotland, in a letter to the *Lancet* (7 June 1969). "In Hong Kong, for example, the average Chinese diet contains less than 70 I.U. per day, and yet osteomalacia is excessively rare, owing to the generous exposure to sunshine enjoyed in that part of the world."

But he cautioned that the disease is on the rise in temperate climates: "Since we have become aware of this situation in recent years, nearly 150 cases of osteomalacia have now been recognized in this area alone, and I have little doubt that these represent only the tip of the iceberg."

Later reports confirm Dr. Chalmers' prediction. After finding evidence of osteomalacia in 47 percent of men and 34 percent of women treated for bone fractures, Dr. J. E. Aaron and colleagues at the Leeds General Infirmary expressed their conclusion in the *Lancet* (16 February 1974), "It seems reasonable to suggest that for every case of proven osteomalacia, representing severe vitamin D depletion, there must be others with minor degrees of vitamin D deficiency. In view of the dominant role played by vitamin D in calcium absorption, possibly malabsorption of calcium in elderly people may be a manifestation of a degree of vitamin D deficiency falling short of osteomalacia, and this must at least contribute to senile bone loss."

The best way to avoid those kinds of problems is to take supplementary vitamin D, naturally derived from fish liver oils. Most diets can't be counted on to meet vitamin D needs, and even sunshine, the very best and most natural source, fails us in the winter.

## Vitamin D and Osteoporosis

Osteoporosis is that dread disease of older people, particularly older women, in which porous and fragile bones can crack in response to the slightest bump or compression—even a brief spell of coughing. Many an older woman has found herself hospitalized with a fractured hip, disabled for weeks or even months, all as a result of a minor fall that wouldn't even have been noticed during her youthful years.

Many factors can contribute to the tendency of older bones to demineralize—that is, suffer abnormal loss of calcium and other minerals and thereby become dangerously fragile. At least half a dozen hormones are in one way or another involved with the turnover of minerals in the skeletal structure, and hormonal changes in the late decades of life undoubtedly increase our susceptibility to osteoporosis. Of greater significance, however— and a circumstance we can readily do something about—are physical inactivity and faulty nutrition (particularly deficiencies in calcium and vitamin D). Both of these recognized causative factors are all too often linked to the senior years.

As researchers continue to investigate osteoporosis, we are learning that, in addition to recognized basic factors, other contributing causes also enter the picture—and could spell the difference between sound bones and bones that fracture. In a letter appearing in the *Journal of the American Medical Association* (31 July 1972), Dr. Harry W. Daniell reported his findings that heavy cigarette smoking appears to be a prominent factor in inducing osteoporosis. Dr. Daniell's findings on cigarette smoking provide yet another strong motive for quitting cigarettes and yet another preventive measure for protection against this epidemic geriatric disorder.

How can cigarette smoking affect the bones? Dr. Daniell pointed out that bone minerals (mostly calcium and phosphorus, responsible for the bone's hardness) are "known to be strikingly more soluble in acid solutions," and cigarette smoking is known to increase the acidity of bone tissue. Thus the bone minerals can be expected to dissolve and be absorbed into the bloodstream at a much faster rate when smoking provides the acid environment.

Studies have shown, Dr. Daniell reported, that three consecutive cigarettes cause a prompt transient hypercalcemia—or high content of calcium in the blood. This finding, he said, suggests that the act of smoking is associated with rapid calcium loss from bone structures.

# The Vanishing Minerals

To many people it will come as a shock to learn that it is even possible for bones to lose minerals. But the fact is that bones are not stable but physiologically dynamic. They normally lose minerals all the time, and just as normally take up new minerals. It's only when the mineral loss is greater than the mineral gain that the health and integrity of the bone is in danger. The skeleton can be (and is) constantly and subtly remodeled to accommodate changes in the individual's weight distribution and changed conditions of stress. The bones also serve as a reservoir of calcium for replenishing the bloodstream when serum calcium levels drop. Adequate calcium in the blood, instantly available to nerve cells, is essential for the functioning of the nervous system. Several hormones, plus vitamin D, help both store this mineral in bone deposits and release it as needed to maintain constant serum calcium values.

Once we understand this turnover of bone calcium, the importance of adequate intake of dietary calcium becomes very apparent. Hormone-triggered mechanisms will readily sacrifice your bones on the altar of a dropping serum calcium level, minute by minute. It's much more vital to your life and health to insure that your nerve cells continue to be bathed in circulating calcium than it is to protect the hardness of your skeletal structure. Fragile bones are less threatening than an impaired nervous system. You can't move a muscle, entertain a thought, or even take a breath if the proper nerve cells aren't working.

The trick, then, is to make sure your bloodstream is so well supplied with dietary calcium that your bones needn't be robbed in order to make up for faulty eating habits. But calcium intake is only part of the story. You also need vitamin D. For calcium requires the help of this nutrient in order to be absorbed from the intestinal tract into the circulating bloodstream. Without vitamin D, your calcium intake is useless, eliminated from your system without ever having contributed to nerve cell or bone cell.

No medical authority disputes the importance of calcium and vitamin D in preventing abnormal bone mineral loss. Oddly enough, there is no up-to-date research on the effectiveness of this nutritional team in preventing and reversing osteoporosis. New advanced techniques for bone appraisal and detection of hormone fluctuations have been used to test the efficacy of a variety of medications, including synthetic hormone drugs and the potentially toxic mineral, fluoride. But, as Dr. Jennifer Jowsey and associates at the Mayo Clinic acknowledge in an article in *Postgraduate Medicine* (October 1972), comparable work has yet to be published when it comes to the easy and obvious self-help dietary measure of calcium plus vitamin D supplementation.

Such a study with osteoporotic patients, however, is at last under way at the Mayo Clinic. But Dr. Jowsey said the results cannot be expected for several years. And she added this thoughtful caution: whatever the results of the study, there can be no question that the time to start this supplementation is long before the age when people usually start worrying about osteoporosis.

Osteoporosis characteristically occurs in women after menopause and is presumably related to low estrogen output—the female hormone that dwindles when ovulation and menstruation cease. In men, fragile porous bones typically develop considerably later in life and the disorder is less severe. But though the disease is associated with late middle age and old age, the process probably begins many decades earlier.

# Researcher Advises Early Dietary Supplements

"I would advise women to start calcium and vitamin D supplements at age 30, or perhaps 25," Dr. Jowsey said. With the average American diet, there's apparently a long-term gradual loss of bone mineral exceeding the rate of mineral uptake and bone formation. In later years, when hormonal changes increase the susceptibility to osteoporosis, the skeleton has already lost a good deal of its substance. By then, because of previous loss, the rate of bone formation must not only equal the rate of bone demineralization (the normal condition) but must exceed it if bone strength is to be restored.

It's far more difficult, as Dr. Jowsey warned, to induce new, compensatory bone formation than it is to simply slow down bone demineralization. Adequate calcium and vitamin D in the diet will go far to accomplish the latter. But preliminary findings, according to the Mayo scientist, indicate that lost bone tissue will not automatically be restored by such dietary correction. The evidence suggests that long-term marginal deficiency in calcium and vitamin D is the principal villain in the tragedy of osteoporosis.

# CHAPTER 66

# Regular Heartbeat Requires Vitamin D and Calcium

The fact that vitamin D plays an indispensable role to both deposit and withdrawal of calcium gives to this vitamin a much more important role than was formerly recognized because, besides being necessary to bones, teeth, and nerves, calcium is absolutely essential to every beat of the heart. If for some reason your calcium pool becomes dangerously low, your heart will flutter and fibrillate (twitch) and send out an SOS for more calcium. Vitamin D must be on the job before this calcium can be withdrawn from the bones to come to the aid of your heart.

Calcium is one of the major factors in regulation of the heart. Dr. Winifrid Nayler of the Baker Medical Research Institute describes the process in *Heart Journal* (March 1967). It involves an electrochemical process which takes place in the heart with every beat and within every cell. On the outer surface of each heart-tissue cell there is a thin filament called actin. The actin reaches with a kind of magnetic attraction toward the center of the cell, thereby shortening its length. The result of many cells shortening at one time brings about contraction of the muscle, and it is calcium, fed to the actin by the bloodstream, that provides both the stimulus and the means by which the actin does its work. A shortage of calcium must inevitably result in a weakened heartbeat or an irregular heartbeat or an arrhythmia. So vital is calcium to the heart, that when the heart is short of calcium, the bloodstream will withdraw calcium from the bones and carry it to the heart. But, if vitamin D is lacking, the blood is unable to complete this lifesaving maneuver.

The amount of calcium in your bloodstream is small but critical. The body strives simultaneously to keep the heart muscle supplied and at the same time to keep the bones well mineralized and strong. But, to sustain all these delicate adjustments and readjustments, you must have enough vitamin D going for you.

# CHAPTER 67

# Vitamin D Combats
# Harmful Drug Effects

"Bone is a living substance that depends on a constant supply of nutrients for the manufacture of osteoid matrix and its subsequent mineralization," said Dr. Ronald A. Barrett, D.D.S., in the *Journal of Periodontology-Periodontics* (March 1968).

"Under physiological conditions," Dr. Barrett explained, "adult bone is constantly and equally being formed and destroyed. Hence, two major groups of mechanisms are operative. . . ." Both of these mechanisms depend on vitamin D. Because of pronouncements on the part of the medical profession and the FDA that adults do not need vitamin D, many, many people are fearful about including this vitamin in their daily regimen. This might be a factor which is raising the incidence of such diseases as osteoporosis, rheumatism, and osteomalacia, which is adult rickets.

This attitude may soon change because, as pointed out by Samuel Vaisrub, M.D. in the *Journal of the American Medical Association* (28 May 1973), " . . . recent developments in vitamin D research are truly portentous. They are currently engaging the attention of physicians concerned with calcium metabolism and the treatment of its disorders."

Indeed, investigators from Washington University School of

Medicine, and Jewish Hospital (both located in St. Louis, Missouri), have found that vitamin D may help to solve a problem that has been plaguing physicians and patients, by reversing the bone loss that produces disabling fractures and vertebral collapse in patients being treated with steroids.

Physicians do, of course, make every attempt to treat such painful conditions as rheumatoid arthritis, for instance, without corticosteroid therapy because, for relief that doesn't last, the price is so high in terms of side effects. Dr. Tom Spies said long ago that at least the minor pains of arthritis could be helped with vitamin therapy and that he used hormone treatment only for the "big pains." While the steroids do the job of reducing swelling and relieving pain, too often the patient trades his aching joints for broken bones.

But according to the results of the St. Louis study, broken bones do not have to be the toll for patients on steroids. Not if the patient is also given large doses of vitamin D. In fact, the process of bone resorption triggered by the steroids can, according to Dr. Bevra Hahn, assistant professor of medicine at Washington University, be reversed with the administration of vitamin D which, it is well-known, facilitates intestinal absorption of calcium.

Because steroid therapy blocks intestinal absorption of calcium, it induces a sort of hyperparathyroidism (overactivity on the part of the parathyroid glands), Dr. Hahn told the Arthritis Foundation in Los Angeles, according to *Medical World News* (13 July 1973).

Patients on steroid therapy frequently suffer compression fractures of the spine. Sometimes it takes only a good healthy sneeze to break a few vertebrae. It is believed that this painful and disabling consequence occurs because steroid therapy causes the loss of more trabecular bone (supporting strands of connective tissue) than cortical bone (the long outer bones). This same phenomenon, Dr. Hahn realized, is characteristic of primary hyperparathyroidism, a condition which is controlled with vitamin D. Since vitamin D corrects the trabecular bone loss caused by the overactive parathyroid gland, will vitamin D also help restore the trabecular bone loss suffered by the patient on steroid therapy?

Dr. Hahn set up an experiment to find out. Using a relatively new procedure called osteodensitometry, she was able to measure both the cortical and trabecular bone mass in several different groups of patients. Some had osteoporosis, some were rheumatoid arthritis patients who were not receiving steroids, some were receiving steroids, and some patients were suffering with primary hyperparathyroidism.

It is interesting to note that both osteoporosis patients and patients with rheumatoid arthritis, who were not receiving steroids, showed a decrease of 20 percent in both cortical and trabecular bone. However, those arthritics who were receiving steroids and those patients who had primary hyperparathyroidism both revealed much greater losses of trabecular bone over cortical bone. In fact, most patients had lost 40 to 50 percent of their trabecular bone.

## Vitamin D for Bone Density

Dr. Hahn and her team then started treatment with 50,000 I.U. of vitamin D orally on Mondays, Wednesdays, and Fridays, for a period of 13 weeks. Then the osteodensitometry readings were repeated. Just as Dr. Hahn anticipated, there were some amazing improvements. In fact, nine of the 10 patients studied showed an increase in trabecular bone density. The effect of vitamin D was further confirmed when measurements were repeated on five arthritic patients who were receiving steroids and no vitamin D. The ratios were worse in all five. There was a further loss of trabecular bone in each case.

## Common Foods Rich in Vitamin D

No standard food composition tables are available as yet from the United States Department of Agriculture for this vitamin, but the following foods are generally recognized as the richest sources.

| | |
|---|---|
| Cod liver oil | Milk (vitamin D-enriched) |
| Halibut liver oil | Salmon |
| Eggs (yolk) | Tuna |

# VITAMIN E

## CHAPTER 68

# The Great Vitamin E Controversy

*By Richard E. Passwater*

*Richard A. Passwater, of Silver Springs, Maryland, is a biochemical researcher and a consultant in gerontology. His technical work has been widely published in the scientific press. He is also the author of* Supernutrition: Megavitamin Revolution *(New York: Dial Press, 1975).*

Vitamin E, a most intriguing vitamin, has puzzled and embarrassed scientists for years. It has become a popular topic for the public and scientists alike. Vitamin E is an enigma to scientists because they can't agree exactly how it works. Scientific interest is at an all-time high as evidenced by the nearly 500 research reports appearing in 1973. Yet, even with more than 15,000 previous reports, the basic questions are still unanswered to everyone's satisfaction. The American Medical Association, the Food and Drug Administration, and a number of university researchers ridicule the claims made for vitamin E. Newspaper reporters often refer to the controversy as the "vitamin E war." The public is confused because each group seems convincing, but which is right?

In 1959, the FDA first recognized that vitamin E was essential. It wasn't until 1968 that a recommended daily allowance was estimated by the National Research Council.

In 1971, the *Medical Letter* claimed "Vitamin E is of no value for *any* human ailment." Yet, a report from the National Research Council in 1972 concedes that premature babies (especially those with hemolytic anemia) and people who have faulty absorption of fats need extra vitamin E. The latter condition includes steatorrhea, cystic fibrosis, liver cirrhosis, postgastrectomy, obstructive jaundice, pancreatic insufficiency, and sprue.

In 1973, an "establishment" conference, chaired by Dr. Max Horwitt, added intermittent claudication (calf pain while walking due to poor circulation) to the list of diseases benefited by vitamin E. The conference reports suggested supplementing infant formulas with vitamin E and endorsed further research into vitamin E's use as a protection against air pollution. It seems that a little more is accepted each year as to what vitamin E definitely does.

## Scientists Resist Unwelcome Ideas

Controversy exists throughout science, but particularly in nutrition. Human biochemistry, especially as it pertains to each individual, is a most complex subject. It is difficult to get two nutritionists to agree on many issues unless they have been taught at the same school.

There can be honest disagreement about the effectiveness of any therapy, new or old. Human emotion, however, becomes a factor even with scientists and physicians. If a physician receives extensive publicity, his methods and motives become suspect. This is true especially if his methods are greatly different from current practice. Funding committees hesitate to grant funds to such controversial scientists.

Scientists, like everyone else, have some prejudices and occasionally have to play politics. Consider the following extract from the *Christian Science Monitor* (18 December 1973) by R. C. Cowen: "Scientists are committed to an open-minded study of the universe. But don't count on it. They can resist an unwelcome idea as stubbornly as any other establishment. Referring to this, Harvard University's evolutionist, Aranson

Meyer, has observed. 'It happens almost invariably when new facts cast doubt on generally accepted theory. The prevailing concepts have such a powerful hold over the thinking of all investigators that they find it difficult, if not impossible, to free themselves of this idea.' "

Even open-minded scientists have been baffled by the complicated behavior of vitamin E. Part of its strange behavior can be attributed to its interrelationships with other nutrients. When you consider that vitamin E is dependent upon nutrient partners such as the microtrace element selenium, vitamin A, sulfur-containing amino acids, and vitamin C, you wonder about some of the negative reports which attempt to discredit vitamin E.

## Why Some 'Scientific' Studies Prove Nothing

For example, consider the studies often cited by the skeptics. Their most popular study was conducted by Dr. S. Rinzler and his cardiovascular research associates at Cornell Medical College. They conducted a proper double-blind test, giving 19 patients 300 I.U. of vitamin E daily for about four months. The second group of 19 patients received placebos. No "significant" differences between the two groups were noted.

This is reminiscent of the early reports on vitamin C and the common cold. Researchers used small quantities of vitamin C (typically 100 or 250 mg.) and found only minor improvements. And so, for many years, the "experts" declared over and over again that the idea that vitamin C could protect against colds had been *disproven*. However, just within the last year or so, there have been three or four new major studies conducted by outstanding researchers. But instead of using small amounts of vitamin C, they all used 1,000 mg. a day. And without exception it was found that people receiving a gram of vitamin C a day had either significantly less colds and other upper respiratory ailments, or had significantly less total days of disability—in some cases, they enjoyed both benefits. Suddenly, we are not hearing very much from all those "experts" who had been insisting for all those years that vitamin C was just a big hoax.

Getting back to the Rinzler study, we must now ask: what would have happened if the vitamin E intake had been the 1,600 I.U. that Drs. Evan and Wilfrid Shute recommend to recover from heart attacks? What would the results have been even at the 800 I.U. level that they recommend (in general) for prevention of heart problems in apparently healthy people? What would have happened if the patients were studied for six months? What would have happened if more than 19 patients had been given vitamin E?

The experimental error may have been even more serious and complicated than the relatively weak dosage and small number of patients. Had this test, which was conducted in the late 1940s, been conducted today, the researchers might have understood the importance of the critical interrelationship of vitamin E and selenium. Vitamin E can act alone in many functions, but for other functions it requires partners. Heart disease now appears to have involvement with vitamin E and selenium in concert. The evidence is more than preliminary, though far from conclusive.

Biochemists attempting to create vitamin E-deficient diets in experimental animals may coincidentally create selenium deficiencies, we now know. When they add vitamin E, the selenium deficiency prevents any improvement. Medical researchers may have tried to reverse the progress of disease with vitamin E and had no success simply because the person was also deficient in selenium. If the 19 test subjects in the Rinzler experiment developed heart disease because of a poor diet, they may have been deficient in selenium also. Feeding them 300 I.U. of vitamin E alone would not correct the selenium deficiency. Therefore, there could be no improvement.

## Vitamin E Efficiency Linked to Selenium

Why do I consider this so significant? For one thing, we know that vitamin E and selenium act in a synergistic way to help produce antibodies. We learned this from an experiment in which laboratory animals were all given a vaccine, and some of them were also given vitamin E or selenium or both. The group given vitamin E had the same antibody production as the control group which had received nothing but the vaccine. The animals receiving selenium had about a 12 percent increase in antibody production. But the group which got vitamin E and selenium *together* had more than double the antibody formation of the other groups. This powerful synergistic action has been confirmed by several experiments carried out by different investigators.

With relation to the health of the heart, my feeling that selenium is important is influenced largely by clinical trials of a vitamin E and selenium combination conducted in Mexico. According to the *Wall Street Journal* (13 March 1973), similar clinical trials are underway in the United States. The Mexican tests showed a reduction of angina pectoris (a form of heart disease) with the combination of vitamin E and selenium. Would you believe that this same formula has been used successfully for angina pectoris by veterinarians for more than ten years? In fact, a handful of U.S. scientists have been taking the same formulation. It is not recommended that anyone pursue this themselves until the safety and efficiency has been confirmed, particularly because selenium in large doses can be extremely toxic. However, it is perfectly safe and healthful in foods, so it is recommended that people eat a balanced and varied diet, rich both in vitamin E and selenium. Selenium can be found in many foods, especially in brewer's yeast, eggs, and tuna.

If earlier reports indicated no medical value in vitamin E, why did so many scientists continue to study it? Speaking for myself, I have two reasons: Scientific curiosity as to just how vitamin E works, and the many clues that vitamin E does indeed have important medical usefulness. What are some of these clues?

First, there is the epidemiological link between the increase in heart disease and the disappearance of vitamin E from our diets. Today's typical vitamin E consumption is only a fraction of what it was 50 years ago. Degermination, bleaching, processing, and longer storage periods have depleted foods. Meanwhile, our consumption of polyunsaturated fats has increased, and very recent findings (1973) show that people eating diets high in polyunsaturated fats need more vitamin E, not less, to protect the polyunsaturated fats from dangerous peroxidation reactions.

Then there is the work of Dr. N. DiLuzio, who has shown that diene fats, formed when insufficient vitamin E is present to prevent peroxidation of fats, were found in 78 of 81 persons, indicating that an antioxidant-deficient state existed in 96 percent of those studied. The concentration of these dienes has been correlated with heart disease.

Another reason for believing that vitamin E has a profound effect on the heart is the report by Dr. W. M. Toone in the *New England Journal of Medicine* (280:18, 979, 1973). Dr. Toone found that 400 I.U. of vitamin E given four times a day reduced nitroglycerin need in a significant number of patients.

I am also impressed with the 1971 findings of Dr. M. Fedelseva and colleagues of the faculty of medicine at the University of Manitoba. They've proven that a vitamin E deficiency produces marked alterations in heart metabolism. This abnormality is due to changes in both energy conduction and utilization.

## Personal Experience Must Be Considered

Aside from the scientific literature, there is the evidence of personal experience. A colleague, Dr. J. Rinse, has received more than a thousand letters which attest to heart disease reduction after a change to a balanced diet including vitamins C and E, lecithin, and other supplements.

My personal experience is similar. After reading my technical articles, many scientists have written telling of their better health obtained by increasing vitamin E and vitamin C intake.

I remember seeing the slow-healing incision of Redskin quarterback Sonny Jurgensen's Achilles' heel operation heal after two weeks of vitamin E therapy. I watched an 80-year-old colleague, Dr. A. K. Brewer, rapidly recover to a normal electrocardiogram and excellent blood chemistry by taking vitamins C and E following his second heart attack. I've watched burns heal, warts disappear, and many other wonders due to this curious vitamin. In the words of *Science News*, vitamin E seems to do some "nifty things." I agree with that.

But there are still more clues. Additional evidence shows that vitamin E regulates the levels of ubiquinone (also called coenzyme Q). Ubiquinone is of interest because deficiencies exist in human diseases such as muscular dystrophy, cancer, heart disease, and periodontal disease. Ubiquinones are required for proper heart function. Ubiquinone has been successfully used in two young boys in the early stages of muscular dystrophy by Dr. Karl Folkers of the University of Texas.

Recently, vitamin E has been shown to reduce concentrations of the inflammatory prostaglandins. Prostaglandins are messengers between the hormones and cell membranes. This helps explain why vitamin E may be involved in so many diseases.

## Why Vitamin E Won't Cure Sterility

New findings about sterility show why vitamin E deficiency may cause sterility—though the vitamin will not cure it. Physicians often assume that if the lack of a substance causes a disease, then adding it will cure the disease. Therefore, they reason that if large doses of vitamin E are given to a patient and sterility isn't cured, then vitamin E deficiency wasn't the cause in the first place. But new findings by Drs. Raychaudhuri and Desai show that when there is a shortage of vitamin E, irreversible damage to the reproductive organ tissues occur from lipid peroxidation (the process of making rancid fats). After the tissue fats are oxidized, adding vitamin E will not undo the damage. This example could be applied to heart disease, cancer, or many other diseases. If damage is done by even a slight shortage of vitamin E, that particular damage may not be corrected when more vitamin E is taken. If the researcher looks only for a change related to the irreversible damage, other important changes, if they occur, will be missed.

New evidence has also been found showing that vitamin E is a regulator of blood formation. Also, its effect on thrombin (a clotting agent) and the role of thrombin in heart disease is being re-evaluated. In addition, new evidence tells us that many of the old measurements of vitamin E in the blood may not accurately be reflecting what is happening in the tissues of the body. Since the blood beta-lipoprotein fraction transports vitamin E, the blood vitamin E level is primarily dependent upon the fats in the blood, and may not accurately reflect the immediate vitamin E content of the tissues. This was always assumed to be the case previously. Dienes in the blood may indicate vitamin E deficiency better than blood levels of vitamin E itself.

Vitamin E has even been found to reduce damage to chromosomes and DNA by carcinogens and radiation. Thus it may be a deterrent to damage that possibly would otherwise lead to cancer. Vitamin E has reduced the incidence of cancer in laboratory animals fed carcinogens.

Several investigators, including myself, have found increased lifespans in laboratory animals fed greater than "nutritionally required" amounts of vitamin E. But other investigators have found no increase in lifespan.

Dr. Max Horwitt, who helped prove that vitamin E is essential to humans, has spoken against over-supplementation. He says that "over-supplementation may not be all bad, but it probably benefits the mind more than the body." He also has said there are people "who are accomplishing no more than enriching the sewers of the country." In a letter to me, Dr. Horwitt said "Perhaps one is better off with higher doses of vitamin E, but I wish I had the facts or any good evidence to prove it."

In answer to Dr. Horwitt, I call attention to the concept that I published suggesting that the "excess" vitamin E in the colon protects against colon cancer. I listed supporting observations in an article in *American Laboratory* (June 1973). This is preliminary evidence, but rather than enriching the sewers, excess vitamin E may be interfering with harmful free-radical reactions from bowel carcinogens. The carcinogens are formed in the bowel by decaying and slow-moving wastes. As far as benefiting the mind, there is evidence from a double-blind study that vitamin E increases alertness and learning ability.

Critics are generally not aware of these new findings, having written off the usefulness of vitamin E decades ago. Until they become familiar with the current research, they should not enter into discussions of the subject.

While scientists continue their research and debate, there does come a time when prudent decisions can be made by lay people. This is disturbing to the scientists, who feel that non-experts do not have the background to make qualified decisions about a highly technical matter. However, these scientists are oriented toward general laws, and are not familiar with individual experiences to the extent that some practicing physicians are. They do not consider that lay people can experiment with vitamins and diets to find what is best for their own health.

If you know that reasonable quantities of vitamins give you better health over long periods of time, because you can feel and see the difference, don't worry about debate. On the other hand, do not become fanatical and take exceedingly large amounts of vitamins until the question of long-term safety is established. Vitamin C appears to be safe in daily quantities of five grams or more in many people, but that amount may very well cause problems with *you*. A safe approach would be to take gradually increasing amounts of a vitamin, while working with your family doctor, until an optimum state of health is reached. Move cautiously, in moderation, and let your body be your guide.

# CHAPTER 69

# The Vitamin E Story

*By Wilfrid E. Shute, B.A., M.D.*

*Wilfrid E. Shute, B.A., M.D., a pioneer in the study of vitamin E research, graduated in biological and medical sciences in 1929 and earned his M.D. in 1933 at the University of Toronto. He followed this with five years of postgraduate training at the University of Chicago clinics and the University of Toronto. He practiced in North Dakota and in Iowa before returning to Canada, where he became the cofounder and codirector of the Shute Institute for Clinical and Laboratory Medicine. He is the author and coauthor of many medical publications on hyperthyroidism, nephritis, and cardiovascular disease. Dr. Shute is also author and coauthor of four books on the medical application of vitamin E. He is retired from active medical practice.*

That vitamin E will save lives from myocardial infarction and from heart failure must now be accepted by all physicians—this since the acceptance by even the most recalcitrant of our critics, of its usefulness in treating intermittent claudication, or leg pains, when walking.

In 1936, Dr. Evan Shute treated a patient with angina pectoris with vitamin E, with complete relief of his angina. He then asked me to try the same treatment on heart patients under my care in the hospital. My patients failed to respond so we abandoned it and actually forgot about it until Floyd Skelton, a medical

410

student, spent the summer of 1945 doing research under Evan's direction.

Looking back on the 1936-37 episode, it becomes all too obvious why our one success was not followed by others. The first patient was unique in his ability to take a large dose of wheat germ oil—cold-pressed through burlap and tasting like a burlap bag—without gagging or vomiting; he actually rather liked it! More particularly, he was one of the very few patients whose angina left him completely on a minimal dose of vitamin E.

My patients were given too small a dose and I abandoned the experiment after two or three weeks—too short a period as we now know for coronary artery insufficiency to show a response.

For the next 10 years (1936 to 1945), vitamin E in the form of wheat germ oil (a product especially prepared for us) kept refrigerated and used soon after preparation, did give continued evidence of its effectiveness as we now know. However, we did not see this effect even though it was presented to us regularly. Some of our obstetrical patients had definite evidence of rheumatic heart disease, and since all of our obstetrical patients were given vitamin E prophylactically to maintain their pregnancies and to avoid complications, especially prematurity and miscarriage due to *abruptio placentae,* they were, in fact, being treated for their rheumatic heart disease.

Many times we marvelled at how well their hearts withstood the strain of the pregnancy. My own wife was a case in point. Although she had been Canada's outstanding woman swimmer, representing Canada at two successive Olympiads, she nevertheless was a victim of rheumatic heart disease. Both of her pregnancies were maintained with the greatest difficulty with heroic doses of vitamin E. Fortunately, by this time a potent product, well tolerated, had become available. Her heart gave no trouble until some time later after she had stopped her vitamin E. The role of vitamin E in sustaining the heart still went unrecognized.

# A Lucky Accident

It was not until 1954 that we treated what we thought were our first heart patients with vitamin E. Again, it was to some extent a lucky accident. Floyd Skelton's research project concerned *purpura hemorrhagica*—a condition in which blood from the vessels escapes into various tissues of the body. Using dogs as experimental animals, Skelton was able to produce *purpura* with estrogen, and to both clear it up completely and alternately to prevent it by giving the dogs vitamin E in megavitamin quantities.

This led to two important discoveries. The first, that the dosage range in humans was much larger than anyone had previously realized. Equating the dog dose with the human dose in the usual way, the result arrived at was 200 to 300 I.U. a day. Second, it confirmed the antagonism of vitamin E and estrogen—a much earlier observation, deduced from the well-known antagonism of thyroid and estrogen. Thyroid and vitamin E reduce the estrogen in the body and vice versa.

Again, chance worked in our favor. The first human case of *purpura hemorrhagica* which we treated with alpha-tocopherol was in deep heart failure. His physician had discussed surgery, a splenectomy, but he was so sick that he was considered a serious operative risk. On vitamin E, the heart failure cleared up completely as well as the *purpura*. We then recalled our patients of 1936, especially the one whose severe angina had completely disappeared.

# Doctor's Mother Saved

At the same time, two other patients were desperately ill, one our mother. She had suffered from hypertension for years with numerous episodes of paroxysmal auricular fibrillation which were very incapacitating. Lately, she had developed a permanent auricular fibrillation with increasing peripheral edema and shortness of breath. She grew steadily worse in spite of rest and digitalis, and had reached the stage of extreme swelling of the legs and shortness of breath. A determined woman, she still lived alone, but now had a chair in the middle of each room and in each doorway and she moved from chair to chair, still looking after herself and her home.

This was in 1946—for my brother and I discussed putting her on vitamin E while he was attending my wife, in labor with our second child.

On vitamin E therapy, mother began to improve slowly until suddenly one day she began a violent diuresis with the loss of nearly 20 pounds of fluid over 48 hours, with a subsequent complete loss of both her shortness of breath and swelling of the extremities. After three weeks of vitamin E, she dug up her flower garden and planted her spring flowers. She remained well for nine years thereafter, finally succumbing to an illness unrelated to her heart condition.

The third patient had suffered a heart attack and had been cared for by the university cardiologist. He survived the attack but after discharge from the hospital he began to develop heart failure. His condition became extremely serious, with massive peripheral edema. He was so short of breath that he could no longer sleep in bed. The only rest he could get was by sitting in a chair leaning on three pillows tied to the top of a table. He could no longer get his shoes on but wore heavy socks and his big son's big slippers.

The day Evan was called to see him, the cardiologist had visited him to give him an injection of a mercury diuretic. When there was no obvious effect, the patient's wife called the cardiologist again, who stated that he had no further help to offer and that it was too bad the patient's mind was so clear, since he was therefore so aware of his discomfort.

This man was a member of our church and the wife then called Evan, who suggested vitamin E. Three weeks later this patient was free of all symptoms, back at work and playing in the little symphony orchestra.

You can, perhaps, imagine our surprise, then our exhilaration and delight at the prompt and thorough response of these patients to vitamin E. All three were terminal, desperately ill, very near death, and all three became almost, if not quite, perfectly well. Truly these were miracles in the true sense of the word.

What to do? Obviously, the first thing to do was to share our find with the rest of the world. This we did immediately with a short note announcing this discovery to the two appropriate, recognized scientific journals in this field: *Science* (10, 3:762, 1946 and *Nature* (157:772, 1946).

## Proceeding With Caution

Then, of course, the next step was to enlarge our series as quickly as possible. Since Evan was an obstetrician and gynecologist, the only patients immediately available were mine, and to a degree those of Dr. Vogelsang.

Again, I would ask the reader to realize the situation at that time. When one makes a discovery of this magnitude, he stands alone and lonely with no one to turn to for help or advice, with the responsibility of treating human patients with an entirely new mode of treatment, whose modes of action are relatively unknown and obscure. These were the first human patients treated with megavitamin therapy. Obviously, in a dosage range in the neighborhood of up to 100 times that previously used, this material was no longer acting as a vitamin but as a biochemical therapeutic agent to reverse serious untreatable conditions with results never before obtained by any available means.

Fortunately for our patients, the Shute brothers had early come under the influence of the great Joseph B. DeLee, the founder of the Maxwell Street Dispensary, followed by the Chicago Lying-In Hospital. I had interned at the former and Evan had trained for three years at both, ending up as chief resident. One of the well-known DeLee precepts set in stainless steel letters in his delivery room walls, in Latin, was *"First do no harm."* We have always accepted this motto as our own.

Therefore, we proceeded cautiously to treat heart patients with vitamin E. It was essential that we should not withdraw any medication that they had been taking. In every case we merely added vitamin E, making no change in their environment save this one factor. In this way we were able to assess the exact effect of the vitamin E. When we had treated some 25 patients and were sure most patients would respond to the treatment to a very worthwhile degree, we prepared a paper for publication. It had to be complete, unassailable by any critical reader; an accurate reporting of the diagnosis, treatment, and results obtained. To make sure that our diagnoses were correct and our reporting of the patients' response factual, we assembled all these patients together and had them examined and questioned by two internists; their histories minutely scanned and our medical paper thoroughly reviewed.

One or two amusing episodes resulted. One of my patients who, unknown to these two doctors, had been a professional wrestler, and at the time was the coach of the world's champion, was highly incensed at the medical workout he was being submitted to. I had to calm him down and explain that we had asked these internists to examine and criticize our work as harshly as possible.

The result was a paper which has stood up for over 30 years as factual and accurate to the smallest detail. This paper was read by Dr. Vogelsang to the regular monthly meeting of the St. Thomas and East Elgin Academy of Medicine, thus fulfilling the ethical requirements of correct medical and scientific procedure, and then released to the press.

## Learning More About Vitamin E

Gradually, we began to understand more fully just how vitamin E worked. Reading all the literature available on vitamin E, we began to map out its modes of actions, substances which interfered with or decreased its beneficial effects, and how to use substances which enhanced its value. We applied knowledge gained from the years of use of wheat germ oil by my father and ourselves.

We had known that inorganic iron, if it came into contact with vitamin E, reduced its effectiveness or completely neutralized it. Indeed, in the early days of research with animals, the method used to obtain vitamin E-free diets was to use food which contained as little as possible, and then to wash it with an iron solution. The diets so obtained, thought at the time to be vitamin E-free, were really only vitamin E-poor. When molecular distillation was used, it was possible to remove still more of the vitamin from the "vitamin E-free diets." We have always insisted that if iron must be given to a patient, that they be separated by at least eight to 12 hours.

We knew that estrogen and vitamin E were antagonists. Indeed, all of us had used this knowledge in the effective treatment of several obstetrical and gynecological conditions for years.

We knew that mineral oil dissolved vitamin E but did not release it readily in the body, while the vegetable oils, on the other hand, did release their vitamin E readily.

We knew that polyunsaturated fats increased the normal requirements for vitamin E, and therefore reduced the amount of vitamin E available to the body in treating patients.

Gradually, we were able to list the actions of vitamin E in megavitamin dosage range. Later, as we became bolder, we slowly and carefully raised the daily intake. All this we had to do by ourselves without any help except a few reports of animal experiments and biochemists' papers.

We had to contend with a lot of incorrect information, published or verbally offered. The two most unfortunate ones were that vitamin E probably acted as vitamin C in the treatment of scurvy and vitamin D in the treatment of rickets. Treatment in both these conditions requires large daily quantities of the vitamin to arrest the disease—but then the dosage could be radically reduced to a "maintenance level." We found out the hard way that this was not so of vitamin E. The dosage level at which improvement was obtained with vitamin E *was* the maintenance level.

# A Word of Caution

The second erroneous bit of knowledge—an error perpetuated in many "reports" as well as in articles in the popular press—is that "It can do you no harm." The truth is that there are two special situations in which vitamin E therapy must be used carefully.

Chronic rheumatic heart disease responds exceedingly well to vitamin E therapy, but it is necessary to use a much smaller dosage schedule. For example, where a patient with coronary artery disease should take 800 to 1,600 I.U. a day, we start patients with chronic rheumatic heart disease on 90 I.U. a day for a month, then 120 I.U. a day for a month, and then 150 I.U. Worthwhile response may take as long as three to three-and-a-half months to become established, and most such patients need never exceed the 150 I.U. a day regime.

Similarly, when the patient has a serious elevation of blood pressure, we first treat that blood pressure if his doctor has not already done so and *then* begin vitamin E therapy. Usually it is possible to achieve very significant improvements in such cases, but the presence of elevated blood pressure does require careful supervision.

Proper knowledge of the method of treatment in these two instances will produce an excellent response in virtually all such patients.

One of the peculiar attributes of vitamin E therapy is the slowness with which it works in many conditions for which it eventually proves to be of great value. In acute nephritis, acute thrombophlebitis, and acute rheumatic fever, it may and often does, give complete recovery in a matter of days. However, in coronary heart disease, it usually takes five to 10 days to start to act, and four to six weeks before its effects are definite and obvious. Yet, in cases of intermittent claudication it may take weeks to months to show its great value, as has been mentioned specifically by many authors, notably Boyd and Haeger.

# Encouraging Success

May I stress again that the responses of our first three cases were miracles—absolutely! We early began to investigate its power to heal and sustain tissue life and health in many other fields—notably in acute nephritis, acute thrombophlebitis, huge varicose ulcers, diabetic gangrene, intermittent claudication, and burns, to name but a few. In these fields also, the use of megavitamin E resulted in absolute miracles. It saved legs from amputation, healed huge intractable ulcers, healed burns without the contraction of scars which normally make skin-grafting mandatory.

Soon, our original reports were being confirmed in medical journals in Europe, the British Isles, the United States, and eventually in Canada.

For example, our first case of acute thrombophlebitis was treated in May of 1946, our second in February of 1947. In 1949, the eminent surgeon, Alton Ochsner, reported successful treatment and prevention of thrombophlebitis at the International Congress of Surgeons and in the *Journal of the American Medical Association* in 1950 (42: 533, 1950). There are now over 60 papers in the medical literature confirming its value in this condition.

Our first ulcers of leg and ankle were treated in the fall of 1946; its use in this situation has since been confirmed in 61 medical papers.

Our first case of incipient gangrene of the extremities was treated in June of 1946; its usefulness here since confirmed in nine medical papers.

Since 1946, I have supervised or treated directly many thousands of heart patients. They have come from pretty well all over the world, from every state in the union including Hawaii and Alaska, every province in Canada, from Ireland and England, Switzerland, the Isle of Capri, Australia and New Zealand and Bermuda. Some of the more spectacular cases come immediately to mind, although they are not necessarily by any means the best.

One of the early ones was a war veteran who belonged to the Royal Scottish Regiment. He had survived a heart attack but had very severe angina easily evoked by almost any exertion. After six weeks of vitamin E, he went on a long route march with his regiment.

More spectacular was the railwayman from northern Ontario, who was similarly greatly limited in activity by severe, easily induced angina on exertion or excitement following recovery from an acute heart attack. After eight weeks of vitamin E he went hunting, shot a deer three miles into the bush and dragged it out to the camp all by himself.

Or the farmer who was unable to do any work for the same reasons as the two above. His nephew was trying to keep both his own farm and his uncle's going. After four or five weeks on vitamin E the uncle felt so much better that he thought he could at least hitch up the team of horses for the nephew. One of the horses was a young one and apparently not at ease with the farmer, and just as the man was about to attach the whiffletree to the wagon tongue the horse bolted suddenly. The farmer grabbed the reins and see-sawed the runaway team to a halt just as they reached the gate. Then he realized what he had done!

I will never forget the first case of acute rheumatic fever I was called upon to treat. The man had developed a strep throat when 11 years old, followed by acute rheumatic fever. He was taken to the Hospital for Sick Children in Toronto—a very famous institution—and kept there for seven months. Then he was sent to the convalescent hospital for 15 months more before being allowed to return home to the farm. At first, he was allowed to feed the chickens, later to participate in gentle farm chores. Three days before I saw him he had a recurrence of his rheumatic fever. Three joints were involved; one was red hot and swollen but subsiding, one was at its worst, and a third beginning. Although he had had a tonsillectomy in the hospital, he had red swollen tonsil tags. I had never tried vitamin E in such a case before, of course, but knowing the usual course of the disease, I found it hard to reassure the mother when she asked me if this meant another 22 months in hospitals. You can imagine my utter amazement when this boy walked into the office three days later, completely well. I nearly literally "fell over!" Examination showed a badly damaged heart but no evidence of rheumatic activity, clinically or by laboratory investigation. This boy has not had a recurrence since; has grown to manhood, is a particularly tall and handsome man, has married, is a father, and has lived a normal vigorous life otherwise. He has done all types of farm labor. He went west one summer for the annual grain harvest, and finally settled down to work in a grist mill.

Two interesting aspects of this case must be mentioned. Some four months after I first saw him in November, 1946, he was seen, along with several other of my original patients, by a group of cardiologists appointed by the College of Physicians and Surgeons, including the professor of medicine at our university. They remarked on the large size of his heart and the evidence of gross valvular damage. He told them he had just spent four days in the fields pulling turnips! The second feature of this story is the story of another big heart—his mother's. He was an adopted child, the thirteenth in the family.

## An Illustrative Case

Finally, I want to relate a story which illustrates not only the results that can be obtained in treating the victims of chronic rheumatic heart disease—the late results of heart damage from rheumatic fever in childhood—but also the predictability of vitamin E treatment. It is a tricky, vicious, and unpredictable disease. Often after recovery from the acute attack, the patient remains apparently well for years; may even be a top athlete, and yet suddenly one day he begins to develop, very gradually, symptoms of heart damage. We have had many examples in our practice, one a famous world champion figure skater; a man who had appeared in many movies as the partner of one of the great female skaters of all time. We have had a professional football player and an Olympic swimmer to mention three. Sometimes the original acute episode is so mild that it goes unnoticed, and it is only by a chance examination or by the late appearance of symptoms, that the diagnosis is made.

To introduce the story of my friend, I should tell the reader that one of my many hobbies has been the breeding, showing, and most recently judging of pure-bred dogs. I am the only Canadian who has held various offices in the Doberman Pinscher Club of America, including that of vice-president, and for two years I was its president. One of the interesting friends I made through the club is one who has had a unique job at our annual meetings. We usually meet in motels, overcrowded by our club, with the usual cafeteria quick-order meals available. His job has been to seek out excellent dining places in the city in which the meetings are being held. Our small group of friends and gourmets has never yet been disappointed in the places he picks.

Three years ago, while in Florida, I received a telephone call from him wanting to see me immediately. I knew he had had rheumatic fever but it hadn't bothered him for many years. However, the usual symptoms of progressive shortness of breath on exertion, a cough, and the need to sleep propped up on a couple of pillows had begun. At the University cardiac clinic they had done a thorough investigation, including a heart catheterization. After completion of this examination he was told that his mitral valve—the valve between the two chambers on the left side of his heart—was seriously diseased and narrowed, that his only hope was surgery, and so they booked him for the first available bed. Meanwhile, he was allowed home. This was when he telephoned me. I asked him if he was still able to work and he said "yes." I asked if he had been working every day and he said "yes." I told him that this being so, he didn't need surgery, that vitamin E would restore him to the condition that he was in 10 years before. He said, "That's why I phoned you."

I said there was no need to see me; that he had told me all I needed to know and that if he would do what I told him, he would be well in three and a half months. He was to be careful, reducing his activity but very little, continuing to work but not to overexert, and to begin on vitamin E—90 I.U. a day for the first month, 120 for the second month, and 150 for the third month.

I promised him that he would be as well as he had been 10 years ago after six weeks on 150 I.U. a day. He asked me then if he could see me if he did not respond as predicted, and of course I agreed. He was well in three and a half months. I saw him two years later in February when I judged at the Westminster Show, in Madison Square Garden in New York. He had been out dancing the night before, worked daily on the third floor of an office building, and usually ran up two flights of stairs, two steps at a time, just for fun.

## A Doctor's Shrug

This is not the end of the story. When I saw him in New York he told me he had suffered a heart arrest during the original heart catheterization. In spite of this, when he was called back to the clinic for a follow-up check (they hadn't heard from him since he turned down the original operation), they suggested another heart catheterization. In spite of his unfortunate experience, he agreed. He said he was curious to see whether or not there was real demonstrable improvement to match his clinical improvement. Once more he suffered cardiac arrest, once more its beat was restored, and once more he survived.

After the examination, he was told that he had mitral valve disease, and that—note this—"some day" he would "probably come to surgery." He asked how it could be that at the first examination, surgery was needed immediately and now just sometime in the future. The doctor's answer was a shrug!

At that dog show, after I'd judged the Doberman pinschers, the dog editor for the *New York Times,* Walter Fletcher, entered my ring with pad and pencil for an interview on my assessment of the quality of the dogs. I never did get to answer him, for my ring was immediately filled with patients and would-be patients. The owner of the Best of Breed dog and his wife came in to thank me and to tell me how well they were on their vitamin E. The very well-known handler of the dog had had a disc operation on his back some years before, followed by disabling muscular spasms and pain, until he was put on vitamin E with complete relief. If he gets careless and misses or cuts down on his dose, his backache and muscle spasms return.

Mr. Fletcher was quite amazed at the turn of events. Then it transpired that someone had presented him with a copy of my book *Vitamin E for Ailing and Healthy Hearts* (New York: Pyramid House, 1969), which he had not yet read. He forgot all about the dog interview and asked instead for an interview on the subject of vitamin E! It's hard to guess how many show dogs and their owners are using vitamin E.

## Vitamin E and Heart Attacks

We have marveled at the initial rejection of our work, its gradual acceptance by the profession, and the enormously wide acceptance of its value on the part of the reading public. It was reliably estimated some three or four years ago that between 30 and 35 million Americans were taking vitamin E in megadoses. The inevitable result has been the sudden halt in the rise, and actual decrease in the incidence of deaths from heart attacks. It was announced that nearly 10,000 fewer deaths from heart attacks—correctly named myocardial infarctions—occurred in middle-aged Americans in 1974.

For years there has been a mild decrease in deaths from rheumatic heart disease, due to the use of antibiotics to knock out the streptococcal infections that cause it. Similarly, there has been a 55 percent decrease in deaths from hypertensive heart disease, due to the discovery some 25 years ago of effective and relatively safe antihypertensive drugs.

However, nothing, absolutely nothing, has been able to halt the steady increase in coronary deaths, until the massive use of vitamin E.

The acceptance of vitamin E therapy by physicians and a small percentage of cardiologists has increased to an important degree in the last very few years. The confirmation of our clinical work has multiplied rapidly in the world's medical journals. However, it remained for two relatively recent controlled experiments to make a really worthwhile impact upon the medical world: that of Boyd and coworkers in 1963, and that of Haeger, with his double-blind controlled study reported in *Vascular Diseases* in 1968. Boyd has stated that severe arteriosclerosis, in which the process had been going on for years, could be shown by serial x ray to lose the calcium deposited in the walls after vitamin E therapy. Haeger showed that the local tissues which had suffered a chronic decrease in blood supply, due to arteriosclerotic narrowing of the arteries supplying that area, had a measurable marked increase in blood supply after vitamin E therapy.

We had reported this in 1946 as did Dr. Keith Stuart of London and Dr. George Dowd of Worcester, Massachusetts. In addition to these three and Boyd, the value of vitamin E in treating intermittent claudication (leg cramps while walking) had been reported in some 32 papers!

Dr. Haeger also confirmed what we had published many times, namely that there was no other effective treatment. In his series, the patients treated with anticoagulants or vasodilators showed no more improvement than those on a general vitamin capsule, one that did not contain vitamin E.

## The Versatile Vitamin

One of the early biochemists working with the then new concentrates of vitamin E, obtained by molecular distillation from vegetable oils, called this the most versatile of the vitamins. Professor Comel called it the "angiophilic vitamin." Indeed, its very versatility is one of its greatest drawbacks in the matter of medical "acceptance."

Medical practitioners have accepted several antibiotics as

"broad spectrum antibiotics," meaning that used therapeutically, they act to combat infections in many and various areas of the body caused by any one of many infective organisms. Similarly, cortisone seems to hold in check a whole "spectrum" of human pathological states. However, for the most part, doctors expect one therapeutic agent to work specifically for one specific abnormal state, as for example, insulin for diabetes mellitus, or diphtheria antitoxin for diphtheria only.

Vitamin E, however, is specifically useful for many apparently unrelated conditions, and doctors find it hard to accept this.

It really all falls into place when one realizes that all these conditions have one thing in common—cells which are not functioning normally, but which could do so if their blood supply could be increased somehow. Vitamin E in megadoses accomplishes this in several ways.

First of all, it has been shown in whole animals, in isolated hearts, and in heart muscle strips, to decrease the need for oxygen. Thus, when heart muscle is unable to get its full quota of blood because the coronary arteries supplying it are narrowed, the ability of vitamin E to decrease the muscle's need for oxygen allows that muscle to function normally or nearly so.

Similarly, in the diabetic whose arteries in his legs are so narrowed that the tissues of his great toe no longer have enough blood supply to survive, the toe dies. When the arteries of the leg have reached this degree of narrowing, it is seldom possible to save the leg. Usually, the leg must be amputated above the knee, since it is necessary to go high enough to ensure adequate blood supply to the flaps, so that the stump may heal.

In virtually all such patients, the use of 800 to 1,600 I.U. or more will allow the leg to be saved. In most cases, only the tissue actually dead when treatment is instituted will be lost. The need for oxygen in the cells immediately proximal to the dead cells is decreased and the cells can now survive. By normal processes, the dead cells separate off and the amazing result is the complete healing of the proximal tissues.

## Increases Effective Blood Supply

This, then—the decrease of oxygen-need of cells, and tissues in general—is one of the principal actions of vitamin E, and so this general principle can now be enunciated: In any condition where there is a decrease in blood supply or oxygen, vitamin E-therapy will help to some degree, and in most such cases to a degree sufficient to allow worthwhile improvement. Remember that Knut Haeger demonstrated that the continuing use of this therapy brings about a very real increase of blood supply. We have seen the blood supply in many legs return to the point where the pulsation of peripheral arteries which could not be detected at the outset of treatment has returned to normal or nearly so.

Ochsner and his group have published their results in treating fresh clots in the peripheral veins. Vitamin E will dissolve these fresh clots and, of great importance, without the danger of having the clot break loose and travel upwards to the lungs—a condition known as pulmonary embolism. Pulmonary embolism is accompanied by a death rate of approximately 50 percent.

Again, it should be noted that this condition is rapidly increasing—in one 10-year period increasing by five times. Of great importance is Ochsner's successful use prophylactically of vitamin E—thus preventing clots in peripheral veins.

Then we can expand our general principles to say that in any condition in which intravascular clotting is threatened or has occurred, or in which there is a decrease in blood supply or increased oxygen need, vitamin E will help to some degree, and in most cases to a sufficient degree to solve the problem completely or nearly so.

## Other Uses of Vitamin E

Besides these two principal actions of vitamin E, there are several others, more useful in some pathological conditions than in others. One is the ability of vitamin E to restore abnormal capillary permeability to normal—the main action that allows rapid and complete return to normal in acute rheumatic fever and acute nephritis. With normal capillary permeability restored, the oxygen-sparing action of the vitamin allows the body defenses to act effectively.

Vitamin E allows burns and traumatically denuded tissues to heal with scars that are not tender and do not contract. All scars contract and are tender, except these.

Vitamin E speeds up the opening of collateral circulation around occluded or seriously narrowed veins or arteries.

An understanding of all these various unique and useful actions of vitamin E will cause, then, no amazement when Drs. Samuel Ayres and Richard Mihan of Los Angeles report its usefulness in several recalcitrant skin conditions. Dr. Ayres states that it is practically a specific for nocturnal cramps, as well as a variety of other muscular problems, including the restless leg syndrome, nocturnal rectal cramps, exercise cramps, some cases of intermittent claudication and one spectacular case of polymyositis (inflammation of several muscles) after the total failure of three immunosuppressive drugs (*Journal of the American Medical Association,* 10 January 1972).

Ayres and Mihan became interested in vitamin E therapy because of the presentation by Milton Stout before the Los Angeles Dermatological Society in 1950, of the case of a woman with *pseudoxanthoma elasticum* (a rare skin disease) whose cutaneous and visual impairment were restored to near normal following administration of vitamin E for a period of one year (*Archives of Dermatology,* 60: 310, 1951). "This astounding therapeutic accomplishment in a hitherto untreatable disease" alerted them to this potential substance. Their results in treating a number of skin abnormalities have subsequently been published in several medical journals.

Haeger reports that his initial interest in vitamin E therapy "was aroused by a distinguished member of the Faculty of Medicine at the University of Malmo." He reported that "his walking had been much improved" after taking vitamin E.

No doctor can use a potent product of vitamin E, following

our published dosage routine, in a suitable case, without duplicating our results, and becoming an enthusiastic user of this fantastically useful treatment.

Finally, I would like to point out that there are nearly 150 papers now completely confirming our original observations in 1936, that vitamin E was a specific in the treatment of heart disease.

# CHAPTER 70

# How Much Vitamin E Do You Really Get from Food?

According to the *FDA Consumer* (July–August 1973), "The amount of vitamin E needed by most people appears to be satisfied by the average well-balanced diet, even though some vitamin E is lost in food processing. Many common foods contain some vitamin E, and it is present in large quantities in leafy vegetables, whole-grain foods, and vegetable oils."

An analysis of this statement suggests that the FDA should spend as much time doing research as it does demeaning vitamin supplements and "health foods."

## How Much Vitamin E Do We Really Get from Vegetables?

First, consider the vitamin E in vegetables. In one of the most complete studies analyzing the alpha-tocopherol content of foods as they are eaten, R. H. Bunnell, Ph.D., and associates writing in the *American Journal of Clinical Nutrition* (July 1965) conclude that ". . . fruits and vegetables do not contribute significant amounts of a-tocopherol to the diet." (Alpha-tocopherol is that fraction of vitamin E which is the most biologically active.) Furthermore, they say, "The tocopherol content of canned vegetables is low in comparison to fresh or frozen vegetables, e.g. fresh, frozen, and canned peas contain 0.55 mg. (.82 I.U.), 0.25 mg. (.37 I.U.), 0.02 mg. (.03 I.U.) percent a-tocopherol, respectively." That's a 96 percent decrease in tocopherol content due to commercial processing.

Some time ago two British researchers, V. H. Booth and M. P. Bradford, analyzed the alpha-tocopherol content of store-bought fruits and vegetables and those in their raw state at the University of Cambridge in Great Britain (*British Journal of Nutrition,* vol. 17, 1963). Their findings, which are translated here from milligrams per kilogram to international units (I.U.) per pound, are very revealing. Remember that these values are for an entire pound of fresh, raw produce. Here are some examples from their list, beginning with the vegetables which are most rich in vitamin E. Keep in mind also that the U.S. Recommended Daily Allowance (RDA) for vitamin E is 30 I.U. for adults.

| Vegetable | Alpha-tocopherol per pound |
|---|---|
| Nettle leaf | 98.2 I.U. |
| Cabbage, outer leaf | 40.7 |
| Mint leaf | 33.8 |
| Carrot leaf | 20.3 |
| Dandelion leaf | 17.0 |
| Nasturtium | 17.0 |
| Spinach | 17.0 |
| Asparagus | 17.0 |
| Broccoli | 13.6 |
| Celery leaf | 4.8 |

Now, how many of these foods does the typical American eat? Notice that the *best* sources of vitamin E are probably not part of many diets. The outer leaf of cabbage has a goodly amount of vitamin E, but the inner portion, the part usually eaten, has less than one I.U. of vitamin E per pound.

Researchers Booth and Bradford underlined this point when they said, "In many plants there was much less tocopherol in the 'edible part' than in the discarded portion." Some poor vegetable sources of vitamin E include the more commonly consumed carrots, celery stalks, cucumbers, mushrooms, onions, peas, potatoes, radishes, and turnips.

That leaves only spinach, asparagus, and broccoli as dependable sources — unless you're in the habit of dining on nettle leaf or nasturtium.

But even with these vegetables, there may be problems. Booth and Bradford noted that if fresh raw vegetables are dropped into water which is already vigorously boiling, losses of vitamin E are minimized. But if you buy frozen spinach and then place it in a pan of water which is brought to a boil over a period of minutes, the loss of vitamin E may be great. As for broccoli, the vitamin E is all in the leafy portions. The "flower," which is the portion most people eat, contains not even a trace of vitamin E! The same holds true for cauliflower.

Turning now to whole grains, we find that, just as the FDA says, they are a relatively good source of vitamin E. Unfortunately, they don't play a significant role in the diets of most Americans. It's only the "health-food faddists" who seem to use and enjoy whole grain products. Most people eat "enriched" white bread, not knowing that almost every trace of the vitamin E that nature put into the wheat has been lost in the refining and bleaching processes.

## The Trouble with Vegetable Oils

The question of vitamin E content in vegetable oils is critical. On the one hand, these oils *are* the major source of vitamin E in the American diet. But at the same time, many vegetable oils actually *increase* the need for vitamin E above and beyond the extent that they supply it! Here's why:

Vegetable oils provide polyunsaturated fatty acids (PUFA), many of which we need for normal growth and general well-

being. They are troublesome, however, because of their susceptibility to change by the radiation which constantly bombards us
from natural and man-made sources. A. L. Tappel, Ph.D.,
professor of nutrition as well as food science and technology
at the University of California at Davis, explains that when these
rays strike a fat molecule, they knock loose a hydrogen atom and
initiate the *peroxidation* of polyunsaturated lipids. In this
process of peroxidation, free radicals are formed. According to
an article by Dr. Tappel in *Nutrition Today* (December 1967),
"The free radical flies about within the cell under terrific force
and without any pattern to its movement until it strikes another
molecule and causes all sorts of damage." Constant free radical
damage is one of the theories by which the process of aging is
explained. There is also the possibility that this same effect may
be involved in the genesis of many cancers, although this has
never been proven.

Here is where vitamin E comes in. As Dr. Tappel explains,
"This vitamin offers primary biochemical protection against the
excessive oxidation of cellular lipids." By doing this, vitamin E
helps prevent the formation of the dangerous free radicals. For
this reason, vitamin E needs are based on the amount of PUFA
eaten.

But how much vitamin E do you need to protect against the
formation of these dangerous free radicals? In 1963, Philip L.
Harris, Ph.D., and Norris D. Embree, Ph.D., suggested a convenient way to determine the amount of vitamin E which is desirable to occur along with polyunsaturated oils. They came up
with a rating expressed as E: PUFA—the ratio of the number of
milligrams of d-alpha-tocopherol (natural vitamin E) to the
number of grams of polyunsaturated acids. The dietary ratio
they believed to be desirable and protective is 0.6 (*American
Journal of Clinical Nutrition,* December 1963). Today, it is
generally agreed that this ratio of 0.6 is the *minimum* ratio
necessary for protection.

But what is the *actual* ratio which exists in vegetable oils
which we consume?

## Most Oils Create a Need
## for More Vitamin E

David C. Herting, Ph.D., and Emma-Jane E. Drury at the Health and Nutrition Research Division of the Tennessee-Eastman Research Laboratories in New York, reported their work on the vitamin E content of various vegetable oils in the *Journal of Nutrition* (vol. 81, 1963). Their analysis of refined, unhydrogenated oils gave these average E:PUFA ratings:

| | |
|---|---|
| Cottonseed oil | .65 |
| Safflower oil | .45 |
| Corn oil | .36 |
| Soybean oil | .28 |

From these figures, it appears that only cottonseed oil is a wise choice, since it is the only oil in which the polyunsaturated fatty acids are compensated for by sufficient vitamin E. Concerning the other oils, the researchers state: "The possibility cannot be ignored that an appreciable increase in consumption of such oils, whether as supplemental or replacement fat, could result in gradual depletion and eventual deficiency of vitamin E." These are words to the wise for those who have been taking large amounts of polyunsaturated oils in hopes of reducing blood cholesterol levels.

As shown in the preceding analyses, the E:PUFA ratio of soybean oil is very low. Since soybean oil is used in many foods advertising themselves as high in polyunsaturated fats (such as margarine and imitation mayonnaise), its corresponding lack of sufficient vitamin E could make it an unwise dietary staple for those who aren't getting supplemental vitamin E.

The point is driven home by Dr. Bunnell and his associates, who warn: ". . . there is a general trend toward increased consumption of vegetable oil and decreased consumption of animal fats. Particularly marked is the large increase in the use of soybean oil. . . . A resulting imbalance in the vitamin

E-polyunsaturated fatty acid (E:PUFA) ratio is therefore possible in many foods which are based on soybean oil which has not been hydrogenated (solidified)."

The authoritative text *The Biochemistry of Clinical Medicine* (Chicago, Illinois: Year Book Medical Publishers, Inc., 1970) declares: "With the present vogue for diets high in unsaturated fatty acids, the requirement for tocopherol should be increased. It is true that natural unsaturated fats are rich in tocopherol, but most of it is destroyed in the processing of the oil. Perhaps tocopherol should be added to the finished oil."

It seems that vegetable oils, despite what the FDA says about their being a rich source of vitamin E in the diet, are more apt to create a deficiency of vitamin E than anything else. This isn't the kind of deficiency that your doctor can spot while he's taking your blood pressure, or a deficiency that would be noticed by researchers using the usual method of finding signs of nutritional deficiency. The harmful products of lipid peroxidation are believed to cause very subtle, long-term injuries usually associated with "aging."

## Lipid Peroxides Linked to Breast Cancer

Fluid found in the breasts of women with a high risk of breast cancer often contains high levels of lipid peroxides—the very same deteriorated fats that occur in the absence of vitamin E. That's the finding of Nicholas L. Petrakis, M.D., professor of preventive medicine and international health at the University of California in San Francisco.

Using a special breast pump to examine 2,500 women, Dr. Petrakis discovered that (a) fluids are more likely to occur in the breasts of women in populations known to be cancer-prone and (b) these stagnant fluids may contain cigarette smoke by-products, chemicals, and peroxidized fats that may cause cancer in the cells lining the breast ducts.

Dr. Petrakis told an American Cancer Society seminar for science writers that the amount of lipid peroxides in breast fluid was seven times higher in Caucasian women than in women of

Chinese descent, who are relatively free of breast cancer (*New York Times,* 23 March 1975).

## Bringing the E:PUFA Story Down to Real Life

That's the story for vegetable oils. But what about the rest of the diet? Is it possible that people are getting enough vitamin E from other sources to protect against the peroxidation of polyunsaturates?

The answer to this question comes from John G. Bieri, Ph.D., and Ritva P. Evarts, D.V.M., who analyzed the food obtained from the employees' cafeteria at the Clinical Center of the National Institutes of Health, Bethesda, Maryland. A composite of three meals a day revealed the average content of alpha-tocopherol per day to be only 9.0 mg. (13.4 I.U.) with a range from 4.4 mg. (6.6 I.U.) to 12.7 mg. (18.9 I.U.) (*Journal of the American Dietetic Association,* February 1973).

When these figures are compared against the RDA for vitamin E, 30 I.U., it is apparent that the average diet is deficient.

# Ratio of Vitamin E (mg.) to Polyunsaturates (grams)

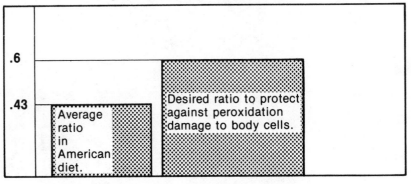

More to the point, their study also revealed that the daily average E:PUFA ratio was 0.43, with ranges from 0.16 to 0.71. And that average turns out to be more than 28 percent below the safety limit of 0.6 for peroxidation damage protection. Some people are as much as 73 percent below the safety point.

Now, let us consider the FDA pronouncement on vitamin E again: "The amount of vitamin E appears to be satisfied by the average, well-balanced diet, even though some vitamin E is lost in food processing."

It seems clear that this statement leaves something to be desired in terms of scientific accuracy. But the FDA frequently operates this way, and we often hear apologists for the FDA making these same meaningless declarations about how wonderful the "average" diet is.

Many people do take supplements of vitamin E, and it appears to be a wise idea—in large part because we get so little from today's processed foods. But that is only part of the reason. Most of us know that there is a great body of clinical information about the benefits of vitamin E in a variety of human diseases and abnormal conditions. The fact that the FDA does not recognize this evidence as valid is regrettable but not surprising, in the light of this agency's evaluation of our vitamin E supply in food and the importance of the vitamin to normal life.

# CHAPTER 71

# Special Requirements of a Low Cholesterol Diet

When your electrocardiogram shows the slightest irregularity, or your cholesterol is what your doctor terms "too high," he becomes deeply concerned and cautions you sternly to cut out those saturated fats. "Use margarine" is standard medical advice. "No butter. No eggs or maybe two a week. Use polyunsaturated fats."

Your doctor is no doubt deeply concerned for your health, but this advice might be dangerous. When a doctor prescribes the high use of polyunsaturated fats without also prescribing the high use of an antioxidant (vitamin E) he is putting his patient on a fast train to a dangerous disturbance in cell metabolism.

According to Dr. T. W. Anderson of the University of Toronto, writing in the *Lancet* (11 August 1973), "Nutritional muscular dystrophy is a disease that develops in a number of animal species when dietary unsaturated fatty acids are inadequately protected by antioxidants. Under these circumstances, highly reactive lipid peroxides are formed that affect both skeletal muscle and the myocardium, and the animal is liable to die suddenly of a 'heart attack,' especially when stressed."

You may find this news puzzling, disturbing, and contradictory. After all, aren't polyunsaturated fats helpful because they reduce cholesterol levels? True, but Dr. Anderson warns that unless those unsaturated fats are protected by antioxidants they will make you more vulnerable to ischemia (deficiency of blood due to constriction).

"A subclinical form of this disease may have developed in man (especially males) during the past few decades, and by increasing the vulnerability of the myocardium to atherosclerotic ischemia," Dr. Anderson suggested, "the unprotected polyunsaturates may well have increased the incidence of myocardial infarction."

He was not just guessing. The Canadian doctor based his ideas on a study of the sex ratio changes that have occurred in cardiovascular mortality rates during the past fifty years.

"These changes are compatible with the appearance of a myocardial disorder due to developments in food processing that have disturbed the normal ratio between unsaturated fatty acids and biologically effective antioxidants in the human diet," said Dr. Anderson.

## Natural Antioxidants Lost in Processing

In the raw state, most fats and oils that are high in polyunsaturated fatty acids also contain enough natural antioxidants (mainly vitamin E) to keep them from combining with oxygen in the bloodstream and forming poisonous peroxides. But, as Dr. Anderson pointed out, this antioxidant "umbrella" can itself be destroyed by oxidation during prolonged storage or processing. "Thus even such an apparently innocuous procedure as heating corn oil in air results in such a serious loss of antioxidants that if the oil is then fed to pigs the animals develop acute and fatal myocardial degeneration." This would certainly indicate that frying foods in oil or margarine is a dangerous practice, as is the common practice of extracting them at high temperatures.

Ironically, the very oils that doctors strongly advocate are potentially the most deadly. According to Dr. Anderson, the extent of the disruption of cell metabolism is "directly related to the ease with which the unsaturated fatty acids form peroxides, and this increases sharply with their degree of unsaturation.

Linoleic acid, with two double bonds, has approximately seven times the toxicity of oleic acid, with one double bond." Thus, the more polyunsaturated the fatty acid is, the more disruptive it is to your cell metabolism if oxidized, and the more it needs antioxidant protection.

How does your doctor's advice measure up against the data? Did he advise you to avoid butter? Butter contains only a trace of linoleic acid, and four grams of oleic acid per tablespoon, according to the *Home and Garden Bulletin No. 72* compiled by the U.S. Department of Agriculture. Did he advise you to substitute margarine? One tablespoon of margarine gives you three grams of linoleic acid and six grams of oleic per tablespoon. Margarine is 21 times more liable to form peroxides, while butter, being a natural food, also contains vitamin E, a natural antioxidant which prevents the formation of peroxides. Margarine, a highly processed food, loses its vitamin E during processing.

Let's take a look at corn oil which is so frequently touted as the optimum food for heart attack victims. One tablespoon gives you seven grams of linoleic and four grams of oleic acid. The commercial corn oils have been so processed that any vitamin E that was in them originally is completely destroyed so that corn oil, instead of protecting your heart, actually endangers it with unchecked peroxides.

It is unfortunate that both doctor and patient become smugly satisfied that they are on the right track to heart health with a diet rich in polyunsaturates, because cholesterol levels do tend to stabilize or go down on such a regimen. But, in the *Journal of Atherosclerosis Research* (7: 647, 1967) Drs. D. Kritchevsky and S. A. Tepper revealed that, in a series of studies with rabbits, only a slight addition of .25 percent linoleic, stearic, or free fatty acids increased the formation of atheromatous lesions in the arterial walls, and that while serum cholesterol levels were not necessarily increased by the addition of free fatty acids, the aortic deposition of lipids was accelerated. Dr. Kritchevsky and his colleagues also discovered that when an oil was added to a standard ration of cholesterol in the rabbit diet, atherosclerotic lesions were more pronounced than when cholesterol alone was given. They found that this startling result occurred only when oils were first heated to 200° C. for a period of 15 minutes. Heat-treated oils increased the severity of the atherosclerotic lesions.

Dr. Roger Williams in his book, *Nutrition Against Disease,* (New York: Pitman Publishing Corp., 1973), draws from these data the same inference as does Dr. Anderson in Canada: "It strongly indicates to us that, once again, the mistaken notion of increasing one's daily intake of vegetable oils in line with the current fad of eating lots of polyunsaturated fats may expose the consumer to even greater risk of atherosclerosis and coronary heart disease." Dr. Williams warns that, "the indiscriminate eating of polyunsaturated vegetable oils must be strongly condemned."

Did your doctor warn you not to cook with the polyunsaturated oils? The longer these fats are heated, the more dangerous they become, and the danger is not limited to heart attacks in the male. According to *The Cholesterol Controversy* (Los Angeles, California: Sherbourne Press, 1973), Dr. Henry Eyring of the University of Utah maintains that anything that generates "free radicals" as polyunsaturates do, also causes chromosome damage which may well lead to cancer.

## Butter is Better for Cooking

When it comes to cooking and baking, you are much better off with a saturated fat like butter. When animals fed heated polyunsaturates were compared with animals fed heated butter, those fed heated corn oil had lower growth rates, developed diarrhea and rough fur, and every single one developed tumors. Only one animal survived the 40-month experimental period. But none of the animals fed the heated butter developed tumors and every one survived (*Critical Reviews in Food Technology,* September 1972, and *Nutrition Today* January 1972).

Even if you take your oil straight from the bottle, as in salad dressing, without submitting it to heat, unless you are using an unrefined oil or one that has been truly cold-pressed, you are not safe from the peroxides. The commonly available polyunsaturated vegetable oils, unless specified as unrefined, have been subjected to extraction by chemicals and high heat, bleaching, refinement to neutralize the free fatty acids and finally, and what Dr. Williams terms "most disastrously," a deodorization process in which the oils are held above 215° C. for a period sometimes as long as 12 hours.

As the ratio of antioxidant to polyunsaturated fatty acids declines, there comes a point at which there are not enough antioxidants in the human diet to prevent the formation of lipid peroxides in the body. This point was reached, Dr. Anderson believes, in the British and North American diets about 1920, causing an increased vulnerability of the myocardium (heart muscle) to atherosclerotic ischemia, and a consequent rise in the incidence of myocardial infarction.

It is interesting to note that the major change in the British and North American diet around this time was the widespread adoption of what Dr. Anderson calls "oxidative processing of bread flour." It was at this time that wheat germ was removed from the flour which went into commercial bread. The germ of wheat contains an unusually large amount of tocopherol relative to its polyunsaturated fatty acid content so that whole-grain wheat products normally contribute a surplus of antioxidant to the diet.

Towards the end of the nineteenth century, this surplus had been considerably reduced by the general change from whole meal to highly refined white bread. This was bad enough, but the industry also introduced oxidizing agents which finally eliminated every bit of dietary antioxidant that had once been in the bread.

## Less Dangerous to Women

For some reason which is not yet apparent, damage to the heart muscle as a result of the decline in the ratio of antioxidants to polyunsaturated fatty acids affects males more severely than females and is responsible for the appearance of a rising cardiac sex ratio. This sex ratio is an important clue to dietary factors causing myocardial infarction. For instance, bread has been an important constituent of the Italian diet for many years. Until 1947 there was a low cardiac sex ratio in that country. That is, just as few men as women died of heart attacks. Italian bread was relatively unrefined until after 1945. In 1967, after 20 years on refined flour, the Italian cardiac sex ratio rate was two to one. That is, twice as many males as females were succumbing.

Coronary thrombosis—the major cause of heart attack death—is taking the lives of over one million people a year in the United States alone. Yet, and this may surprise you, coronary thrombosis was unknown as a disease entity in 1900. The medical profession has singled out saturated fats and cholesterol as the villains in this sad saga. Warning against the use of eggs, cream, and butter and other high cholesterol goodies is standard procedure by doctors and even some nutritionists.

Actually, the intake of animal fat in the American diet has been reduced over the past 15 years to about one-third of what it was, yet the coronary rate has gone up considerably every year. During this same period, the intake of animal fats in Canada remained unchanged.

Yet, although the average Canadian ate three times as much saturated fat as his American counterpart, the incidence of coronary thrombosis in Canada leveled off, came to a halt, and began to decrease during that same period.

There has to be a more rational explanation than the animal fat-atherosclerosis theory to explain why a disease entity that was not common enough to be medically recognized prior to 1910 has become a greater ravager of human life than any plague recorded in history.

The polyunsaturated fatty acids do play a seesaw role. On the one hand they do help to reduce atherosclerosis. On the other hand, unless they are protected against peroxidation, they may interfere with myocardial metabolism and make the heart more vulnerable to the ischemia that results from the atherosclerosis.

What to do about it?

"It would seem prudent to suggest," said Dr. Anderson, "that when attempts are made to reduce human serum cholesterol levels by prescribing diets high in polyunsaturated fats, steps should be taken to insure that there is a correspondingly high intake of biologically effective antioxidants." Another name for biologically effective antioxidants is, of course, vitamin E. Has your doctor suggested that you include it in your health plan?

# CHAPTER 72

# A Dynamic Weapon
Against Wrinkles
and Aging

Is it possible that premature aging of the skin sometimes has nothing to do with environmental causes such as harsh weather or too much sunbathing, but rather the accelerated aging of the entire body? No one really knows for sure, but one doctor has suggested that premature wrinkling may be related to internal chemical reactions resulting from undesirable dietary patterns. And although this report is based more on an informal survey than a rigorous study, it fits in very well with recent scientific research which shows that: (1) vitamin E is intimately related to youthfulness, and (2) much more of this vitamin seems to be needed than anyone previously suspected to put the brakes on deterioration that would otherwise be inevitable.

## Premature Wrinkling and Polyunsaturates

Writing in *Medical Counterpoint* (February 1973), Edward R. Pinckney, M.D., describes a lengthy scientific study in which more than one thousand patients were examined by a plastic surgeon for signs of premature aging. A dietary survey was also taken. The examiner, Cadvan O. Griffiths, Jr., M.D., professor of surgery at the University of California at Irvine, graded each patient on the basis of the degree of wrinkling, crow's-feet, frown lines, and on other signs of skin degeneration, such as changes in coloration and elasticity. Of 1,093 patients studied, 76 percent were women. The patients' ages ranged from 17 to 81. All were scored to see if they looked older than they really were.

When the results were tabulated, Dr. Griffiths found a striking correlation. Of those who said they regularly and frequently included polyunsaturated fats and oils in their diet, 78 percent showed marked clinical signs of premature aging. *Some actually looked 20 years older than they really were,* Dr. Pinckney wrote in *The Cholesterol Controversy* (Los Angeles: Sherbourne Press, 1973). But among those subjects who made no special effort to eat more polyunsaturates, only 18 percent showed any outward signs of early aging.

How could such a link be explained? "Polyunsaturated fatty acids, in themselves, are very unstable compounds," Dr. Pinckney explained. "A polyunsaturated lipid (fat) . . . when exposed to the slightest trace of a catalytic agent automatically begins the process of auto-oxidation." As a result, "the polyunsaturated fatty acid molecule breaks down to furnish free radicals. . . ."

Free radicals are highly reactive particles that, if left unchecked, will go on a destructive rampage inside our bodies. According to Dr. Pinckney, free radicals in the presence of available oxygen molecules will form toxic peroxides that can damage and destroy cells.

"When there is destruction of a body cell by a free radical," he says, "the end result is a lipofuscin pigment granule, sometimes called a 'clinker' by pathologists. And it is known that with aging the amount of lipofuscin pigments (ceroid bodies) increases; each one representing the death of a body cell. Or, to put it another way, the body becomes one cell older with each cell that is destroyed by a free radical from a polyunsaturate."

Under certain conditions, the more polyunsaturated oils we eat, the more "clinkers" we can expect to form in our bodies, and presumably, the more signs of premature aging that will appear. Of course, once such damage is done, it is very unlikely that it can ever be undone. According to Denham Harman, M.D., Ph.D., of the University of Nebraska College of Medicine, "Free radical reactions are almost invariably irreversible. . . . " Increasing the amount or degree of unsaturated fat fed laboratory animals decreases the average life span by as much as 10 percent, Dr. Harman told the Fourteenth Annual Symposium of the International College of Applied Nutrition in Los Angeles in April, 1974.

Cutting down on polyunsaturate consumption is not the answer, however. This would not only be impractical, but undesirable as well. The body needs polyunsaturated fatty acids for healthy skin and good metabolism. Some outstanding foods such as sunflower seeds, safflower oil, and wheat germ contain generous amounts of polyunsaturated oil. And many doctors and medical researchers believe that eating more polyunsaturated oils, and less saturated fats (found in animal products), may reduce the risk of heart disease.

## Vitamin E Helps Keep Polyunsaturates 'Honest'

Here we arrive at the connection between wrinkles, aging, and vitamin E: fortunately, there is much evidence that polyunsaturates will not enter into nearly as many destructive free radical reactions if adequate amounts of vitamin E are present. Vitamin E is nature's own antioxidant. That is, it acts to block the oxidation that can turn lipids into harmful peroxides. In a sense, vitamin E could be called a free radical scavenger. It latches on to these troublemakers and puts them out of action. Vitamin E "can minimize the damage done by free radical chain reactions because it can act as a chain-breaker," said Irwin Fridovich, Ph.D., a biochemist at the Duke University Medical Center (*American Scientist,* January–February, 1975).

As Dr. Harman told the Los Angeles symposium, free radical reactions can never be stopped entirely, but vitamin E and other antioxidants can significantly reduce the rate at which they occur.

Most natural foods that contain polyunsaturated oil also contain some vitamin E. But the nutrient is largely used up in protecting the food from peroxidation. Finally, when all the vitamin E has been "sacrificed," chemical degradation occurs: vegetable oils turn rancid, for example. Thus, the premature aging Dr. Griffiths observed could be more accurately described as the result of vitamin E deficiency, rather than polyunsaturate toxicity.

The more polyunsaturates we consume, the more extra vitamin E we need. And not just to protect our skin against premature aging. Antioxidants like vitamin E can prevent free radicals from doing all sorts of dirty work.

"Accumulating evidence implicates free radical reactions in the pathogenesis of cancer, amyloidosis (an abnormal starch-like formation in body tissues), senility, atherosclerosis, and hypertension—all disorders and associated with aging," says Dr. Harman. "Smog-related pulmonary disorders may also be due, at least in part, to free radical reactions."

Two researchers at the Lawrence Berkeley Laboratory in California reported that vitamin E can more than double the life of human cells cultured in an artificial test-tube environment. Normally, these cells reproduce, or double, about 50 times before dying. But when Drs. Lester Packer and James R. Smith added vitamin E to the culture medium at about 10 times the normal level in human tissue, the cells reproduced through the one-hundred twentieth generation (*Medical World News,* 25 October 1974).

It is significant to note that the Berkeley researchers didn't even try the additional vitamin E until the cells were already about two-thirds of the way through their normal life span. Apparently it is never too late to start taking advantage of vitamin E's natural abilities as an antioxidant.

## Doctors' Feelings About E as a Supplement

Can vitamin E slow down the biological clock for living human beings, as well as cultured cells? Dr. Packer hesitated to jump to any such conclusions as a result of his experiment, but he said, "Even if vitamin E can't prevent aging, it may prevent an early death, senility, or heart attack that results from environmental factors." Presumably, that's why he personally takes a daily supplement of vitamin E.

Dr. Harman is more outspokenly optimistic about the potential benefits for humans from adding an antioxidant like vitamin E to the diet. "This approach offers the prospect of an increase in the average life expectancy to beyond 85 years and a significant increase in the number of people who will live to well beyond 100 years, along with accompanying increases in the period of healthy, effective living," he says.

How much vitamin E you should decide to try may depend heavily on your age. L. H. Chen, Ph.D., of the University of Kentucky's Department of Nutrition and Food Science discovered that, in laboratory animals at least, vitamin E-needs increase sharply with age.

Eighty mice were divided into two groups. Both received the same modified commercial rat chow diet including refined corn oil that contained some vitamin E. But one group also received extra vitamin E; their diet was supplemented with 100 I.U. of vitamin E per kilogram of food. Then, at regular intervals for the next 20 months, mice from both groups were sacrificed and their liver tissue analyzed for signs of peroxidation damage. The liver was chosen because this organ is especially vulnerable to free radical damage.

## Vitamin E Needed Most with Advancing Age

"Vitamin E supplementation lowered significantly liver lipid peroxidation of mice at all ages," Dr. Chen noted in an article in *Nutrition Reports International* (December 1974). But most important, he continued, "The data indicates that the amount of vitamin E which is adequate to protect liver from peroxidation in young and adult mice is not adequate to protect the liver from peroxidation in very old mice." The amount of vitamin E in the refined corn oil was not nearly enough.

If other nutritionists are aware that vitamin E needs increase with age, they certainly don't show it. "In many reports," Dr. Chen said, "the age of the animal is not even considered when the minimum requirement for vitamin E is discussed. And in this connection, the recommended daily allowance (RDA) for vitamin E for adults as suggested by the Food and Nutrition Board of the National Research Council is the same for all age groups." RDAs have always been routinely established on observations of young, healthy people—not older people with health problems. Therefore it is quite possible, in Dr. Chen's view, that older people need much greater amounts of vitamin E.

The amounts of vitamin E that researchers Harman, Chen, and others are talking about for protection against free-radical-induced aging represent modest supplementary amounts. Dr. Harman suggests increasing our vitamin E intake to approximately 450 to 750 I.U. of natural vitamin E (d-alpha-tocopherol) per week, or about 100 I.U. a day. Of course, many people take more than this amount, because of all the evidence that vitamin E has more jobs to do than preventing peroxidation damage.

# CHAPTER 73

# How Vitamin E Works to Keep Cells Younger Longer

*By Jeffrey S. Bland, Ph.D.*

*Dr. Bland is associate professor in the Department of Chemistry at the University of Puget Sound in Tacoma, Washington.*

The evidence that vitamin E can produce dramatic improvements in health problems continues to mount, even while debates rage over the reliability of this evidence. But in the midst of the controversy over the clinical or medical applications of vitamin E, biochemical research has focused on understanding how vitamin E acts.

In our laboratory at the University of Puget Sound, we have been carrying out research aimed at understanding the effective mechanism of vitamin E at the molecular level. And we are now convinced that our studies place the medical indications of vitamin E's reported effectiveness on a much firmer scientific basis, and significantly increase our understanding of how it works.

In a nutshell, our results indicate that greater amounts of vitamin E in the diet can help to prevent the cells of our bodies from aging faster than is necessary. The implication is that while vitamin E might not necessarily cause anyone to live longer, it can at least help prolong the useful life of the cells of which our bodies are formed.

The study actually began when we found that human erythrocytes—or what are more commonly known as red blood cells—could be "aged" rapidly by exposing them to light and oxygen, producing strange "budded cell" types or cells which appear convoluted in comparison to smooth, normal, healthy cells. What we wanted to do was determine how and why this aging occurred. We reasoned that the budded cells were a result of exposure to what chemists call oxidizing conditions, which would weaken the cell membranes, causing the cell to bulge, much as a weakened bicycle tire does under pressure. We also learned that the number of budded cells increased rapidly with the time of exposure to light and oxygen as shown in Figure 1.

Abusing red blood cells in this way might seem to be completely unnatural, but it is only an exaggeration or speeding-up of a process which occurs normally in the body under many conditions. One powerful oxidant which reaches the body tissues of many people is ozone, a principal ingredient of photochemical smog—and a powerful oxidant. Drs. Goldstein and Balchum of the University of Southern California School of Medicine at Los Angeles have already demonstrated that exposing red blood cells to ozone causes them to become extremely fragile, a result of cell membrane destruction.

But even oxygen as it circulates through the body can produce oxidation, and in the presence of intense sunlight, the process may occur even more rapidly.

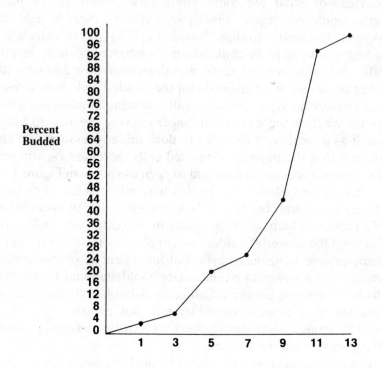

Figure 1                                Hours of Exposure

*Without vitamin E protection, the number of normal cells which budded when subjected to light and oxygen increased rapidly as the time of exposure lengthened.*

# Defusing Molecular Bombshells

When cells are subjected to oxidative damage, it is as if they have been hit with a tiny hand grenade. It's difficult to say exactly what kind of damage is done. It probably varies a great deal depending on what portion of the cell is damaged. But there is little question that damage is done, and that as the years and decades pass, it's possible that these accumulating submicroscopic injuries could hasten the onset of many degenerative diseases.

Our studies were directed particularly at understanding the relationship between vitamin E and oxidative damage to the cell membrane. These membranes are one of the most exciting areas of current biochemical research, and for a good reason.

There is a popular idea that the membrane is simply a kind of bag surrounding a cellular "soup" in which all the activities of the cell are carried out. Actually, recent discoveries have shown that cell membranes are of critical importance in the health and longevity of cells. First, there is not simply one membrane surrounding the cell, but a number of them, which compartmentalize various functioning units from each other. As a whole, the cell is a kind of tiny biochemical factory, which at any one time is involved in thousands of different chemical reactions, each of them vital to health and life. And it is the cell membranes which are largely responsible for the success of these functions. That's because it's the membranes which actively transport all the vitamins, minerals, trace metals, nutrients, hormones, and other chemical messenger substances on which the cell depends for its very existence. These vital substances don't merely "ooze" through the membrane to reach the places within the cell where they're needed. We now feel there is a kind of "push-pull" mechanism in which the membrane actively selects what it is going to take in and what it is going to expel. There also seem to be particular "ports" on the cell membrane which are programmed to recognize various substances—kind of like molecular doormen. In other words, without the active cooperation of the cell membrane, the cell is not going to get what it needs to go on leading a useful life.

And in fact, it now appears that many disease processes ranging from cancer to diabetes are associated with altered or abnormal cell membrane structure. In the case of diabetes, it appears that for some reason the cell membranes will not take up glucose or blood sugar. In the case of cancer, it seems that something happens to the cell membrane which prevents such abnormal cells from being attacked and destroyed by the phagocytes of the immune system. Therefore, maintaining healthful function in these membranes can be considered one of the most important aspects of health at the biochemical level.

## Vitamin E Protects Cell Membranes

Vitamin E enters the picture through the beautiful work of Dr. A. L. Tappel of the Department of Food Science at the University of California at Davis. His findings suggest that antioxidants, including vitamin E, reduce the rate of "peroxidation," or oxidative damage, caused by chemicals such as the ozone in smog.

Vitamin E has a great affinity for cell membranes, because these membranes contain large amounts of unsaturated fatty acids and other fats, and vitamin E is a fat-soluble vitamin. Our work shows that the cell membrane is a kind of sandwich or bilayer of fat-like molecules with cholesterol between them, and selected proteins trapped in this system. Vitamin E sits in the very middle of this fatty bilayer and, we have found, protects the fats from reacting with oxygen in a manner that damages the cell.

To get back to our strange "budded" blood cells, we wondered if we could retard the rate of their formation by placing the blood donors on a vitamin E regimen. We therefore had the same 24 volunteers who gave blood for the first study take 600 I.U. of alpha-tocopherol a day for 10 days. Then we checked their blood for its tendency to "age" by exposure to light and oxygen.

We were amazed to find that exposure of the cells to light and oxygen for 16 hours, conditions which, in the absence of the vitamin E regimen, would have led to totally budded cells, gave only a very small number of budded cells.

This observation of the extension of human cell vitality under stress conditions by vitamin E is similar to the effects observed by Dr. Lester Packer and Dr. James R. Smith of the Department of Physiology at the University of California at Berkeley. They found that human cell cultures grown in a medium containing extra amounts of vitamin E were able to divide and live much longer than cells grown in ordinary culture mediums.

At that point in our study, we wanted to make certain that the active agent was vitamin E itself, and not a secondary reaction formed as a result of vitamin E ingestion. We therefore took blood from donors who were not being supplemented with vitamin E and exposed their blood in the test tube to known concentrations of the vitamin. We were gratified to see that upon exposure to light and oxygen, the cells resisted membrane destruction at the same rate as the cells taken from those donors on the augmented vitamin E diet. That demonstrated that the effects we observed were most likely due to vitamin E itself, and not a secondary reaction.

We also found that there seemed to be an optimal level of vitamin E in the red blood cell to lend it maximum protection against membrane destruction. Amounts below this level or even above it seemed to reduce the protective efficiency. We have not completed this work, but at present we believe the optimal level to be between 400 and 600 I.U. a day. Situations which would lead to rapid utilization of vitamin E, such as exposure to photochemical oxidants (smog), ionizing radiation (sun or x-rays), smoking, or other factors which lead to increased cellular oxidation, should be met with somewhat greater intakes of vitamin E.

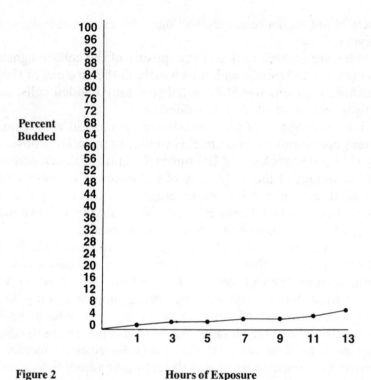

**Figure 2**　　　　　　　　**Hours of Exposure**

*When normal cells were protected with vitamin E and then exposed to the same conditions as those in Figure 1, the percentage of cells which budded remained amazingly low.*

Our studies support the mechanism of function of vitamin E proposed originally by Dr. J. Lucy of the Department of Biochemistry, Royal Free Hospital of Medicine, London, about a decade ago. He proposed that vitamin E is incorporated predominantly in the fatty acid rich cell membrane and inner membranes. The vitamin E there serves as a powerful "sink," trapping oxidants which, in the absence of vitamin E, would chemically alter the unsaturated fatty acid membrane components. That, in turn, would distort and weaken the membrane and therefore the entire cell.

Our findings were also consistent with those of Dr. D. Warshauer and his associates at the Section of Infections and Immunologic Diseases, School of Medicine, University of California at Davis, who found that vitamin E deficiency increases susceptibility to ozone-induced lung damage, by reducing the pulmonary defense mechanism to infection and making the organism more susceptible to invasion by bacteria. Weakened membranes of cells could easily explain the easier penetration by bacteria or viruses in vitamin E-deficient lungs. The membrane, after all, is the cell's first defense barrier, and its integrity is essential for warding off potential threats to the cell's biochemical machinery. A weakened membrane means weaker resistance to disease. Vitamin E is essential to protect this defense barrier.

Specifically, we have found that the presence of additional vitamin E in the red blood cell membrane greatly reduces the rate at which cholesterol, an important component in the red blood cell membrane structure, is peroxidized by oxidants to a product known as cholesterol hydroperoxide. If formed, that compound greatly weakens the membrane. That is one more corroborating piece of evidence to support our new concept of vitamin E's mechanism of action.

In addition to our other laboratory work, we are also in the preliminary stages of testing a small group of long-distance runners. Our early results, which need to be confirmed by longer observations of a larger group, show that with 600 I.U. of vitamin E a day, the peroxidative damage to the blood cells of these runners is decreased by as much as 50 percent.

Earlier, in our laboratory, we had observed that when vitamin E is introduced into blood plasma, nearly all of it rapidly disappears into red blood cells, indicating that supplemental amounts of this vitamin are indeed selectively taken up by cells. And our observations of the runners—although strictly preliminary—suggest that the cells make good use of this additional vitamin E.

It seems reasonable to conclude that an essential biochemical role can be defined for vitamin E. While doubts and controversy about its clinical or medical usefulness still rage, the insecurity associated with not knowing how it acts at the cellular and subcellular level is waning.

And while there is still no evidence that a person taking vitamin E will live longer, the work outlined in this report suggests that a person with the optimal level of the vitamin in his or her system should be able to avoid unnecessarily rapid cellular aging which results from ongoing peroxidation.

The importance of that benefit could conceivably amount to considerable protection against the stresses in our modern polluted world that might bring on premature weakness and disease.

# CHAPTER 74

# Improving Your
# Energy and Endurance

Unlike the situation in the United States, vitamin E has long been accepted by the medical establishment in Russia and some of the most impressive research on its efficacy has come from there.

According to a report in the *Medical Tribune* (12 April 1972), investigators at the Soviet Academy of Medical Sciences Nutrition Institute and the Central Institute of Physical Culture have found that supplementary vitamin E gives a definite boost to the performance of athletes such as skiers and racing cyclists.

The Russian investigators carried out a three-week study on 34 cyclists and 37 skiers between the ages of 15 and 25, to determine how much vitamin E could profitably be used under training and competitive conditions. How much would improve performance? Would more help to make a winner?

The athletes were divided into groups. All groups went through the same stiff training regime and all partook of the same high-calorie diet to provide ample energy for demanding activity. The only variant was the amount of vitamin E given to the various groups.

The control group received no supplemental E at all. As a result, even though they ate a high-calorie diet (up to 4,200 calories daily) they obtained only 15 to 20 mg. of vitamin E. In this control group, the blood levels of vitamin E fell during the training period to a point below the lower limit determined in people not doing heavy physical work. There are two points here of vital interest to every athlete and anyone starting an exercise program or a physical activity to which he or she may be unaccustomed—like shoveling snow in winter, mowing the lawn in summer, or even running after a toddler. The first point is: demanding physical activity uses up vitamin E much more quickly than ordinary accustomed activity. The second is: no matter how much you eat of the usual foods, you can't get enough vitamin E to see you through.

The difference in the other groups which used the supplemental E was dramatic. The level of the vitamin in their blood was maintained and even increased which means that they emerged from their training sessions with no oxygen deficit. They might feel physically tired—but not depleted.

## Optimum Amounts

The Russian researchers determined that the optimum daily addition of vitamin E was 100 to 150 mg. for a training period of one and a half to two hours. For a training period between three and four hours, the optimum daily supplement was determined at 250 to 300 mg. When these amounts were taken, the levels of vitamin E in the blood serum could be maintained without excessive depletion. (It was assumed that reduced vitamin E levels would indicate inability to perform as well, even after thorough rest.)

What factors in vitamin E make it the athlete's best friend? There are many but one of the most important is its antioxidant effect. It keeps more pure oxygen available to the tissues for the production of energy. Oxygen is, of course, the breath of life to every one of us. In an athlete or anyone engaged in competitive sports—in a swimming program, a gym or jogging program—

when the oxygen supply gives out, that's it. In other words, you can measure the extent of your activity or your endurance potential in terms of available oxygen. Vitamin E, due to its antioxidant effect, can give the use of more oxygen. Therefore— more wind and more endurance.

A corroborating study on "Alpha-Tocopherol and Oxygen Consumption in Healthy Men During Work" was done in Czechoslovakia and published in the *Acta Universitatis Palackianae Olomucensis* (vol. 42, 1966). This study by Dr. Z. Jirka, head of the Institute of Sports Medicine of the Medical Faculty of the Palacky Institute in Olomouc, Czechoslovakia, was undertaken to ascertain if vitamin E had some positive effect on maximal sporting performance.

"Vitamin E, and especially its most active component alpha-tocopherol," said Dr. Jirka "has a wide-spread activity taking part in a great number of biological processes. Its participation in enzymatic processes in glycogenesis and glycolysis influences the activity and metabolism of the muscle and therefore experiments dealing with this problem are in the foreground of the interest of many laboratories." To get an answer to their question—"Does vitamin E affect performance on the athletic field?"—Dr. Jirka summarized the available knowledge about the complexity and extent of the activity of vitamin E in different biological processes before he conducted his own.

Some of these studies shed light on the areas of misunderstanding as to what vitamin E can and cannot do. For instance, it has often been claimed by those who use vitamin E, and just as often disclaimed by doctors in this country, that there is a direct, specific effect on the female reproductive organs and that vitamin E will help to avert miscarriage in women.

"Vitamin E has not a direct specific effect on the female sexual organs in the human," said Dr. Jirka. "However, it has a great reduction effect necessary to the metabolism of cells. Deficiency of this vitamin causes a disturbance of the metabolism and it is this disorganized metabolism which is responsible for sterility or habitual abortion."

# Horses Thrive On It

The effect of vitamin E on stamina has long been known to many swimmers and athletes. It is also known to those who breed race horses. Herbert Bailey, in his book, *Your Key To a Healthy Heart* (Philadelphia: Chilton Books, 1965) tells of experiments with vitamin E undertaken at Windfields Farm, Toronto, and the National Stud Farm in Oshawa, Canada. The report on the results of a two-year study was issued by F. G. Darlington, manager of the farms and the experiment and J. B. Chassels, Doctor of Veterinary Medicine, both of whom supervised the experiments.

You may go to the track just for fun and diversion, but horse racing is a serious business. This horse-breeding enterprise began its study of vitamin E supplementation midway in the racing season of 1955 as a possible method through which to increase its earnings. The experiment proved that the smart money goes on the horse that's getting lots of E. Earnings are determined by the number of wins.

The percentage of wins per horse jumped as much as 66 percent in the first year of vitamin E supplementation, but the horses actually hit their peak of efficiency the following year when their dosages were doubled or tripled. In 1956 the stable increased the number of animals taking vitamin E. The farms' income more than doubled. It went from $88,000 to over $196,000. The number of winners increased from 80 to 95. The number of seconds (place) increased from 25 to 40 and the number of horses running third (show) increased from 17 to 30.

Not only did the farms greatly improve their earnings using vitamin E, but there were many other nice side effects. Race horses are notoriously highstrung and some refuse to eat properly. Under vitamin E therapy, almost all of these nervous horses were gradually quieted and began feeding normally. Mr. Bailey notes that this calming effect was first discovered on human beings by German researchers who called vitamin E "nature's own tranquilizer."

The horse-racing experience with vitamin E gives some clues as to how the vitamin can best be used not only by those engaged in competitive sports, but by those who want the best of everything as far as optimum health is concerned. It was found that the vitamin extended the animals' lease on vigorous youth. It was found, too, that results are much better when the vitamin is taken all year around and not just during the training season.

Who benefits most from vitamin E? Everyone benefits, but according to Dr. Jirka's study, those who need it most benefit most. The effect of alpha-tocopherol was greater on those who were unaccustomed to muscular work or those who were untrained. This is explained by the fact that those who are untrained must put out more effort and therefore use more oxygen. As Dr. Jirka described it, "The greater effect of alpha-tocopherol in untrained subjects was perhaps a result of an insufficient adaptation on body effort in these men. The trained subjects, according to stress theory, were in resistance phase and this resistance in the well-trained is supported by other mechanisms."

The powerful endurance-building effects of vitamin E are well known to many athletes and their trainers. It was first utilized en masse by the Australians, who surprised everyone, particularly their American opponents, when they won all the swimming medals at the XVI Olympics some years ago. The Australians had been getting their vitamin E in the form of wheat germ oil and wheat germ cereal every day.

The record shows that six months before they were to compete, the Australian team was put on a supervised program of physical training, in which heavy emphasis was placed on scientific eating. In addition to their regular meals which included everything except fried foods, their diet was heavily fortified with vitamins and minerals with the emphasis on wheat germ oil and wheat germ cereal.

## Spectacular Results With Wheat Germ Oil

Dr. Thomas K. Cureton, head of the renowned Physical Fitness Laboratory at the University of Illinois, is convinced that wheat germ oil can not only change "chumps into champs" but can restore the vigor of youth to sedentary middle-aged men. He personally obtained dramatic results with a group of sagging, bagging, falling-to-pieces middle-aged executives by putting them on a teaspoon of wheat germ oil each day in conjunction with an exercise program. The regimen increased their physical capacity and endurance by as much as 51.5 percent.

The treadmill was one of the many tests in which their performance was measured. Eight middle-aged professors who combined the wheat germ oil with physical training were able to run on a treadmill twice as long at the end of the 12-week training period before becoming exhausted. They had no opportunity to practice on a treadmill between tests. They were tested for a first time, given 12 weeks of other types of exercise along with wheat germ oil, and then tested again. They did not go near the treadmill in the interim.

At the same time, a matched group of men—matched in age and run-time after the initial test—gained only 19.4 percent after receiving the same physical training without the wheat germ oil. Dr. Cureton was able to obtain equally convincing evidence in tests with athletes already at the peak of training, like varsity wrestlers and swimmers. "It is well established," said Dr. Cureton, "that men cannot be kept at a peak of physical condition indefinitely—that most of them reach a plateau after about 12 weeks of hard training and then begin to slump."

However, when the athletes were given wheat germ oil after they began their slump, the scientific measurements of their performance jumped up to new peaks. At the same time a control group which did not receive the wheat germ oil continued to slump.

Dr. Cureton himself was amazed. "Never before in any experiment," he said, "have I seen a subject train hard for 12 weeks, reach the plateau, and then go on to a higher peak."

Dr. Cureton stresses the importance of combining the wheat germ oil with physical training. They go together like love and marriage. His explanation is that exercise opens up the tiny blood vessels (the capillaries) of muscles and heart tissues, increases the blood flow of arteries, and allows the nutrient to reach the muscle and tissue where it is needed.

Since vitamin E has been processed out of most of our foods, a sure way to get a steady, reliable intake is to take supplements of vitamin E and wheat germ oil daily. Experiments indicate that there is in the wheat germ oil some as yet unknown factor which seems to enhance energy and stamina.

# CHAPTER 75

# A Valuable
# Antianemia Agent

The red blood cells in your bloodstream have an important job to do, and only they can perform it—carrying oxygen-bearing hemoglobin to every other type of cell in the body. They have been specially designed to do that one job and do it well. Without them and their life-giving oxygen, our tissues would "starve" and die.

But red cells don't go on working forever. After about 120 days they break up and their hemoglobin is lost. Fortunately for your body's "factory," however, not all of the workers leave at the same time. Such turnover, although seemingly on a grand scale, is perfectly normal. In *The Living River* (New York: Abelard-Schuman Publishers, 1959), biochemist Isaac Asimov reassures us: "If our average adult has 25,000,000,000,000 (twenty-five trillion) red cells altogether and 1/125 (or 0.8 percent) of them break up each day, then 200,000,000,000 (two hundred billion) are being destroyed daily, or 2,300,000 each second. Of course, this should not be at all disturbing. The body can, and does, replace the quantity being broken down as fast as they are being broken down."

But such a happy state of equilibrium doesn't always prevail. Sometimes the red cells quit prematurely. When they disintegrate in the bloodstream before their time is up, the bone marrow can't replace them fast enough, and the result is hemolytic anemia. Iron supplements, recommended for some forms of anemia, won't help here; iron is vital to the formation of hemoglobin-rich cells, but the problem now is one of cell longevity, not quantity. There may be plenty of iron on hand to manufacture hemoglobin, but if that hemoglobin and the red cell that contains it meet an early end, it won't do your body much good.

## Vitamin E Preserves Red Cells

A report in the *American Journal of Clinical Nutrition* (April 1971) indicated that only vitamin E can maintain healthy red cells. The link between vitamin E and the health of red blood cells was demonstrated by Drs. Patrick J. Leonard and Monty S. Losowsky of the Department of Medicine, St. James' Hospital, Leeds, England. They selected eight patients with vitamin E deficiency, as indicated by low plasma vitamin E levels and the abnormal susceptibility of their red cells to hemolysis (breakdown) by hydrogen peroxide in the test tube. (This hemolysis test is a standard diagnostic procedure for detecting vitamin E deficiency in man.)

To find out just how long the subjects' red cells were holding up they were "labeled" with tiny amounts of radioactive chromium and reinjected into the bloodstream. Then, by measuring the rate of disappearance of the radioactivity, the researchers could tell just how fast the tagged red cells were being destroyed.

After a three-day wait to allow for an initial rapid loss of radioactivity from the cells, blood samples were taken at regular intervals, the radioactivity measured, and the results plotted on a graph. Normally, the injected chromium could be expected to lose half of its radioactivity every 25 days, but in this case the chromium half-life for all eight subjects averaged out to only 19.2 days. This could mean only one thing: their red cells were breaking down much too soon.

Aware that "in vitamin E deficiency, the red cell is known to be abnormally fragile in the response to hydrogen peroxide," the doctors decided to try vitamin E therapy. After an interval of from five to 15 days, they began giving the subjects a daily dose of alpha-tocopherol (vitamin E)—200 mg. orally and 100 mg. by injection.

They didn't have long to wait for results. In from one to four days, the plasma vitamin E level shot up to normal or above in all eight subjects, remaining "significantly higher" than before treatment in all but one.

But even more startling was the abrupt change in the plotted curves of the falling radioactivity. Following the start of vitamin E therapy, and coincident with the attainment of normal plasma vitamin E levels, the rate of radioactivity loss in five of the eight subjects dropped markedly—the chromium-tagged red cells were no longer disappearing as fast. In fact, the half-life of the radioactive chromium was now averaging 24.9 days, well within the normal range. Somehow, the vitamin E was protecting the red cells, allowing them to survive longer. As Drs. Leonard and Losowsky put it, the results could only be interpreted as "suggesting a direct effect of circulating tocopherol . . . in maintaining the integrity of the red cells," resulting in "an actual improvement in red cell survival."

## Mechanism Is Not Yet Certain

How does vitamin E promote the health and long life of the red cells? Many scientists have suggested that because the vitamin is a natural antioxidant in the body, it protects the cells by preventing the formation of hydrogen peroxide. In the absence of vitamin E, they explain, some of the essential fatty acids in our diets—notably linoleic acid—are permitted to combine with oxygen and form hydrogen peroxide, a known destroyer of red cells. In fact, the rate of formation of hydrogen peroxide in the blood has been used as an index of vitamin E deficiency.

Other researchers have suggested that without enough vitamin E, there may be a greater fragility of the outer membrane of the red cells, resulting in more frequent ruptures and the spilling of valuable hemoglobin. Or perhaps certain intracellular enzymes needed for membrane integrity are more readily oxidized in the absence of vitamin E. Whatever the case, vitamin E's protective effect on the red cells is obvious, even though the exact mechanism has yet to be agreed upon by scientists.

Particularly in the case of premature babies born with vitamin E deficiency and accompanying anemia, doctors have successfully employed vitamin E therapy, even after iron supplementation has failed. In the *New England Journal of Medicine* (28 November 1968), four California investigators, Drs. J. Ritchie, M. Fish, V. McMasters, and M. Grossman, reported that they gave 75 to 100 I.U. of vitamin E to five of seven premature infants. Even though the babies were on a commercial formula supplemented with 15 to 30 mg. of iron daily, their anemia failed to respond until vitamin E was added to their diet. Then, after a few days, their plasma tocopherol levels rose, their red cell survival time lengthened, and the anemia was corrected.

Both in the test tube, and then in the babies themselves, vitamin E had stopped the accelerated destruction of red cells. "The critical factor in both circumstances is that there must be, in the fluid bathing the erythrocytes (red cells), a level of tocopherol adequate to protect the red cells from oxidative damage and resultant hemolysis," they concluded.

## Deficiency Often Unidentified

But how common is this vitamin E deficiency anemia? Apparently it is much more widespread than generally suspected. As the four researchers cautioned, "The frequency with which this syndrome is observed will depend on the level of awareness of its existence, and the care with which it is sought. Some of the manifestations such as anemia, puffy eyes, and firm legs with shiny skin, not unusual in premature infants and often called 'physiologic' or 'characteristic of prematures,' may prove in many cases to represent vitamin E deficiency."

Similar findings were reported three years earlier by two pediatricians at the University of Pennsylvania Hospital in

Philadelphia. Drs. Lewis A. Barness and Frank A. Oski told a meeting of the American Pediatrics Society in May, 1965, that "A vitamin E deficiency appears to be a common nutritional disturbance that manifests itself as a hemolytic anemia in the premature infant of low birth weight."

The pair successfully corrected the condition in eight infants at the University hospital in an average time of 10 days, with vitamin E taken by mouth. "Vitamin E, unlike other nutrients, does not readily cross the placental barrier to nourish the fetus," Dr. Oski reported. Thus, infants often start out in life with low stores of the vitamin: serum tocopherol levels of newborns are only about one-fifth of maternal blood levels. In such a situation, the expectant mother might be well advised to increase her intake of the nutrient to make sure the infant gets enough.

Premature infants aren't the only ones likely to suffer from hemolytic anemia, however. Back in the late 1960s, astronauts on Gemini orbital missions in outer space were returning to Earth with the same malady. It was found that the oxygen atmosphere aboard their spacecraft led to faster consumption of vitamin E, exposing the red cells to damage from hydrogen peroxide. In 1969, vitamin E supplements were added to the astronauts' diets and the problem cleared up.

You and your family may never be exposed to the same kind of risks and demanding situations as the astronauts, but the evidence is growing that the amount of vitamin E in your diet can make the difference in protecting you from hemolytic anemia. And with the nutrient readily available from wheat germ oil, sunflower seeds, and natural supplements, why risk a deficiency?

Your red blood cells are "dying" every minute. It's natural and there's nothing you can do about it. Under normal conditions, your bone marrow will go right on turning out enough replacements to keep the body's supply line manned. But vitamin E can help to insure that these vital workers won't be destroyed before they have a chance to finish the job they started.

# CHAPTER 76

# Vitamin E Also Reduces
# the Danger of Blood Clots

The ability of blood to clot is one of the most basic protective devices of the human body. Hemophiliacs, who suffer from a defect in the blood-clotting mechanism, live in constant fear of any mishap that might puncture the skin. But for many more Americans, the problem is exactly the reverse. Their health and even their lives are endangered because their blood clots too quickly.

People with such a strong clotting tendency sometimes develop spontaneous clots inside their very arteries and veins even when there is no cut or wound to act as a trigger. That can lead to a heart attack, stroke, or pulmonary embolism (when a clot breaks away and is carried to the lungs).

Adding extra unsaturated oils to the diet can significantly increase platelet aggregation time, or the time in which blood platelets attach themselves and stick together (aggregate) in a clump, attracting long strands of fibrin in the blood to form a small net-like cobweb which sometimes stretches across the blood vessel.

When L. J. Machlin and four other researchers at Hoffmann-La Roche's Department of Biochemical Nutrition in Nutley, New Jersey, fed extra vitamin E to a group of laboratory rats, blood platelet aggregation was markedly reduced (*Proceedings of the Society for Experimental Biology and Medicine*, 149, 1975). Something else happened also. The platelet count, which tended to be higher in vitamin E-deficient animals, dropped into a more normal range when vitamin E was administered. (Any increase in the total number of platelets circulating in the blood might tend to enhance the blood's stickiness, the authors reasoned.) "It will be of considerable interest to determine whether the effects of vitamin E on platelet aggregation and platelet count are involved in the etiology of vascular pathology found in vitamin E deficient states . . . or in the development of thrombosis in humans," they concluded.

A similar effect *does* appear to be occurring in humans who take vitamin E supplements. P. M. Farrell and J. W. Willison, two researchers with the National Institutes of Health in Bethesda, Maryland, have reported that platelet counts were slightly reduced in about one-third of a group of adults consuming between 100 and 800 I.U. of vitamin E daily. Their results were released in April 1975, at the annual meeting of the Federation of American Societies for Experimental Biology (FASEB) in Atlantic City, New Jersey.

In a Swedish study, long-term supplementation with vitamin E (approximately 400 I.U. daily) prolonged blood-clotting time in nine men recuperating from heart attacks. This potentially life-saving effect was observed after six weeks and became significant after 18 weeks, according to Dr. K. Korsan-Bengtsen and two colleagues in the Blood Coagulation Laboratory of Goteborg's Sahlgren's Hospital (*Thrombosis et Diathesis Haemorrhagica*, 1974, 31, 505). Earlier, the same researchers found that patients suffering with atherosclerosis have shorter clotting time than the population at large.

# CHAPTER 77

# Now You Can
# Breathe Easier

About a quarter of a century after medical tests revealed that air "purifiers" and "deodorizers" which generate ozone are not only useless, but potentially very dangerous, the Food and Drug Administration has finally seen fit to take some action. "Action" may not be the right word, because all the FDA has done is to limit the amount of ozone which can be released into the air, and the figure they've chosen—.05 parts per million of ozone by volume of air—is at the very borderline of the point at which ozone is known to begin destroying cells of the respiratory tract.

To the millions of Americans who live in large cities, however, this limit on ozone generation doesn't mean very much. Because of industrial and automotive pollution, everyone in such cities is already breathing considerably more ozone than .05 parts per million. In Los Angeles, which is the ozone capital of the U.S.A., the typical concentration of ozone is .4 parts per million (ppm). It is frequently higher than this figure and levels of .9 ppm have been recorded.

The obvious moral of these unsettling facts is that Los Angeles and other big cities had better do something fast to reduce the ozone level in their air. The not-so-obvious moral is that people who live in such cities had better be quite positive they are getting enough vitamin E. Laboratory experiments show that vitamin E is absolutely essential if we wish to keep the damage wrought by ozone to a minimum. In fact, it is probably the next best thing to walking around city streets with a gas mask on.

The truth is that wearing a gas mask to protect yourself against ozone in the city air is not quite as silly as it sounds. In announcing their new regulations for ozone generators (*Federal Register,* 17 April 1974), the FDA cited a standard chemical reference text which lists the toxicity of ozone as "comparable to phosgene and chlorine," Phosgene was introduced as a war gas by the Germans in 1915, and was generally acknowledged as responsible for more than 80 percent of all the gas fatalities in World War I.

The FDA document stated that, "although undesirable physiological effects on the central nervous system, heart, and vision have been reported, the predominant physiological effect of ozone is primary irritation of the mucous membranes. Inhalation of ozone can cause sufficient irritation to the lungs to result in pulmonary edema. The onset of pulmonary edema (collection of fluid in the lungs) is usually delayed for some hours after exposure; thus, symptomatic response is not a reliable warning of exposure to toxic concentrations of ozone. Since olfactory fatigue develops readily, the odor of ozone is not a reliable index of atmosphere ozone concentration."

## Vitamin E Fights Ozone Damage

A research team consisting of Drs. D. Warshauer, E. Goldstein, P. D. Hoeprich, and W. Lippert, from the School of Medicine of the University of California at Davis, reported that respiratory infections are a major complication of exposure to ozone, even at weak concentrations (*Journal of Laboratory and Clinical Medicine,* February 1974). It's not that ozone itself causes infections; rather, it appears to markedly reduce the activity of the phagocytes in the lungs which fight and actually kill the germs which all of us breathe into our lungs. The University of California doctors conclude that the crippling of the phagocytes is a result of the formation of free radicals and lipid peroxides. These latter two substances are highly unstable chemicals created by the unusual oxidizing power of ozone. And they in turn attack cells they come in contact with by combining in unnatural chemical bonds with constituents of the cells, such as fatty acids and enzymes. On a short-term basis, such changes are associated with crippled and dying cells; on a long-term basis, some investigators believe, such changes are associated with cancer.

How did vitamin E enter the picture? The answer to that one is simple. Ozone does all its dirty work by nature of the fact that it is an extremely potent oxidative agent. Vitamin E, the researchers said, is "a major biologic antioxidant." So vitamin E tends to block the oxidation caused by ozone, and is therefore a natural defense against this poison gas.

To determine if vitamin E helps protect against ozone toxicity not just in theory, but in practice, Dr. Warshauer and his colleagues ran a series of experiments using mice. Basically, one group of mice was given a diet deficient in vitamin E, and another received a diet supplemented with generous amounts of vitamin E. They were then exposed to concentrations of ozone ranging from just above the average level found in Los Angeles to just higher than the greatest amount ever measured there. Exposure was made for various lengths of time. Meanwhile, a control group of mice was exposed to plain air.

After being exposed to ozone-polluted air for a week, the animals deficient in vitamin E were discovered to have a concentration of bacteria in their lungs twice as great as those which received the vitamin E. This was clear evidence of the extent to which vitamin E protects the body's natural defenses from being knocked out by ozone.

Another important difference was that during this exposure to ozone, the vitamin E-deficient animals lost more than twice as much weight as the supplemented animals. This shows that vitamin E not only protects against ozone locally, in the lungs, but helps protect the whole system.

The doctors also observed that animals exposed to ozone

without the protection of vitamin E suffered hemolysis (destruction of the red blood cells) at a rate of 80 percent or more. Animals which were fed a standard laboratory chow which contained some six times more than the minimum amount of vitamin E that is known to be required for mice, suffered a rate of hemolysis of only 38 percent. Animals supplemented with eleven times the minimum required amount of vitamin E had the lowest hemolysis rate of all—just 30 percent.

No group of mice was fed only the minimum required amount of vitamin E for mice. But it appears to be highly significant that supplementation at the rate of 11 times the minimum requirement for mice had a greater protective effect than six times the minimum requirement. We can only imagine that if another group of mice were fed only the minimum requirement, they would have suffered considerably greater destruction of their red blood cells.

Here is a clear indication that in this polluted world, the minimum required amount of protective nutrients can be far less than the optimal level.

## Symptoms Vary, But Everyone Suffers

Besides what we normally think of as pollution sources, you may be dismayed to learn that any equipment you have around the house or shop that produces sparks, arcs, or static discharge, as well as ultraviolet or other ionizing radiation, also produces ozone. Many "air purifiers" also generate sufficient ozone to be hazardous under certain conditions, and although you may be unaware of it, such units may be in operation in hospitals, offices, and elevators.

In the *Journal of Environmental Health* (May–June, 1969), warnings against these unsuspected sources of ozone contamination were issued by N. Balfour Slonin, M.D., Ph.D., and N. Karen Estridge of the Cardiopulmonary Diagnostic Laboratory in Denver, Colorado. They also revealed that some producers of distilled water actually add this poisonous gas to their product without informing the purchaser, and without regard as to whether it is for use in a baby formula or the chemical laboratory. Since baby formulas are usually made with distilled water, and since ozone causes pulmonary problems, certainly the relationship between this distilled water and crib deaths should be investigated. Unless a baby is nursing, he or she gets very little vitamin E and therefore does not have any significant defense against the ravages of the highly oxidative gas.

## Fight Ozone on the Civic and Cellular Levels

There are two ways that all of us can fight ozone pollution. One is by imposing ever-stricter rules on every smokestack and tailpipe in the country. But as damaging as ozone is, very little progress has been made in this direction. As an article in *New Scientist* (27 April 1972) noted, "The results (of ozone experiments) suggest that a walk on a busy street at midday may leave a person's lungs in less-than-normal working order, even if no symptoms are apparent." These facts, the journal reported, also "make a restriction on its production worthy of thought; yet none is contemplated, even in America's ambitious antipollution program for automobiles." So it looks like ozone is going to be around for a while.

A way to defend ourselves on a personal basis, is to make sure that we have enough vitamin E to combine chemically with ozone when it reaches our lungs to render it harmless. The new experimental evidence reviewed here—as well as common sense—suggests that to get the maximum degree of protection, more than the minimum requirement of vitamin E is necessary. This vitamin is called upon not only to perform its normal duties, but to do double duty as a detoxifier of an extremely powerful pollutant. It is also a fact that vitamin E is used up as it combines with invading ozone—so to the extent the air you breathe is polluted with ozone, you need that much more vitamin E.

# CHAPTER 78

# Women Feel Better with Vitamin E

By now, nearly everyone interested in his or her health knows that vitamin E can help protect against a premature heart attack. And because heart attacks afflict American men with a vengeance, while for unknown reasons posing much less of a threat to women, more and more men are taking vitamin E every day in hopes of closing the wide gap in life expectancy between the sexes.

But now there is evidence that women, too, may be able to forestall some of the most dreaded diseases to which they are uniquely vulnerable, by placing as much emphasis on vitamin E as their husbands do.

This hope was expressed at the annual meeting of the Gerontological Society in San Juan, Puerto Rico on December 20, 1972 by Dr. Denham Harman. Dr. Harman, of the University of Nebraska College of Medicine in Omaha, holds both M.D. and Ph.D. degrees, and has been focusing his research attention upon the relationship between unsaturated dietary fats and cancer.

He reminded his audience of physicians who specialize in the problems of aging that x rays are used to treat cancer, but they can also cause cancer. Presumably, he said, both these effects are "mediated in some way by free radical reactions . . . arising from the disassociation of water by the radiation." Free radicals are peculiar atoms whose electron structure is such that they very easily combine and react with other structures, producing abnormal compounds. When these destructive forces are unleashed within the confines of a tumor, that growth may be destroyed. By the same token, they can disrupt healthy tissue to the extent that cancer begins.

If this presumption is correct, Dr. Harman speculated, it ought to be worthwhile to try to prevent the creation of free radicals in the body from sources other than x rays. And among the major sources of these dangerous atoms are unsaturated fats and oils, which are very easily oxidized within the body, yielding damaging peroxides and the highly suspect free radicals.

## Cancer Tied to Oil Consumption

In agreement with this theory, said Dr. Harman, is a correlation found in no less than 23 countries between the consumption of fats and oils and the death rates from leukemia and cancer of the breast, ovaries, and rectum in persons over 55 years old. Two of these forms of cancer, of course, afflict only women. In a study of female mice, Dr. Harman said, it was found that increasing either the amount of unsaturated fats fed, or the degree of unsaturation, led to significant increases in the incidence of mammary tumors.

The question is how to short-circuit the chemical wiring between unsaturated fats (which people are eating more of these days) and the development of cancer. If oxidation of fats, which produces free radicals, is in fact a major cause of cancer, it should then be possible to reduce cancer by stopping the oxidation. And this—blocking oxidation—is rather easily done by introducing into the system extra amounts of substances called—logically enough—antioxidants.

Two very powerful antioxidants are chemicals called BHA and BHT. You may have seen these shorthand names listed at the end of the ingredients in products such as breakfast cereals, where their antioxidant properties are put to work to retard rancidity, which is just another name for oxidation. But both these chemicals are unnatural, synthetic, and like virtually all other food additives, under suspicion of being biologically toxic.

There is another antioxidant, though, which is entirely natural and entirely safe: vitamin E. It is not quite as powerful as BHA and BHT, but its status as a safe and essential nutrient makes it vastly preferable to chemicals. And it was vitamin E which Dr. Harman chose to use in his experiments.

To test his hypothesis that an antioxidant can reduce cancer formation, Dr. Harman worked with closely inbred rats. Some of the rats were given diets consisting of five percent by weight of safflower oil as the sole source of fat, while others received a diet in which safflower oil consisted of 20 percent of the total volume. In addition, each of these groups was divided into those animals which were given alpha-tocopherol acetate (vitamin E) supplements and those which were not supplemented. The experiment was carried out for several years, so the animals would live into extreme old age.

A periodic examination of the animals revealed that both sex and vitamin E made a big difference in terms of cancer development. As a group, the male rats developed very few gross tumors, and the numerical difference between the supplemented and unsupplemented animals was small. However, it did seem to be significant that the first tumor was noted after nine months in the group which did not receive vitamin E supplements, while those which were supplemented did not show evidence of tumors until after 25 months.

## Females Develop Far More Cancer

Likewise, the unsupplemented female rats also developed tumors before those which were supplemented. But the females suffered a much greater incidence of tumor formation, and the difference between those receiving and not receiving vitamin E was highly significant.

Among those on a five percent safflower oil diet, the unsupplemented animals developed 20 tumors, as compared to only 14 for those who got the vitamin E. Among those on the 20 percent safflower oil diet, the unsupplemented group developed 21 tumors, as compared to 13 for those getting the extra vitamin E.

Interesting? Of course. But applicable to human beings? That remains to be seen. But unlike most other researchers and physicians who make such discoveries, Dr. Harman chose not to simply let the question lie there until someone else can come up with positive proof, maybe 50 years from now.

This is how he put it to his audience of fellow physicians: "Whether or not the data are applicable to man remains to be demonstrated; one recent study of the effect of polyunsaturated fat on cardiovascular disease suggests that it is. However, it would seem desirable *now* to try to lower the level of more-or-less random free radical reactions in man. Methods can be employed, such as the addition of a moderate amount—say 300 to 500 I.U. per week—of vitamin E to our diet, which we can be absolutely certain will not have any adverse effects when employed over the lifespan."

Dr. Harman added that, while this prescription may ultimately prove to be of little value, it is at least one defensive step that we can take, and offers hope that "we may see a marked decrease in our cancer incidence as well as in that of other diseases and nonspecific effects in which free radical reactions play a role."

## Pollution Aggravates Problem

The study concerning the effect of polyunsaturated fat on man which Dr. Harman referred to was carried out at a Veterans' Administration hospital in the Los Angeles area, and showed that hospitalized men eating a diet high in polyunsaturated fats and low in cholesterol had fewer heart attacks than those who ate a typical diet, but the overall death rates were about equal, largely because those eating the polyunsaturated fat had a very high incidence of cancer.

It may be highly significant that this study was conducted in Los Angeles, the smog capital of the United States. Ozone and oxides of nitrogen, two of the chief components in smog, have been repeatedly shown to vastly accelerate the oxidation process of polyunsaturated fats, even when these pollutants are present only in trace amounts.

Further, the speed of oxidation is directly dependent upon the amount of vitamin E present in tissues. The more vitamin E, the less oxidation, according to researchers Menzel, Roehm, and Lee in their article, "Vitamin E: the Biological And Environmental Antioxidant," *Journal of Agriculture and Food Chemistry,* (May–June 1972). But reserves of vitamin E are wiped out as they come into contact with pollutants, and the vitamin must be continually replaced. Menzel and his colleagues pointed out that once depletion has occurred, oxidation proceeds even when test animals are breathing pure, filtered air, underscoring the need for vitamin replacement on a regular basis.

Perhaps you have read that the effect of tocopherol depletion on human beings is not really known. Writers who set out to "debunk" this vitamin are fond of making this point. Here's what Menzel and his colleagues, all experienced and distinguished researchers, have to say about that: "The complexity and, unfortunately, the catastrophic nature of tocopherol deficiency may well preclude human experimentation for some time, but our data suggest that it might be well to recommend the provision of adequate levels of tocopherol for the inhabitants of air-polluted areas."

From what these scientists have learned with animals, and from the epidemiological evidence with human beings, they suspect that it is far too dangerous to experiment with induced states of vitamin E deficiency. And, like Dr. Harman, they believe that an ounce of vitamin E is worth more than a pound of drugs. For those who wonder just who these scientists are, here are their affiliations at the time of writing: Daniel B. Menzel, Duke University Medical Center in Durham, North Carolina; Jeffery N. Roehm, the famous laboratories of Battelle-Northwest in Richland, Washington; Si Duk Lee, U.S. Environmental Protection Agency's National Environmental Research Center in Cincinnati, Ohio.

## Menopause Pains Can Be Relieved

Vitamin E has also shown its value to women in less catastrophic illnesses, although with these conditions, the evidence is not theoretical, but based on considerable clinical experience.

Several studies show that vitamin E is often effective in alleviating the most distressing symptoms of menopause. One such report came from Henry A. Gozen, M.D., who described his treatment of 66 patients with menopause trouble. In the *New York State Journal of Medicine* (15 May 1952), Dr. Gozen reported that vitamin E eliminated serious symptoms in 59 patients out of the 66. W. H. Perloff, writing in the *American Journal of Obstetrics and Gynecology* (vol. 58, pp. 684–94, 1949), reported on the treatment of 200 women with vitamin E in doses of 75 to 150 I.U. daily. This therapy completely relieved the undesirable symptoms of 26.1 percent of the women, and another 26 percent were improved. Dr. Gozen believed that higher doses might well relieve some of the patients who did not respond to 150 I.U. He also noted no unpleasant side effects.

Dr. N. R. Kavinoky, writing in *Annals of Western Medicine and Surgery* (vol. 4, pp. 27–32, 1950), described the treatment of 92 patients with vitamin E in doses ranging from 10 to 25 I.U. daily. Thirty-four subjects had a very heavy menstrual flow; in 16 it diminished. Thirty-seven of the patients complaining of hot flashes were relieved. Sixteen of those who suffered from backaches were relieved. Using vitamin E in larger doses, 50 to 100 I.U. daily, Dr. Kavinoky reported that even better results were obtained in another group of 79 patients. Fatigue, nervousness, restless sleep, and insomnia were reduced in more than half. Nearly all the patients were relieved from dizziness, heart palpitation, and shortness of breath. In some cases, results became apparent only after two or three months, but in others it took only two weeks.

484—The Complete Book of Vitamins

# Varicose Veins Often Helped

Varicose veins are not confined to women, but they seem to afflict more women than men. Varicosities are not a mere cosmetic problem. The walls of the veins may become inflamed in a condition known as phlebitis. A dark red solid mass of fibrin and blood cells may plug up the vein in a more serious condition known as thrombophlebitis. The danger here is that the clot may break loose from the wall of the vein and be swept along to the lungs or heart, where it may obstruct a crucial blood vessel and precipitate a heart attack. Varicosities of long duration are often accompanied by ugly, itching eczema, and ulcerations which can become so large as to involve the entire leg structure, even down to the bone.

Dr. Evan Shute told the Second World Congress of Obstetrics and Gynecology in Montreal, Canada, on 6 June 1958, that vitamin E helps in two ways. Vitamin E, he said, "produces collateral circulation about the obstructed deep veins by calling into play the unused networks of veins lying in wait for emergency utilization. We have such venous reserves just as we have reserves of brain, lung, and liver. Alpha-tocopherol (the most active part of vitamin E) mobilizes them. It does more. It has the unique power of enabling tissues to utilize oxygen better and hence the devitalized and congested leg tissues of the chronic phlebitic who is given alpha-tocopherol are receiving the equivalent of more oxygen." Alpha-tocopherol, he has stated elsewhere, also acts to dissolve fibrin in the blood, fighting the formation of blood clots while interfering only slightly or not at all with the clotting of blood to seal a wound.

He said that in his own experience with 166 patients who had chronic phlebitis, 32 enjoyed excellent or complete relief, 79 experienced good relief, 20 obtained moderate relief, and 35 had only slight relief after treatment with vitamin E. Most of these patients suffered from one to five years and some of them had had phlebitis for longer than six years.

Dr. Shute's brother, Dr. Wilfrid Shute, in his book *Vitamin E for Ailing and Healthy Hearts* (New York: Pyramid House,

1969), describes many cases of success using vitamin E for varicose veins. He tells of a woman who had suffered from varicose veins for 30 years and came to Dr. Shute after suffering an acute thrombus. There was swelling of feet and ankles during the past 20 years, and in the last two years both legs had become badly discolored with "a dead, heavy feeling in them." On 300 I.U. of alpha-tocopherol a day, the aching was gone in six weeks. But when she decreased her dose, her legs started to ache again. On 600 I.U. a day, her legs ceased to bother her at all, Dr. Shute reports.

# CHAPTER 79

# The Pill Is a
# Vitamin E Antagonist

To much of the modern world, "The Pill" is synonymous with contraception. Hailed as a scientific breakthrough by some, and damned as a contaminant of morals and probable cause of cancer by others, the Pill has become the most widely used contraceptive in America.

As early as 1962 scientists named the Pill as a probable factor in pulmonary embolism. Today the connection is generally recognized by the medical community. The Pill contains relatively large amounts of estrogen, or progestogen to prevent ovulation, and if it occurs, to stop implantation of the fertilized egg on the uterus wall.

How does it happen that estrogen administered in a pill can cause blood clots in the recipient? There is little hard knowledge and much speculation. Doctors write learnedly about "pseudo-pregnancy" and the fact that embolisms occur also in true pregnancy. But in true pregnancy, it is a body inside the womb putting pressure on the portal vein that interrupts the flow of blood and permits clots to form. This condition does not occur in the false pregnancy of birth control pills.

A far more plausible reason for internal blood clotting—even though one that appears to be completely overlooked by the researchers—is that estrogen is a vitamin E antagonist; that is,

486

estrogen neutralizes vitamin E and reduces the circulating level in the blood. Noted Canadian heart specialist, Wilfrid E. Shute, M.D., wrote in Harald J. Taub's *Vitamin E for Ailing and Healthy Hearts* (New York: Pyramid House, 1970), that there are "at least four estrogen antagonists, namely: progesterone, thyroid extract, alpha-tocopherol (vitamin E), and testosterone. . . . " Of the four it is vitamin E that reduces the blood's formation of thrombin, a clotting agent, and thus prevents thrombosis.

Vitamin E also regulates or controls the formation of fibrin, the protein in the blood which normally hardens when blood leaves its usual channels—a visible example of fibrin at work is the coagulation of a surface wound. Vitamin E dissolves fibrin, preventing its buildup in the form of an internal blood clot, whereas estrogen, by nullifying vitamin E, allows fibrin to collect resulting in thromboembolism.

"Currently," Dr. Shute said, "there is much in the medical literature about the increased dangers of thrombophlebitis in women taking contraceptive pills and the case has been fairly well made out, at least in England. . . . These women and their physicians ought to know that, just as every patient whose doctor has put him on a polyunsaturated fat diet needs increased vitamin E, so does the woman who takes the Pill. With the simple addition of a vitamin to her diet, she reduces virtually to zero the dangers of thrombophlebitis complications."

## Other Functions of the Vitamin

Estrogen, by destroying vitamin E, leaves the patient unguarded against a number of ailments in addition to embolism. Acting primarily as an antioxidant, vitamin E works to keep the oxygen in our blood pure, so every cell and fiber can function normally, helping the body to resist disease and maintain maximum health. Without an adequate supply of vitamin E, cellular wastes and lipids in the blood combine with oxygen to form toxic compounds such as hydrogen peroxide. The result means adverse effects for all parts of the body.

Side effects laid to the Pill (many of them markedly resembling symptoms created by a shortage of vitamin E) are legion. Hardly a week passes that some new study doesn't reveal ills traced to the Pill. High blood pressure is said to be aggravated by the Pill. An English study linked jaundice with the Pill. The University of Minnesota reported an increase in blood glucose and plasma insulin levels among women after 19 days on the Pill. Western Reserve University School of Medicine found a link, in a limited number of cases, between the Pill and strokes. A study out of the Netherlands Institute of Nutrition revealed the Pill can cause a rise in serum cholesterol levels. One study of patients in 19 British hospitals showed that 45 percent of the women suffering from venous thromboembolism had been taking the Pill the month before the onset of their illness.

Oral contraceptives are powerful drugs and there is serious risk. Yet millions of women rely on the Pill in spite of all its hazards. These women should recognize that, at best, the American diet with its processed food falls short of the normal requirements of vitamin E. With estrogen robbing the meager supply, women using oral contraceptives need additional vitamin E and should take a natural supplement. Vitamin E will not eliminate the risk of all the Pill's side effects but according to Dr. Shute, it will reduce "virtually to zero the danger of thrombophlebetic complications."

## Common Foods Rich in Vitamin E

No standard food composition tables are available as yet from the United States Department of Agriculture for this vitamin, but the following foods are generally recognized as the richest sources.

|  |  |
|---|---|
| Green leafy vegetables: | Cabbage |
|  | Spinach |
|  | Asparagus |
|  | Broccoli |
| Whole grains: | Rice |
|  | Wheat |
|  | Oats |

Wheat germ oil
Cottonseed oil
Safflower oil
Peanuts

# VITAMIN K

## CHAPTER 80

## Vitamin K—It Keeps You from Bleeding to Death

The world's most versatile do-it-yourselfer is the human body. It excels at mending and patching flaws without closing for repairs. Its workshop is usually the bloodstream, since most of its tools are right there. A prime example of the body's self-reliance is the coagulation of blood to close a wound, or rupture. While you might be able to care for a cut from the outside by applying an antiseptic and Band-Aid, the body busily weaves a gauzy covering inside to stop the bleeding. However, there is an ingredient, without which the work cannot proceed—a small portion of the vitamin most associated with *blood clotting*, vitamin K. But that's usually no problem. A person normally gets enough vitamin K from a varied and balanced diet plus vitamin K stores that are manufactured by the body as well.

The average person does not require vitamin K supplementation. However, there are times when additional vitamin K is needed. Some body illnesses, certain medications, and, especially, a combination of them can reduce the amount of vitamin K inside the body; also they inhibit the body's ability to absorb and utilize vitamin K.

The importance of vitamin K, known as the antihemorrhagic vitamin, is expressed in its very name, which was derived from its ability to assist in blood clotting. The Danish scientist Henrik

Dam discovered the vitamin in 1935 and named it from the Danish word *Koagulation*.

Inability to coagulate blood is a serious matter, for it can result in hemorrhaging. If vitamin K levels are extremely low, blood clotting time may be so prolonged that it is possible to bleed to death from a slight wound. If we had none of this vitamin at all, every one of us would ultimately die of hemorrhages.

## Infants Need Vitamin K

Elderly people are not the only ones vulnerable to vitamin K shortages. Bleeding becomes an equally serious problem under such conditions as prolonged menstruation, a major cause of anemia in women. Even newborn infants risk hemorrhaging, since it takes several days after birth for their intestinal flora to synthesize vitamin K. Because of this, small amounts of the vitamin are routinely administered to newborn infants. But the need for assuring sufficient vitamin K intake does not stop there.

Two doctors who investigated bleeding in infants *more than* 10 days old have recommended a minimum dietary intake of 10 mcg. of vitamin K per kilogram of body weight. Doctors Herbert I. Goldman and Peter Amadio reported in *Pediatrics* (November 1969) that a combination of low vitamin intake and a diminished supply of vitamin K in the intestines of babies may result in hemorrhages, and recommended relieving the situation through elevated dietary intake. Even small hemorrhages in infants can have a serious adverse effect if they involve a key organ such as the brain.

They found that each of 15 infants who were more than 10 days old and had bleeding was receiving a diet in which vitamin K was low or absent. Twelve of the infants had received antimicrobials, and nine had diarrhea, both of which could curb normal intestinal production of the vitamin in children of that age. Two of the bleeding infants, however, had neither diarrhea nor antimicrobials. Their symptoms appeared to be caused by vitamin K deficiency alone.

# Sources of the Vitamin

Normally the body gets its vitamin K in two ways: from certain foods (especially spinach and green cabbage) and through intestinal bacteria which manufacture or synthesize additional vitamin K. These kinds of vitamin K are natural and fat-soluble. They are the materials on whose presence the body depends for blood clotting.

The vitamin K must then be absorbed through the intestines along with dietary fats in the presence of bile salts. From there they go to the liver, where the vitamin mysteriously performs the function which is so vital to the body, and which, without the presence of the vitamin, cannot be accomplished—the production of coagulation factors in blood plasma.

Four out of the five blood coagulation factors are proteins whose production in the liver requires minute amounts of vitamin K. In the blood plasma these proteins are needed for the factor prothrombin to be changed into the enzyme thrombin. Thrombin in turn responds to wounds by converting fibrinogen in the blood into fibrin, a protein net which catches corpuscles at the site of a wound or rupture to bring about clotting.

Under normal circumstances the body dispatches vitamin K unerringly, getting it to the liver where it does its work. But there are potential pitfalls all along the vitamin's route that can stop it from reaching its destination. Without enough vitamin K, the blood becomes deficient in prothrombin, and then the whole human organism is endangered by hemorrhage, most often apparent as easy bruising.

For fat-soluble vitamin K to be absorbed by the intestine, bile salts are needed. In case of fat-absorption defects, gallstones, and liver disease such as obstructive jaundice, bile flow may be inhibited and absorption of the vitamin reduced. Dietary restrictions, diarrhea, colitis, and antibiotics are additional obstacles that may stand in the road of normal vitamin K intake.

Even if enough of it is received and absorbed by the body, vitamin K relies on a properly functioning liver for its utilization, or prothrombin will not be formed. In this organ a disease such as cirrhosis, as well as antagonists that include anticoagulant drugs, may render the vitamin useless.

Often when poor absorption is the defect, water-soluble, synthetic vitamin K can get through the intestinal walls since it does not depend upon bile salts which the natural fat-soluble vitamins require in the intestine. However, while the naturally occurring forms of vitamin K are nontoxic, even when given in huge doses, the synthetic form, which possesses only the basic vitamin K nucleus, may have adverse effects on the body if taken in large doses.

## How Much Is Required

In an attempt to establish a "minimum daily requirement" for vitamin K, P. G. Frick, G. Riedler, and H. Brogli, reporting in the *Journal of Applied Physiology* (23, 387, 1967) studied four patients who had a deficiency of vitamin K, testing their ability to coagulate blood as evidence of the effectiveness of vitamin K. As stated in *Nutrition Reviews* (June 1968), "The minimum daily requirement was taken as that dose of vitamin K which elicited a sustained elevation of clotting factors sensitive to vitamin K. This effect was achieved by a dose of 0.03 mg. of vitamin $K_1$ per kilogram of body weight," which should be the amount of the vitamin needed for normal clotting. ($K_1$ is one of two naturally occurring forms of vitamin K. Both are soluble in organic liquids, but in nature $K_1$ is found as a yellow oil and $K_2$ as yellow crystals.)

What are the chances and consequences of an overdose of vitamin K? Many people have taken very large doses, up to several hundred milligrams, without toxic effects, according to Sebrell and Harris in *The Vitamins* (New York: Academic Press, 1954). These elevated doses were taken under abnormal conditions, however, and for the purpose of counteracting the possible damage from anticoagulants. Under normal conditions, far less is required and in the synthetic form, should never be used. Vitamin K supplements, synthetically made, may cause undesirable excessive clotting and coagulation. However, there are no reported cases in which people have been harmed by natural vitamin K from food.

Obviously, vitamin K therapy is no job for the layman. Even people trained in the sciences have had difficulties evaluating vitamin K needs.

For some time many scientists believed that a deficiency was impossible, since the intestinal bacteria synthesize the vitamin, and that there was no need to be concerned about the vitamin K content of the diet. Yet, it has been found that people do suffer from such a deficiency, frequently with drastic results. One reason is the widespread use of antibiotics, which in killing the bacteria of the intestine, greatly reduce the amount of vitamin K in the system. Another reason is that anticoagulants, often prescribed for heart patients, dangerously reduce the clotting ability of the blood.

Vitamin K has been used successfully to offset the risks of anticoagulants. The *Journal of the American Medical Association* (14 March 1964) reported a study in which heart patients, who had been treated with anticoagulant drugs (to prevent clots), ate high amounts of spinach and other green vegetables for two weeks. Their "free prothrombin had returned to normal," and prothrombin time (length of time it takes for blood to clot) decreased. The dangers of the anticoagulants had been eliminated.

Today, vitamin K is widely used to counteract the effects of anticoagulant drugs, which tend to bring on hemorrhage. Dr. Armand Quick of Marquette University notes, however, "While it is well known that vitamin K given parenterally (by injection) strikingly reverses the action of the coumarin drugs, the effect of the vitamin content of the diet has been given little consideration."

This is especially true in the case of the pregnant woman. Normally, the mother should obtain enough vitamin K from foods during pregnancy to protect herself against excessive bleeding at childbirth and her child against hemorrhaging after birth. Unfortunately, many women simply do not eat enough of the foods rich in vitamin K, or else take too many aspirins or sedatives that actually reduce vitamin K synthesis.

As a safeguard, synthetic vitamin K, a water-soluble substance, used to be injected into mothers at labor to protect the newborn, whose prothrombin levels are often very low in the first days of life. It has been found, however, that injections of synthetic vitamin K could damage the infant liver. This possibility has properly caused many doctors to become wary of this particular therapy. Certainly a much better solution is for the mother to be fortified with natural vitamin K from food, which is a superb safeguard against hemorrhaging and has never been found to injure anyone.

Doctors K. Hazell, M.B., and B. H. Baloch, M.D., recommended in *Gerontoligica Clinica* (Basel, Switzerland, 12: 10, 1970) that "Antibiotics should not be used for long periods in the elderly without a thrombo-test being given. Anticoagulant therapy, in particular, is extremely risky and extremely unstable when factors are present suggesting vitamin K deficiency. Careful consideration should be given to all these factors before using anticoagulant drugs in patients over 60, and the sooner they are abandoned in the elderly, the better."

If you are taking anticoagulant drugs, and you suspect a vitamin K deficiency, should you supply the needed vitamin through supplements? The answer is simply and emphatically "no." Check with your doctor. He will probably withdraw the anticoagulant drug immediately, and give you vitamin K supplements in the proper dosage.

However, there is nothing to stop you from getting as much vitamin K as possible into your diet. That way there is no risk of an overdose, and you will be helping your body to raise its prothrombin level naturally.

A study by John Udall, M.D., of the Maricopa County General Hospital in Phoenix, Arizona, appeared in the *Journal of the American Medical Association* (11 October 1965). He found that when healthy volunteers ate nothing but polished rice, black coffee, granulated sugar, and a multivitamin tablet (without vitamin K) for three weeks, blood-clotting time rose from 14.8 seconds to 16.0 seconds. When pork liver and fresh spinach were added, one man showed "three sharp falls in prothrombin time, almost to normal." Dr. Udall concluded, "Foods, rather than bacterial synthesis, probably provide most vitamin K for humans."

For best results, the food you eat should be fresh. Cooking will not easily destroy vitamin K, but frozen foods tend to be deficient. So concentrate on fresh meats and vegetables. Since your body under normal conditions makes its own additional supply, it should never be too difficult for you to obtain enough of this vitamin that may one day be responsible for saving your life.

# CHAPTER 81

# Unseen Causes of Vitamin K Deficiencies

Since much of our supply of vitamin K is manufactured by bacteria in our intestines, it is extremely important that we maintain our colonies of benign intestinal flora in good condition. Unfortunately, in an effort to keep us healthy, the medical profession sometimes uses antibiotics so liberally as to make this more difficult and sometimes impossible. Antibiotics do not distinguish between good and bad bacteria. They kill them all.

In the *Canadian Medical Journal* (3 November 1973), researchers from St. Joseph's Hospital and McMaster University in Hamilton, Ontario reported many patients deficient in vitamin K.

Led by Dr. G. F. Pineo, an assistant professor of the Department of Medicine at St. Joseph's Hospital, the research team studied 27 patients who were hospitalized over a period of 24 months. The patients were in the hospital for a variety of reasons, all of which involved operations.

Their study confirmed previous findings that showed a decreased food intake, and treatment with antibiotics contributed to vitamin K deficiencies in all patients. This, in turn, created hemorrhaging problems in surgery. Postoperative bleeding stopped rapidly when the coagulation defect was corrected with doses of vitamin K.

"Vitamin K deficiency, often resulting in serious bleeding, may occur unexpectedly in the early postoperative period and in patients with renal failure," the study said. "It is likely that the more rapid onset of vitamin K deficiency in our postoperative patients was due to a combination of multiple antibiotic treatment and poor oral (food) intake."

The Canadian researchers noted that some of the patients may have been marginally deficient in vitamin K before their admission to the hospital but didn't think that was the cause since there was no abnormal bleeding encountered during surgery. In addition, no abnormal bleeding occurred before the patients were admitted. This suggests, the researchers say, that the vitamin K deficiencies developed during hospitalization.

This study confirms a host of other studies which outlined the inherent dangers of being on antibiotics over a long period of time. One doctor, John Ham, of the Prince Henry Hospital in Sydney, Australia, said in *Medical World News* (16 June 1972), that any patient on long-term intensive care should be given doses of vitamin K regularly.

## Vitamin Should Be Standard in Hospital Practice

Dr. Ham believes that hypoprothrombinemia (lack of prothrombin) is probably more common than is generally recognized. It could be the cause of major hemorrhages. He thinks that vitamin K should be given to *all* patients who are on intravenous fluids for more than seven days as well as to those on long-term antibiotic therapy. Describing the effects of vitamin K therapy on five patients, he said that when given the vitamin, bleeding was stopped in four or five patients with hypoprothrombinemia that developed during extended care. In addition, he said, prothrombin times (length of time it took for blood to clot) returned to normal in three patients and to near normal in the other two.

If any one group of hospital patients needs vitamin K more

than another, it is newborn infants. Dr. Herbert I. Goldman, coordinator of Community Neonatology at Long Island Jewish-Hillside Medical Center, said in *Medical World News* (December 1972), that he first became aware of a vitamin K deficiency in children in 1963.

# Food the Best Vitamin Source

Vitamin K has two sources—either intestinal flora or dietary intake, Dr. Goldman explained. Intestinal disturbance by way of diarrhea or antibiotics can produce deficiency—if dietary sources are not great enough to offset the lagging flora source. But physicians may not consider vitamin K deficiency a problem—nor dietary supplementation as a therapy—because the dietary source of vitamin K has been more or less ignored in medical literature, the doctor said.

"I believe the literature dating back 35 years was the primary source of the problem. It stressed intestinal flora as a vitamin K source and underemphasized dietary sources," he said.

He saw a week-old baby who had diarrhea and was dehydrated. The child was given intravenous fluid and put on a diet which consisted of a milk substitute. Two weeks later, however, the infant came down with convulsions, and exhibited a tendency to bleed. These signs, coupled with a long prothrombin time, led him to suspect that vitamin K deficiency was at the root of the problem. The baby recovered quickly after being put on vitamin K therapy.

Dr. Goldman began adding up the signs of deficiency over the years. Decades ago, vitamin K was recognized as a factor in blood coagulation. All babies were prone to bleeding. The milk substitutes that were given to the infants at that time were very low in vitamin K content. When the infants were put on cow's milk instead of a milk substitute, the signs of vitamin K deficiency disappeared.

Since the early 1960s, Dr. Goldman's theory on vitamin K deficiency in bleeding babies has been accepted by the medical profession. Researchers at the University of Cincinnati College of Medicine found, for example, that prothrombin times of infants not given vitamin K were extremely low compared to those who received vitamin K. The investigators concluded: "In view of the common occurrence of hypoprothrombinemia—and the danger of potential hemorrhage, *a small prophylactic dose of vitamin K should be given to every newborn infant shortly after birth.*

"This is a worldwide problem," Dr. Goldman told doctors attending a New York City seminar. "But it hasn't been recognized as such. I'm trying to stimulate awareness of the idea. A minimum daily requirement of vitamin K has to be discovered and set."

Many elderly patients are deficient in vitamin K, too. In a report that appeared in *Geriatrics* (July 1970), two British researchers, K. Hazell (M.B.) and K. H. Baloch (M.B.), from St. Mary's Hospital in Colchester, England, stated point-blank that a vitamin K deficiency seems to be present "in the majority of elderly patients with serious disease, despite production of the vitamin in the intestine by bacteria."

The two point out that in elderly patients with liver disease, vitamin K is not absorbed or utilized and there are consistent indications of vitamin K deficiency.

They point out that many drugs used in the elderly cause hypoprothrombinemia, and this does not improve with vitamin K therapy unless the drugs are stopped. They also point out that antibiotics should not be used for long periods in the elderly without tests to make sure that clotting time has not dropped. In addition, anticoagulant therapy in particular is extremely risky and extremely unstable when factors are present that suggest a vitamin K deficiency, they said.

"Careful consideration should be given to all these factors before using anticoagulant drugs in patients over 60, and the sooner they are abandoned in the elderly, the better."

The researchers performed clotting tests on 110 patients selected at random whose ages ranged from 56 to 100. The patients all suffered from a variety of conditions ranging from cerebral thrombosis, to bronchial pneumonia, to myocardial infarction.

Of 81 patients with low clotting times who were given vitamin K therapy, only 19 responded inadequately or gave no response at all. These were found to have liver damage or to have been on a program of antibiotics.

At this time you may be asking yourself, "How can I get vitamin K?"

Vitamin K does not come in a food supplement form. It would be much too dangerous, even in a very small dose as low as one mg. The reason for this is simple. Taking a supplement that would induce faster-than-average clotting would be not only dangerous, but it would be foolhardy. Internal blood clots are as dangerous as hemorrhages, and supplemental vitamin K should be administered only under the direction of a doctor. If the vitamin is obtained from normal food, however, there is virtually no danger of getting too much. Make sure your diet frequently contains vitamin K-rich food.

Vitamin K is far from being the only benefit of a fresh, natural diet, but it is a substantial one. These days, when traces of antibiotics appear in all sorts of food, you may need vitamin K more than you realize.

## Common Foods Rich in Vitamin K

No standard food composition tables are available as yet from the United States Department of Agriculture for this vitamin, but the following foods are generally recognized as the richest sources.

| | |
|---|---|
| Spinach | Lean meat |
| Cabbage | Peas |
| Cauliflower | Carrots |
| Tomatoes | Soybeans |
| Pork liver | Potatoes |

BOOK III

# VITAMIN THERAPY FOR DISEASE

# CHAPTER 82

# The Antianemia
# Action of Vitamin C

For many young women the price of beauty is poor health. In pursuit of better figures they diet, cutting down their nutritional intake. All too often the results are listlessness, headaches, irritability, and other unpleasant symptoms. The reason is that these women fail to safeguard against the additional loss of nutrients during menstruation.

The combination of blood loss from menstruation and a lowered intake of essential foods often results in a deficiency of the nutrients necessary for good health. And of all such deficiencies, the most common among women of childbearing age is a lack of iron which can result in anemia.

The body normally retrieves iron for new red blood cells from its own supply of old red cells that have broken down. But when these old red blood cells are lost in menstruation, the body's need for iron increases. Then the body must get and absorb additional iron from outside sources.

The National Research Council estimates that two-thirds of menstruating women and a majority of expectant mothers have very limited iron stores, or are without them completely. No authority knows the exact number, but hundreds of millions of the world's people suffer from iron deficiency at any given time.

Moderate to severe anemia is common in young children and

in the elderly, and it is now reported to be on the rise in adolescent girls and in boys in their late teens. Anemia occurs often in men, but women are far more susceptible to it, due to menstruation and pregnancy.

Iron deficiency is the major cause of anemia, and in turn anemia is among the body's most common danger signals. There is more to anemia than a pallid face and tired eyes. It can cause palpitations, severe headaches, vertigo (dizziness), spots before the eyes, and, in some instances, psychotic behavior. Even mild cases can cause weakness, irritability, stomach pains, and other symptoms.

The standard medical treatment for iron deficiency is iron salts, called hematinics. These salts improve the quality of the blood by increasing the hemoglobin level, which enables the red blood cells to distribute oxygen throughout the body.

Unfortunately, in all too many cases as soon as the patient stops getting injections, the anemia returns, even though in many of the cases the doctor has prescribed daily dietary supplements of iron pills. In this case, and actually in most cases of iron deficiency anemia, it is not so much the lack of an adequate supply of iron in the diet, as the lack of another biochemical element that makes it possible for the body to absorb the iron it consumes. The additional needed element is vitamin C.

## Vitamin C Needed for Iron Absorption

Emil Maro Schleicher, Ph.D., the director of hematology at St. Barnabas Hospital in Minneapolis, recently found in experimental studies that vitamin C is necessary to the body's absorption of iron. According to an article in *Minnesota Medicine* (February 1970) Dr. Schleicher warned, "While clinicians may be aware that iron salts such as ferrous sulfate and ferrous gluconate are effective hematinics, they may not fully appreciate the reason for compounding ferrous salts with ascorbic acid."

Dr. Schleicher reported his findings after treating 30 female patients, aged 14 to 42, who suffered from iron deficiency in the blood plasma in excessive uterine bleeding. Each of the patients was given one tablet twice daily containing 200 mg. of ferrous fumarate (another iron salt) and 600 mg. of ascorbic acid. Iron deficiency "was alleviated within 60 days," said the report.

It was found that the use of vitamin C helped the body to absorb the iron contained in the therapeutic tablet far better than without the vitamin. Besides that, 21 of the patients were examined a year after the therapy was discontinued. All of them experienced normal menstrual discharges and blood tests revealed that their iron stores remained normal.

Earlier researchers, Drs. Israel and Simmons, who had experimented with a combination ferrous sulfate-ascorbic acid tablet, recommended using 700 mg. of vitamin C along with the iron salt, according to the *Minnesota Medicine* article mentioned above. Dr. Schleicher added that a chronic deficiency of iron in the blood is often complicated by side effects of scurvy, a condition which results from prolonged depletion of vitamin C. This fact, he said, justifies the apparently large dose of the vitamin. On the other hand, severe anemia is also one of the symptoms of scurvy. So it is clear that vitamin C and iron do complement each other and that a lack of one can lead to a deficiency in the other.

In another study, reported in the *American Journal of Clinical Nutrition* (April 1968), by Dr. Paul R. McCurdy of Georgetown University School of Medicine and Dr. Raymond J. Dern of Loyola University Stritch School of Medicine, vitamin C was shown to enhance the effects of iron absorption. Drs. McCurdy and Dern found that with doses of ferrous sulfate ranging from 15 to 120 mg., ascorbic acid in 200 to 500 mg. amounts nearly doubled the absorption of the iron. With all quantities of iron, they found that 500 mg. ascorbic acid had a better effect than 200 mg.

# Recommended Daily Allowance
# Too Small for Effect

Men who volunteered for the study were tested with various combinations of iron and ascorbic acid. One of the facts that had already been established in earlier Scandinavian studies by researchers H. Brise and L. Hallberg was that what is considered a normal intake of vitamin C (from 10 to 50 mg.) had no effect whatsoever on the absorption of iron. In order to influence absorption, the dose of vitamin C had to be substantially larger. It took at least 200 mg. of the vitamin to initiate absorption of iron while the best possible absorption was achieved with doses of 500 mg. Using 500 mg., it was found that 1.88 times as much iron—nearly twice as much—was absorbed.

The authors pointed out the therapeutic implications of these findings—that it may be possible to administer less iron and still secure greater absorption by adding vitamin C to the compound.

Even though maintaining a diet rich in iron, we are not guaranteed our minimum requirements of this important mineral. According to Dr. Clement A. Finch, professor of medicine and head of the Division of Hematology at the University of Washington, "Measurements in man indicate that food-iron absorption usually ranges from five to 15 percent of that available from intake. Studies of various food substances show two to 10 percent of iron in vegetables can be absorbed; from animal protein, 10 to 30 percent of the iron can be absorbed." (*Nutrition Today,* Summer 1969.) By getting enough vitamin C daily, however, we can greatly increase the amount of iron absorbed from our food. The difference, for many, could be critical.

# CHAPTER 83

# Arthritics Need Vitamin C

Americans spend an estimated one billion dollars annually for medical care and treatment of arthritis, which afflicts 50 million people, and claims 250,000 new victims every year. The brunt of that cost is paid by the 17 million persons whose arthritis is severe enough to warrant medical attention, but the greatest suffering brought on by this disease is felt by the five million victims of rheumatoid arthritis, which destroys and disfigures the joints of the body, particularly those of the fingers, hands, and feet.

The person suffering from rheumatoid arthritis would give practically anything to get even temporary relief from the agony. Yet despite billions spent researching a lot of different things to relieve the pain of arthritis—such as gold salts, phenylbutazone, antimalarial drugs, indomethacin, or cortisone, and related steroid drugs—by far the most successful weapon against its torment is common aspirin. While aspirin may not help the condition, it does make life bearable for millions of people who have arthritis.

Any doctor will tell you that when you take aspirin for arthritis, however, you do not take it the same way you might if you wanted to relieve a headache with that drug. If you take aspirin for a headache, you stop taking it when the pain goes away. Not so when you are on aspirin therapy for arthritis. For then you must take aspirin at regular intervals throughout the day, and continue to take it even when the pain subsides. But there is one other aspect of aspirin therapy for arthritis that your physician may never have heard about, and therefore hasn't told you. It is this: if you must take aspirin regularly to relieve the pain of arthritis, you should also be taking supplementary vitamin C to relieve some of the side effects of high-dosage aspirin treatment.

Doctors Marvyn A. Sahud and Richard J. Cohen of the University of California's Department of Medicine and the Paul M. Aggeler Memorial Hematology Research Laboratory reported in the *Lancet* (8 May 1971), that patients who took 12 or more aspirin tablets per day over a long period of time to relieve the pain of arthritis were found to have significantly lower blood platelet and plasma levels of ascorbic acid than patients who supplemented a high dosage of aspirin with vitamin C.

According to the report, "It appears that a high dosage of aspirin in patients with rheumatoid arthritis is associated with tissue ascorbic acid depletion. Administration of supplemental ascorbic acid to rheumatoid patients receiving a high dosage of aspirin as primary therapy seems warranted."

The researchers selected 34 patients who had rheumatoid arthritis and 48 healthy subjects to serve as controls. The patients were split up into five groups according to the sort of therapeutic regimen they had followed for the treatment of arthritis for three months prior to the experiment. Seven of them had taken a high dosage of aspirin, that is, twelve or more tablets per day; seven others had taken a high dosage of aspirin plus corticosteroid drugs; 10 of them had taken fewer than 12 aspirin per day; eight had taken a high dosage of aspirin supplemented by vitamin C; and the remaining two patients had been on indomethacin therapy.

## All Drugs Depleted Vitamin C

When blood samples were taken of the 34 patients and 48 controls, and measured for concentrations of ascorbic acid in blood plasma and in platelets, the results showed that ascorbic acid levels of both plasma and platelets were below normal in patients who had taken high doses of aspirin with or without corticosteroids, and even lower in those patients on indomethacin therapy, while the ascorbic acid levels of both platelets and plasma were within the normal ranges measured in the control subjects for patients who supplemented high doses of aspirin with vitamin C.

The report said that regardless of how severe the arthritis was in the individual patients, "the major determinant of reduced ascorbic acid concentration in platelets appears to have been the daily dosage of aspirin." Drs. Sahud and Cohen added that, "It seems reasonable that patients receiving large doses of aspirin for the treatment of rheumatoid arthritis should take vitamin C supplements."

Aspirin's newly discovered effect of lowering ascorbic acid levels in blood plasma and platelets underscores the previously known detrimental effects of aspirin on blood platelet functioning.

Dr. Theodore Spaet of the Albert Einstein College of Medicine and Montefiore Hospital in New York reported findings that bear out the dangers from aspirin when he spoke before the Federation Of American Societies for Experimental Biology's Fifty-third Annual Meeting, and then explained to reporters later the significance of aspirin's effect on the body's platelets.

"First of all," he said, "the body contains three kinds of blood cells: red cells which carry oxygen; white cells which fight foreign substances that infect the body (we are familiar with them as pus cells); and third, fragments of cells called platelets."

## Platelet Clumping Stops Bleeding

The main function of the platelets is to keep people from bleeding to death. When an injury occurs which breaks a blood vessel wall, collagen tissue, which makes up the "basement" membrane of the blood vessels, is exposed. As the blood rushes out through the injury wall, platelets come into contact with the collagen. The collagen affects the platelets so that they release a mineral substance called adenosine diphosphate (ADP) which makes the platelets very sticky. They stick to the collagen surrounding the wound, then new platelets attach to the old ones until finally a clump of platelets have sealed off the wound.

The second mechanism whereby the body stops bleeding is, of course, clotting. This happens at a wound site when a liquid protein called fibrinogen is transformed into solid, thread-like strands of connective tissue called fibrin. Hundreds and hundreds of strands of fibrin mat together to form a clot and later a scab if the wound is on the outer surface of the body.

When the clotting process doesn't function adequately, as in hemophilia and other blood diseases, only platelet clumping can bring bleeding to an end. In most of us both clotting and clumping work hand in hand, and so effectively that even in serious injuries, bleeding to death is not common. Yet a simple thing like aspirin can dramatically affect the normally smooth functioning of the process. For that drug seems to have an unusual ability to bind with the sticky platelets, rendering them no longer capable of adhering to one another. The astounding fact is that only one or two aspirin tablets can have this effect on every platelet in the body.

What's more, the platelets remain thus affected for about seven days—which seems to be the lifespan of an individual platelet. According to Dr. Spaet, one ordinary dose of aspirin seems to destroy permanently the ability of the body's platelets to clump together when necessary. Of course, the body is constantly manufacturing new healthy platelets, but, said Dr. Spaet, "the person who takes two aspirin tablets twice daily is probably maintaining a permanently ineffective platelet system."

While aspirin may cut down your body's normal response to an external injury, it can actually be the cause of internal bleeding. Dr. James Roth, professor of gastroenterology at the University of Pennsylvania Graduate School of Medicine, demonstrated in 1963 that aspirin makes 60 to 70 percent of all people bleed internally in small amounts, no matter what the form of the aspirin. The usual loss of blood is about a teaspoon or so, and an occasional patient loses as much as three ounces internally. However, occasionally the result may be a severe hemorrhage, according to Dr. Roth.

While vitamin C will help to relieve your body of the strain put on it by aspirin, if you are taking that drug for arthritis therapy, doctors have recently recognized that a person who gets adequate amounts of vitamin C and other nutrients might very well never encounter arthritis to begin with.

## Only Good Nutrition Prevents Arthritis

In 1967, Dr. Robert Bingham, a California orthopedic surgeon specializing in rheumatism and arthritis, told the annual seminar of the American Nutrition Society that to any specialist in disorders of the bone it is apparent that nutrition plays a major role. He said he agreed completely with a pioneering dentist named Weston A. Price who said, "Applied nutrition in everyday life is the only way a human being may avoid arthritis and it is the first and best step a patient may take to treat his arthritis."

He said that it is impossible to dispute Dr. Price's findings which have since been confirmed by independent studies. Dr. Price noted that wherever there is a group of isolated people, whether primitive or otherwise, whose diet is abundant in natural, unprocessed foods and sufficiently varied to supply all necessary nutrients, there is not a single case of arthritis to be found. This, in itself, is not conclusive proof since the way of life of such isolated and usually primitive people is in many respects besides diet different from that of more civilized and arthritic people. But Dr. Bingham feels that the major portion of the medical profession would be amazed to learn how many arthritics can be helped by nutritional measures.

He said, "Diseases of the bones and joints which are due to deficiencies in a single nutritional factor are many. They include scurvy, a vitamin C deficiency; osteoporosis, from a lack of calcium and protein; neuropathy, from vitamin B complex deficiency; and degenerative joint disease due to a combination of nutritional deficiencies.''

He pointed out that these same nutrition deficiencies open the door to many of the infectious diseases by lowering the natural resistance of the body to bacteria, viruses, and parasites. This further emphasizes the relationship of nutrition and arthritis, he said, because "secondary arthritis is often caused by diseases which interfere with the absorption, digestion, metabolism of certain vital nutritional factors." Such diseases include disturbances of the digestive system, food allergies, glandular diseases, and the changes in body chemistry associated with the menopause and the aging processes of the body.

## Arthritics Are Low in Vitamin C

While the San Francisco researchers advise taking vitamin C supplements simply to counteract the detrimental side effects of aspirin therapy, previous reports have shown that vitamin C in many arthritic patients was either lacking in the diet, or at least that the diet did not contain enough of this nutrient to cope with the body's condition.

The *Journal of The American Dietetic Association* (May 1954) described a survey involving 131 children with rheumatic fever (called acute rheumatism) compared with 131 carefully paired children who did not have the disease. The rheumatic fever children were eating less vitamin C-rich foods than the healthy children. Many of the sick children did not get as much as one serving per day of food that contained even moderate amounts of vitamin C.

Elderly persons, particularly those in institutions, eat very little fruit and have correspondingly low blood levels of vitamin C. When chronic arthritic patients were given high doses of vitamin C every day, they reported that their pain was less and they had improved appetite and sense of well-being (*Geriatrics,* vol. 9, 1954). Massive doses in this case meant four grams (4,000 mg.) daily.

When arthritis strikes, its most common symptom is a combination of restrictive stiffness in the joints and excruciating pain. Therefore, arthritics welcome anything that will reduce these symptoms. For most arthritics, the most common treatment is aspirin, which we know, too, lowers the body's ascorbic acid level.

But E. Abrams and J. Sandson recorded in the *Annals of Rheumatic Disease* (23: 1964) that synovial fluid (the lubricating fluid of the joints) becomes thinner (allowing easier movement) when serum levels of ascorbic acid are high. The *American Journal of Clinical Nutrition* commented, "Whether or not this finding will eventually indicate that the amount of vitamin C in the arthritic patient's diet should be increased remains to be seen."

It seems sensible that any person who must wake up every day to face the persistent pain and stiffness of arthritis, should be getting extra vitamin C, just on the chance that it might give him freer movement and relieve his pain.

It is worth noting here that ascorbic acid is drained from the system by prolonged treatment with ACTH or cortisone, according to the *Archives of Internal Medicine* (December 1951). Both of these, of course, are used heavily in the treatment of arthritis, although aspirin is far and away the most common treatment, and now we know that aspirin, too, in high doses, uses up the body's vital vitamin C stores.

Therefore, it is clear from accumulated evidence, that if the body doesn't have enough vitamin C at its disposal—and remember that vitamin C is a water-soluble nutrient which the body cannot store—a victim has little hope of recovery from arthritis. And the San Francisco experiment shows that doses of 12 or more aspirin tablets per day, which are to many millions of Americans representative of their daily therapeutic dosage for arthritis, are the prime factor in reducing the vitamin C levels in the platelets and blood plasma of arthritic patients. In most cases people who are taking aspirin for arthritis are reducing their pain but making the arthritis worse.

Of course, the pain of arthritis is too severe to ignore. If your physician has put you on aspirin therapy for arthritis in order to reduce pain and inflammation in your joints, it's best to comply. Just remember the recommendation published in the prestigious British medical journal, *Lancet:* "It seems reasonable that patients receiving large doses of aspirin for the treatment of rheumatoid arthritis should take vitamin C supplements."

# CHAPTER 84

# Vitamin B₆ Brings Relief from Rheumatism

*by John M. Ellis, M.D.*

*The discomfort and crippling pain of rheumatism has plagued mankind for many centuries, but medical men still do not know exactly what rheumatism is or what causes it. However, after years of extensive clinical research, John M. Ellis, M.D., believes he has found an effective treatment, and possibly a preventive, for rheumatism—B₆. Dr. Ellis is an acknowledged authority on B₆, and has been treating patients with the vitamin since 1961. Here, taken from his own book,* Vitamin B₆: The Doctor's Report *(New York: Harper & Row, 1973), pp. 39–56, is an account of Dr. Ellis's success against rheumatism with B₆.*

Rheumatism—"any of various painful conditions of the joints and muscles"—goes back at least to the ancient Greeks, who named it, and perhaps even farther. It has been speculated that Neanderthal man of the Paleolithic period was afflicted with it. For the first mention of paresthesia, the medical term for the numbness and tingling we have already discussed, one goes back at least to Galen, a Greek physician in the second century more than 1,800 years ago. In his early twenties Galen treated gladiators, learning his anatomy from the severely wounded. Later he became court physician to the Roman emperor Marcus Aurelius. One of his patients, who had fallen from a horse, had numbness in the fourth and fifth fingers of one hand. Galen grew intrigued

517

with the belief that nerves came from a central nervous system, and in this patient he reasoned that the numbness had been caused by an injury to the neck vertebrae.[1] However far back in history it may be traced, without a doubt rheumatism has brought pain and suffering to millions of persons in many lands.

But what, exactly, is rheumatism? What causes it? What will relieve it? How can it be prevented?

These are large questions, so large that an entire specialty of medicine, rheumatology, is devoted to them. By and large, the questions remain unanswered. This chapter, however, will attempt to answer the questions at least partially.

A precise definition of rheumatism is extremely difficult to arrive at—a problem encountered by the rheumatologist as well as the general practitioner. It has come to be thought of, broadly, as any disease condition of a chronic recurrent nature that involves the connective tissues of the muscles, tendons, bursa, joints, and nerves in the shoulders, arms, hands, hips, legs, neck, and back. In more recent times another term, arthritis, has been vaguely and loosely associated with rheumatism and rheumatism-like conditions.

Although "arthritis" is a commonly used term today by both doctors and patients, I hesitate to use it without very carefully describing what I mean. Arthritis has inspired more controversy, probably, than anything else in medicine. Books purporting to possess the cure for arthritis are numerous, and because of the desperate nature of the persons afflicted with arthritis, the books are almost invariably assured a healthy sales. Over the years arthritis has drawn into its orbit more food faddists, steam parlors, masseurs, bath houses, mineral springs, red springs, warm springs, hot springs, charlatans, and just plain quacks than, possibly, any other disease. There have been more patented drugs for arthritis than for almost anything else in medicine. Yet I know of no drugs that significantly help hypertrophic and degenerative arthritis, outside of a few analgesics for pain and adrenocorticotropic hormone. Some doctors have administered a female hormone and claimed some success, but there seems to have been little more than temporary relief.

Rheumatic and arthritic conditions may come from a number of causes, such as bacterial infection, which masks itself as rheumatism. Because these various disease conditions sometimes arise from different causes even though the signs and symptoms are very similar, separating and distinguishing them has been a tedious, laborious task for scientists in different countries, treating different people in different areas. Bacterial infections can cause painful, swollen, and inflamed joints, which is diagnosed as inflammatory arthritis. Rheumatic fever, a condition that may treacherously affect the heart, can also mask itself as rheumatism.

However, the signs and symptoms of the rheumatism I will be discussing in this chapter are of the idiopathic—or spontaneous and primary—rheumatism that has been a painful experience of *Homo sapiens* for centuries. It does not come as the result of a germ or an injury or a secondary infection. It is, primarily, a *nutritional* disease that my patients referred to as "rheumatism." It was because of the patients with rheumatism that I gained my earliest and deepest insight into the effectiveness of B₆ therapy.

The range of treatment for rheumatism is amazingly limited. Before 1961, as many another doctor had done, I treated the disorder with aspirin and buffered aspirin. Once in a while I would prescribe guarded doses of cortisone, held to a minimum—if the patient was begging for something to stop pain. Although gold salts have been used with some success in treatment of rheumatoid arthritis, buffered aspirin and aspirin therapy is the conventional method of treatment that is commonly used today.

## Rheumatism Responds to B₆ Therapy

What I learned about B₆ therapy and rheumatism I learned by moving gradually from one patient to the next, from one symptom to another, from one sign to another, slowly and laboriously until the relationship was obvious. For four years I did very little reading in the medical literature about rheumatism because I wanted to have an open mind on the subject. I was trying to see the whole clinical picture. After I had formed my clinical judgments I could then read the literature with far more understanding of what the researchers had found in the laboratory. It was, for me personally, an experience characterized by a theme of serendipity, of seeking one thing and happily finding something else, as valuable or more so.

The first patient who drew my attention to these related disease conditions was an oilfield worker with tingling fingers. All of my work with B6 eventually grew from that seminal case. Soon I treated a number of cases of rheumatism. While questioning patients about diets that seemed to contain excessive amounts of fat, I learned that numbness and tingling of the fingers (paresthesia) were common symptoms.

This paresthesia of the hands was most noticeable when the hands were at rest or while the patient was driving an automobile or lying in bed. When he moved his fingers and rubbed his hands, the numbness and tingling would subside, only to return later. Occasionally a patient would awaken to find an arm temporarily paralyzed. He would have to rub it or shake it with the other, unaffected hand to "get the circulation going again." Adults of all ages complained of this. Some of those who seemed worse off would tell me that they had pain in the finger joints when the fingers were flexed or "bumped" on objects. The sensitivity was so exquisite that even "bumping" the fingers on a bed cover would bring pain. As the symptoms got worse in both men and women, hand-grip strength began to fail. There seemed to be a failure of motor power in the hand, somehow, so gradual in its onset that the patients themselves were not aware of it until, suddenly one day, they could no longer wring water from a dishcloth or squeeze milk from a cow's teat. Their disability became more noticeable at such times, with a corresponding reduction in the speed of finger movement, especially in flexion and range of flexion.

Invariably I would find numbness, tingling, and loss of sensation to be in agreement with the anatomical distribution of the digital nerves arising from the trunk nerves in the arm. Quite frequently, in early cases, disturbed sensation was limited to the little finger and the adjacent side of the ring finger. This, for instance, is the exact terminal distribution of the ulnar nerve in the hand. In other cases the tingling and numbness would follow the exact distribution of the median nerve.

The most characteristic sign of this form of rheumatism was the patient's failure to perform perfectly what I later came to call the QEW (Quick Early Warning) test. Before therapy there was an obvious disturbance of tendon action, which was caused by swelling of synovia in the hands. Synovia are thin lining membranes of bursa, joint cavities, and tendon sheaths. The two finger joints of the hand could not be flexed completely because of three other evident factors: impaired nerve, muscle, and tendon motor powers; swelling of the soft tissues, as well as the joint capsules, of the fingers; and pain in the finger joints. This, a syndrome known as "rheumatism," was a condition I was to see over and over through the years, and it responded to vitamin B₆.

The case history of L.G., a sixty-year-old deputy sheriff, is instructive. On 20 January 1967, he complained, "Doc, I've got arthritis in my hands, feet, back, and spine." His hands and fingers were swollen. His legs felt so weakened that he could hardly climb the steps of the county courthouse, a daily routine for a deputy sheriff. For the past two years he had been troubled with a swelling and pain in both knees, and his fingers had been painful longer than that. While driving his automobile he frequently noticed a numbness and tingling in his fingers and hands.

He had been having pains for twenty-four years now, since 1942, the deputy explained to me. His hands and feet had become so swollen that he had been discharged from the Army with a diagnosis of arthritis. From time to time over the years he would improve; then he would have relapses. Now his legs were so stiff and painful that he couldn't cross one leg over the other at the knees while he was sitting. He had been having nocturnal muscle spasms in his legs about two or three nights a week.

A childhood bout with pneumonia had been the extent of his serious illness in the past. Except for the extremities of which he complained, my findings were negative. But there the signs of disease were large enough for any man to see. His hands and fingers were so swollen that he could barely screw off his ring. Both knees were swollen; there appeared to be a slight amount of fluid in both knee joints. Both feet were marked by slight, diffuse edema. In the interphalangeal joints of his fingers he had lost his flexion by about 50 percent. I gave him 100 mg. of pyridoxine daily and told him to return in two weeks.

By 3 February the swelling had subsided in the knees, and when he sat down he could cross one leg over the other at the knee—comfortably. He had no pain in the fingers, and his finger flexion, at the interphalangeal joints, was remarkably improved. Numbness and tingling had subsided in the fingers and hands. The swelling in his hands and feet had subsided; now he could more easily remove the ring from his finger.

"I thought I was going to have to retire," he proclaimed happily, "but I can climb the steps of the courthouse without any trouble now."

Three years later, on 23 March 1970, after he had taken pyridoxine (100 mg. daily) throughout the intervening period, I examined him again. He had no paresthesia of the hands, no swelling in either hands or feet, no swelling in the knees. He did have some tenderness in the finger joints, but it was not to the extent he had had it three years before. His flexion at the interphalangeal joints was much better than before treatment back in 1967.

His, it appeared, was a case of the idiopathic, *nutrition-related* rheumatism that has brought agony to millions over the centuries. At his age, 100 mg. of pyridoxine was used to dispel his symptoms and signs; perhaps at an earlier age half that much would have been sufficient; if he had received an adequate daily supply of pyridoxine as a child—who can say that he would have later suffered his "arthritis?"

## B$_6$-Responsive Rheumatism Has a Definite Pattern

There appeared to be a pattern in my patients. As deformity of the finger joints increased, along with disturbed sensation in the fingertips, there eventually was a pronounced impairment of shoulder function and, to some extent, elbows. They commonly complained of pain at both pressure and movement of the shoulders. Yet it was difficult, if not impossible, to determine if the pain about the shoulder came, in a given case, from the synovia of the joint or a nerve or bursa near the joint. In some cases most of the pain was in the arms and was located between the elbows and the shoulders. Simultaneously and insidiously, stiffness tended to develop as the fingers became more deformed. The index finger was affected more than its neighbors. In advanced cases, even when there was little or no edema present, the tip of the index finger could not be made to touch the tip of the thumb. Because of this, housewives became unable to sew, for the thumb and finger could not be approximated enough to use needle and thread. For a woman who was a seamstress by trade or who made some of the family's clothing herself, this presented very serious economic consequences, aside from the pain.

Particularly in women who were near the age of menopause, the finger joints became very painful. Little reddened and exquisitely tender burrs or knots, described by William Heberden in London in 1802 and since called "Heberden's nodes," appeared on the sides of the finger joints. While these also affected the fingers of older men, the condition seemed more attracted to women at or past the age of menopause. Degree of pain and swelling seemed to go together, although some individual joints were more involved than others.

Coordination of finger and hand movement was directly influenced by the degree of impaired flexion. Mechanics dropped screwdrivers, carpenters dropped hammers, and housewives dropped and broke their dishes. Clearly there was, in these instances, an involvement of the nervous system. Patients spoke of the condition as a weakness in the hands; there was a slight tremor and reduced speed when they tried to flex their fingers, and then the fingers were only partially flexed.

Sensation in the fingers was so disturbed in many of the

patients that they could not distinguish one substance from another by touch. Housewives could not feel or guide the movements of thimbles on their fingers. Craftsmen often sacrificed employment because of their disabled fingers; they could not meet the requirements for production.

Cramps and muscle spasms were common and were not limited to the hand. In fact, my patients suffered some of their most brutal and forceful muscle spasms in the backs of the legs and arches of the feet. . . . Most of the time these cramps occurred at night and were preceded by what was described as a "restless" feeling in the legs. The patients would bolt from their beds in agonizing pain to massage or rub the contracted and knotted muscles in the legs or feet. Aged people sat many nights by their heaters or ran hot water over their feet and legs in efforts to halt the vicious leg cramps.

From time to time a patient was seen—usually a woman near middle age—whose fingers were miserably tight. The skin of the fingers was shiny and glistening white, more so than the rest of the hand, and without wrinkles and quite thin. Frequently she— or he—would grimace, point to the particular finger joint that was the culprit and complain that the joint would lock so that she had to unlock it with the other hand. Some called it a "trigger finger." The patient usually feared that exercising it would set off an involuntary cramp or spasm in the hand or forearm.

Swelling, or edema, usually accompanied the aches and pains. Frequently it was diffuse and barely detectable except by the trained eye. Housewives often complained that their wedding rings had become too tight or that they had to be removed forcibly from their ring fingers. In the more severe cases, the veins and tendons in the backs of their hands were indistinct and the hands appeared "puffy" or "fat."

Younger women experienced an increased amount of swelling in the soft tissues of the hands during the week prior to menstruation. Women frequently told me of discomfort in their hands a day or so before menstruation. In medical circles this has been called "premenstrual edema." Along with it came varying amounts of swelling in the eyelids and the cheeks. Women patients who already had finger and joint pain usually had increased finger and joint pain during the day or so before menstruation.

Because of a possible relationship between it and the elastic connective tissue in the body, one more sign should be described. Some patients suffering from a long-standing rheumatic disease in the hands had no wrinkles there. This held true even in some of the aged. Instead, in the cheek of the face there was this same glistening, shiny sheen that characterized the skin of the tight, stiffened, and almost fixed fingers. The relationship here between edema and the connective tissue of both hands and face is of particular interest to us. Histologists long ago demonstrated that the cheeks of the face, not the whole face, are composed of cells that contain a remarkably high percentage of elastic connective tissues. It seems probable that the same mechanism that made the hands tight and glistening also was at work in the tissues of the face—and perhaps elsewhere, as we will see in subsequent chapters.

In dealing with these various conditions that can be lumped generally under the diagnosis of "rheumatism," after a few months of clinical study I began prescribing oral doses of pyridoxine. Usually 50 mg. were given daily, and all the symptoms I have listed here responded to the therapy. Pain was relieved or eradicated. Function was restored. After a period of time I was able to establish a timetable for improvement or recession of symptoms. Some patients experienced a return to health within a week or two; some, in six weeks; others, usually the elderly, had gradual improvement, up to six and eight months.

Hand grip, for instance, was usually restored dramatically. One well-dressed woman with expensive rings could not touch the tips of her fingers to her palm when she first came in. After eight days of B6 therapy she could do this exercise with facility. Disabled dairymen, who could no longer squeeze the teats of a cow, took 50 mg. of B6 and by the end of two weeks were milking, by hand, a half-dozen cows a day. These cases undoubtedly also involved an improvement in motor-nerve physiology, related to the reduction of swelling at the wrist. Let us examine in detail the case of L. C. S., aged fifty-six.

# Excruciating Finger Pain Relieved

L. C. S. had been a successful dairyman for twenty-five years and a swine grower for the past five years when I first observed him on 15 March 1966. His signs and symptoms were numerous. They included, in the sometimes technical medical language that I used on his chart, bilateral numbness and tingling in the fingers and hands; swelling of fingers and hands; "trigger finger" of ring finger of the right hand; failure to flex tips of the fingers to touch metacarpophalangeal crease in either palm (QEW test); painful interphalangeal finger joints; weakness of hand grip in his right hand; painful elbows; periarticular swelling around both knees; occasional nocturnal paralysis of the entire left arm such that, on awakening, the unaffected hand would be used to massage and shake the affected arm and hand to return of function; and point tenderness near the tips of the acromion (the outer extremity of the shoulder) in both shoulders.

He had been assaulted, it seemed, by a plague of painful, abnormal conditions, whether one called them arthritis or "just plain ol' rheumatism." Although each of the signs and symptoms was enough to cause complaint, his finger joints were quite painful even when they were only passively squeezed or massaged. In most cases this could be used as a general index of the severity of a patient's condition.

Treatment began with daily oral doses of 50 mg. of pyridoxine, with no discussion of diet. No other medication was prescribed.

On 4 April, three weeks later, L. C. S. reported an overall general improvement. An increased wrinkling of the skin on the hands and fingers indicated a reduction in edema. He passed the QEW test by flexing *all* his fingers to touch the metacarpophalangeal crease of each palm. His right hand grip had returned to normal, and the numbness and tingling in his hands and fingers had subsided. The nocturnal paralysis of his left arm had been relieved. The "trigger finger" problem in his right ring finger had disappeared. The pain in his shoulders was improved but not completely relieved. The pain in his knees, as well as the periarticular swelling of the knees, had lessened. In all, he had enjoyed about as much improvement as a doctor is likely to hope for in such a short period of time. . . .

Six weeks after initial therapy with pyridoxine had begun, the pain and swelling had subsided around all joints except that of the right knee. There, the swelling was less, but pain continued, although there was considerably less than before treatment.

In an informal follow-up examination six years later, on 24 April 1972, I saw L.C.S. at a cattlemen's meeting. During that six-year period he had taken 50 mg. of pyridoxine daily. Still actively employed in livestock production, he had better use of his shoulders, arms, and hands. He had no edema in his hands, and he could flex his fingers perfectly.

L.C.S.'s case is not an isolated one. I have seen patients, time and time again, who could not pull open the front door of my office because of the excruciating pain in their fingers. Within three weeks a daily dosage of B₆ would enable them to open the door by themselves. Most frequently these patients were of middle age. There is something about middle-aged persons that is different, probably a hormone imbalance or deficiency in both men and women, and it responds to pyridoxine.

It seems likely that the pain in the fingers is caused by actual degeneration, or melting away, so to speak, of the coverings of the little nerves that go to the nerves—the myelin sheaths. It has been proved that dogs subjected to B₆ deficiency actually develop a sloughing or degeneration of myelin sheaths of the sciatic nerves in the backs of their legs. This indicates, as do the reported signs and symptoms, that patients with painful fingers have a nerve, as well as bone, disease. Tingling is the first signal that B₆ is needed; pain develops later, followed by edema and stiffness of the joints. In association with it there is both swelling and deformity of the joints, and this is usually diagnosed as osteoarthritis. . . .

While the outlook is optimistic for most rheumatism sufferers treated with B6, . . . I hasten to emphasize that two disorders of the joints have not responded to B6, in my experience: traumatic arthritis, caused by injury, and rheumatoid arthritis. For purposes of distinction I prefer to set traumatic arthritis (due to injury) to one side, and then to divide the remaining cases into rheumatism and rheumatoid arthritis. Rheumatoid arthritis has a different etiology that is unrelated to B6.

In my experience clear-cut and distinctive rheumatoid arthritis did not respond to vitamin B6. Interestingly enough, however, some relationship seems to have been established between rheumatoid-arthritis patients and B6 deficiency by other investigators. Patients with this disorder did excrete increased amounts of xanthurenic acid and kynurenine, two of the abnormal metabolites of the amino-acid tryptophan, which would indicate an increased need for pyridoxine in order to handle tryptophan properly. This is one of the puzzling aspects of this particular form of arthritis. Dr. H. Spiera, chief of the Arthritis Clinic at Mt. Sinai Hospital in New York, stated: "It is impossible to assess the significance of the abnormal excretion of tryptophan metabolites by patients with rheumatoid arthritis. It does not seem to be related to tissue destruction, pyridoxine deficiency, inflammation, gamma globulin turnover, or to drugs used in the management of rheumatoid arthritis."[2] But, adds Dr. Spiera, because nothing is known of the etiology or pathogenesis of rheumatoid arthritis, any differences such as the increased xanthurenic-acid excretions should be explored.

Isobel M. Bett of the Rheumatic Diseases Unit of the Northern General Hospital in Edinburgh has noted that pyridoxine restores normal metabolism of patients who had excreted elevated metabolites. Nonetheless, as in the experience of others, excretion of these metabolites did not correlate well with the disease's clinical activity. In one series of clinical studies, Bett reported results that tended to support earlier investigators who suggested that low urinary pyridoxine did not necessarily mean low availability in the body and that it could be used up at an unusually rapid rate in these patients by some other metabolic or immunological process. Bett thought that any pyridoxine deficiency in patients with rheumatoid arthritis was probably a relatively mild one. However, there were other puzzling sides to the whole question. "Patients whose tryptophan metabolism became normal on pyridoxine did not necessarily improve clinically," wrote Bett. "On the other hand, in those who did improve, kynurenine excretion tended to fall."[3] Kynurenine is another metabolite of tryptophan, the high excretion of which indicates a pyridoxine need.

In an earlier study, Bett had reported that prolonged administration of pyridoxine to patients who had rheumatoid arthritis had brought about a fall in kynurenine in tryptophan-load tests. When pyridoxine was withdrawn, kynurenine was again excreted in increased amounts. These results occurred in a majority of patients. [4]

Before that, in 1961, investigators A.B. McKusick and J.M. Hsu had reported a syndrome similar to the shoulder-hand syndrome of rheumatoid arthritis in patients with tuberculosis who were being treated with the drug isoniazid and PAS, or para-amino-salicylic acid. When the drug was removed, or else was accompanied by pyridoxine, the patient improved.[5] It should be noted that pyridoxine had earlier been used in tubercular patients as a means of counteracting some side effects of the drug isoniazid.

Parents of children with rheumatoid arthritis have asked me if B₆ might help them. I have explained very carefully that I recommend, with children having rheumatoid arthritis, that they be given 25 mg. of B₆ morning and night, with the expectation that the signs and symptoms will not change unless they also have these other signs and symptoms that are not necessarily associated with rheumatoid arthritis. In other words, B₆ can do no harm, but by the same token it may do no good either, unless the patient also has one of the other conditions that I have earlier described as "rheumatism." I have had patients who had two different conditions—rheumatoid arthritis, which did not change, and rheumatism, which did change when B₆ was given.

Despite the fact that B₆ has not achieved clinical success with rheumatoid arthritis, it must be remembered that laboratory data based on the tryptophan-load test and subsequent excretion of kynurenine and xanthurenic acid indicate that B$_6$ is needed by the majority of those patients suffering from rheumatoid arthritis.

Because the objective findings in the hands of these patients I successfully treated for rheumatism were so apparent to patients and doctors alike, I would like to outline briefly the results obtained by pyridoxine. The ten main features include:

1. Reduced edema
2. Reduced pain
3. Improved range of flexion
4. Increased speed of flexion
5. Eliminated locking of finger joints
6. Increased strength of grip
7. Improved sensation
8. Improved coordination
9. Reduced stiffness
10. Sustained flexion

These changes in the hands could usually be related to improvement elsewhere in the body. Reduction of edema, for example, invariably occurred over the rest of the body as well as the hands. Almost without fail, hitherto tight wedding rings became looser; many women feared they would lose their rings down the kitchen drain pipe. On the average there was a weight loss from five to seven pounds following pyridoxine treatment. The reduction of edema was also evident in other ways. Before treatment, a patient's cheeks often were shiny, almost glistening, and devoid of wrinkles, just as the fingers were tight and shiny. After pyridoxine, the skin in both the hands and the cheeks gradually relaxed, in time forming tiny wrinkles and losing the characteristic shiny skin coloring.

Although it was found in only a few cases, the cold perspiration of the palms indicated a severe abnormality in some patients. Paroxysms of palm sweating would appear for a few minutes and then wane. This was most likely caused by pressure of swollen synovia on the median nerve. The patients had cold, moist fingers at normal room temperature. After pyridoxine, the fingers became warm and dry and remained so.

Pain is an experience difficult to gauge and difficult to trace. Obviously the patient is the best judge of where and how a portion of his body hurts. It is simple for him to determine *if* he has pain, but it is not always so simple to pinpoint precisely where the pain is or how it may have come about. He is certain, however, when the pain appears—and when it disappears. Painful interphalangeal joints, common among my patients, were relieved to some extent within three weeks of beginning treatment. Most were substantially improved at the end of six weeks. Elderly patients who already had deformity of their fingers improved gradually for months and even years. In hands where there was no deformity to begin with, pain was relieved in the fingers more completely, in both men and women. Heberden's nodes, the painful little burrs or knots, became less painful and, in some instances, smaller.

Shoulder pain was an important symptom in patients who had severe pathological changes in their hands. However, it was quite hard to locate exactly where the pain stemmed from, because the nerves, bursa, and capsule of the shoulder joints are in such close proximity. Yet this shoulder pain—to be distinguished from traumatic bursitis, which would not respond— responded to pyridoxine. Elbow pain also had a vague, indistinct location, making it difficult to determine if the pain was in the synovia or nerves or both. I entertained suspicion that it came from the synovia. Pyridoxine relieved elbow pain in about six weeks. Hip pain seemed to be in the hip joint, and to some extent it responded to pyridoxine. Knee pain, even more difficult to evaluate, showed some response to pyridoxine. A few patients showed reduction of swelling in the area of the knees within two weeks; as swelling subsided, knee pain improved.

Paresthesia—numbness and tingling—was the most frequently mentioned symptom that was treated with B₆, and it was the one most successfully relieved. When 50 mg. of pyridoxine were given daily, paresthesia was relieved within two weeks. Nocturnal paralysis of an arm was relieved completely within two weeks, and nocturnal muscle cramps, a very common complaint with patients who had pathological changes in their hands, were usually relieved within one week.

Hand grip was restored within two weeks and often dramatically in less time. By some unexplained means there was a restoration of motor power, probably as a result of improved motor-nerve physiology.

Definite improvement of sensation in the fingertips usually came within two weeks. As paresthesia got better, so did sensation. Patients previously unable to feel the weave of cloth could do so after treatment; a seamstress then could close her eyes and distinguish what type of cloth was between her fingers merely by touch.

Improved sensation, speed of flexion, and range of flexion seemed to lead to better coordination of finger movements. Mechanics and carpenters no longer dropped their screwdrivers and hammers; housewives held onto their teacups and dishes; elderly women resumed sewing with thimble, needle, and thread. Finger stiffness was improved within six weeks, with the fingers becoming more pliable. This also seemed to accompany other, generalized improvement. For example, elderly women could get in and out of bed or the bathtub easier than before. There was more power and strength in their legs.

A key to success in treatment was the index finger. The index finger was the stiffest, most difficult finger of all to improve. It was the last finger that could be made to flex completely. The reason for this lies in the fact that the anatomy of the index finger is remarkable in its difference from its three neighbors. The muscle bellies of the flexor digitorum profundus tendons that insert into the little, ring, and long fingers of the hand are all grouped in a common muscle sheath, and motor power is supplied by the ulnar nerve. But the flexor digitorum profundus of the index finger is separate; it is supplied by the median nerve for motor power, and the median nerve also supplies sensation for the index finger. Spontaneous compression of the median nerve at the carpal tunnel is probably the reason why the index finger is stiffer than the other fingers. Also, this anatomical difference explains the longer wait for the index finger to improve. Motion pictures I took of several patients, before treatment and six weeks afterward, clearly revealed that improvement in the flexion of the index finger was slower and required a longer period of therapy than did the others. Index fingers normally required six weeks of therapy before improving.

Exercise seemed to make symptoms and signs worse. For instance, after twelve or fourteen days of treatment with pyridoxine, a patients's finger pain and swelling would substantially subside. Yet if the fingers were repeatedly flexed, after a night of rest, within minutes one or two of the affected fingers would become swollen and painful. After pyridoxine had been used long enough, exercise failed to cause this discomfort.

It is a simple solution to a medical problem that has plagued patients for ages; yet it has proved itself to be effective without harmful side effects. This is what the patient hopes for and needs.

The ancient Greeks—and Neanderthal man, no doubt—would have called it miraculous.

---

1. Bender, George A., and Thom, Robert A., *A History of Medicine in Pictures* vol. 2, (Parke, Davis & Co., 1958).
2. Spiera, H., "Excretion of Tryptophan Metabolites in Rheumatoid Arthritis," *Arthritis and Rheumatism* (April 1966, pp. 318–24).
3. Bett, Isobel M., "Urinary Tryptophan Metabolites in Rheumatoid Arthritis and Some Other Diseases," *Annals of the Rheumatic Diseases* (vol. 25, 1966, pp. 556–62).
4. Bett, Isobel M., "Effect of Pyridoxine on Tryptophan Metabolism in Rheumatoid Arthritis," *Annals of the Rheumatic Diseases* (vol. 21, 1962, p. 388).
5. McKusick, Anne B., and Hsu, Jeng M., "Clinical and Metabolic Studies of the Shoulder-Hand Syndrome in Tuberculosis Patients," *Arthritis and Rheumatism* (vol. 4, 1961, p. 426).

# CHAPTER 85

# An Answer for
# Those Aching Backs

For the millions of people in this country who suffer from various forms of backache, happiness is simply a back that stops aching. The excruciating pain of an aching back seems to be a consequence of achieving middle age. Annually some two million adults are initiated into the "bad back" club: total membership, seventy million Americans, or one out of every three. According to the Public Health Service, at any given moment seven million Americans are undergoing varying forms of therapy for bad backs.

Only about one out of twenty people with bad backs will ever require surgery, according to Dr. Leon Root, a New York orthopedic surgeon and coauthor with Thomas Kiernan of the book *Oh My Aching Back* (New York: David McKay, 1973). However, such reassurance is of little solace to someone doubled over with a bad and painful back. There are nutritional steps anyone can take right now to avoid a life with backache, or to help those who have one to handle it with common sense, so that a single episode of backache does not lead to a lifetime of agony.

## Vitamin C Plays a Big Role

Vitamin C is one of the nutrients which can prevent or come to the aid of an aching back, says Dr. James Greenwood, Jr., of Baylor University College of Medicine, Houston, Texas. Dr. Greenwood insists on more vitamin C for all patients with back problems. "We have seen that large doses of vitamin C help patients with back, neck, or leg pain due to spinal disc injuries. Some people have been able to avoid the necessity for surgery and others have been able to avoid returns of the syndrome when their vitamin C intake was greatly increased."

The relationship between vitamin C, the building of bones, blood vessels, cartilage, and collagen has, in fact, been long established. The late W.J. McCormick, M.D., international expert on vitamin C, pointed out that one of the most definite physiological functions of vitamin C is that of assisting in the formation of collagen for the maintenance of stability and elasticity of connective tissues generally. And this would include the bones, cartilage, muscles, and vascular tissues, Dr. McCormick said in *Archives of Pediatrics* (January 1954).

It was this relationship of vitamin C to the building of collagen which first prompted Dr. Greenwood to try vitamin C for his own personal stab in the back which had been keeping him on and off the heating pad for a period of 10 years while his pain grew more excruciating with each attack. About four months after he started taking 100 mg. of vitamin C three times a day, he noticed that he was comfortable and able to exercise without difficulty. Serving as his own control, Dr. Greenwood cut the vitamin C out of his daily schedule. He was promptly back on the heating pad. When he resumed taking vitamin C, his back improved.

Then the Texas neurosurgeon applied the benefits of his own experience to more than 500 patients with back pain who reported gratifying relief even when the pain was caused by a slipped disc. Dr. Greenwood recommends 250 mg. three times a day with an increase to 1,000 or 1,500 mg. daily if there is any discomfort, or if heavy exercise is anticipated. Some patients, he said, need 1,500 to 2,000 mg. a day.

# Exercise and Vitamin C

Further evidence of the value of vitamin C as a preventive of muscle stiffness comes from Dr. I.H. Syed, a London physician who wrote in the correspondence columns of the *British Medical Journal* (30 July 1966) that, "Muscle stiffness which arises after exercise or unaccustomed work can be prevented or treated by taking massive doses of ascorbic acid."

Dr. Syed found that 500 mg. of vitamin C before exercise and 400 mg. after exercise, together with plenty of fluids, was usually sufficient to prevent stiffness developing next morning. "But if it does develop, it is usually very slight and is easily cleared up by taking an additional 400 mg. of vitamin C and extra fluids, and if required, one or two hourly doses of 200 mg. As Dr. Syed explained, "Vitamin C looks after the endothelial lining of the capillaries. Therefore it may prevent damage or puncture of these capillaries in muscles during exercise. It may also help detoxification of metabolites and by its diuretic effect help with excretion."

If your doctor has determined that your problem is muscular, you should avoid the rigid posture that many backachers assume, say Ellen B. Lagerfwerff and Karen A. Perlroth, authors of *Mensendieck Your Posture and Your Pains* (New York: Doubleday, 1973). Generally the reaction to a sensation of discomfort is to hold the body rigid, the authors point out. But a rigid body cultivates muscular pains. "As a rule, if you sense discomfort in your muscles, move. Usually, this will bring about the longed-for relief immediately." At first it may be agony to break through the barrier of pain. But movement in and around the affected area will eventually release the muscular pain. Any on-and-off muscular activity is better than no movement at all, say the authors.

There's a difference between relieving symptoms and taking care of the problem. Good nutrition, lots of vitamin C, and the correct alignment of your body, whether you are sitting, standing, walking, or resting, can do more than you realize to get at the basic causes of the ache in your back that makes you so happy when it goes away.

## Vitamin C Can Help In Stress-Related Aches

Many patients with a pain in the back or neck try to ignore it. They drive themselves beyond their endurance until they suffer from general fatigue. The fatigue itself, instead of inducing sleep, produces nervous energy and tension. This nervous tension drives the patient on to greater endeavor, resulting in more fatigue, and this vicious cycle continues with more pain as the result, say Drs. William K. Ishmael and Howard B. Shorbe of Oklahoma City in their booklet, *Care of the Back* (New York: Lippincott, 1964).

"Life situations provoking grief, resentment, guilt, anger, or other emotional reactions may initiate or aggravate these nervous and muscular tension states," according to the Oklahoma physicians.

An emotional strain is a stress situation. While vitamin C helps the body to meet its stresses, it is used up in the process so that stress situations can therefore cause a depletion of this vital substance making you a candidate for many physical ailments including the excruciating stab in the back.

Vitamin C is only one of the nutrients involved in this aching back syndrome. "A lack of calcium, protein, vitamins, and other essential nutrients may produce fatigue rendering the back susceptible to strain," say Drs. Ishmael and Shorbe.

Studies done many years ago by Dr. Henry A. Gozan indicate that nutrition can effect a change in the hormone balance and that the body, including the bony structure of the back, will take care of itself if given the proper nutrition, according to an article in the *New York State Journal of Medicine* (15 May 1952).

# CHAPTER 86

# Weak and Brittle Bones

We need ultraviolet radiation, which is a component of sunlight, to maintain the health of our bones. The problem is that between us and the sun, there are too many "filters" which prevent that portion of the sunlight from reaching us. This is especially true in winter.

When natural sunlight reaches our skin the ultraviolet portion activates a lipid substance just below the surface called 7-dehydrocholesterol. We cannot see ultraviolet light, but 7-dehydrocholesterol knows it's there and responds by forming cholecalciferol, which is natural vitamin D, or $D_3$.

Without vitamin D, the body cannot properly utilize calcium. As a result, bone health suffers. The bones themselves deteriorate, lose calcium, and grow weaker and more prone to fracture. Two bone disorders which result from inadequate calcium utilization are osteomalacia and osteoporosis. Osteomalacia, the adult form of rickets, is a direct result of vitamin D deficiency. The bones, particularly those of the spine, pelvis, and lower extremities, become demineralized. And as the bones become softer, the body's weight causes the long bones to bow, the vertebrae to compress, and the pelvic bones to flatten.

Osteoporosis also involves the loss of minerals from bones. Rather than softening, however, the bones become porous and brittle. Pain eventually develops in the back, and loss of height occurs as weight-bearing vertebrae weaken and fracture. Both of these disorders can lead to the kind of serious bone fragility that makes every slip or fall a potential disaster.

Falls are the leading cause of non-transport related accidental deaths, and the leading cause of all accidental deaths in elderly white females, according to Albert P. Iskrant, M.A., F.A.P.H.A., chief of Epidemiology and Surveillance Branch, Injury Control Program of the Public Health Service, writing in the *American Journal of Public Health* (March 1968).

Fractures are the most common injuries involved in these tragic episodes, responsible for over 75 percent of deaths from falls. Age and sex are definitely important factors. In a localized study reported by Dr. Iskrant, 85 percent of the accident injuries to elderly persons requiring hospitalization were the result of falls. Females outnumbered males three to one. Most of the men were injured outdoors, while most of the women were injured indoors. Interestingly, almost two-thirds of the hip fractures had "no apparent cause."

## Ordinary Actions Can Snap Bones

Further investigation uncovered that large numbers of hip fractures are associated with such ordinary actions as walking or getting out of a chair. Fractures of the thigh bone were also studied and found to be "associated with moderate trauma (slight bumps), with advancing age, and 'femaleness'." Data from the National Health Survey, considering all fractures, said Dr. Iskrant, "show the peak rate in males in the 15 to 24 age group with a declining rate with increasing age. In females, however, the rate increases with age, reaching its peak in the 65 and over age group. Moreover, the fracture rate is higher in elderly females than in elderly men. When only fractures of the femur (thigh bone) are considered, the rate for females 65 and over is almost eight times that of the males 65 and over (9 to 1.2). The rate for females 65 and over is higher than for any other age-sex group."

Dr. Iskrant and his colleagues believe that osteoporosis-related bone fragility increases the likelihood of fracture in conjunction with "moderate trauma." Early findings in a study at Ford Hospital, Detroit, designed to investigate this belief, have shown "that there is a positive association between the incidence of fractures and the degree of osteoporosis in females over 45. There is also a positive association between the incidence of fractures and increasing age. The age-adjusted fracture rate of women with severe osteoporosis was about three times the rate of 'nonosteoporotic' women."

Osteomalacia, the second threat to bone strength, was discovered to be "not uncommon" in elderly men and women in a 1971 British study conducted by B. E. C. Nordin (*British Medical Journal*, 1, 571). And osteomalacia was associated with 50 out of 134 patients who had suffered suspicious fractures of the thighbone in another British study conducted by Jean Aaron, of the Mineral Metabolism Unit at the General Infirmary at Leeds, England, reported in the *Lancet* (13 July 1974).

Of course, *anyone* who's not getting enough vitamin D is in danger of developing osteomalacia or osteoporosis. But the elderly, the house-bound, and the long-staying hospital patients are especially susceptible.

The introduction of new, highly sensitive means of determining blood levels of vitamin D enabled Dr. D. Corless and his colleagues from the Department of Geriatric Medicine, St. Bartholomew's Hospital, London, to compare vitamin D status accurately in a number of different situations. Four groups of elderly patients were classified according to the amount of exposure to sunlight and amount of vitamin D supplementation. These in turn were compared to a "control" group of younger subjects.

The main finding, reported in the *Lancet* (28 June 1975), was the very low level of vitamin D in the long-stay patients compared with the younger group. The group of long-stay patients never exposed to sunlight had a median level of vitamin D only one-seventeenth as much as the younger subjects. The group occasionally exposed to sunlight had a median level one-fifth as much as the younger subjects. A third group, consisting of patients treated with 1,000 to 1,500 I.U. of synthetic vitamin D daily, had blood levels one-seventh as great as the younger group. But when the dosage was increased to 50,000 I.U. daily in a fourth group, the level of vitamin D in the blood reached or exceeded the upper range of that reached by the younger control group. Apparently, a little bit of sunshine is better than a low dose of synthetic vitamin D.

Dr. Corless determined through further tests that blood levels of calcium were the same for all patients, treated or not. But without vitamin D or vitamin D-producing sunshine, the calcium is not deposited where it belongs, in the bones.

## The Sun, the Lamp, or D₃

A study conducted by Richard J. Wurtman and Robert Neer, mentioned in Wurtman's "The Effects of Light on the Human Body" in *Scientific American* (July 1975), measured the effect of sunlight on calcium absorption. "The study, conducted among elderly, apparently normal men at the Chelsea Soldiers Home near Boston, suggested that a lack of adequate exposure to ultraviolet radiation during the long winter months significantly impairs the body's utilization of calcium, even when there is adequate supply in the diet."

During the first seven winter weeks of Wurtman's study, two groups of men remained indoors during daylight hours. At the end of the seven weeks, the men in both groups were found to absorb only about 40 percent of the calcium in their diets. In the next four weeks, one group remained indoors, while the other group was exposed for eight hours per day to a special fluorescent lamp (Vita-Lite) which is designed to simulate the solar spectrum in the visible and near ultraviolet regions. While the control group's ability to absorb calcium fell another 25 percent, that of the experimental group, receiving light from the special lamp, rose by 15 percent.

"The additional amount of ultraviolet radiation received by the experimental subjects was roughly equivalent to what they would get during a 15-minute lunchtime walk in the summer," according to the study.

Unfortunately, no one can take a 15-minute summer lunchtime walk in the winter. In winter, because of the change in the angle at which the earth receives the sun's radiation, only a tiny fraction of the summer levels of ultraviolet radiation reaches the earth. In December, the amount is one-fifteenth the amount present in June, in the northern third of the United States.

The body can store vitamin D, but after a month or so of winter "darkness," unsupplemented vitamin D levels sink dangerously low. Jean Aaron, who led the mineral metabolism study in Leeds, England, found that osteomalacia is far more prevalent in autopsy samples collected during winter than it is in samples collected during summer.

Of course, more than decreased amounts of vitamin D-producing sunlight threaten bone health in winter. Even if it were practical to spend more than half of each winter day outdoors to stimulate enough vitamin D production, the ice and snow would make dangerous falls more likely.

The surest way to guarantee adequate vitamin D is through natural vitamin $D_3$, usually obtained from fish liver oil. As mentioned in Wurtman's *Scientific American* article, researchers at the Washington University School of Medicine, found that 70 to 90 percent of vitamin D activity in blood samples was accountable to vitamin $D_3$ or its derivatives. Fortification of foods with artificial vitamin D is not as effective nutritionally as the vitamin D formed by sunlight.

But when winter makes it next to impossible to get all the vitamin D our bones need from a walk in the sun, you can get natural vitamin $D_3$ from fish liver oil to make up the difference.

# CHAPTER 87

# Asthmatic Children
# Can Turn to Vitamin B₆ for Relief

At the Nassau County Medical Center a team of five physicians, headed by Platon J. Collipp, M.D., chief of the Center's Department of Pediatrics, presented convincing evidence in *Annals of Allergy* (August 1975) that vitamin B₆ or pyridoxine is a remarkably safe and effective source of relief for many asthma victims.

Dr. Collipp and his colleagues first took note of vitamin B₆ levels in asthmatic children because of the results of a standard diagnostic test—the tryptophan load test. Clinicians use this technique to determine whether the body is getting enough vitamin B₆ and is using it properly. The patient is given an oral dose of tryptophan, an essential amino acid that requires B₆ for proper metabolism. If B₆ levels, for whatever reason, are inadequate, metabolic breakdown products are formed in abnormally large amounts. The presence of high levels of the metabolites xanthurenic and kynurenic acid in the patient's urine after swallowing tryptophan is usually a warning signal that the patient is not getting enough B₆.

Tryptophan load tests administered to 32 children with bronchial asthma had indeed resulted in high levels of xanthurenic acid and kynurenic acid. Dr. Collipp and his colleagues decided to step up the B6 intake of five of the children to see what would happen. The children first received 50 mg. of B6 for three months, and then 100 mg. for six more months. Tryptophan load tests were repeated periodically. At the end of the nine months, levels of excreted xanthurenic and kynurenic acid in the children's urine had dropped to near normal levels, indicating that they were finally getting enough B6.

But something much more dramatic also happened while the youngsters were taking the vitamin: their asthma symptoms (these five subjects all suffered from severe asthma which had required frequent hospitalization) were reduced, and they showed definite clinical improvement. In fact, the more vitamin B6 the children received, the better they felt.

## Results Come After One Month

Encouraged by these results, Dr. Collipp and his coworkers prepared a more elaborate clinical study. Seventy-six young asthma patients, ranging in age from two to 16 years, were selected. All suffered from moderate to severe asthma. The children were divided into two groups: half received two 100 mg. tablets of vitamin B6 daily; the other half took two placebo or dummy tablets. Neither doctors nor patients knew who was receiving the pyridoxine—a true double-blind study.

During a period of five months, parents evaluated their children's condition every day. Using special forms, all symptoms, such as wheezing, difficult breathing, cough, tightness in the chest, and number of asthma attacks, were carefully recorded. Each month the children were examined by doctors and the forms were collected and analyzed.

The results were astonishing. During the first month of the trial both groups fared about the same. However, beginning the second month, the group receiving 200 mg. of B6 daily experienced fewer asthma attacks than the controls. These children had significantly less wheezing, coughing, tightness, and breathing difficulty. As a result, they required less medication—in the form of oral bronchodilators and cortisone—than children not receiving the vitamin. These differences continued until the trial ended, being most significant during the second and fifth months.

"The data from these patients suggest that pyridoxine therapy may be a useful medication which reduces the severity of asthma in many, but not all, asthmatic children," Dr. Collipp and his colleagues concluded.

## B₆ Safer Than Many Asthma Drugs

The success of the B₆ therapy is enhanced by the fact that other, more widely used asthma therapies can involve some risk. For example, prednisone, a steroid drug commonly prescribed for bronchial asthma, may produce such serious adverse reactions as convulsions, glaucoma, peptic ulcer, and psychic derangements. Steroids are even capable of suppressing growth in children. Another popular medication, isoproterenol, which is inhaled through the mouth when an acute bronchial attack strikes, can actually cause increased airway obstruction in certain individuals. In some instances, misuse of such inhalers has resulted in abnormal heart rhythm and even death.

Pyridoxine, however, produced no side effects at all, according to the Nassau County Medical Center researchers, even at the 200 mg. dosage level—more than 100 times higher than the Recommended Daily Allowance for B₆ set by the National Academy of Sciences.

Dr. Collipp and his associates pointed out that the asthmatic children who were helped by vitamin B₆ apparently suffered from B₆ *dependency,* not deficiency. That is, some uniqueness in their biochemical makeup dictates an abnormally high pyridoxine requirement for optimum health.

The researchers could not fully explain how extra B₆ helps such individuals. Perhaps, they theorized, the key is pyridoxine's influence on the production of serotonin and epinephrine, two imperfectly understood body chemicals that very probably play a role in asthma. On the other hand, B₆ might simply benefit asthma sufferers by calming the central nervous system.

In any event, there is no denying the fact that relief does follow B₆ supplementation, at least for some asthma victims. "The beneficial results were generally apparent by the second month of treatment if improvement was going to occur," the researchers concluded.

# CHAPTER 88

# Vitamin C and Cancer

Can vitamin C really do anything to combat an already-established cancer? Answering that question is difficult, even now that there is a detailed report from Scotland, where two doctors, one a surgeon, gave large doses of vitamin C to 50 consecutive advanced cancer patients. The general impression, though, of Dr. Ewan Cameron and Dr. Allan Campbell is that "Our clinical findings support the general contention that large doses of ascorbic acid enhance natural resistance to cancer. Further, we have found this form of medication to have definite palliative (symptomatic relief) value in the management of terminal 'untreatable' human cancer" (*Chemico-Biological Interactions,* 9, 1974, 285–315).

The first question that needs to be asked is why vitamin C should even be tried in treating cancer. Was this study a mere "fishing expedition"? Did the doctors get a government research grant on the wild guess that vitamin C might be helpful in treating cancer?

Not exactly. In another article in the same issue of *Chemico-Biological Interactions*, an international science journal, Dr. Cameron and Linus Pauling, Ph.D., director of the Linus Pauling Institute of Science and Medicine in Menlo Park, California, reviewed some of the highly suggestive bits of evidence that vitamin C, or ascorbic acid, may act in several ways to increase resistance to cancer. Chiefly, it's believed that vitamin C strengthens the natural defense mechanisms that help protect us not only against cancer, but against all disease.

Drs. Cameron and Pauling underline the importance of this natural resistance to cancer by mentioning a 1973 study published in the journal, *Cancer*. That report showed that while malignant cells were detected in the circulating blood of about half of all patients undergoing resection of colon and rectal cancers, this finding appeared to have no significance at all in predicting which patients were going to be alive at the end of five years. That's important, because some people have the idea that to treat cancer, every last cell in the body which is cancerous must be destroyed. Obviously this isn't the case, Drs. Cameron and Pauling point out. If it were, every one of those patients in whom malignant cells were found in the circulating blood would have been dead from cancer at the end of five years. Somehow, their bodies must have been able to cope with those malignant cells in such a manner as to prevent them from establishing new malignancies.

## The Rationale Behind Trying Vitamin C

How does vitamin C fit into the picture of increasing these natural defense mechanisms? First, say the authors, the ability of the organism to encapsulate the spreading cancer in a "relatively impermeable barrier of dense fibrous tissue" may depend on the dietary availability of ascorbic acid, because this nutrient is necessary to build fibrous tissue. Vitamin C is also needed to give lymphocytes enough vitality to effectively attack invading foreign bodies in the system. And cancer may be one of the foreign bodies lymphocytes attack. Another area of possible importance for vitamin C is in the functioning of the adrenal and pituitary glands, which normally have a very high concentration of ascorbic acid. Under stress, however, the vitamin C is quickly depleted—and cancer certainly stresses the system to its very limits. By feeding these glands all the vitamin C they need to produce their hormones, the body may be better able to cope with such stress, Drs. Cameron and Pauling suggest.

Moving from theory to laboratory experiences, the authors point out that when laboratory animals are challenged with a powerful cancer-causing chemical, methylcholanthrene, this triggers a sudden upswing in their natural synthesis of ascorbic acid. In rats that develop tumors, the production of vitamin C goes even higher. On a body-weight basis, they produce the equivalent, in a 154-pound man, of 16 grams (16,000 mg.) of vitamin C a day.

Man, of course, has lost the ability to synthesize vitamin C, and must get it in his diet. But under the challenge of cancer, the dietary intake of vitamin C does not necessarily increase in man as the production of vitamin C does in most animals. In fact, two British doctors recently reported in *Medical World News* (24 February 1975) that patients with malignant disease are apt to have extremely low intakes of vitamin C, to the point where they may develop scurvy. They therefore urge that all cancer patients be given vitamin supplements.

Scientists believe that a number of cancers may be caused by viruses, and if this is true, vitamin C may have an important role here, because several studies have shown that vitamin C tends to have a general antiviral effect. An antibacterial effect has also been described, which Drs. Cameron and Pauling point out could be important, because many tumors become ulcerated, making the patient vulnerable to a secondary bacterial invasion, which weakens him.

Finally, there are a few studies, mostly German, and published during the forties and fifties, indicating that there is "some clinical improvement" in cancer patients who are given vitamin C. However, because these patients were also being given drugs or radiation, it is difficult to assign much importance to them, except to note that the doctors who reported the studies seem impressed with the potential value of vitamin C in such cases.

## Fifty Patients, All 'Beyond' Therapy

That brings us to the series of 50 patients treated by Drs. Cameron and Campbell. Dr. Cameron is a consultant surgeon at Dunbartonshire Hospitals in Scotland and a nonresident Fellow of the Linus Pauling Institute of Science and Medicine. Dr. Campbell is a consultant physician at Lanarkshire Hospitals, also in Scotland.

Although only 50 patients are included in their current report, the doctors actually gave vitamin C to many more patients, but excluded them from the study for various reasons. For example, because J.U. Schlegel, M.D., of the Department of Surgery of Tulane University, has reported that extra vitamin C can prevent bladder cancer in animals and is a "possible preventive measure" in regard to bladder cancer in man, all patients with bladder cancer were given vitamin C. However, they were also given standard methods of cancer treatment, so they were not included in the current study.

In some cases, patients who had originally been diagnosed as being "untreatable," and who were given vitamin C, improved so much on the vitamin regimen that it became ethically imperative to immediately give them established forms of cancer treatment as well. All these patients were therefore excluded from the study. That left only those patients who were considered by Drs. Cameron and Campbell, as well as at least one other independent clinician, as not having any chance at all of benefiting from any form of therapy. In most cases, they were considered "terminal." At best, they suffered from advanced cancer, and were beyond the hope of any known therapy.

Most of the patients received 10 grams (10,000 mg.) of ascorbic acid daily, in four divided doses. Some received more. In the beginning, the vitamin C was administered by injection, but eventually, the doctors decided that this was no better than giving it orally.

# Vitamin C Isn't 'Harmless' to a Cancer Patient

One of the first surprises in this study was not a pleasant one. Long experience with vitamin C has led to the general impression that it is amazingly harmless, even in large amounts. In cancer patients, it turned out, this is not always true. Some patients proved not to be able to tolerate high doses of vitamin C in their stomachs, particularly those whose disease involved the upper alimentary tract. Some of these patients suffered from heartburn, nausea, and acid regurgitation. On the other hand, although fears have been expressed that when more than four grams of ascorbic acid are taken daily there is an increased risk of developing oxalate kidney stones, not one patient out of 50 developed any problems along these lines.

The biggest surprise, though, was that in four patients the large doses of vitamin C produced a catastrophic deterioration in a matter of days. In all cases, it seemed that the vitamin C had actually caused the tumor to hemorrhage and become necrotic (dead). Although the bleeding produced by this process proved fatal because the tumors were so large, Drs. Cameron and Campbell point out that this reaction "is in fact a manifestation of the very strong defense reaction, and would certainly be regarded as a very favorable response indeed in patients suffering from earlier and more localized lesions."

That was the outcome in four patients out of 50. In 17 other patients, nothing much of anything happened that could be attributed to vitamin C. Actually, that's not exactly true, because the majority of the patients in this study felt better after beginning vitamin C, and suffered less from pain. But right now, we're just talking about the progress of the disease itself and not the subjective symptoms. For this purpose, then, the 17 patients had "no response."

Ten patients had what Drs. Cameron and Campbell call a "minimal response." Some patients in this group seemed to take a slight turn for the better before going downhill, as expected. In other cases, the improvement was more dramatic, but was eventually followed by a surprisingly swift state of deterioration.

In 11 patients, the development of the tumor or tumors seemed definitely to be slowed down. Case No. 29, a 67-year-old man, was typical. Suffering an inoperable cancer of the gallbladder and liver, he was expected to live not more than a few weeks. A week after beginning the vitamin C regimen, his appetite returned, he gained weight, and his obstructive jaundice problem improved. He died at home 209 days after starting on vitamin C.

## The Eight Most Interesting Cases

In three patients, the megadoses of vitamin C brought cancer to a standstill. A 56-year-old woman with adenocarcinoma of the colon underwent surgery but her condition had already spread to her liver. Curiously—perhaps significantly—when she began taking vitamin C, she experienced discomfort in the region of the liver, but was encouraged to keep taking it, and the side effect eventually went away after about two months. "Now," the two physicians reported, "some 18 months later, (she) remains clinically well, with no evidence to suggest progressing malignancy."

Two other patients responded similarly; although they were hardly "cured," they simply stopped getting worse. In five patients there was actual regression, or shrinking, in size of the tumor. But this didn't always mean that the patient recovered.

A 55-year-old man with cancer of the kidney that had spread to his right shoulder and left hip was put on ascorbic acid after undergoing surgery. At the time, he was not in severe pain, but was unable to work. He began taking 10 grams a day of vitamin C on 10 April 1972. There was steady symptomatic improvement with pain relief, and he was able to return to his job. Even more encouraging, x rays showed that his bones seemed to be fighting off the cancer, and were becoming recalcified where they had been eaten away with cancer growth. After one year, however, his condition took a turn for the worse. At this time, his vitamin C dose was doubled to 20 grams a day, and he again improved for a number of months. Following this improvement, however, the disease once again flared up and he died on 25 January 1974, 656 days after beginning ascorbic acid treatment. Two other patients also died eventually, but not because of cancer. In both cases, autopsies showed that there had apparently been significant regression of cancerous growths.

Another patient had an extremely dramatic response to treatment. In a matter of weeks, his enlarged liver and spleen returned to normal size and there were other signs of very significant regression found in x rays and biopsies. Eventually, his dose of ascorbic acid was reduced and finally eliminated. Unfortunately, a few weeks later, the malignancy began to return and he was again put on ascorbic acid therapy—which at the time of their report, the doctors say, seemed to be inducing a second regression.

Another man, 69, was operated on in 1969 for cancer of the colon. In 1972, he was readmitted to the hospital, deteriorating, with numerous signs that the cancer had returned in his liver. Six months after beginning the ascorbic acid therapy, all his liver function tests returned to normal. "More than 2.5 years later, (he) continues with his ascorbic acid and remains fit, active, and well in all respects with no clinical or biochemical indication of neoplastic disease," Drs. Cameron and Campbell write.

## What It Means—And What Must Be Done

The big question at this point is whether or not the survival times of this group of patients were significantly longer than they would have been without taking vitamin C. The only way to pin down such an effect would have been for the doctors to have not treated another group of 50 patients whose conditions closely matched those of the treated patients. This wasn't done. And if it had been done, the doctors report, they would have broken the "control," because as their clinical experience increased, "we felt it to be ethically wrong to withhold ascorbic acid in otherwise hopeless situations, merely for the sake of obtaining observations of dubious significance for statistical comparison.

"However," they declare, "it is our opinion that most clinicians familiar with the practical realities of terminal cancer . . . would be inclined to agree that many of these patients survived much longer than reasonable clinical expectation."

Beyond the question of survival time, Drs. Cameron and Campbell report that in a number of patients they treated, giving ascorbic acid "produced quite dramatic relief from pain and opiate dependence in a matter of days." There were other benefits as well, one of which was that all patients who had malignant disease of the urinary tract experienced a significant reduction in the amount of blood in their urine, and a reduction in pain and distress as well. In at least six cases, the doctors say, "there is indisputable clinical and biochemical evidence to show that reversal of terminal malignant jaundice was induced for significant periods of time."

The doctors who made this report consider it to be a "pilot study" designed to see if there is any reason for conducting a more extensive and more carefully controlled test of vitamin C in cancer patients. The answer to this question, they believe, is definitely affirmative. If it does nothing more than relieve pain, it would be of great value. But there is good evidence to indicate that vitamin C may do more than this.

Drs. Cameron and Campbell say that they "expect it to have even greater value when used in the treatment of earlier and more favorable patients." Looking ahead, they state, "We believe that, in time, ascorbic acid supplementation will come to be accepted as a standard measure in most, if not all, forms of cancer treatment. We conclude that large-scale clinical trials along such lines are now clearly indicated."

## Prevention is Still the Greatest Hope

Findings in a number of scientific laboratories suggest that supplemental amounts of vitamin C might help protect against a number of cancers which arise from environmental toxins. But the protective action of vitamin C is not universal—it only applies to a limited number of carcinogens. And it is only one possible means of protection. Other nutrients are also important: vitamin A, thiamine, and magnesium are among those which have been mentioned by scientists as being of possible importance. Even more important, no doubt, is avoiding as many dangerous chemicals as you can, and this means no smoking, no steady or heavy drinking, no chemical aerosols or cosmetic preparations, and perhaps filtration of the air if you live near an industrial complex.

But with regard to vitamin C, the distinction between preventing malignancy and fighting one which is already established may turn out to be artificial. Irwin Stone, in *The Healing Factor* (New York: Grosset and Dunlap, 1972), has put forward the thesis that human beings lost the ability to produce their own vitamin C through an evolutionary accident, and came to depend upon eating large amounts of fresh natural foods which were rich in this vitamin. If you put this theory next to the fact that laboratory rats with tumors increase their production of vitamin C to a higher level, you could postulate that getting extra vitamin C at the time of serious illness is like restoring a natural protection which we lost somewhere in our long evolutionary history.

Drs. Cameron and Pauling cite a medical report published in 1972 indicating that routine autopsies frequently find small cancers which have evidently been completely controlled for many years. Such cancers may outnumber actual clinical cases of cancer by as much as 40 to one, they say. This lends further credence to the idea that our bodies do have a very powerful natural protective mechanism against cancer, and that when this disease becomes frightfully evident, the "fault" is not so much the presence of cancer, but the failure of these natural mechanisms to keep it in check.

When Dr. Linus Pauling gave his dedication speech at the opening of Ben May Laboratories for Cancer Research at the University of Chicago in 1971, he predicted that an adequate intake of ascorbic acid might reduce cancer-related illness and death by some 10 percent, with a possible saving of some 15,000 to 20,000 lives in the United States alone each year. Here is where our greatest hope lies—in primary prevention. If the further clinical trials which Drs. Cameron and Campbell call for produce some positive results in the early stages of malignancy, it will point the way to transforming Pauling's prediction into reality, and perhaps even exceeding it.

# CHAPTER 89

# Nonsurgical Treatment of Precancerous Polyps

We usually think of vitamin C as being a valuable help in a number of ordinary and moderately troublesome disorders—the common cold being the most obvious example. But new research coming to light strongly suggests that something as simple as vitamin C may also play an important role in preventing diseases generally regarded as incurable.

The first of these, familial polyposis, is a hereditary disorder in which large numbers of polyps or growths develop on the lining of the patient's colon. Any one of these polyps has a high probability of developing into a cancerous tumor.

The standard medical procedure in treating familial polyposis is drastic but apparently necessary; the entire colon is surgically removed. In some cases, the rectum is left in place and surgically connected to the small intestine to permit more normal bowel evacuation. Unfortunately, in most of these patients the dangerous polyps will reappear on the remaining section of rectum.

The standard procedure has required the surgical removal of the rectal polyps. But a team of five physicians at a well-known midwest cancer clinic, the Vince Lombardi Colon Clinic, Milwaukee, Wisconsin, has succeeded in eliminating or reducing the number of polyps in five out of eight polyposis patients by administering 3,000 mg. of vitamin C daily. This breakthrough in treating a relatively rare disease, by Jerome J. DeCosse, M.D., Ph.D., and his four colleagues in the Medical College of Wisconsin's Departments of Surgery and Pathology could ultimately lead to new hope for all those who live in fear of colon cancer, the number-two-cancer killer of American men and women.

Dr. DeCosse's patients were all men and women whose condition warranted the operation, called *ileorectal anastomosis,* in which part of the colon is removed and the ileum, or last section of the small intestine, is connected to the rectum. But the first five subjects chosen by Dr. DeCosse had undergone surgery anywhere from six to 21 years before the study, ruling out the possibility that any improvement now was due to spontaneous regression. Two people who were added to the study in progress had their operations less than a year previously. And an eighth and final subject was a woman who had not as yet had the operation.

## Results Very Promising

Treatment consisted of one gram of vitamin C taken three times each day in the form of a timed-release capsule. At varying intervals during the 13-month study, patients were examined and the number of polyps counted. The results were reported in *Surgery* (November 1975). In one of the initial five subjects, the number of polyps increased from 15 to 28 in six months of treatment. But in the remaining four people, the polyp count was substantially reduced: from 45 to 17 and eight to two in two patients, and from 29 to zero and ten to zero in the remaining two. Among the three people added to the study, two experienced an increase in their polyp count after four to six months of treatment. But the woman whose colon was still intact went from six polyps to three in four months.

Dr. DeCosse's attempt was the first serious effort to treat precancerous polyps without surgery. He said that follow-up examinations have confirmed the initial results: "Complete disappearance of polyps in two of our patients and a major reduction in three others, beyond the time limits of spontaneous regression and in excess of any errors in counting. We attribute this effect to ascorbic acid (vitamin C)."

The promising implications of the Wisconsin study are bound up in the reasons Dr. DeCosse used vitamin C in the first place. He believes polyps and colon cancer may be caused by chemicals in the colon which, when oxidized, become carcinogenic. Statistical studies, according to Dr. DeCosse, show that intestines of people living in areas with a high incidence of colon cancer have a larger proportion of the kind of bacteria that begin the oxidation process, than people living in low-incidence areas. Dr. DeCosse reasoned that since a chemical coming in contact with the walls of the colon might be causing the polyps, perhaps a chemical that could detoxify the carcinogens could be added to the contents of the gut. Such a chemical would have to prevent or reverse the oxidation process.

Because of vitamin C's known antioxidizing and antitumor properties, Dr. DeCosse chose it for his study. Timed-release capsules were used because the researchers wanted as much of the vitamin C as possible to reach the end of the digestive system intact, without being absorbed into the blood.

Dr. DeCosse explained that he chose people with familial polyposis for his study because the relatively high rate of spontaneous regression among people undergoing *ileorectal anastomosis* suggested that some element from the gut contents coming in direct contact with the remaining piece of rectum might be causing the improvement. Furthermore, with these patients, observation of the total "target" area for polyp formation was relatively easy.

Someday, vitamin C may be the first line of treatment for people with polyps.

## Regional Enteritis—A New Clue

Another study demonstrates that vitamin C apparently has a role in preventing serious intestinal lesions of another kind, those that occur in regional enteritis. Unlike polyposis, regional enteritis is not considered a precancerous condition, although the symptoms—cramps, diarrhea, fever, loss of appetite and weight, anemia—do mimic those of intestinal cancer. In this disease, the membranes of the lower section of the small intestine, the ileum, become inflamed. As the disease progresses, this vital tissue becomes swollen with fluid, abscessed, perforated, and fibrous. Fistulae, or abnormal channels from one organ to another, develop in a substantial percentage of sufferers. Until lately, doctors could not even come close to a real clue as to what causes regional enteritis. But now, it appears, they can.

Charles D. Gerson, M.D., and Eva M. Fabry of the Division of Gastroenterology, Mount Sinai School of Medicine, New York, measured the level of vitamin C in the blood and in the intestinal tissue of patients with regional enteritis. They discovered that patients with the inflammatory disease had significantly lower blood levels of vitamin C than control patients without the disease.

What's more, patients whose illness was aggravated by fistulae had tissue levels of vitamin C which were not only lower than those of people without enteritis, but also significantly lower than those of the patients with enteritis, but without fistulae. In other words, the less vitamin C, the worse the disease.

Dr. Gerson feels that the fistulae are most likely a result of the low levels of vitamin C in the blood and tissue of the patients. Without sufficient vitamin C, collagen—which is the "glue" that maintains the integrity of every single cell in the body—cannot be manufactured rapidly enough to repair ulcerations in the bowel wall. More than half of the patients with fistulae had blood levels of vitamin C which were actually lower than the levels at which the first signs of scurvy usually appear. But none of these people had what the medical establishment would acknowledge as scurvy. In *Gastroenterology* (September 1974), Dr. Gerson noted, too, that patients with regional enteritis are usually told to avoid raw fruits and vegetables, some of the highest food sources of vitamin C.

Some orthodox medical men would have the public avoid supplementary doses of vitamin C entirely. These critics say vitamin C interferes with the absorption of vitamin $B_{12}$. But the usual charge is that taking more than the government-dictated Recommended Daily Allowance of vitamin C is just wasteful since the excess is eliminated.

Dr. DeCosse's study answers both these charges. During the course of the clinical trials, Dr. DeCosse tested the blood of his patients for vitamin $B_{12}$. If the large doses of vitamin C he was giving them were rendering them deficient in $B_{12}$, he wanted to know about it. He found that they weren't. All blood levels of $B_{12}$ were normal—and none of the patients was receiving $B_{12}$ supplementation.

As for the idea that large doses of vitamin C are a waste, Dr. DeCosse's results demonstrate that vitamin C anywhere in the body can help maintain better health.

# CHAPTER 90

# Vitamins Against Skin Cancer

Months before the earth tilts toward the sun to bring summer to northern climes, millions flock to southern shores in search of a "Florida tan," the souvenir most proudly displayed on the wintry streets of the north. When summer finally embraces the entire land, tanning, which at one time was done only to leather to make it tougher, becomes the most fashionable pastime.

Those millions of seekers of "fun in the sun" don't realize it, but they are laying themselves open to the most common form of cancer: skin cancer. Each year, the over 300,000 recorded new cases of skin cancer make up almost one-third of the estimated new cases of cancer.

The majority of skin cancers are either basal or squamous cell cancers. Basal cell skin cancer begins as a small, red, raised sore which slowly enlarges and eventually displays a gray or pearly translucent border. The center of the lesion becomes depressed or ulcerated and sometimes heals. Basal cell carcinoma sometimes resembles a patch of psoriasis or seborrheic dermatitis. Slow to invade surrounding tissue, this form of skin cancer is relatively less deadly.

Squamous cell carcinoma begins as a raised red sore with a hard surface which eventually grows inward in a circular fashion and may ulcerate. This cancer is more deadly because it has a greater tendency to spread to vital body organs. Together, these two skin cancers account for about 97 percent of all cases of skin cancer, and about 30 percent of the deaths from skin cancer.

A third type of skin cancer, malignant melanoma, is the least common, with around 9,000 new cases expected in 1976. But melanoma is by far the most deadly, accounting for 70 percent of all skin cancer deaths. Melanomas begin as birthmarks and moles. While most of these heavily pigmented dots, taken for granted by most people, are not cancerous, one in a million does develop into a malignant melanoma. While dermatologists are certain that excessive exposure to sunlight is the primary factor in basal and squamous cell skin cancers, they have only recently begun to suspect sunlight's role in melanoma.

This suspicion is growing as researchers see more and more of these deadly cancers occurring on parts of the body, such as women's legs and upper backs of men and women, which have been exposed to sunlight more and more as fashions have grown "less modest" over the past half-century. Along with the change in fashions to more revealing, less protective clothing, the incidence of malignant melanoma has increased at a rate greater than any other human cancer, except lung cancer. Melanomas are practically nonexistent in areas of the body never exposed to sunlight.

While the incidence of skin cancer is high, the death rate is relatively low, about 5,000 people or one percent of the yearly cancer death toll. Doctors attribute this to the comparative ease of diagnosis—the cancer is usually obvious in its early stages—and simplicity of surgical removal. But its relatively benign nature should not lull us into ignoring the very real hazards of skin cancer.

Yet people will, of course, continue to worship the sun in the manner of their choice and, except for the 300,000 or so who will become cancer statistics, most will escape unscathed—or will they?

# Wrinkles From Sunburned Skin

According to leading dermatologists, such as John M. Knox, M.D., who is chairman of dermatology at Baylor College of Medicine in Houston, there are plenty of other reasons to avoid excessive exposure to the sun. While it may accelerate social acceptability, tanning can also accelerate aging. Year after year of soaking up free sunshine takes an expensive toll on the skin, leaving it with a tough, weather-beaten look usually associated with farmers and cowboys. Even cowboys, though, have the sense to wear ten-gallon hats.

Very little external aging is caused by genetic changes, says Dr. Knox. Constant exposure to the sun can multiply wrinkles and toughen the skin. "Gross changes in actinically (by sunlight) damaged skin take the form of a dry and leathery appearance, slackness with wrinkling and pigmentary changes."

This process is called *solar elastosis* and *senile elastosis* by others. The skin loses its elasticity because sunburn has damaged the collagen fibers in the upper part of the skin. These lesions often take the form of horny, calloused, wart-like growths called actinic or senile keratosis. Dry, leathery skin may be bad enough, but keratotic lesions are frequently forerunners of squamous cell skin cancers. Even when they don't develop into cancer, reported Albert K. Kligman, M.D., professor of dermatology at the University of Pennsylvania, they "can be more painful and disfiguring than cancer itself" (*Medical World News,* 12 January 1976).

As an example of what a difference the sun can make, dermatologists point out that it is hard to determine the age of most black people by examining the texture of their skin. This is because the skin of black people, protected as it is by its high content of pigment, does not suffer the aging—or the cancer-causing—effects of sunlight.

The natural response of white skin to sunlight, tanning, is a step in the right direction. But black people, who evolved in sunny climates, have had countless generations to adapt, so they are protected from birth. White-skinned people evolved in parts of the world where the sun was dangerous for only a few months out of the year, if at all. They have a relatively meager—and apparently inadequate—defense mechanism: upon exposure to sunlight, the outer skin thickens, and melanin, a brown pigment, is produced at an increased rate. The durable, sought-after, and to some extent protective tan, however, does not develop until days later.

Most people don't make it that long. Those who have had too much, too soon, usually know it from two to eight hours later, when the redness, the blistering, the pain, and the fever of sunburn strike. A false tan, brought about by the oxidation of melanin already present, may accompany sunburn. But it fades in a few hours, leaving behind only suffering.

Among white-skinned people, the ability to tan early, and therefore, resist burning, varies considerably. Those who burn easily, blister, and tan badly are higher risks for developing skin cancer and other adverse effects of sunlight, said Dr. Kligman. Blonds, redheads, and people who freckle easily are at the top of the list. "These people should stay indoors constantly, or they should use the best sunscreen they can find and use it every day."

## Why PABA Is the Best Protector

Since few people are willing or able to stay indoors when the sun shines, they need "the best sunscreen"—especially between the hours of 10 A.M. and 2 P.M. when ultraviolet radiation is most intense. "The best sunscreen available, confirmed by laboratory tests and outdoor trials, is para-aminobenzoic acid, or PABA," noted Dr. Kligman.

PABA is called, among dermatologists, a sun*screen,* not a sun*shade*, because rather than merely act as a physical barrier to sunlight, it has the ability to absorb those portions of the ultraviolet spectrum of sunlight which produce sunburn and skin cancers. A Harvard team of researchers, reporting in the *New England Journal of Medicine* (26 June 1969) showed that PABA in a solution of ethyl alcohol is the most effective sunscreen available.

The Harvard scientists tested a large number of suntan lotions in the Arizona desert and high in the Swiss Alps. They found that the PABA solutions "after a single application, can protect fair-skinned persons undergoing long exposure (over four hours) under natural sunlight, and are more effective than 24 of the commercially available products tested.

"Furthermore, after a single application, the three formulations (all of PABA or its related esters) afford excellent protection when subjects undergo exercise accompanied by profuse sweating, and tend to remain on the skin after bathing or swimming and exert a partial yet very satisfactory protection."

The Harvard team discovered that when the PABA solution is applied, it clings to the epidermis with a peculiar attraction, and actually enters into a chemical reaction with the stratum corneum layer of the skin. That's why it keeps on giving protection even after a brief swim or hours of perspiration. In contrast, nearly all the other preparations were found to be "ineffective," particularly when the person using them went for a swim or did a lot of exercise that produced perspiration. As if that weren't enough, the PABA preparation is also reported to be invisible, odorless, and colorless. Also, while it does prevent burning, it permits tanning. Its only drawback is that if not applied carefully, it can stain bathing suits.

The most recent laboratory tests to confirm PABA's protective abilities were performed by researchers in Washington, D.C. and Miami, Florida.

In the University of Miami study, groups of hairless mice were exposed to ultraviolet light in the dangerous wavelengths and treated with a chemical that produces cancer when the skin is exposed to light. One group of mice was also treated with a solution containing PABA. By the end of the study, it was evident that PABA afforded virtually complete protection from sunlight-induced skin cancer. The study results, reported in the *Journal of Investigative Dermatology* (December 1975), showed that while the mice not treated with PABA were afflicted with an average of six squamous cell tumors per animal, only one PABA-treated animal developed as much as a single tumor.

After two months without further ultraviolet light treatments, the PABA-treated mice had no additional cancers, while cancers on the untreated group grew to involve an average of more than 50 percent of each animal's skin. Furthermore, a follow-up examination of the surviving animals found the untreated animals to have thickened, yellow, wrinkled skin, while the skin of the PABA mice was remarkably normal.

The second study was conducted by a dentist concerned about sunlight-induced damage to the sensitive tissue of the lips. Lip cancer strikes over 4,000 people each year. Over 90 percent of its victims are men, who don't wear protective lipstick. Thomas F. Payne, D.D.S., M.S.D., tested the abilities of various commercial sunscreening preparations on the lips and forearms of 23 volunteers, and reported his results in the *Journal of the American Dental Association* (February 1976). Dr. Payne found that "agents containing PABA or its esters gave superior protection on both lip and skin when compared with all other agents." He recommended hourly application, although some preparations gave complete protection three hours after initial application.

# Two Vitamins Help Prevent Dangerous Oxidation

Two antioxidants, vitamins C and E, show promise that they can help prevent sun-induced skin cancer, according to recent findings of Dr. Homer S. Black and Dr. Wan-Bang Lo, dermatology researchers associated with the Baylor College of Medicine, Houston, Texas (*Nature,* 21–28 December 1973).

The Texas researchers studied the mechanism by which sunlight triggers skin cancer and discovered a very interesting phenomenon. After human or animal skin is exposed to ultraviolet light, cholesterol in the skin oxidizes and forms by-products (*Nature,* 3 December 1971). One of the by-products of this oxidation process is a substance called cholesterol alpha-oxide, a known cancer-causing chemical.

Since vitamins C and E are known to reduce the oxidation of fats, Drs. Black and Lo wondered if adding extra antioxidants to the diet might block the formation of the cancer-causing cholesterol oxide in the skin.

The first step was to determine if antioxidants taken orally would affect the concentration of antioxidants in the skin. To find out, they fed one group of mice an ordinary diet and another group the same diet supplemented with vitamins C, E, and other antioxidants of a chemical nature. Skin was obtained from animals sacrificed at intervals of two weeks, and irradiated for 30 minutes to simulate the effect of several hours of ultraviolet light.

The researchers discovered that those animals which had received a supplemented diet had 64 percent more antioxidants in their skin after two weeks than the other animals. The level decreased somewhat after this, but was maintained at about 18 percent above the control level for the next 24 weeks.

The really important finding, though, was that as the antioxidant content of the skin increased, the formation of cholesterol alpha-oxide decreased. In fact, complete protection against formation of this carcinogen was observed in those animals which had received the vitamin supplements during the first two weeks of the study, when the maximum increase of antioxidant content of the skin occurred. Approximately 50 percent-protection against formation of cholesterol alpha-oxide was afforded those animals fed the supplemental diet for four to 24 weeks, at which time the experiment ended.

This study shows that when supplemental antioxidants are consumed, they *do* get to the skin, and they *do* act as a deterrent to the formation of a carcinogenic substance induced by ultraviolet light. Your need for vitamins C and E tends to increase with time, and as you are repeatedly exposed to sunlight. They won't give you complete protection, but there's every reason to believe that they will help significantly.

# CHAPTER 91

# Folic Acid Treatment
# Combats Circulatory Problems

As people get older, many experience the consequences of indifferent nutrition by developing circulatory problems. Their arteries begin to thicken and lose their youthful elasticity, slowing the normal flow of blood throughout the body. Fortunately, nature has provided numerous collateral channels for the blood to flow through, but these channels must often be opened or dilated before they can handle the new blood flow.

By successfully using folic acid to treat arteriosclerosis and leg ulcers, two of the most common circulatory problems facing older people, Tibor L. Kopjas, M.D., Ph.D., demonstrated that this harmless vitamin is an effective means of improving circulation when given therapeutically. Dr. Kopjas' first study, which appeared in the *Journal of the American Geriatric Society* (November 1966), dealt with the treatment of arteriosclerosis, commonly known as hardening of the arteries.

Since folic acid seemed to be an effective dilator for small arteries, Dr. Kopjas was intrigued with its possible potential in the treatment of diffuse chronic arteriosclerosis where the small arteries are called upon to play a vital role. He undertook a study of 17 patients whom he divided into three groups according to age, duration of disease, and the degree of arterial damage.

In the first group, folic acid was administered intravenously to determine its immediate effects on the small arteries. About 40 minutes after the injection, the patients in this group, who were already suffering impaired vision as a result of insufficient circulation to the eyes, showed marked improvement. On a standard eye chart they were able to read two lines below the lines recorded before medication.

The second group consisted of seven patients who had had chronic diffuse peripheral vascular disease for at least 10 years. Most of them responded well to the folic acid. After the injection, all experienced the manifestations of improved circulation—pleasant warm feelings in the face and head within five minutes, in the hands within 10 minutes.

Six patients comprising the third group had diabetes mellitus, with diabetic retinopathy, where eyesight is greatly diminished, and arteriosclerosis obliterans (almost complete blockage of the arteries). Each took a five mg. folic acid tablet daily for four weeks. Improvement in vision and in skin temperature of affected limbs was observed by four patients. In two of these cases, there was healing of pregangrenous toe ulcers—dramatic manifestation of improved circulation. At no time did Dr. Kopjas note any increase in blood pressure or pulse rates. There were no side effects either during or after the study.

## Leg Ulcers Treated Successfully

As circulation in the legs becomes more and more restricted, tissue begins to deteriorate and even a small injury like a bump or any continuing pressure may result in an open sore that just won't heal. Many geriatric specialists feel that these chronic leg ulcers are among the most severe and disabling conditions of the lower extremities in older people.

Continuing his work on improving circulation with folic acid treatment, Dr. Kopjas reported his successful treatment of leg ulcers in the *Journal of the American Geriatrics Society* (March 1968). Dr. Kopjas explained that since all the nutritive elements, the oxygen supply, immunizing substances, and defensive cells are carried by the blood, patients with constricted blood passages are being deprived of the very healing power leg ulcers must have. He reasoned that widening the blood vessels would speed the healing of the leg ulcers, so he decided to try folic acid.

The average age of the three men and seven women selected for a test was 61. Four of them had moderate to advanced hardening of the arteries with resultant leg ulcers. One of these four had had a leg amputated above the knee because of advanced hardening of the arteries and gangrene with ulcers of the leg. Although the usual pharmaceutical vasodilators were used continuously on this patient, the stump had responded very slowly. Another of the patients with hardening of the arteries had vascular surgery for vein grafts because of severe arterial changes in the legs, but only two months after the operation a dime-sized ulcer developed on one of the legs. The other two patients suffering from advanced arteriosclerosis had small ulcers on each toe; the legs were cold, the pulse in the legs was slow, and skin color was bad. The six remaining patients had poor circulation in their legs with chronic ulcers of varying sizes.

## Results Excellent

Dr. Kopjas did no more than prescribe five mg. tablets of folic acid three times a day for three months. Four of the most seriously affected patients received, in addition to the regular dosage of folic acid, 20 mg. of folic acid twice weekly by injection. All of the patients but two dressed their ulcers every day with plain sterile gauze pads. The two exceptions suffered with infection and edema, so antibiotics and diuretics were prescribed until these conditions improved. Five of the patients continued with a previously prescribed maintenance dose of digitalis. Aside from this, no other medication was used during the three-month study period.

In six to eight weeks complete repair was achieved in the patients with the smaller ulcers (one to three centimeters in diameter). For patients with larger sores, healing took 12 weeks. After only two months of folic acid therapy, satisfactory repair of the ulcer was observed even in the stump of the amputee who previously had healing difficulties. His other leg also showed definite improvement in the skin color and temperature. For the patient who had earlier vascular surgery, the ulcer that appeared near the graft was completely healed in six weeks; both legs became noticeably warmer and walking improved. Only one out of the ten cases did not show complete healing of the ulcer in the 12 weeks, although it was reduced to about half its size. Dr. Kopjas believed that in this case, chronic atrophy in the toe, plus poor foot hygiene was responsible.

## How Folic Acid Works

X rays published with the article showed how folic acid works, apparently creating auxiliary routes for blood transmission when the major arteries are clogged. Dr. Kopjas explained that "In older patients with generalized vascular disease, the poor blood supply does not provide enough hydrodynamic pressure to dilate the small arteries and develop collaterals. . . ." That's where folic acid's effective vasodilation of the smaller blood vessels comes in.

Among the usual treatments for chronic leg ulcers and pains due to varicose veins are surgery, aspirin, antibiotics, cortisone, and pain killers that are known to have potentially dangerous side effects. No ill effects occurred with the folic acid treatment.

Equally important as a clear highway for the blood to travel, is having worthwhile elements for it to carry. "The state of nutrition is important for the efficiency of the healing process," according to Dr. Kopjas. "For instance, the protein depletion in malnourishment, chronic wasting disease, or avitaminosis C has a profound effect upon wound healing. Collagen formation is depressed, the integrity of the capillary wall is altered, and capillary rupture and hemorrhage hinder the healing process." So good diet counts heavily in speeding recovery.

# CHAPTER 92

# Vitamin E
# for Varicose Veins

Male doctors enjoy proclaiming that women enjoy a life expectancy which is considerably greater than that of men. What they almost never mention is that women of mature age are much more likely to develop chronic conditions which can make those extra years of life far from enjoyable. Most of these conditions involve the lower half of the body, particularly the legs. And most of them are a direct result of impaired blood circulation. The trouble appears to stem from the fact that during childbirth, fantastic pressure from the baby's emerging head distorts veins in the pelvic area which drain blood from the legs. As a result, blood tends to back up in the veins of the legs, disabling the venous valves whose job it is to fight the effects of gravity by preventing blood from lying stagnant in the veins or even slipping backwards when it should be pumped back to the heart. With these valves disabled, it is more difficult for the blood to run up the legs, and the result is that the veins stretch and expand under the increased pressure, making swift return of the blood even more difficult.

Following childbirth, a woman typically lies in bed for a number of days and thereafter spends an unusual amount of time "taking things easy." This aggravates the problem considerably, because even under normal conditions, the veins depend on muscle contractions in the legs to force the blood upward. The longer the period of immobilization, the greater tendency there is for the leg veins to become distended and incapacitated. And frequently, there is a period of constipation before and after childbirth, as a result of pressure on the lower bowel. But as waste matter collects in the colon, still more pressure is exerted on the portal vein, further retarding the return of venous blood from the lower extremities.

The result of all this—at least the most immediate and obvious result—is the development of varicose veins. But the unsightly blue cords popping out of the calves and ankles are only a superficial sign of deeper distress. That's because the veins that run near the surface of the skin normally transport only a small fraction of the venous blood. It is the veins deep inside the leg muscles which are designed to carry about 80 to 90 percent of the returning blood up and out of the legs. And it is these deep veins which are first affected by pressure against the large pelvic veins which they feed. What you are seeing in visible varicosities is nature's way of bypassing or at least easing the burden of invisible varicosities deep within the leg. Unfortunately, the superficial veins are all too often disabled themselves as they are forced to carry this extra burden.

Moreover, simple varicosities are only the beginning of the ordeal in many cases. The walls of the veins may become inflamed in a condition known as phlebitis. A dark red solid mass of fibrin and blood cells may plug the vein up in a more serious conditon known as thrombophlebitis. The danger here is that the clot may break loose from the wall of the vein and be carried swiftly to the lungs or heart, where it may obstruct a crucial blood vessel and precipitate a heart attack.

These complications of varicose veins are found more frequently in the aged than the young, and in many cases, according to Philip H. Rakov, M.D., of the Department of Surgery at the State University of New York at Syracuse, the diagnosis is difficult because the varicosities are not visible or discoverable by touch (*Geriatrics,* August 1970).

Varicosities of long duration are often also accompanied by ugly, itching eczema, and ulcerations, which can become frighteningly large and involve the entire leg structure, even down to the bone.

Still another condition which may result from the tremendous pressures of childbirth is hemorrhoids. And like varicose veins, hemorrhoids are further aggravated by both the pressure of an overloaded colon, and the subsequent straining at stool which may be necessary to empty it.

## How Vitamin E Can Help

There is something you can do about varicose veins besides ask a surgeon to strip, inject, cut, or freeze them. That something is to take vitamin E. According to numerous medical reports it is very often effective in alleviating or curing these results of impaired circulation. Not that vitamin E is the best or only preventive measure you can take or that it is always the best or only treatment. Lots of exercise, a minimum of chair sitting, and a bulky diet which prevents constipation are probably more important as primary preventive agents. However, vitamin E can be of very significant help, both as a preventive measure and as a treatment.

The pioneers in vitamin E therapy are Doctors Evan and Wilfrid Shute, of the world-famous Shute Foundation in London, Ontario, Canada. The Shute brothers are best known for their work in treating cardiovascular disease, but the beneficial action of vitamin E in the veins is, for all practical purposes, identical to its action in the arteries. And as we have seen, a blood clot which tears loose from a vein in the leg is as dangerous as one in an artery, and can easily bring about a heart attack. So the use of vitamin E for phlebitis is very intimately associated with its use in controlling heart disease.

Specifically, Dr. Evan Shute on 6 June 1958, told the Second World Congress of Obstetrics and Gynecology in Montreal, Canada, that in a group of 166 patients, all of whom had chronic phlebitis, 32 patients got excellent or complete relief, 79 cases good relief, 20 cases moderate relief, and 35 cases slight relief after treatment with vitamin E. Most of these patients had suffered from one to five years and some of them had had phlebitis for longer than six years.

One man of 47 had suffered for six years with the usual swelling and soreness. He was given 300 mg. and later 400 mg. of vitamin E daily. The trouble in one of his legs cleared four days after the dosage was raised to 400 mg. At his last visit he could walk half a mile each day and there was no tenderness in his leg. His feet swelled very slightly and ached a little on rare occasions.

Dr. Shute went on to explain to his colleagues why vitamin E should have such a striking beneficial effect on all these patients. Vitamin E, he said, "produces collateral circulation about the obstructed deep veins by calling into play the unused networks of veins lying in wait for emergency utilization. We have such venous reserves just as we have reserves of brain, lung, and liver. Alpha-tocopherol (the most active part of vitamin E) mobilizes them. It does more. It has the unique power of enabling tissues to utilize oxygen better and hence the devitalized and congested leg tissues of the chronic phlebitic who is given alpha-tocopherol are receiving the equivalent of more oxygen." Alpha-tocopherol, he has stated elsewhere, also has a clearcut fibrinolytic (fibrin-dissolving) potency. This ability eliminates internal blood clots while interfering only slightly or not at all with the clotting of blood to seal a wound.

More results achieved using vitamin E for impaired circulation of the legs are reported by Dr. Wilfrid Shute in his book *Vitamin E For Ailing and Healthy Hearts* (New York: Pyramid House, 1969). Dr. Shute writes "we have treated patients with varicose veins, with and without previous surgery, with gratifying results. However, the reasons for treatment have not been to shrink the varicosities but to reduce the symptoms. The distended and torturous veins cause a chronic venous stasis which produces edema, stabbing and aching pain, and, if severe enough and prolonged enough, indolent ulceration, overgrowth of connective tissue, and occasionally, hemorrhages or ecchymosis, leakage of blood under the skin.''

# Relief After 50 Years

Here is one case which Dr. Shute presents: A woman, age 65, had varicose veins in both legs since her first pregnancy. For four years there had been marked discoloration of both ankles and the lower halves of both legs, aggravated by the development of varicose eczema and an episode of infection which set in as a result of the woman's scratching. This woman, who lived on a western prairie farm in Canada, had 16 children, and by the time she saw Dr. Shute, her legs bothered her constantly, with severe cramping in bed.

On alpha-tocopherol, Dr. Shute writes, "these varicose veins of nearly 50 years' duration, aggravated by numerous pregnancies, not only ceased to cause symptoms of venous stasis but diminished greatly in size. She now wears her normal nylon stockings and has a nice pair of legs, just like her eight daughters."

The Shute brothers are both the pioneers and leaders of research and therapy using vitamin E for improving circulation, but they are not the only ones who have reported success using alpha-tocopherol for circulatory diseases of the legs. *Arizona Medicine* (16:100, 1959) carried an article by Dr. R. F. Bock, concluding that postoperative and postpartum thrombophlebitis responded well to 1,100 I.U. of alpha-tocopherol per day. Usually, Dr. Bock reported, the patient notices subjective improvement in 12 to 24 hours, while clinical results are apparent in 24 to 48 hours.

Varicose ulcers are also cured by alpha-tocopherol, according to Dr. Bock. It can be used prior to surgery as a preventive against dangerous blood clots, and is characterized as safer and just as effective as the drugs dicumarol and heparin and is never accompanied with hemorrhage complications. Dr. Bock saw no side effects from alpha-tocopherol use.

Dr. Wilfrid Shute has reported on many cases of varicose ulcers helped with vitamin E. One case he mentions in his *Vitamin E for Ailing and Healthy Hearts* is that of a woman who had an ulcer on the right leg which almost completely girdled the lower third of that limb, while the ulcer on the left leg was equally wide but even larger, extending beyond the natural crease between the foot and ankle into the upper part of the foot. After a course of treatment with oral vitamin E and vitamin E ointment, the ulcers healed, for the first time in 13 years.

Dr. H.T.G. Williams and his associates at the University of Alberta Hospital in Edmonton, Canada, tested a total of 59 patients. Thirty patients had poor circulation in their legs, and suffered from extreme pain when they had to walk any distance. Another 29 patients also suffered pain after walking, but not as a result of poor circulation in the small blood vessels of the legs. All of the patients with bad distal circulation were given vitamin E, but only half of those with good circulation received it. The dosage was 1,600 mg. of alpha-tocopherol daily in divided doses over an extended period.

Of the 30 patients with impaired circulation who received vitamin E, 19 were able to walk greater distances, with an average gain of about 250 percent. But only two of the 29 who did not have impaired circulation were able to walk a greater distance, according to a report in *Surgery, Gynecology, and Obstetrics* (133:662-66, 1971). Although no placebos were used in these tests, the striking difference in therapeutic effect between the two groups shows that the benefit from vitamin E is not a result of the power of suggestion but specifically its ability to open new channels of blood flow in the vessels of the lower legs.

None of the conditions we've talked about so far is limited to women, although they do seem to plague women more than men. But there are some clinical situations which are found exclusively in women and are, according to the medical literature, helped by vitamin E. They are abortion, miscarriage, and menopause.

In an article appearing in the *Urological and Cutaneous Review* (April 1943), Dr. Evan Shute described how he used vitamin E to treat 122 women with symptoms of threatened abortion and 87 women threatened with miscarriage. Symptoms in both cases were severe pain or considerable bleeding, often but not always, signs that the fetus is in grave danger.

Dr. Shute reported that 60 percent of the threatened abortions and 86 percent of the threatened miscarriages were handled successfully with the help of vitamin E. He added that "large doses are often needed and the therapy should continue till term."

Here are two notes of caution. First, because vitamin E often has a dramatic effect upon blood circulation, it can produce troublesome symptoms in patients with high blood pressure. These patients must begin with relatively small doses (no more than 90 I.U.) of vitamin E and work up to larger doses only gradually. It should also be stressed that many of the conditions that are discussed here, however common, are potentially very dangerous. Obstructed blood vessels and ulcers should always receive careful medical attention, and the desirability of taking vitamin E in conjunction with other therapy should also be discussed with one's physician.

It is most desirable, however, not to develop obstructed vessels and their complications in the first place, and from all the evidence which we have reviewed here, it would seem that vitamin E can play an important role in achieving this goal. Combined with an excellent total diet, which includes ample amounts of roughage or fiber, and as much exercise as you can fit into your life, vitamin E should be at least one of a woman's best friends.

# CHAPTER 93

# Vitamin E
# for Painful Legs and Feet

Rare is the person who marches into his Medicare years with happy feet, judging by the findings of Dr. Robert B. Rakow, chief of Podiatry Service at Coney Island Hospital and Dr. Sandor A. Friedman, chief of the Chronic Disease Unit.

The frequency of foot problems in the older set was brought to light by Drs. Rakow and Friedman when they examined 201 patients admitted to the Chronic Disease Unit of the Coney Island Hospital over a three-year period (*Geriatrics,* May 1969). Bear in mind that these patients were not in the hospital because of foot trouble. They were older people who needed nursing or custodial care. And yet, when the shoes came off, it was revealed that nine out of 10 of these patients had one or more of the following conditions: thick, dystrophic, or ingrowing toenails; hyperkeratoses, either thick corns or excessive callus; and dry skin.

All of these conditions are potentially dangerous, especially when they are associated with another condition which the doctors found in as many as 161 of the 201 patients: no pulse in the pedal extremities. This indicates poor circulation. In medical parlance it is called arterial insufficiency. A foot without a pulse is vulnerable to a host of problems. It has no defense. Any break in the skin may lead to infection or gangrene because the increased requirement for blood flow cannot be met.

Poor circulation is a condition to guard against no matter what your age. If you get cramps in your feet or legs at night, or even if you have a tendency to have cold feet, if your feet hurt when you walk, all these warn of trouble ahead. It is not just a matter of comfort or relief from an annoyance. Playing the martyr and enduring these annoyances stoically is not being noble. It is foolhardy because these problems indicate poor circulation and poor circulation can trigger many other problems, some of them very serious.

Some of the ensuing problems of poor circulation as demonstrated by the Rakow-Friedman study are thickened toenails, which are hotbeds for infectious problems, hyperkeratotic lesions which are painful corns or calluses, areas of ulceration and necrosis, leading to gangrene and amputation.

## Vitamin E Is the Best Answer

The effectiveness of vitamin E in problems involving peripheral circulation has been demonstrated many times at the Shute Institute in Canada. In his book, *Vitamin E for Ailing and Healthy Hearts* (New York: Pyramid House, 1969), Dr. Wilfrid Shute describes the case of a 61-year-old woman brought to the Institute with gangrene involving the heel of her right foot. It had begun as a small ulcer some 10 months previously. She had been a known diabetic for 33 years. Dr. Shute considers this case of particular interest because it has been so positively stated in several textbooks and medical journals that diabetic gangrene involving the heel cannot be conservatively treated, but means that above-the-knee amputation must be done. "I remember that we told the daughter that we thought the condition too advanced, but would try to help." By the end of four and one-half months on a dose of 1,200 units of alpha-tocopherol daily, not only did her insulin requirements drop from 35 to 10 units daily but her gangrenous heel was showing definite signs of healing.

Here, Dr. Shute points out, there occurred an example of the unique and most valuable characteristic of the healing of wounds under alpha-tocopherol treatment. The epithelial tissue healed without contracture, and so the healed wound showed no shrinking and no tenderness and the patient was able to walk in perfect comfort on a rubber pad in her shoe—and her own two legs.

## Intermittent Claudication

You may not know it, but the conditions which affect the health of your feet don't necessarily originate there. Any condition which tends to obstruct the flow of blood to your extremities can be the source of pulseless feet. One of the most common clinical manifestations induced by a deficient blood supply to the peripheral blood vessels is called intermittent claudication. Claudication means limping or lameness. It's called intermittent because in the beginning it only hurts when you walk.

Intermittent claudication is a condition which can sneak up on you. You might feel a slight pain when you walk. Not an extreme pain—just a slight annoyance that hardly registers. Maybe you'll feel it in the foot or thigh, but the calf of the leg is the most common site of discomfort. Gradually, you start finding excuses for not walking.

Sometimes you feel a sharp constricting pain like a muscular cramp in one or both legs, sometimes accompanied by severe fatigue.

Some people find that they can walk no more than 50 paces and then will suddenly feel the symptoms and be unable to go further. Rest at this point will promptly relieve the symptoms.

In heavy smokers intermittent claudication is frequently the initial complaint in what develops into Buerger's disease or *thromboangiitis obliterans*. In Buerger's disease the leg pains are not long limited to times of exercise, but soon begin occurring at rest as well. The patient is awakened by severe cramping that can involve both calves and feet and feels he must either get up and walk about or at least hang his feet over the edge of the bed in order to secure relief.

Many of these conditions can be headed off at the pass with vitamin E, according to Dr. Shute. In *Vitamin E for Ailing and Healthy Hearts,* he says, "Alpha-tocopherol increases the extent and speed of the opening up of collateral circulation, and this is of great importance in the treatment of intermittent claudication and of chronic thrombophlebitis, indeed, of any condition involving the peripheral circulation, venous or arterial."

Doctors at the University of Alberta Hospital found that when intermittent claudication was caused by arterial blockage in the thighs, vitamin E brought decided relief to eight out of 10 patients, while in a control group there was no improvement in any of the 10 patients (*Canadian Medical Association Journal,* 8 September 1962).

This condition frequently begins as phlebitis (inflammation of a vein and formation of a thrombus or blood clot). Where there is phlebitis, there is frequently ulceration and sometimes gangrene in the toe or of an entire foot.

"During the last 20 years, we have seen many such cases and have done, on more than one occasion, something which most textbooks and most scientific medical articles have said cannot be done," Dr. Shute says. "We have restored life to dying tissues proximal to large areas of gangrene on the heels of patients with severe degrees of atherosclerotic ischemic peripheral artery disease. This allowed the gradual sloughing off of the dead tissue and the healing, without contraction, of the tissues underneath."

"Most patients get satisfactory results," he says, "some do not. However, even in the most extreme cases, results can be excellent and very, very few of our patients have come to amputation."

The matter of dosage of vitamin E, according to Dr. Nelson George of London, Ontario, is one the Shute brothers have long stressed, but is often ignored.

Dr. George, who is a diabetic and suffered gangrene and subsequent amputation of his right leg, had been taking 75 mg. of alpha-tocopherol daily for several weeks prior to amputation.

When, several months later, his left leg became ulcerated with discharge from several toes and the heel, he called in Dr. Wilfrid

Shute who prescribed a daily dose of 400 I.U. of alpha-tocopherol. "In about one week the pain subsided and I was able to sleep without sedatives, something I had not done for many months," Dr. George said. The healing process was gradual but definite and in a few months his foot was completely healed. "There has been no return of pain. Considering the pathological changes reported in my amputated extremity," says Dr. George, "this healing seems quite remarkable."

## Feet Need Exercise

Good circulation, it seems, is the key word when it comes to staying in circulation as you get older. Exercise is one of the simplest and most effective measures to improve circulation to the feet and legs and is probably the least practiced in our motorized society.

But if your legs hurt, or if you have corns or calluses in your pulseless legs, walking can be torture and all your good intentions about "taking a nice long walk" are soon abandoned.

Vitamin E can help put you back in circulation. It has a profound effect in maintaining the tone and health of the cardiovascular system.

Not everyone, of course, has diabetic foot problems; not everyone suffers with intermittent claudication or Buerger's disease. But, if you are old enough to dandle grandchildren on your knee, chances are you're having some kind of trouble with your feet. And if you're young enough and healthy enough to have feet that feel great, you couldn't do yourself a better favor than to keep your feet that way. In either case, vitamin E and sensible exercise to improve your circulation, plus, of course, well-fitted shoes that let your toes move and your feet breathe, will only do you good.

# CHAPTER 94

# A Surgeon's Success Story: Vitamin E as a Treatment for Intermittent Claudication

*by Knut Haeger, M.D.*
*(Chief Surgeon in the Department of Vascular Surgery at Malmo General Hospital in Sweden until 1973)*

My own interest in vitamin E for peripheral arterial disease was aroused by a distinguished member of the Faculty of Medicine at the University of Malmo (in Sweden). He suffered from diabetes mellitus and had considerable claudication due to arterial occlusion in both legs. As a gynecologist, he was familiar with vitamin E, but had abandoned the nutrient in his practice. However, he said that after taking vitamin E himself for some years as his sole medication, his walking had been very much improved.

The medical literature at that time was not particularly encouraging. At the urgent request of my elderly friend we started, however, a very limited open clinical trial at the Department of Vascular Diseases as a pilot study. When five out of six gentlemen with rather severe claudication reported marked subjective improvement, we decided to go on.

We wanted to have a reliable control series, and also a sufficiently long period of observation. Since the symptoms of occlusive arterial disease of the leg have a tendency to come and go, and also are clearly dependent on the time of the year, it is imperative that the period of observation must be at least two years, preferably longer.

In our first clinical study, we compared the effect of alpha-tocopherol with that of vasodilator agents, anticoagulant therapy, and vitamin tablets without vitamin E. Vasodilating agents are drugs which tend to dilate blood vessels, permitting more blood to flow through them. Anticoagulant agents fight the tendency of the blood to form abnormal clots and are often given to patients with obstructed blood circulation and the tendency to form clots or thromboses.

We further divided the patients in each therapeutic group into two subgroups, one subgroup being instructed to exercise regularly and the other group not told to exercise.

We found that the patients who received vitamin E were able to increase their walking distance much more than any other group of patients. Fully 38 percent of patients receiving tocopherol were able to double the distance they could walk before having to halt in pain. In contrast, only 3.5 percent of the other patients showed an increase. In the vitamin E group, 36.7 percent increased their walking distance between 50 and 100 percent; in the other group, only 16.5 percent showed such an increase. We should add that those patients who took vitamin E and also exercised by walking regularly improved most of all.

There was no significant difference in degree of improvement between those who took the various drugs or the vitamins without the vitamin E; whether or not they exercised also made no difference.

## Patients Felt Much Better

We then asked the patients to rate their own improvement in terms of how far they could walk, how much their legs bothered them, and to what extent they were troubled with coldness and numbness of the feet, both of which are symptoms of impaired peripheral circulation. Once again, the patients who took the vitamin E scored much higher, particularly those who also exercised. In the other groups, regardless of whether they exercised or not, there was very little difference between the groups using the various regimens.

During the years in which we conducted this study, it was necessary to amputate 12 legs because of intractable pain and/or gangrene. This was, of course, done as a last resort, only after more conservative treatment and operative techniques had failed. In the group of patients who were taking vitamin E, there was only one amputation case out of 95 surviving patients. But of 104 patients who did not receive vitamin E, there were 11 amputations. This difference is very significant.

During the course of this work, we also learned that the clinical effect of vitamin E therapy does not appear until after three to four months of administration. It seemed to us that this is the amount of time needed to load depleted muscles with tocopherol, and this observation has been corroborated by several other Swedish physicians. Nowadays, we always warn the patient not to expect any relief within the first three months on alpha-tocopherol.

## The More Vitamin E in the Muscles, the More Improvement

In a following investigation, in collaboration with the biochemist Hans Larsson, we discovered that older men with peripheral arterial disease have a lower content of alpha-tocopherol in their skeletal muscles than healthy men. We also observed that the increase of alpha-tocopherol in the muscles after supplementation was proportional to the clinical improvement—another definite sign that vitamin E was really working. In fact, the highest percentage of increase in walking distance occurred in those patients who were capable of storing the most alpha-tocopherol, and vice versa. In a way, this may be regarded as correlated drug-response curve—if the dose is taken as the amount of the given drug which really reaches the reacting organ.

So far, we had reasonable proof that vitamin E was helpful in intermittent claudication, and also some theoretical evidence to support this claim. Furthermore, our results corroborated those of the British and Canadian investigators. However, we felt that one important link was missing. We wanted to know if the significantly increased walking distance in claudicators on vitamin E also corresponded to an increase of the arterial flow in the muscles of the calf.

At that time, the best and most reproducible method of measuring blood flow was venous occlusion plethysmography. Using this technique, we followed 47 patients (mean average age, 67 years) with intermittent claudication for from two to five years. Their disease was rather severe. All patients had been proven by x ray to have total occlusion or blockage of a major artery. The arterial flow in all patients was lower than 14 ml/100 grams of tissue per minute, while the normal range is from 22 to 30 mg.

## High Potency Natural D-Alpha Tocopherol Used

Thirty-three patients received d-alpha-tocopherol acetate, and 14 served as controls. The patients took three tablets of vitamin E a day, each tablet containing 100 mg. of a highly purified natural vitamin E with a higher biological activity than synthetic alpha-tocopherol. It was equal to 400 to 500 mg. daily of older preparations which contained synthetic dl-alpha tocopherol acetate.

As expected from our earlier experience, the walking distance improvement caused by alpha-tocopherol was again much better than that in the control group. Our tests stopped at walking for 1,000 meters (about .6 of a mile) but many patients were able to walk much longer without pain or stopping.

When we measured arterial blood flow, the difference between patients who took vitamin E and those who did not proved to be highly significant.

The initial value of blood flow was 7.6 in the vitamin E group, and 7.7 in the control group. After 20 to 25 months of treatment with vitamin E, patients improved their average blood flow to 10.2, while during the same span of time, patients who did not receive the vitamin experienced a *decrease* of blood flow down to 5.7. In the vitamin E patients, there was an average improvement of 34 percent; in the other patients, an average deterioration of nearly 26 percent.

Altogether, 29 out of 33 patients who took vitamin E experienced an improvement of blood flow. Only three patients of 14 in the control group improved.

## Improvement Is Gradual

Another finding was that the improvement in blood flow did not come at the same time as the improvement of walking distance. In fact, the effect on blood flow was delayed for 12 to 18 months after the beginning of the treatment. This may be interpreted to mean that vitamin E in some way improves walking ability, and that the increased muscular capability causes a favorable development in vessels which permits a greater flow of blood.

The truth is that we do not know exactly how vitamin E works. Its action is probably associated with the known fact that it is intimately concerned in the metabolic cycle. It is a cofactor in the synthesis of ascorbic acid; it is necessary for normal oxidation in the liver enzyme system; and—probably most important from the viewpoint of intermittent claudication—alpha-tocopherol is concerned with the biogenesis of coenzyme Q. Dr. J. Marks of Britain (1962) noted that the greatest benefit from tocopherol is derived by patients with definite but not severe claudication, "i.e., in those patients in whom there is a definite gap between the muscle demand for blood (i.e., oxygen) and the supply, but a gap which is not too wide to close." The enzymes dependent on alpha-tocopherol take a very active part in the energy synthesis of skeletal muscle, and coenzyme Q is a particularly essential component.

In normal, healthy, and vigorous individuals, there is apparently no saving of oxygen consumption when they are given an extra supply of vitamin E. Watt and colleagues could not demonstrate a difference of maximum oxygen consumption in two groups of ice hockey players, one of which received vitamin E. One assumes that such athletes are in superb physical condition. The observation by Larsson and myself that patients with atherosclerotic disease appear to be depleted of vitamin E in their muscles might offer an explanation of the beneficial effect of vitamin E in patients with this condition.

It should also be recalled that deficiency of vitamin E in animals may cause a peculiar type of muscle degeneration. Muscular dystrophy in tocopherol-deficient cattle and sheep has been reported from several countries. Obel (1953) reported a waxy degeneration of skeletal muscles of pigs, and demonstrated the ability of vitamin E to prevent it. Horse race enthusiasts will be very interested to learn that the percentage of wins per horse was increased after addition of large doses of vitamin E to the forage, and that five animals with muscular disorders were healed by vitamin E. Vester and Williams (1963) reported on a case of muscle degeneration in association with vitamin E deficiency in man: after 100 mg. of alpha-tocopherol three times a day, there was a striking return of muscle strength.

It might very well be possible that the properties of vitamin E are better utilized if the skeletal muscles are more or less inactive, or degenerated, as the case may be in states of disturbed arterial supply.

A further possibility of action is the antithrombotic effects of vitamin E. Adamstone reported obstruction of the blood vessels in vitamin E-deficient hens. Zierler demonstrated that alpha-tocopherol has antithrombotic activity both in living and test-tube tissue. Kawahara, of Nagoya, Japan, reported 28 cases of venous thrombosis treated with vitamin E with excellent results.

The final word about the action of vitamin E remains to be said. It is not unlikely, though, that the clinical effect is due to multiple mechanisms.

# CHAPTER 95

# Vitamin E
# Calms Restless Legs

Since the seventeenth century, when the syndrome was first described by Thomas Willis, the medical profession has been puzzled by "restless legs." Not quite a cramp, it is spasm in the leg muscles which comes upon a person during sleep and is described as a sensation of pulling, stretching, and twisting that is "awful, dreadful, tormenting. . . ." People get rid of it by walking or moving the affected leg, but often, as soon as the sufferer gets back to sleep or even lies still, the spasm returns.

Medically unimportant in itself, restless legs induce so many nights of pain and sleeplessness that it can lead to far more serious afflictions. The medical profession does take it seriously, and periodically bemoans its lack of any effective therapy for the condition. The *British Medical Journal* (26 December 1970) devoted two articles and an editorial to the unsolved problem. *Medical Tribune* (August 1971) called it a medical puzzle.

Two California physicians, Dr. Samuel Ayres and Richard Mihan, reported in the *Journal of Applied Nutrition* (Fall 1973) that treatment of this ailment with vitamin E has brought an end to the despair and misery for hundreds of victims of this most annoying syndrome. The problem of muscle spasms is hardly an area of concern for dermatologists, which is the specialty of both

Drs. Ayres and Mihan. Their interest was triggered by an incidental observation in the course of a clinical investigation into the possible value of vitamin E in certain skin conditions whose cause was obscure. Early in this investigation, several patients mentioned that since taking vitamin E, they had ceased suffering from nocturnal leg cramps which had plagued them for several years. Dr. Ayres and his wife were both longtime victims of the "restless legs" syndrome, so naturally their interest was aroused. Sure enough, they, too, found that vitamin E brought them relief.

The dermatologists then started a systematic investigation. In taking the history of every new patient, regardless of his dermatological complaint, they included questions regarding various types of muscle spasms. After several years, they published a preliminary report documenting 26 patients, all of whom were benefited by vitamin E, and most of whom experienced complete control of nocturnal leg cramps, "restless legs," exercise cramps, intermittent claudication, and nocturnal rectal cramps. This report was published in the journal, *California Medicine* (11: 87-91, 1969).

Since the publication of this first report, the California dermatologists have successfully treated over one hundred patients who suffered muscle spasms. Their observations on the control of muscle spasms by vitamin E have been confirmed by an orthopedist, Dr. R.F. Cathcart, III, who also reported successful treatment of approximately 100 cases of nocturnal leg cramps and other types of muscle spasms in his private practice, according to a report in the *Journal of the American Medical Association* (219: 216-217, 1972).

Drs. Ayres and Mihan concede that the mechanism by which vitamin E controls the "restless legs" syndrome and other types of muscle spasms is a mystery to them, and they have made no attempt to investigate the problem since they are engaged in the practice of dermatology. But, they say, the prompt response of various types of muscle spasms to adequate doses of vitamin E suggests that these conditions are due either to an inadequate supply, a defective absorption, or defective utilization of the vitamin. They made no attempt to conduct double-blind controlled studies, but the initial prompt response, the relapse upon discontinuing treatment, and the immediate response upon resuming and continuing treatments serve as their own controls.

## Attacks Return When Vitamin is Discontinued

One of the California doctors' subjects, a nurse, had suffered with restless legs almost every night for approximately 10 years and had tried the usual medical prescriptions without avail. She experienced no true cramps, but had the uncomfortable feeling that she had to keep her legs moving and occasionally they would jerk. Vitamin E in the form of d-alpha-tocopherol acetate in a dose of 100 I.U. three times a day before meals was prescribed. Within two weeks, she noticed that her legs were comfortable at rest. The dosage was later changed to 400 I.U. once daily which has been continued for three years with complete control of symptoms, except for a period of one month about a year ago when she discontinued taking the vitamin E. The "restless legs" gradually recurred, but ceased again when the vitamin was resumed.

Another of the patients had suffered with restless legs for a year and a half. Sometimes her legs remained restless for three or four hours at a stretch. She also suffered nocturnal leg cramps which gripped her about twice a week for a few moments of agonizing pain. And on some nights she suffered from both restless legs and leg cramps. When she took 100 I.U. of vitamin E three times a day, the whole scene changed. She was at last able to enjoy a whole night of restful slumber. She reported 15 months later that she had reduced the dose to 100 I.U. twice daily and had had no further episodes of either restless legs or leg cramps except for one occasion when she discontinued the vitamin for one month. Both problems promptly subsided when vitamin E was resumed.

A gentleman who had suffered with "restless legs" for 13 years, would sometimes have to get up out of bed and soak in a tub of hot water to get some relief. He tried oral and intravenous calcium, tranquilizers, sedatives, and muscle relaxants. But nothing helped until he tried vitamin E—100 units three times a day, before meals. Later he increased to one 400-unit capsule once a day. His symptoms gradually diminished during a three month period and he was now able to sleep uninterrupted for the first time in 10 years. Subsequently he reported that he had had an occasional episode of restless legs after strenuous tennis matches played late in the afternoon or evening. He was advised then to increase his dose of vitamin E to 400 I.U. twice daily.

In contrast to the usual dismal outlook for victims of this syndrome, those patients treated by the dermatologists experienced dramatic relief when they were treated with vitamin E in doses that ranged from 300 to as much as 1,600 I.U. daily. Seven patients experienced prompt and practically complete relief of symptoms. The other two patients, while not completely controlled, experienced about 75 percent improvement in one instance and about 50 percent improvement in the other.

While restless legs and nocturnal leg cramps are usually dealt with as separate entities, they frequently torture the same patients. Since both conditions responded to vitamin E, the dermatologists postulated that there is perhaps a close relationship—that they have a common cause. Despite the fact that nocturnal leg cramps are a fairly common complaint, the dermatologist found that most current texts on internal medicine and orthopedic surgery give scant attention to it.

How does the vitamin E work to alleviate cramps in the legs? Drs. Ayres and Mihan suggest that one possible mode of action might be through improvement of glycogen storage in the muscles. Glycogen is the storage form of glucose, formed by the liver. Blood sugar levels are at low ebb in the middle of the night. Dr. Stephen Gyland of Tampa, Florida, a physician who made hypoglycemia his life study, found that as many as 40 percent of his patients with low blood sugar suffered with twitching, jerking muscles. Dr. H. J. Roberts, writing in the *Journal of the American Geriatric Society* (July 1965), observed that patients affected with spontaneous leg cramps and restless legs have been found to be extremely low in blood sugar levels. The fact that vitamin E improves glycogen storage in the muscles would explain how it can bring relief to a muscle crying for food and would certainly imply that among the many uses for this vitamin, we should include the care and treatment of the millions of people suffering the manifestations of low blood sugar.

Vitamin E is a fat-soluble vitamin composed of many fractions. As Drs. Ayres and Mihan point out, many investigators have shown that the alpha fraction is more physiologically active than all the others.

To get more mileage out of your vitamin E supplements, the doctors suggest that you take your vitamin E on an empty stomach about 30 minutes before meals. They also suggest avoiding medications containing iron, estrogen, mineral oil, or laxatives which tend to counteract the effectiveness of vitamin E. Mixed vitamins containing iron and cereals reinforced with iron should also be avoided, since iron tends to knock out vitamin E. If you are taking both, it would be wise to take them 12 hours apart.

The doctors point out, too, that diets high in polyunsaturated fats increase the requirements for vitamin E. The popular movement toward high polyunsaturates, frequently advised by doctors, may well be one pathway to the whole tormenting condition.

The doctors point out, too, that the frequent use of laxatives interferes with the absorption of vitamin E. Mineral oil, one of the most damaging of all laxatives, decreases the absorption of many minerals and vitamins, including vitamin E, from food in the intestines.

There were no serious side effects from the use of vitamin E in any quantity, the doctors reported. But they suggest that because there is a tendency of vitamin E to improve glycogen storage in the muscles, diabetic persons who are taking insulin which performs the same function should probably start on smaller doses, which can be gradually increased as the insulin dosage is adjusted. Patients with severe hypertensive heart disease should also start on smaller doses, although the hypertension may later be benefited, at which time the dosage can be increased. Drs. Ayres and Mihan start patients who have severe hypertension, severe cardiac impairment, and those receiving insulin for diabetes, on 100 I.U. of vitamin E daily. This dosage is slowly increased. For other patients who do not have these impairments, they recommend one or two 400 I.U. capsules a day.

It should be happy news for those who suffer restless legs and sleepless nights that they can get back to a full night of heavenly repose simply by increasing their dosage of vitamin E and perhaps experience other health benefits at the same time.

# CHAPTER 96

# Phlebitis

Phlebitis can occur anywhere in the body, but it usually shows up in the legs first. When you sit for long uninterrupted periods with your knees bent, blood tends to pool, a condition which is conducive to clotting. When a clot forms in a leg vein, there is an inflammatory reaction. If the clot should disengage itself from the vein and begin traveling through the circulatory system there is no way of knowing just where it will eventually lodge. If it travels to the heart or lungs, the situation can be critical, especially if the clot is large enough and if it lodges in an important blood vessel.

For most people, though, phlebitis or thrombophlebitis means a painful, tender, and swollen lump on the leg. Sometimes the inflammation subsides by itself and collateral circulation develops around the point of blockage. In other cases, medical or surgical treatment is needed. In all cases, however, swift medical attention is imperative.

Failure to move around is not the only cause of phlebitis. In pregnancy, the enlarging womb restricts blood flow to the limbs, and may trigger the condition. Women taking oral contraceptives also run a somewhat higher risk of thromboembolic disease. A pulmonary embolism may occur after surgery when prolonged bed rest slows down the flow of blood to the lower extremities. That's why doctors advise elevating the legs while in bed which prevents the pooling of blood in the lower legs.

Alton Ochsner, M.D., Professor Emeritus of Surgery at Tulane University School of Medicine, refers to phlebitis as "the chair disease," according to an article in *Executive Health* (vol. XI, no. 3, 1974). Phlebitis, states Dr. Ochsner, is especially threatening to the busy executive who spends a good deal of his time sitting—in a car, a train, a plane, at a conference table, or at a desk.

Dr. Ochsner is convinced that to maintain a healthy and vigorous circulatory system it is a sound precaution to include a good supply of vitamin E in your daily diet. Dr. Ochsner reported in the previously mentioned issue of *Executive Health* that he had discovered over a quarter of a century ago that vitamin E in the presence of calcium acted as an antithrombic agent. "It has the advantage over other anticoagulants that it does not produce a hemorrhagic tendency and can be used safely, prophylactically, in patients who are candidates for the development of phlebothrombosis," observed Dr. Ochsner.

In conditions involving blood clots, it is customary for doctors to give drugs which keep the blood from coagulating. This is a first-aid measure which can sometimes be life saving. But it does have complications. Anticlotting agents destroy the substances in the blood which make it clot. If the blood becomes too thin and loses its ability to clot, there is the danger of hemorrhage.

A blood clot is, of course, a serious thing, especially if it occurs in a vessel leading to the brain or the heart. But a hemorrhage into either of these organs can be just as serious. When you tamper with the blood's ability to clot, you can get into serious trouble.

That is one reason why Dr. Ochsner puts his patients on vitamin E. It is a natural constituent of the body—not a drug. It tends to normalize the blood regulating both those substances which cause clotting and those substances which cause hemorrhaging.

# Other Doctors Who Use Vitamin E

Vitamin E has other powers which give it even more life-saving potential. Evan Shute, M.D., pointed out many years ago in an address before the World Congress of Obstetrics and Gynecology that vitamin E "has an extraordinary ability to increase collateral circulation." This is a very important maneuver. When some part of the circulatory system is injured, the body makes an effort to repair it. Let's say a blood vessel is clogged with a clot. Naturally that part of the body to which this blood vessel carries blood is going to suffer from loss of blood. Another blood vessel must quickly be brought into activity so the blood can be detoured around the obstruction. Vitamin E, Dr. Shute pointed out, has the ability to get this extra blood vessel into working order so that normal traffic can resume.

In his book *Vitamin E for Ailing and Healthy Hearts* (New York: Pyramid House, 1969), Wilfrid Shute, M.D., reported that a pregnant woman treated by his brother Evan for thrombophlebitis had a growth the size of a fist in her lower thigh, veins involved extending from mid-thigh to mid-calf with considerable swelling in the tissues surrounding the affected veins. When she was put on alpha-tocopherol, the mass and the inflamed veins disappeared in four days. She was kept on a maintenance dose, and there was no recurrence at delivery. Drs. Evan and Wilfrid Shute treated many such patients and have found that the response is always within 48 to 96 hours and nearly always complete. The longer the phlebitis condition has been present, however, the slower the improvement because the clot has been organized.

One of the most exciting and important effects of vitamin E, according to Dr. Wilfrid Shute, is that patients on it do not throw off emboli, which so frequently travel to the heart and lungs and quickly snuff out the breath of life. Only once did Dr. Shute have a patient throw a pulmonary embolus. This was in the early days of vitamin E therapy when physicians were still following the practice of six weeks in bed for a case of coronary thrombosis. When one such patient was found on a routine check-up to have thrombophlebitis in his left leg, Dr. Shute increased the dosage of alpha-tocopherol. The very next day this patient suffered a pulmonary embolus. But in two days this pulmonary embolus was gone.

Instead of using highly dangerous anticoagulant treatment or, as is the rule when the condition is advanced, radical surgery, physicians can give patients vitamin E and keep them ambulatory, and save many more lives. Dr. Ochsner, who has been using vitamin E therapy in his famous Ochsner Clinic in New Orleans, reports that he has found this form of prophylaxis to be a "very satisfactory" procedure in candidates for venous thrombosis and in individuals who have a clotting tendency.

How much vitamin E do you need to prevent the condition? Dr. Wilfrid Shute suggests 200 I.U. daily for the adult in normal good health. When a patient has thrombophlebitis, Dr. Shute has found that anything less than 600 I.U. daily is inadequate. In fact, Dr. Shute says, he has seen embolisms occur when the dosage was lower. But with 600 I.U. alpha-tocopherol daily, results are consistently satisfactory, he maintains.

Here are some basic guidelines that are simple and effective: Learn to regard habitual chair-sitting as a potential menace. Walk every day to keep the blood flowing smartly through your legs. Get enough vitamin E in your diet.

# CHAPTER 97

# Vitamins That Help
# Clean the Blood

Investigators in a West German laboratory have discovered that two vitamin complexes—one of which is not even recognized as a vitamin in the United States—can counteract a disease condition that blocks the flow of fluid through the vessels of the lymphatic or "second circulatory" system.

At first this research seems remote in its application to our everyday dietary needs. It has to do with surgically induced lymphedema in rats: through surgical procedures, certain lymph vessels were blocked, causing edema (pathological collection of fluid in the tissue) because the lymph vessels were unable to perform their usual function of draining off this fluid and carrying it back to the veins.

In the Lymphological Research Laboratory in Salzgitter–Ringelheim, Drs. Ethel Foldi-Boresok and M. Foldi found that the vitamins of the B complex (particularly pyridoxine, or B6, and pantothenic acid) and the controversial bioflavonoids, or vitamin P, reduced the edema and reduced also the nervous system disturbances experienced by lymph-blocked rats given deficient diets.

Though very cautious about translating their laboratory findings into conclusions about diet and people, the researchers nevertheless suggest that in certain tropical areas where lymphedema is prevalent in a severe form (when it is referred to as lymphangitis or elephantiasis and causes gross enlargement of tissue primarily affecting the legs and scrotum), dietary deficiency "may play an aggravating role" (*American Journal of Clinical Nutrition*, July 1973). In certain types of mental retardation, too, where faulty lymph drainage is indicated, Drs. Foldi-Boresok and Foldi say their laboratory findings "strongly suggest" that unbalanced nutrition will worsen the situation (*American Journal of Clinical Nutrition*, July 1973).

The investigators do not claim that faulty lymph drainage is caused by a dietary deficiency. Their rats, after all, were made diseased by a surgeon's knife—not by withholding B vitamins and the bioflavonoids. But their demonstration that these vitamins are important to the health of the lymph system provides us with one more good reason for eating whole foods and dietary supplements that enhance our intake of these two nutrients.

## Lymphatic Function? What's That?

Most of us, if we ever bother to think of the lymph system at all, think of its role in fighting infectious disease. Our children get "swollen glands" under the ears and we are informed that these are lymph nodes responding to the invasion of a cold virus. Or we become aware of a painful swelling in the groin in conjunction with a faraway infection in the foot, and again we learn that this is a lymph node combating the infecting organism.

But, besides its contribution to the body's defense against infection, the lymph system is a vital adjunct to the main circulation of blood. Alone, the veins and arteries of the vascular system are unable to perform the total job of sending blood plasma to all cells in the body, retrieving the used fluid, and returning it to the heart and lungs (where red blood cells pick up oxygen prior to the next "round trip"). The lymphatic vessels, which are laced into the tissue in almost every area of the body, are indispensable "helping hands."

Let's try to get a picture of how the lymph system is set up to accomplish these two functions—to fight infection and keep blood plasma circulating properly.

Think of the arteries and veins as a closed, pressurized, fluid-flow system leading to and from the heart. Arterial blood (from the heart) is pressured by heartbeats into branches of smaller and smaller arteries, each of which finally empties into a network of tiny capillaries. These, in turn, lead into branches of veins that (becoming larger and larger, fed by many tributaries) carry the blood back to where it started from—still under pressure from the heartbeat—though the force is greatly diminished by the end of the return trip.

It's at the capillary level that the lymph system comes into play. Because of the capillaries' thin permeable walls (as distinguished from all other blood vessel walls, which in health are watertight), pressure of the blood flow forces fluid, or plasma, to "leak out," along with a varying amount of plasma-carried nutrients, including quite large molecules of fats and proteins. This "escaped" fluid merges with the tissue fluid that constantly bathes the cells—and it is at this point in circulation, and this point only, that cells receive from the bloodstream all that they need in the way of oxygen, nutrients, hormones, certain enzymes, antibodies, and all other blood-delivered biological needs.

After dispersion in the tissue, some of the plasma seeps back into the capillaries at the venous end (that is, the end leading into a small vein). This return flow is activated by osmotic pressure, caused by a larger quantity of protein in the capillary fluid than in the surrounding fluid. But the mechanics of the situation are stacked against re-entry because, while diminished, pressure from blood flow is still exerted against the inside capillary walls and hence against inward flow. Large molecules that have leaked out of the capillaries, plus the waste material discarded by surrounding cells, plus excess fluid, have to be drained off by another mechanism—that mechanism being the lymphatic system.

The lymph vessels, or lymphatics, that first pick up the intercellular fluid and its contents, are closed at one end of the tiny tube, the other end leading to a larger lymph vessel. More permeable than the capillaries, and lacking counter-pressure, these smallest and most thin-walled of lymphatics apparently permit the free in-flow of intercellular fluid, along with the fluid's particles and large molecules. But what prevents the equally free out-flow? What heads the fluid (now called lymph) on its journey away from the tissue? Why doesn't it linger indefinitely, with the porous walls of lymphatics permitting constant in-flow and out-flow?

Though nobody has pinned down the certain answer, in the opinion of Hymen S. Mayerson, Ph.D., Sc.D., writing in *Scientific American* (July 1963), both in-flow and out-flow *do* take place; but every time the small lymph vessel contracts, the contents are squeezed in all directions—one direction being the desirable one that leads to fluid drainage. At least some of the lymphatic's contents, Dr. Mayerson explained, would thus be forced into the larger lymphatic vessels, whose thicker walls prevent leakage. Because larger lymphatics (like veins) have valves to prevent backflow, contractions of these vessels can send the fluid only in the one (and desired) direction. Again like veins, lymphatics branch into ever-larger vessels, the largest ones emptying into the veins just before these blood vessels carry their cargo back into the heart.

"One can argue," Dr. Mayerson commented, "that this seems a rather inefficient and even casual way of getting the job done. Indeed it is, and this physiological casualness is a characteristic of the lymphatic system as a whole. There is no heart to push the lymph. . . . The flow of lymph depends almost entirely on forces external to the lymphatic system: rhythmic contraction of the intestines, changes in pressure in the chest in the course of breathing, and particularly the mechanical squeezing of the lymphatics by contraction of the muscles through which they course."

## Move Your Muscles to Move Your Lymph

You can see that one requirement for a healthy lymphatic system, quite apart from any nutritional needs, is at least a minimum amount of daily exercise. Far more than the veins (which themselves are partially dependent on exercise to move blood uphill on the return trip to the heart), this second circulatory system "presupposes," you might say, its existence in an active animal. In a chapter on the lymphatic system in *Medical Physiology, Vol. 1* (St. Louis, Missouri: C. V. Mosby Company, 1968), William R. Milnor, M.D., described how carbon particles introduced into the thigh of a rat travel through the lymph vessels to the chest in 20 minutes when muscular activity is induced in the animal; however, if the rat is kept at rest, there is no evidence of lymphatic transport even after 24 hours.

So far we have been talking about the lymphatic system solely in terms of its role in making possible the continuous circulation of blood plasma. And, indeed, this seems to be its primary purpose. As the more complex higher vertebrates developed, Dr. Mayerson said, it was essential that some mechanism come into play to compensate for the capillary's inability to retrieve its leakage. It is believed that the specialized lymphatic vessels evolved from veins.

Nature has a way of making use of available mechanisms for sundry purposes. As the lymphatic system developed, its vessels became the means whereby certain fats (the long-chained variety) are absorbed from the intestines and passed to the bloodstream via the thoracic duct—the site where the major lymphatic empties into the veins. Cholesterol, too, enters the bloodstream by this route, as do the fat-soluble vitamins A and K. A number of internally produced products, too, are believed to be first picked up by lymphatic vessels rather than capillaries. "At least some hormones," Dr. Mayerson claimed, "and probably certain enzymes, such as histaminase (which breaks down histamine) are carried to the bloodstream by the lymphatics."

## How Lymph Nodes Battle Infection

But the most fascinating "extra function" of the lymphatic system is that of body defense. On their homeward trip to the large veins, lymphatics travel through a series of glands, or lymph nodes. Each of these is, in effect, a fluid treatment plant.

"The lymph nodes serve, first of all, as filtering beds that remove particulate matter from the lymph before it enters the bloodstream," Dr. Mayerson wrote. "They contain white cells that can ingest and destroy foreign particles, bacteria, and dead tissue cells."

Additionally, white blood cells that manufacture antibodies (the lymphocytes), stored in the lymph nodes, begin to proliferate and increase production of appropriate antibodies if the lymph flow brings in bacteria, viruses, or any foreign biological substance that triggers the immune response. (Lymphocytes are manufactured in the bone marrow and multiply by cell division in the thymus, the spleen, and the lymph nodes—all three of which are composed of lymphatic tissue and are part of the lymphatic system.)

It's when the lymph nodes are overworked in combating infection that your child will get "swollen glands," or the nodes in your own groin will swell because the lymph flowing upward from an infected foot carries harmful bacteria that must be trapped and destroyed. It's also because lymph nodes trap harmful substances that surgeons, when cutting out a malignant tumor, often also remove lymph nodes into which the lymphatics drain from the tumor site—for example, lymph tissue in the armpit in cases of breast cancer. The lymph node traps the cancerous cells but then becomes vulnerable to cancer spread.

## How Nutrition Hurts or Helps

Research is beginning to reveal many ways in which nutrition may affect the health of the lymphatic system for better or worse. Severe malnutrition, as in the protein-calorie deficiency disease of kwashiorkor, is known to gravely reduce the immune response and also the phagocytic, or destructive, power of white blood cells. Likewise, there is evidence that phagocytic activity by white cells is dependent on adequate vitamin C. Additionally, the findings of a team of researchers at the Albert Einstein College of Medicine, New York City, (reported in *Federation Proceedings,* March 1973) indicate that under stress, the body must have an extra supply of vitamin A to prevent shrinkage of the thymus—the lymphatic organ where a large part of the body's lymphocytes are produced through cell multiplication.

And now the West German researchers have shown us that not only the defense function of the lymphatic system but its primary function too—that of playing an indispensable role in circulation—can be weakened or strengthened by subtracting or adding specific nutrients.

There are many good reasons for adding the vitamin B-rich supplements of wheat germ, nutritional or brewer's yeast, and desiccated liver to your diet. Drs. Foldi-Boresok and Foldi have demonstrated that, in addition to all other benefits, these nutrients may also help to keep excess fluid from collecting in the tissues. Vitamin P, or the bioflavonoids, which the researchers found effective in their animal experimentation, are most plentiful in buckwheat, citrus fruits (especially the white pulpy core), green peppers (again, especially the white pulpy portions), and also in any vitamin C product made from natural sources, such as rose hips or acerola cherries, since in nature, vitamin C and vitamin P are closely associated. Bioflavonoids are also available as a supplement under their own labeling (though the Food and Drug Administration, denying any vitamin activity, prohibits claims of nutritional value).

There's no system in the body that doesn't require proper nutrition. The lymphatic system, with its complex structure of vessels and glands and stored ammunition for body defense, is surely no exception to this hard-and-fast rule.

# CHAPTER 98

# Niacin Therapy Lowers Blood Cholesterol

While doctors are still undecided as to the exact role of cholesterol in relation to heart attacks, most agree that excess cholesterol in the bloodstream is unhealthy. Doctors also agree that a carefully planned diet is the best method of controlling cholesterol levels.

Eating properly and getting the proper amount of exercise is better, say doctors, than any new drug or crash diet that has been developed to control cholesterol. Proper cholesterol levels have been achieved in high-cholesterol patients by the use of various nutrients added to a stock diet. If a daily diet is planned to include such nutrients as a matter of course, the likelihood of a cholesterol pile-up is diminished. Nutrients help the body to work smoothly. A body working as it should can make proper use of the cholesterol it needs and eliminate the rest naturally.

## Megadoses of Niacin Used to Treat Cholesterol Patients

When cholesterol levels do get out of control, research has shown that megadoses of niacin, or nicotinic acid, successfully reduce cholesterol in the bloodstream. As far back as 1956,

*Scope Weekly* (15 August 1956) told of work done at the Mayo Clinic resulting in favorable findings in nine out of 13 patients observed for 12 weeks, during which time they were given large daily doses of niacin. Even over the relatively short period of four weeks, niacin (three grams per day) was shown to lower cholesterol in the bloodstream in three out of five cases. In cases where cholesterol levels failed to respond, dosage was upped to four to six grams daily.

A two-year study by a group of Saskatchewan scientists on niacin and its effect on cholesterol, appearing in the *Canadian Medical Association Journal* (15 December 1957), secured the relationship once and for all, and a report in the *Canadian Medical Association Journal* (15 March 1958) reinforced the principle. In the *British Medical Journal* (20 September 1958), Drs. Rudolf Altschul and Abram Hoffer wrote: "It seems well-established that nicotinic acid in relatively high doses decreases serum cholesterol in healthy and sick human beings."

An eleven-year study at the Dartmouth-Hitchcock Medical Center, Hanover, New Hampshire, recorded results from 160 patients who were treated for high plasma cholesterol levels with nicotinic acid. The nicotinic acid therapy was started at a level of 100 mg. given after each meal, and was gradually increased over 11 days to a level of one gram after each meal, or three grams a day. According to a report of the study in *Modern Medicine* (26 June 1972), "The average decrease in plasma cholesterol was 26 percent in the patients who took the drug for at least a year, and this initial response was maintained for as long as the drug was continued."

When given in megadoses to reduce cholesterol levels (usually three grams daily), researchers feel that niacin no longer operates as a vitamin but as a drug, and should be administered at those levels only under the supervision of a doctor. Researchers have noted mild, but definite, reactions in some patients given niacin in large amounts. In general, flushing of the skin and dilation of blood vessels commonly occur. Some patients may experience gastrointestinal upset and itching of the skin. However, according to the researchers at the Dartmouth-

Hitchcock Medical Center, "In the 106 patients followed who were on the drug for more than one year, no irreversible side effects occurred."

## Niacin May Help Heart Attack Victims

Researchers at the Royal Infirmary, Edinburgh, found that by using a form of niacin which they termed a nicotinic acid analogue, they could reduce ventricular arrhythmias (fluctuations in the rate or force of heartbeats) in patients who had just suffered heart attacks. Reporting in the *Lancet* (27 February 1975), Dr. Michael J. Rowe and associates explained that free fatty acid levels in the blood more than double within two hours after a person suffers a heart attack. These raised free fatty acid levels can cause serious ventricular arrhythmias and threaten the heart attack victim with increased heart injury. Dr. Rowe and his associates found that by administering the nicotinic acid analogue to patients within five hours of the onset of a heart attack, free fatty acid levels were dramatically lowered and the number of patients suffering arrhythmias was significantly reduced. The researchers also reported that there were no significant side effects resulting from the treatment, and that flushing of the skin rarely occurred.

The possible benefits to heart attack victims from the nicotinic acid analogue are great. While discussing previous experiments with the treatment in the *Medical Tribune* (12 June 1974), Dr. Rowe expressed a hope that the nicotinic acid analogue would soon be widely used to help reduce the damage of heart attacks.

# CHAPTER 99

# A Natural Heart Medicine

Although many people are aware of the role of vitamin C as a protection against infection, few know of its value as a tool for surviving a heart attack. A Scottish medical research team has demonstrated that, following a myocardial infarction, the heart is in such dire need of vitamin C for healing itself that it readily eats up the available supply of the nutrient to the extent that the rest of the body becomes deficient.

Dr. R. Hume and his colleagues at Southern General Hospital, Glasgow, Scotland, reported in the *British Heart Journal* (1972, 34, 238-243) that their patients were 31 individuals (26 men and five women) who were admitted to the hospital shortly after suffering a heart attack. The group's first finding was that within six to 12 hours after the attack, leukocyte ascorbic acid levels dropped precipitously all the way down to levels typical of victims suffering from the vitamin C-deficiency disease, scurvy. (Leukocytes are white blood cells, and their ascorbic acid levels are considered the best measure of the general ascorbic acid sufficiency of the body as a whole. Circulating in the bloodstream, the leukocytes' vitamin C load is always available to tissues in need.)

Continuing their measurements, the team of five Scottish physicians found that circulating levels of ascorbic acid rose very slightly after one day and continued rising gradually for several weeks, "eventually reaching normal levels one month after infarction."

But where did all the vitamin C go during the acute phase of the heart attack? The immediate suspicion was that it went to the heart. Since the earliest days of ascorbic acid research, it has been known that the most obvious function of vitamin C is to participate in the formation of the body's connective tissue. This tissue is actually a variety of substances which are found everywhere in the body, and which literally hold all soft tissue together. If the skeleton is something like the beams in a house, the connective tissue is the mortar between the bricks (the cells)—only more so, because there are billions of times more cells in the body than there are bricks in the largest house. Without vitamin C, there can be no tissue repair, because the proliferation of new cells would be a meaningless jumble of mushy tissue, unable to hold its shape or perform any function.

In a heart attack, the blocking of a coronary artery has caused oxygen deprivation and consequent death or damage to portions of the heart muscle, and tissue repair is exactly what the heart must have following this injury.

## Vitamin C Helps the Heart Heal Itself

To determine if the heart muscle had indeed picked up the ascorbic acid supply of the circulating leukocytes, Dr. Hume and his colleagues undertook a second study. This time they compared 17 samples of heart muscle from patients who suffered noncoronary death.

Their suspicions proved correct. They found that the hearts of the coronary victims contained much greater concentrations of ascorbic acid. *The average level of the vitamin in the injured hearts was 25 percent higher than the presumably normal level found in the noninjured hearts.* The investigators concluded that: "The low leukocyte ascorbic acid for the two weeks after infarction is probably a reflection of (the) healing process, and is due to the deviation of ascorbic acid-laden leukocytes from the circulation to the heart muscle."

This period of healing with ascorbic acid, which lasts for about two weeks, is of special importance, because, as the physicians noted, "Thereafter, healing by fibrous scar formation takes place."

Dr. Hume and his coworkers saw profound implications in these findings, and many intriguing links to other recent research into vitamin C and the heart. They told of a 1966 experiment by S. Gudbjarnason and others involving dogs in which myocardial infarction had been induced. Compared to unsupplemented animals, dogs given ascorbic acid showed a 122 percent increase in protein synthesis in the very center of the infarcted area of the heart muscle. Protein, of course, is the primary substance required for tissue repairs—more specifically, the fibrous protein called collagen, whose synthesis is dependent on vitamin C action.

Dr. Richard Bing of Wayne State University in Detroit, found ascorbic acid to be of great value in promoting healing in experimental animals after myocardial infarction. Because heart failure causes not only vascular incapacity and restriction of capillary blood flow, but also changes in enzyme patterns, Dr. Bing did enzyme studies which showed that the process of repair in the damaged heart muscle can be accelerated by three different treatments: ascorbic acid, the anabolic steroids, and a treatment called the Sodi-Pallares polarizing therapy.

Dr. Demetrio Sodi-Pallares of the National Institute of Cardiology in Mexico used the term "polarizing therapy" to refer to an electrolyte therapy utilizing a combination of diet and a solution of glucose, insulin, and potassium chloride which contributes to repolarization (the orderly arrangement of nuclei and tissue permitting normal life activities, such as cell regeneration and rhythmic contraction and expansion) of myocardial fibers, the first step in the restoration of heart health. Dr. Sodi-Pallares told a meeting of the New York Academy of Sciences in January, 1967, that "digitalis compounds and diuretic drugs in heart failure, the vasodilator agents in angina and coronary insufficiency, the hypotensive drugs and diuretics in hypertension, have yielded their place of honor to this treatment."

## Vitamin Avoids Drug Dangers

In supplementing the work of Dr. Sodi-Pallares, Dr. Bing of Detroit achieved the effect of the "polarizing therapy" using ascorbic acid, which plays a vital role in cellular metabolism. The insulin in the original polarizing solution, Dr. Bing said, acts like a growth hormone, stimulating the growth of new tissue. But insulin can promote dangerous complications, especially where there is diabetes or problems of renal function. Potassium is a valuable adjunct in this therapy because it helps restore the alkaline balance necessary for optimal regularity of the heart beat. Severe heart attack is usually accompanied by severe acidosis. However, potassium intake, too, must be carefully regulated. Over-dosage can produce weakness, confusion, paresthesia, and an irregular heartbeat.

Use of the anabolic steroids, while helpful in providing the adrenal hormone which triggers heart action and promotes the growth of new cells, is riddled with dangerous side effects. Continued use of cortisone, for instance, tends to deplete the system of calcium, another element vital to the health of the heart. Patients on cortisone develop abnormally round faces and abnormal growths of hair. Steroids can also cause ulcers, high blood pressure, and diabetes. Of the three therapies found effective in promoting the regeneration of the heart muscle, the only one without any deleterious side effects is vitamin C.

This is not surprising. What a vitamin helps to prevent, it often helps to cure, and the effect of vitamin C on cardiovascular health is well known. Vitamin C triggers the enzyme which breaks down cholesterol and triglycerides into free fatty acids, thus clearing the blood vessels for healthy circulation. When the tissues are well supplied with ascorbic acid, there is less chance for lipids to accumulate into the kind of fatty plaques that cling to artery walls, clog them, and keep the arteries themselves from receiving an adequate blood supply, a condition which is a precursor of myocardial infarction or heart block.

## Fights Stress Damage

Stress is another condition leading to the formation of blood clots. Stress triggers the adrenal glands to produce more of a substance which uses up vitamin C. It is felt that exposure to the stress of surgery is responsible for blood clots after operations, and some surgeons are prescribing massive doses of ascorbic acid before, after, and even during surgery.

## A Natural, Miraculous Medicine

All of this presents a picture of vitamin C as a natural medicine for the ailing heart. It rushes to the precise scene of the injury, often reaching maximum concentration in less than half a day. It immediately goes to work to spark the natural healing process—something which no drug claims to do. It has several weeks to complete the job. After that, whatever healing takes place is not in the form of new, viable tissue that can help the heart back to its normal function, but merely scar tissue.

These revelations in turn provide a double rationale for vitamin C supplementation as routine for heart patients. First, it makes sense to insure that the absolute maximum amount of vitamin C is available to be carried to the heart by the circulating leukocytes. Second, supplementation would bring the levels of vitamin C in other parts of the body to normal levels, after they have been severely reduced by the migration of the vitamin to the heart. Being flat on your back in a hospital in a weakened condition leaves you so vulnerable to infection that it would be foolish not to try to build up the body's natural defenses with large amounts of vitamin C.

Vitamin C is clearly an emergency first aid for the damaged heart. Of course, the main interest is in preventing an emergency from ever arising. Can vitamin C actually help in accomplishing this goal? The Scottish doctors seem to think it can. They think it's a question that needs some very serious looking into. Here's why:

Atherosclerosis is said to develop in arteries "at sites of mechanical stress," Dr. Hume said. Referring to a study by Willis and Fishman which was published in 1955, he went on to say that when these stressed areas of the arteries were examined at an autopsy, "localized depletion of ascorbic acid" was discovered. Adjacent, healthier segments of the arteries which were not stressed had a higher content of vitamin C. Further, "there was some evidence to suggest that it was possible to replenish the ascorbic acid in the arteries by ascorbic acid therapy."

It would be foolish, of course, to assume that adequate vitamin C is the sole nutrient required for arterial health. Many nutrients—other vitamins, fatty acids, protein, and minerals—are needed for the proper functioning of all body cells, while smoking, lack of exercise, and heredity also undoubtedly play a negative role. But it does seem that, for many people, insufficient vitamin C is likely to be the decisive contributing cause when arteries begin to degenerate.

In this sense, atherosclerosis and its often fatal consequences to heart and brain could be described as a deficiency disease— marginal deficiency in ascorbic acid. Quite apart from research on animals and individual human patients, there's epidemiological evidence to support this concept. A British study showed that deaths from heart attacks and strokes were directly related to low dietary intake of vitamin C. In regions of England and Wales where the typical diet contained few vitamin C-rich foods such as fresh fruits and vegetables, the incidence of death from these diseases was high, researchers from the University of Birmingham discovered. And the reverse was also true: where dietary vitamin C intake was high, there was a low incidence of these fatal disorders stemming from atherosclerotic arteries.

We know from Dr. Hume's work that when a heart attack strikes, vitamin C is rushed to the scene by the body's natural and infinitely complex healing processes, so we know that vitamin C is of vital importance in restoring the injured heart to health.

# CHAPTER 100

# Vitamin E—
# The Better Treatment
# for Angina

Millions of Americans are plagued with the problem of too little oxygen getting to the heart—angina pectoris. Only someone who has gone through the agony of an attack accompanied by the crushing, vise-like pain, shortness of breath, and the sudden, overwhelming fear of death knows what it is really like.

For almost 100 years, doctors have regularly given their suffering patients nitroglycerin to dilate the blood vessels because the coronary arteries of the angina pectoris patient are partially narrowed by the disease. The drug causes the blood vessel walls to relax and expand enough to allow more blood to reach the oxygen-starved heart.

Taken as a pill, nitroglycerin gives relief to the angina sufferer. The organic nitrate causes a veritable blood vessel detonation almost as soon as the tablet is slipped under the tongue. The arteries open wider and wider to allow the life-giving oxygen to be carried freely into the heart.

Unfortunately, one of the known major shortcomings of nitroglycerin is that it rapidly wears off, leaving the angina patient right back where he was, faced with the prospect of another attack and another pill. But there may be other, more serious shortcomings as well.

618

One day in early spring, 1971, a woman who worked in a munitions plant paid a visit to her doctor, complaining about weekend chest pains. A physical exam drew a blank. However, she was ordered into the hospital on a Monday morning for more tests. It was found that 95 percent of her blood passages were blocked. When nitroglycerin was administered, however, the arteries promptly opened.

Further study by Milwaukee, Wisconsin, cardiologist Dr. Raymond L. Lange, showed that over an 18-month period, eight out of 160 women whose jobs involved handling a 37 percent nitroglycerin mixture at the munitions plant developed heart disease symptoms. The report in *Medical World News* (16 July 1971), noted that all eight, whose average age was 45 and who had worked at the plant for at least a year, suffered angina on Monday mornings. Most of them, including a few others who reported suffering chest pains, said the pains disappeared when they returned to work or when they were off the job for at least two weeks.

Dr. Lange speculated that the blood vessels of the workers were dilated until they became acclimated by developing increased muscle tone. This constricted the vessels, returning them to normal diameter. When the workers were away from the nitroglycerin, the dilation stopped, but the increased muscle tone did not. It continued constricting the blood vessels enough to deny oxygen to the heart.

In this situation nitroglycerin exposure actually *caused* angina pectoris and it took more of the same to eliminate that painful condition.

Of the eight women who showed signs of heart disease, Dr. Lange discovered that three had myocardial infarctions, two had coronary insufficiency, and one had died in 1969. This 5 percent incidence of heart disease was 30 times the rate among women of the same age in the general population.

Despite the link between long-term exposure to nitroglycerin and heart disease, angina pectoris sufferers continue to take up to 30 pills a day to relieve the pain, even though the drug gives only momentary relief and does no real good over the long run.

Their doctors continue prescribing them because, apparently, they just don't know of anything better.

Vitamin E is a safe answer to angina pectoris, according to Dr. Wilfrid E. Shute, cardiologist of the Shute Foundation for Medical Research in Canada. He has successfully treated more than 30,000 patients for over 30 years with vitamin E.

According to Dr. Shute, alpha-tocopherol (vitamin E) is unique in its ability to prevent coronary thrombosis, to dissolve fresh venous thromboses, and to decrease or abolish the symptoms that usually follow such disasters. These symptoms are chiefly limitations of exercise tolerance due to dyspnea (shortness of breath) or angina pectoris, or both. Experiments have shown that the administration of alpha-tocopherol to normal animals decreases the oxygen requirements of muscle, both cardiac and skeletal. Clearly, a reduction of oxygen demand would reduce the severity of any attack brought on by lack of oxygen.

Dr. Shute describes the treatment in his book, *Vitamin E for Ailing and Healthy Hearts* (New York: Pyramid House, 1969): "Unless there is some contraindication, such as hypertension, an angina patient is routinely started by me on 800 I.U. of alpha-tocopherol a day and seen at intervals of six weeks for reassessment. If no result has been obtained within six weeks, the dosage is increased by 200 to 400 I.U. for the next six weeks. When we reach the dose in which their symptoms are relieved, it is continued permanently."

He warns, however, that like all his coronary patients, angina pectoris patients are urged to lead normal lives as far as possible. He places only two restrictions on them: They shouldn't try to show how much they can lift or how fast they can run.

But even Dr. Shute, a long-time advocate of vitamin E, cautions: "Like every other patent medication, it doesn't work for everyone. The wide variation in its oxygen-sparing activity in different patients means that some get absolute relief as long as they take the optimum dosage while others get nearly complete relief. Some get definite help but still need occasional nitroglycerin."

Of course the angina patient can't just throw his nitroglycerin pills out the moment vitamin E treatment begins—if ever. The alpha-tocopherol takes effect gradually over the long run. And, as Dr. Shute pointed out, many patients find it necessary to take a nitroglycerin pill occasionally. However, the 30-pill-a-day regimen usually stops.

# CHAPTER 101

# Vitamins Protect Against Childhood Diseases

Antibiotics wage war against bacteria—not viruses. What pediatricians sometimes fail to realize is that when they use antibiotics for the usual upper respiratory infections of infants, they are using heavy ammunition for an enemy that isn't there. According to an intensive Canadian study, these infections, when they occur in children under three, are rarely bacterial in nature.

In fact, according to Drs. D. A. Stewart and H. Moghadam of the Hospital for Sick Children in Toronto, Canada, a child may have a positive culture and yet not be infected with the kind of bacteria which are responsive to antibiotics.

Drs. Stewart and Moghadam are convinced that "Much confusion exists about the necessity of using antibiotic drugs to treat upper respiratory tract infections in children, especially infants," according to a report in the *Canadian Medical Association Journal* (9 December 1972). They conducted a study involving 4,746 children under three years of age. Half of these children showed clinical evidence of infection. The other half did not. But "there was no practical difference between the frequency of positive cultures from infected and noninfected children, suggesting that antibiotics were not required."

Before prescribing any antibiotic drug, the physician should take into account the valuable scientific data which, Drs. Stewart and Moghadam say, indicate that most such infections are not primarily of bacterial origin.

Over a period of a year, the Canadian doctors took throat swabs from more than 5,000 children under three years of age who came to the outpatient department of the Hospital for Sick Children, Toronto, for any reason at all. Swabs were examined within an hour and any bacteria present were identified in the bacteriology laboratory. Every pediatrician should take note of their findings. For example, among 2,193 children with no evidence of infection, 77 or 3.5 percent had a positive culture for Group A beta-hemolytic streptococcus. In 885 children who did have upper respiratory tract infection, only 14 had a positive culture for the same strain of streptococcus.

Although the B-hemolytic streptococcus is the main cause of pharyngitis (sore throat in older children), it is seldom the cause in children under two years of age, it was pointed out by Mortimer and Boxerbaum in *Pediatrics* (36: 930, 1965). Reasoning that this organism might be the cause, physicians usually prescribe penicillin and other antibiotics to treat pharyngitis. Indeed, Drs. Stewart and Moghadam said in a report in the *Canadian Medical Association Journal* (10 July 1971) that, "Today it is rare for an infant with fever to escape being given these drugs for a 'sore throat' regardless of the cause."

Pharyngitis in young children is usually a viral and not a bacteriological infection, and yet the tendency to use antibiotics for these throat infections seems to be increasing. Why? Perhaps, according to the Canadian doctors, it is because of "the doctor's doubts, the parents' anxiety, or the pharmaceutical promotions." Also, because "the physician is so pressed for time he often prescribes an antibiotic without looking for the true cause of the fever, cough, or runny nose. This is common practice but inexcusable and dangerous. It may delay diagnosis of a more serious illness such as meningitis or urinary infection with severe consequences to the child," say Stewart and Moghadam. "A proper history, a complete examination, and appropriate laboratory procedures to facilitate diagnosis are the right of any sick child. In most cases the 24-hour delay necessary to obtain a report of the culture is warranted. Pharyngitis or sore throat is rarely an emergency and delaying the administration of antibiotics for 12 to 24 hours which is all the time that is necessary to identify the bacteria will more often than not demonstrate that the antibiotic is not necessary."

Occasionally, the Canadian doctors say, for a baby who is very ill, prescription of an antibiotic is justified before the results of the culture are known. But, they emphasize, there is no justification for prescribing antibiotics over the telephone to treat coughs, fevers, or colds.

Even worse, sometimes a doctor will administer an antibiotic for a child who is not even sick, simply because he has been in close contact with a child who is. In most cases this practice is to be condemned, say George D. Rook, M.D., and Edward Wasserman, M.D., of New York City in a report in the *New York State Journal of Medicine* (15 January 1969). In the case of measles and possibly other viral infections, secondary bacterial infection is twice as frequent if antibiotics are given prophylactically, it was pointed out by L. Weinstein in the *New England Journal of Medicine* (253:679, 1955).

Of course, it is understandable that a parent who has a sick, cranky, uncomfortable baby will go to a pediatrician in the hope that he will prescribe a wonder drug that will improve the child's condition. Unfortunately, the wonder drugs have their limitations and their dangerous side effects.

What can a parent do? Of course, it is axiomatic that the way to avoid the use of antibiotics is to avoid the need for them. The very first step to take if your child is subject to repeated colds and infections, is to improve his diet. It has been found that when nutrition is adequate, colds occur less frequently, are less severe, and do not hang on quite so long as when the diet is inadequate. When the baby's diet is adequate, he has a built-in resistance to bacteria or viruses which may gain entrance to his body. His lymph tissues will produce antibodies or gamma globulins. Each antibody produced matches an attacking virus or bacteria as a key does a lock.

Once these antibodies have been synthesized, your baby's lymph cells remember the pattern and will reproduce them any time they are needed, if his diet supplies the nutrients required to make them. Without the essential nutrients, antibodies cannot be reproduced even after the lymph glands have the pattern for making them. Any disease in the production of antibodies is one of the first signs of a deficient diet.

Repeated infection is a signal that antibody production has fallen off. If your baby is coming down with repeated colds and infections, take a good look at his diet. Is he getting enough protein?

Is your baby getting adequate vitamins A, C, B₁, B₂, B₆, B₁₂, biotin, niacinamide, pantothenic acid, and folic acid? These vitamins are absolutely essential in the production of antibodies. Foods like nutritional yeast, liver, wheat germ, egg yolk, meat, and milk are particularly effective in increasing the production of antibodies. You can add yeast to your baby's bottle to insure an adequate supply not only of protein but of the B vitamins, iron, and trace minerals. Introduce the yeast in very small amounts and increase it gradually. Since yeast is extremely rich in phosphorus, try to get a balanced yeast which contains added calcium and magnesium.

Many of us have learned to rely on vitamin C to nip a cold at the first sign of a sniffle. But how many mothers take advantage of the tremendous antibiotic power of vitamin C and give it to their infants? Vitamin C in the blood of babies who are bottle fed falls to a very low level within three or four days unless this vitamin is provided. If it is not provided, the baby is susceptible to allergies and infections. Vitamin C is not toxic.

Liquid vitamin C is very convenient for infants. It can be added to the formula or given to the older infant right off the spoon. They usually love it.

## Vitamin A Is a Protector

Another vitamin too frequently overlooked in programs to keep baby free of infections is vitamin A. Vitamin A, sometimes called the antiinfection vitamin, works in many ways. One is by protecting the mucous membranes, your body's first line of defense. When vitamin A is generously supplied, all the mucous membranes are washed with mucus. This mucus is kept moving by tiny hairs or cilia which sweep back and forth at the rate of 250 times a minute. This constant sweeping motion carries invading bodies into the bronchi, where they can be coughed out or moved up the throat and expelled. When vitamin A is adequate, the walls of the lungs and other mucous cells are well protected, and though the viruses and bacteria beat on the doors, they cannot enter. If, however, vitamin A is in short supply, the cells of the mucous membrane become dry. They no longer have the ability to secrete mucus and the cilia dry up and slough off. When animals were made deficient in vitamin A, they suffered infections which brought them to the very door of death. But, when the vitamin was again introduced, the animals made a recovery. And the same thing happens with babies. When cod liver oil is introduced as a source of vitamin A, within five to seven days the enzyme lysozyme increases markedly and is ready to assume its role as a destroyer of viruses and bacteria.

Remember that vitamin A is wiped out as if by a bonfire when there are infections, fevers, stresses, or any type of illness. Drugs also destroy vitamin A and increase the need for it. Nitrates from the chemical fertilizers which contaminate most of our foods, including the foods which go into those little baby food jars, destroy this vitamin.

Vitamin A toxicity is something which every mother should be aware of but not frightened by. The possibility has been blown up way out of proportion. In most recorded cases of vitamin A toxicity, it has been caused by the water-soluble preparations which absorb far more rapidly than do the fish liver oils. In fact, tolerance to excessive amounts supplied by fish liver oils is so high that danger of toxicity is most unlikely. Yet there is never any reason to take more of a vitamin than you can reasonably use. For a small child, 2,500 I.U. a day should be plenty, and perhaps a little more when there is actually an infection in the system.

The bioflavonoids are important, too, in your baby's defense program. The bioflavonoids, which are found in the skin and white inner skin of citrus fruit, protect vitamin C from destruction in the body. They seem to intensify the action of vitamin C as an antihistamine and go to bat as a protector of blood vessels smaller than those that are strengthened by vitamin C, Carlton Fredericks points out in his book *Eating Right For You* (New York: Grosset & Dunlap, 1972). Give your baby several ounces of freshly squeezed orange juice unstrained, so that he can get the bioflavonoids that are in the pulp. Since this will not go through the bottle's nipple, try putting it through the blender in order to smooth the lumps. Bioflavonoid or flavonoid mixtures are also available in liquid form from health food sources.

# CHAPTER 102

# Vitamin E,
# the Other Half
# of Diabetes Control

Some 4,000 years ago, an Egyptian doctor wrote out a group of symptoms to be included in *Papyrus Ebers,* now considered to be the oldest medical textbook in existence. He enumerated such things as weight loss, excessive urine production (which smelled sweet), a searing thirst, and periods of unconsciousness.

When the physician's notes appeared in their final form, they were published under the title "Cardia," meaning literally, the "mouth of the stomach" (in the area of the pancreas). But far from describing some disease which is nothing more than a footnote to antiquity, that physician was actually describing a disease which is all too common today: diabetes mellitus.

Medical science has had these past 4,000 years to come up with a cure for diabetes, but no luck. When people get diabetes the medical men can control it, thanks to the 1921 isolation of insulin by Drs. Frederick B. Banting and Charles H. Best. But control does not mean cure.

Today, diabetes mellitus ranks as the fifth leading cause of death from disease in the United States, and is the second leading cause of blindness, according to the American Diabetes Association. The group estimates that there are nearly three million known diabetics in America while close to two million others have undetected cases of the same malady. In 1973 over 39,000 Americans died from that disease.

Sometimes referred to as the "mystery disease," essentially, diabetes occurs when the body cannot make normal use of sugar which enters the blood as glucose.

There are several different sugars to differentiate when talking about diabetes. The troublemaker is sucrose—ordinary table sugar. It is composed of both glucose and fructose. Its glucose gets into the blood so easily and fast that it quickly overloads the blood, a condition the diabetic cannot control. Fructose, the sugar found in fruits and vegetables, somehow does not create this problem. Neither does lactose (milk sugar) or maltose, the sugar of malt and other germinated grains. These other sugars must be converted into glucose by the liver, which can control the amount of glucose fed into the blood, before the body can use them. The glucose of table sugar enters the blood uncontrolled.

Normally, glucose metabolism is regulated by insulin, a hormone secreted by the pancreas. Depending on the class of diabetes, the quantity of naturally produced insulin drops, or its action is interfered with to the point of becoming less effective in facilitating the entry of glucose into the body's cells. As a result, the concentration of glucose increases in the blood. Some of the surplus "overflows" through the overworked kidneys into the urine, but enough excess remains to be a threat to the brain, which uses glucose as its chief food but can be put into coma by too much. Too much sugar in the blood and urine is a sure sign of diabetes mellitus.

Generally speaking, there are two classes of the disease: juvenile diabetes and maturity-onset diabetes.

The former is much more severe, appearing most often in childhood and adolescence and progressing rapidly. Although most of these patients can be maintained for decades with conventional medical treatment such as insulin and controlled diet, their life expectancy is often shortened.

However, at least three out of four cases are maturity-onset diabetes which is usually diagnosed sometime after the age of 40.

Most of the time, this type of diabetes is less severe than that found in younger people and does not progress as rapidly. It can, however, lead to serious complications, especially in overweight patients who develop it.

Today, diabetics rarely die from diabetic coma because insulin—now derived from the pancreas glands of animals—is readily available. Diabetics use their syringe just as routinely as someone else might use a toothbrush or a comb.

## Arterial Disease Threatens Diabetics

Although diabetics may now go on almost indefinitely on insulin maintenance, diabetics face other challenges to survival. These problems involve the heart. In the *New York Times* (3 October 1971), arteriosclerosis was named the major killer of diabetics by Dr. Edwin L. Bierman, one of the nation's leading researchers into diabetes and arteriosclerosis.

Another researcher into the tremendous problem, Dr. Rachmiel Levine, of the City of Hope Medical Center, in Duarte, California, writing in the *Journal of the American Geriatrics Society* (November 1971), estimated that "Seventy percent of deaths in diabetic patients are the direct result of vascular (blood vessel) disease. This is about two-and-a-half times the proportion of deaths from vascular disease among the nondiabetic population of all ages."

Dr. Levine pointed out that the vascular problems exist on every level from the capillary system all the way up to plaque formation in the aorta.

"The introduction of insulin led to an enormous rise in the life expectancy of diabetic patients and has therefore revealed the width and extent and severity of the vascular lesions," he wrote.

"For diabetes, insulin has shifted the center of gravity from glycosuria (presence of glucose—or blood sugar—in the urine) and coma to the heart, the limbs, the kidney, and the eye," in Dr. Levine's opinion.

But just how bad are heart problems among diabetics?

A study published in 1961 by the New York-based National

Health Education Committee, Inc., stated that 55 percent of all deaths in the United States during 1959 were caused by cardiovascular-renal diseases. A 1964 study prepared by the Metropolitan Life Insurance Company stated that of 2,634 deaths among diabetic patients at Boston's Joslin Clinic, 77.9 percent were due to cardiovascular-renal diseases. Coronary heart disease alone accounted for 53.3 percent of all deaths during this period, states an article in the *New England Journal of Medicine* (26 August 1965).

The authors, Drs. Jean O. Partamian and Robert F. Bradley, point out that the immediate mortality of acute myocardial infarction in the general population is much less, varying from 15 to 47 percent. After acute myocardial infarction—heart attacks—diabetic patients have an immediate mortality comparable to the least favorable results reported for the population at large.

No one knows for sure why diabetics have more heart problems but the well-known English nutritional researcher, Dr. John Yudkin, has a plausible theory. He suggests "there might be a pathway through the pancreas: the glucose load leading to excess circulating insulin and this, in turn, affecting lipid metabolism, a situation resembling a sort of prediabetes. Certainly," he continues, "researchers have known since the 1920s that diabetics suffer from coronary heart disease and vascular disorders far more often than normals do and that these disorders occur at younger ages. And patients with atherosclerotic heart disease often show impaired glucose tolerance."

It seems obvious that present measures to help diabetics are really only half-measures. On one side, the need for insulin to control blood sugar is recognized and dealt with. But on the other hand, the diabetic is running a greater risk from heart disease, is certainly suffering damage to his circulatory system, and his doctor is doing nothing about it.

Diabetics have to face the threat of arteriosclerosis, and especially atherosclerosis (a condition in which the inner layer of the artery wall is thickened and irregular, and in which there are deposits of fatty substances on the interior of the artery), which can and often does lead to myocardial infarction.

In an attempt to give diabetics a better-than-even chance of surviving the heart problems once blood sugar problems are licked—or at least controlled—some medical authorities are starting to take a second look at vitamin E (alpha-tocopherol) in particular. Their search for a way to deal with the heart problem in no way detracts from the value of insulin as a control for diabetes. Instead, they are seeking some way to reinforce the protection of insulin by ameliorating the devastating effects of the heart problems that plague the diabetic.

## Treatment Is Incomplete Without Vitamin E

During a talk to members of the Vermont Natural Food and Farming Association, Inc. (1 May 1971), Dr. Evan Shute, of the Shute Foundation for Medical Research in Canada, pointed out that diabetes is like *two* diseases.

"One disease is high blood sugar, treated by diet and insulin and all that sort of thing. All that does," said Dr. Shute, "is usher in the ugly second half of the disease, degeneration of blood vessels, and this is what kills. This is what knocks out the eyes and the kidneys and the heart and produces gangrene. This is where alpha-tocopherol comes into play. No diabetic is being treated at all unless he takes alpha-tocopherol!"

After a number of years of treating cardiac cases, Evan's older brother, Dr. Wilfrid E. Shute, a cardiologist also with the Shute Foundation, writes in *Vitamin E for Ailing and Healthy Hearts,* (New York: Pyramid House, 1969), "Now we can confidently state that every diabetic must have adequate control of his disease through diet and insulin or another antidiabetic drug so that he will not develop coma or hyperglycemia (high blood sugar) reactions.

"It is of equal importance that he have alpha-tocopherol to minimize the result of his vascular involvement. All three are indispensable for effective treatment."

Although quick to point out that results in restoration of sight to diabetics who have gone blind are not very good, there have been some spectacular results on the vision of diabetics.

Dr. Shute describes results with a 35-year-old patient he first saw in September, 1958.

"He had been a diabetic for 20 years. His eyesight was deteriorating, and he had had hemorrhages in both eyes for the past six years. His left eye was nearly blind. He showed other evidence of arteriosclerosis and had a three-plus albuminuria, for example.

"On 600 units of alpha-tocopherol a day, his eyesight began to improve within six weeks and was nearly normal in six months. His albuminuria was greatly decreased, and he was feeling really well.

"In June of 1962 he suffered a fresh hemorrhage in one eye, and his dosage of alpha-tocopherol was promptly doubled. His eyesight returned to normal within two weeks. He admitted that he had become careless and had decreased his alpha-tocopherol to 400 units a day.

"On 18 April 1963, he suffered an anterior myocardial infarction, this in spite of 1,000 units a day of alpha-tocopherol. While in the hospital, he read for many hours a day, and among his books was one on very poor, cheap yellow stock with relatively poor type. With armchair treatment and an increase in his vitamin E, he made an uneventful recovery. As of the present, he takes 48 units of insulin a day."

Dr. Shute also reports that treating "the effects of vascular changes in the brain and retina is much less satisfactory than treating the relatively simple abnormalities in heart, kidney, and extremity. This is to be expected, since nerve cells are so highly specialized and so extremely sensitive to anoxia (lack of oxygen)."

Any treatment with vitamin E that Dr. Shute prescribes for his diabetic patients is in addition to the insulin the patient normally takes.

# CHAPTER 103

# B₁₂ Prevents
# Tobacco Amblyopia
# (Tobacco Blindness)

Tobacco amblyopia has been a medical puzzle for some time. The disorder, although rare and often misdiagnosed, lessens visual acuity and the perception of colors, and can lead to blindness. Physicians have long known that smoking tobacco can cause partial and even complete blindness, but they had not been able to discover why. As often happens in medicine, a cure was discovered, and by working backwards, an explanation for the cause was developed.

According to the *Canadian Medical Association Journal* (28 February 1970), tobacco blindness is brought about by substantial amounts of cyanide in tobacco. This deadly poison causes degeneration of myelin—the lipoprotein that sheathes the nerves. Under the influence of cyanide, the first nerve to go is the optic nerve. If the demyelination goes too far, the result is permanent blindness, however, "Complete recovery seems possible if treatment is begun before degeneration of nerve fibres and ganglion cells has taken place."

The treatment is simply vitamin B₁₂. In fact, the editors of the *Canadian Medical Association Journal* believed that the reason there is less tobacco amblyopia today than there used to be is that today's diets tend to be richer in this vitamin. Thus, as well as treating the eye affliction, $B_{12}$ apparently can also prevent it.

Cyanide, when mixed with hydrogen, forms the lethal gas used in executions; it is also found (not combined with hydrogen) in our bodies. Food, tobacco, and alcohol are sources, with the latter two capable of providing too much. "There is a small metabolically active biochemical pool of cyanide in the body," said the editorial in the *Canadian Medical Association Journal,* resulting in a "trace of cyanide in the blood at all times. This is essential because of its inhibitory effect on the respiratory enzymes."

## Tobacco Amblyopia and $B_{12}$ Lack

Normally, excess cyanide is excreted in the urine after it has been detoxified by the liver into the compound sodium thiocyanite. However, "it has been shown that in tobacco amblyopia a direct relationship exists between tobacco consumption on the one hand and vitamin $B_{12}$ absorption and serum vitamin $B_{12}$ level on the other. Amblyopia occurred with low tobacco consumption where vitamin $B_{12}$ absorption was poor or the serum vitamin $B_{12}$ level low. A high (tobacco) consumption was necessary where the serum vitamin $B_{12}$ level was high. It is suggested, therefore, that tobacco provides a potent exogenous source of the cyanide radical which by accumulation and potentiation results in chronic cyanide toxicity manifested as tobacco amblyopia."

The association of a vitamin $B_{12}$ deficiency with tobacco amblyopia is hardly the result of chance, for the vitamin has been known to influence the nervous system and various eye disorders for some time. Barbro Bjorkenheim, Ph.D., M.D., reported in the *Lancet* (26 March 1966), that the recognition of progressive visual impairment with optic atrophy is important since adequate treatment at an early stage may save the vision. "The optic neuropathy is believed to be a manifestation of vitamin B$_{12}$ deficiency, and good results of treatment with vitamin B$_{12}$ in large doses have been reported by many workers. . . ."

Tobacco amblyopia can be successfully reversed only if it is detected at a very early stage—which appears to be unlikely. Preventive action, by insuring against a B$_{12}$ deficiency, is the only sound approach. Or better still—quit smoking.

# CHAPTER 104

# A Nutritional Approach to Hay Fever

Each year, thousands of hay fever sufferers resort to a great number of allergy remedies. Many of them, from antihistamines to a long series of allergy shots, can bring about a certain amount of relief. But the extent of relief varies dramatically from person to person—and unfortunately, so do the side effects.

Millions of Americans are all too familiar with the extreme drowsiness that can result from taking antihistamines. Working can become all but impossible, and driving for any distance after taking a potent antihistamine may be taking your life in your own hands. Excessing drying of the mucous membranes in the nose may also result from constant antihistamine use, triggering "rebound" secretions. The net result may be an aggravation rather than alleviation of the symptoms.

Air-conditioning filters and the even more effective air filters designed to remove nearly all particulate matter from the air entering a home have the advantage of not producing any side effect except running up the electricity bill. But even they are limited in what they can do. Hay fever sufferers can't stay inside the house all day and it is not economical to run the air conditioner all day and night in the early fall, when the weather has cooled off.

637

The nutritional approach to alleviating respiratory allergies isn't perfect either. Although there are a number of medical studies showing that certain nutrients can be helpful, in actual practice, the amount of relief that people get via nutrition is highly variable. The one sure benefit of the nutritional approach is that no one will collapse into a chair from the side effects, or dry their nose out so much that they get a rebound effect and have to take antihistamines all day long.

One West Coast doctor believes that diet, in particular the B complex vitamins, holds the key to solving many allergy problems. "I would say that about 95 percent of the patients that walk into my office with allergies have a dietary deficiency," remarked Granville F. Knight, M.D., during an interview from his Santa Monica, California, office. "Most of the time," he added, "those people are deficient in the B vitamins."

Dr. Knight said he often sees manifest signs of B complex shortage in allergy patients. Symptoms include a red, notched tongue, as well as cracking of the skin at the corners of the mouth. Dr. Knight believes that dandruff and seborrhea can be deficiency symptoms, also.

## Nutritional Therapy

His treatment calls for a basic good diet, including between 60 and 80 grams of protein a day, along with B complex supplements in the form of desiccated liver and brewer's yeast. In severe cases of B complex deficiency, Dr. Knight said he uses injections, but this is necessary only in extreme cases.

"I put my patients on a good diet that includes plenty of fresh vegetables, raw milk, and cheese," he said. "They must avoid sugar and white bread as well as all processed foods."

Dr. Knight emphasized that his treatment represents a gradual approach that sometimes takes several weeks to really take hold. But he described his results over the past 30 years as "overwhelmingly favorable," with an extremely high rate of remission from allergies.

"Allergies cover the whole gamut of diseases and I think that many of them are from exposure to the great number of chemicals that have been introduced into our environment,'' he said. ''And once this exposure to these chemicals is reduced, there is an improvement almost always right away.'' Eliminating processed foods and chemical cosmetics are two basic steps to cleaning the personal environment.

Nutritionist Adelle Davis pointed out in her book *Let's Get Well* (New York: Harcourt, Brace & World, Inc., 1965) that the nutritional approach to dealing with allergies received much more attention before the widespread introduction of antihistamine drugs and cortisone drugs. Like Dr. Knight, she found in her nutritional experience that vitamins, particularly vitamin C and the B complex, often played an extremely important role in short-circuiting the effects of allergic reactions.

# The Effect of Pantothenic Acid

Ms. Davis called allergies ''stress diseases,'' and regarded the symptoms as signs that the body was unable to cope with the stress of pollen (or drugs). She believed that the B vitamin pantothenic acid is especially important in building resistance to stress. ''Allergies have been repeatedly produced in animals by injections of numerous foreign substances, and invariably the allergic reaction is particularly severe or fatal when pantothenic acid is deficient; the lack of no other nutrient has a comparable effect,'' the nutritionist wrote.

Tests conducted by Dr. I. Szorady of the Department of Pediatrics at the University Medical School in Szeged, Hungary, demonstrated pantothenic acid's crucial role in moderating allergic reactions. Reporting in *Acta Paediatrica* (IV: I, 1963), Dr. Szorady said that in four different groups of children, administration of pantothenic acid, whether by injection or orally, resulted in a reduction of skin reactions to allergens by 20 to 50 percent. Production of histamine, which elicits the allergic reaction, was reduced accordingly.

Why should pantothenic acid, or the lack of it, have such a dramatic effect on allergies? One obvious possibility is that a natural substance called cortisone cannot be produced in the adrenal cortex without it. In the absence of this natural anti-inflammatory substance, allergic reactions can actually be fatal.

One doctor who has tried pantothenic acid for an allergy problem is Sandra M. Stewart, M.D., assistant director of the outpatient department of Children's Hospital in Columbus, Ohio. Her personal experience with the vitamin is related in a book by pediatrician-allergist William Grant Crook, M.D., entitled *Can Your Child Read? Is He Hyperactive?* (Jackson, Tennessee: Pedicenter Press, 1975).

Plagued with an allergy problem, and with an "unfavorable response to the usual antihistamine decongestants, I decided to experiment and try pantothenic acid," she told Dr. Crook. "I took a 100 mg. tablet at night. And I found my nasal stuffiness would clear in less than 15 minutes. I could breathe. And, rather than waking up at four or five in the morning with cough and mucous secretion, I wouldn't have it. The pantothenic acid appeared to have an antimucus-secreting effect on me personally."

## Maybe Vitamin C Is Your Key To A Comfortable Hay Fever Season

Vitamin C also seems to play a very important role in the allergy world and hay fever picture. In a short letter to the *New England Journal of Medicine* (14 March 1974), Dr. Arend Bouhuys, professor of medicine and director of the pulmonary section of the Yale School of Medicine, suggested that the well-known beneficial effects of vitamin C in respiratory disease might be linked to its natural *antihistamine* properties. In his letter to the prestigious *Journal,* Dr. Bouhuys referred to a carefully controlled study by Dr. John L. Coulehan and others which had been published earlier in the same medical journal.

Dr. Coulehan's study showed that school children supplemented with one or two grams of vitamin C a day didn't have any fewer colds, but the actual number of days in which they had symptoms was reduced by nearly one-third. The supplemented children also coughed less and had running noses less often than other children. From this and other studies, many people have concluded that vitamin C helps protect the body against invading viruses. But Dr. Bouhuys suggested that this may not be the entire story.

Dr. Bouhuys' theory is simply: "If histamine plays a part in promoting mucosal inflammation in acute respiratory illness, the antihistamine action of vitamin C might explain, in part, the reduced symptoms and duration of these illnesses." But where did Dr. Bouhuys get the idea that vitamin C has "an antihistamine action?" The answer is simple: he proved it in his own experiments. Along with colleagues Eugenija Zuskin, M.D., and Alan J. Lewis, Ph.D., he published the results of these trials in the *Journal of Allergy and Clinical Immunology* (April 1973).

## Breathing Easier with Vitamin C

In the first set of experiments, 17 healthy people inhaled identical histamine mixtures. Histamine is a substance which reacts dramatically with the walls of the capillaries, making them more permeable and allowing more waste material from the blood to enter the cells. This, in large part, causes that uncomfortable swelling in the nose and around the eyes which is associated with hay fever. It's also largely responsible for that "drowning feeling" which accompanies bronchial asthma brought on by hay fever. Although the release of histamine by the body in response to an allergen is thought to be a protective reaction, in the case of sensitized individuals the reaction is so exaggerated that breathing can become sheer torture. Statistics tell us that all too many people know exactly what this feeling is, and how terrifying it can be.

After the histamine was taken by the 17 subjects, the doctors measured their breathing ability immediately afterwards, then at three hours, and finally at six hours. Later, they measured breathing ability at each of these times after the subjects had been given either 500 mg. of vitamin C, a placebo, or nothing at all.

They discovered a "significant" increase in the ease of

breathing after the subjects received vitamin C. The doctors said that a "single oral dose of 500 mg. of ascorbic acid inhibits the constrictor effect on airways of human subjects." The beneficial effects lasted for up to six hours, they added.

The doctors point out that large doses of ascorbic acid are excreted for the most part in about four to five hours. To maintain the antihistamine effect, they speculated that it might be a good idea to give smaller doses—they mention 250 mg.—at three-hour intervals throughout the day.

They emphasize, though, that the doses of histamine that the research subjects received were relatively mild: "We have not investigated the action of ascorbic acid against more severe degrees of histamine-induced airway constriction. Thus, at present, the possible therapeutic implications of our study are limited to mild degrees of bronchial asthma."

## Vitamin C Better Than Drugs

A study by Drs. F. Valic and E. Zuskin, of Zagreb University in Yugoslavia, showed that supplemental vitamin C is of great benefit to people who must work in environments polluted with dust, according to the *British Journal of Industrial Medicine* (30; 1973).

Twenty women textile workers were the subjects. As a result of chronically breathing large quantities of flax, 13 of the women were diagnosed as byssinotic, meaning that their lungs and breathing function had been adversely affected over the years from the constant breathing of dust. The other seven were considered nonbyssinotic.

The object of the study was to determine which would help these women most—vitamin C, a chemical antihistamine, or a bronchodilator. Traditionally, the workers showed a significant decrease in breathing efficiency as exposure to their polluted environment continued through the week. To evaluate the comparative effect of the different medications and the ascorbic acid on the loss of breathing ability, the study was conducted on four consecutive Mondays.

The first week, their breathing capacity was measured without any treatment at all. On the following Monday, orciprenaline, a bronchodilator, was administered by inhalation before the work-shift. On the third Monday, the women were given an antihistamine orally before they started work. Finally, on the fourth Monday, one tablet of a placebo was given prior to work and then, beginning the following day and continuing through the remainder of the week, 500 mg. of ascorbic acid were given daily, including the following Monday before the shift began.

Everyone who received some form of medication or the vitamin C showed a better rate of breathing when tested. In addition, those who suffered from byssinosis were helped more than those who did not. But when the doctors looked closer at how the women responded to each treatment, it became clear that vitamin C had been the most effective of the agents.

After taking the antihistamine or bronchodilator treatment, eight of the byssinotic workers said they felt better, with less difficulty in breathing and less tightness of the chest. But after vitamin C, 12 of the women reported that they felt much better. The vitamin C was 50 percent more effective.

Of the seven workers who did not have byssinosis, none felt better after the placebo, three felt better after the antihistamine, and four felt better after either ascorbic acid or the bronchodilator. It seems, then, that those who need help the most get the most help from vitamin C, while those who aren't so bad off get as much help from vitamin C as they do from medication.

The authors noted that the mechanism of the preventive effect of ascorbic acid is not quite clear. Previous studies in textile workers showed that the reduced lung capacity resulted from the bronchial-constricting action of histamine and/or some other active substances. However, other factors such as swelling of the mucous membrane or other changes narrowing the respiratory airways may play an additional role, they speculated.

It has also been reported that ascorbic acid decreases the permeability of small blood vessels. It is possible that ascorbic acid, by decreasing capillary permeability (opposing the effect of histamine), prevents edema or fluid formation and consequent narrowing of the bronchial tubes. The researchers suggested that more study is needed to clarify the exact mechanisms of the working of ascorbic acid. However, the only question is *how* it works—they are positive that it *does* work.

## Vitamin Effective Against Allergy Symptoms

Vitamin E may be a better answer to hay fever, at least for some. A Japanese researcher, Dr. Mitsuo Kamimura of the Department of Dermatology at the Sapporo Medical College in Japan wrote in the *Journal of Vitaminology* (18, 204-209, 1972) that vitamin E has effective antihistamine properties which might help hay fever sufferers through their misery, while avoiding the torpor, raised blood pressure, and other side effects that often render pharmaceutical antihistamines undesirable.

Dr. Kamimura decided to investigate the antiallergic potency of vitamin E in his own tests for two reasons. One, several other Japanese researchers reported significant results using vitamin E. And two, as he pointed out, "It is a well-known fact that vitamin E is often effective in the treatment of various inflammatory skin diseases."

In his own work, Dr. Kamimura used both animals and humans. In every test carried out, vitamin E suppressed symptoms of allergy and the kind of fluid accumulation that characterizes an allergic reaction.

First, the animal studies. Dr. Kamimura injected a group of rats with a chemical (dextran) to produce typically allergic swelling and puffiness such as occur around the eyes and nasal passages of the hay fever sufferer. Some of the animals were then immediately injected with 20 I.U. of alpha-tocopherol, or vitamin E, some with just 10 I.U., and some with only sesame oil, to serve as controls. Twenty-four hours later, the animals that had received no vitamin E developed "severe" edema, or swelling. Those which had been given the smaller dose of vitamin E developed much less swelling, while those receiving 20 I.U. of vitamin E developed no swelling whatsoever.

The dermatologist also tried painting the shaved backs of rabbits with an irritating chemical. On some areas of the skin, Dr. Kamimura also applied either vitamin E ointment or sesame oil ointment, along with the irritant.

Although in this case the vitamin E was applied topically instead of by injection, the results were similar. It was apparent that in the areas treated with alpha-tocopherol ointment, "the inflammation was suppressed and the duration of lesion was shortened." The total area of inflammation was only about one-third of that which occurred when no vitamin E was applied, and the degree of hemorrhage and wound infiltration was much less.

What about human beings? The Japanese researcher injected a group of people with histamine, the substance which, when released in the body in reaction to an allergen, is directly responsible for the swelling and puffiness associated with allergic reactions. Histamine is a substance that causes capillaries to dilate. Some of the subjects had long suffered from chronic hives, while the others had not.

After taking 300 I.U. of oral vitamin E a day for five to seven days, the allergic reactions in those not susceptible to hives decreased by 37 percent, while in those who were very susceptible, the area of the reaction was reduced by up to 33 percent.

In another test, Dr. Kamimura applied preparations containing irritating plaster to various portions of the backs of 100 people. In some areas, only the irritants were used. Other areas contained, in addition to the irritants, either vitamin E or a substance known as glycyrrhetinic acid, which Dr. Kamimura said is "claimed to have antihistaminic action." Without any ointment at all, 37 persons developed either redness or itching. With the glycyrrhetinic acid, 23 persons developed symptoms. But with vitamin E, only 19 developed symptoms.

Dr. Kamimura, who has been studying vitamin E for a number of years, admits that he is not certain exactly how vitamin E works to reduce inflammation. But it works. He believes that it does so in two ways: First, by decreasing the permeability of capillaries, which would prevent the accumulation of fluid outside blood vessels, and second, by directly suppressing the release of histamine. Although vitamin E is not usually recognized as possessing antihistamine activity, Dr. Kamimura feels confident that it does. He points out that this is consistent with his finding that vitamin E is more effective if given before irritation than when administered after the fact.

Summing up, a nutritional approach to allergies would include the entire range of the B vitamins with special attention to pantothenic acid, and vitamins E and C along with the bioflavonoids. Many individuals have also reported some degree of allergy relief with such natural foods as raw honey and comfrey. Liver, wheat germ, and plenty of fresh fruits should be part of everyone's diet, especially allergy sufferers.

# CHAPTER 105

# B₆ Teams Up with Magnesium to Prevent Kidney Stones

Long-term studies reveal that vitamin B₆ and magnesium can eliminate the misery of kidney stones. For little-understood reasons, many people tend to form stones (or calculi) from mineral salts in the urine. Primarily produced in the kidneys, urinary stones must often be removed surgically or, if small enough, they may be passed through the urinary tract, frequently causing excruciating discomfort.

According to two clinical studies conducted at Harvard University, calcium oxalate stones, the most common kind, occur in the vast majority of cases because of a double deficiency in vitamin B₆ and magnesium. Harvard investigators Edwin L. Prien, M.D., and Stanley N. Gershoff, Ph.D., first announced their successful use of supplements of B₆ and magnesium to treat kidney stones in the *American Journal of Clinical Nutrition* (May 1967). Of 36 patients who previously had formed at least two urinary stones a year, the investigators reported, 30 either had no further stone recurrence or markedly decreased recurrence during the five years or more that they were protected by a daily supplement of magnesium oxide and pyridoxine.

However, the most reassuring news is that the same investigators conducted a second study, involving many more patients and doctors than the first, which confirms without a doubt the benefits of B₆ and magnesium in the prevention of kidney stones. Reporting in the *Journal of Urology* (October 1974), Drs. Prien and Gershoff gave an account of the study which involved the cooperation of 64 urologists and, initially, 265 carefully selected patients with long histories of chronic stone formation. In the course of the five-year investigation, 98 patients were lost to the study for a variety of reasons.

Of those who stayed with the program and continued to take the protective nutrients, only 17 were considered failures and continued to form stones as in the past. Eighteen others continued to have pain symptoms (though milder than before) and probably—said the investigators—passed small fragments of stone or "gravel" in their urine. The remaining 132 were symptom-free and stone-free.

This is quite a record. All of 89 percent benefited, and 79 percent found complete protection—simply by taking supplements of two harmless nutrients.

"A number of patients, having become free of stones," wrote Drs. Prien and Gershoff, "stopped treatment and began having stones again within a few weeks, only to become free of stones again when they resumed treatment."

## What's In a Stone?

Before getting a clear picture of just how these nutrients work to protect against urinary stones, it is important to understand something about how stones are formed and what they're made of. The content of stones varies geographically and even with the stage of "civilization" a country has reached. But in North America, the Harvard researchers found, the major substance making up urinary stones is calcium oxalate. "About a third of the urinary calculi are composed of this substance and another third contain major amounts, usually associated with calcium phosphate," they noted. Oxalic acid and calcium—both normal constituents of urine—combine to form this relatively insoluble crystal.

Oxalic acid is commonly associated with several foods. Chocolate, cocoa, tea, rhubarb, spinach, chard, parsley, and beet tops are all noted for their high oxalate concentration. If you eat a lot of these foods without increasing your calcium intake, you run a real risk of calcium deficiency. That's because the mineral binds so readily with oxalic acid, and when it's tied up in this combination, it's mostly lost to the body. The calcium can't be absorbed and passes out uselessly via the intestinal tract.

Oxalic acid from the diet, however, forms only a minute portion of the oxalic acid present in urine. Army research scientists Drs. Louis Hagler and Robert H. Herman, wrote a three-part series on oxalate metabolism in the *American Journal of Clinical Nutrition* (July, August, September, 1973) in which they explained that only about two percent of dietary oxalate is absorbed and eventually excreted in the urine. Most of the urine's oxalate is of endogenous origin—that is, it's synthesized by the body itself. Ascorbic acid and a substance called glyoxylate, are the main—though not the only—precursors that provide raw material for oxalate production.

The two kidneys, where urine is formed, remove oxalic acid from the bloodstream. When blood arrives at the kidneys, complex mechanisms go to work to sort out all the various constituents of the fluid. Materials that the body needs are then restored to circulation. Wastes and other unwanted factors, including surplus nutrients and surplus water, are collected and allowed to dribble down a tube (ureter) to the bladder, from where they are excreted (via the urethra) during urination.

Since both oxalic acid and surplus calcium are directed into the urinary pool by the hard-working kidneys (they process between 400 and 500 gallons of blood a day), you can see that the stage is set for these two urinary components to combine into calcium oxalate. And, in fact, they do just that—not only in chronic stone formers but in normal individuals as well.

"The urine is normally supersaturated with respect to calcium oxalate," Drs. Hagler and Herman stated. When a solution is "supersaturated," even the slightest jiggle can trigger the sudden precipitation of the solid. In light of this uneasy situation, the puzzling question is not why *some* people form urinary stones—but why such stones aren't formed by everyone. Why don't most people get urinary stones, the researchers wondered, and in what ways do stone formers differ from the normal?

It seems very clear that nature must normally provide some protective means so that, despite the supersaturation of urine with calcium oxalate, most people never have kidney-stone trouble. If this natural protection is largely provided by dietary magnesium and vitamin B6, one might guess that stone formers "differ from the normal" in terms of their greater requirement for these two nutrients.

Not that they need extravagant amounts. Not at all. In working with stone-forming patients, the Harvard team successfully used 300 mg. of magnesium oxide—actually less than the Recommended Daily Allowance (RDA) of 400 mg. As for vitamin B6, patients received 10 mg., which is five times greater than the RDA. However, much recent research on this B vitamin suggests that 10 mg. is probably much closer to the human physiological need for the nutrient than the meager two mg. declared adequate by the National Research Council and the Food and Drug Administration.

It is an incrimination of the deficiency of the American diet that these patients needed only relatively modest quantities of two key nutrients to control their stone-forming activity. If the food industry's processed products truly provided all the nutrients you need, there's a good chance many of these patients would never have formed stones to begin with.

## Nutrients in Action

Just how do these two nutrients work to protect against stones?

Magnesium, Drs. Prien and Gershoff have shown, makes the urine more solvent in respect to oxalates. With greater solvency, the fluid can hold the crystals in solution with less risk of precipitation or aggregation—that is, the clumping together of particles.

Vitamin $B_6$, on the other hand, has no effect on the solubility of oxalate in the urine, but appears to help control the body's production of oxalic acid and therefore to limit the amount reaching the kidneys. While human studies are somewhat conflicting on this question, the researchers said, "It has been conclusively shown in animals that vitamin $B_6$ deficiency is accompanied by a marked increase in endogenous oxalate excretion."

Dr. Gershoff, quoted in Dr. John Ellis's book, *Vitamin $B_6$: The Doctor's Report* (New York: Harper and Row, 1973), made this comment on the human need for vitamin $B_6$: "It would appear that for many, if not all, individuals, the dietary level of vitamin $B_6$ needed to insure minimal oxalate excretion is greater than the amount needed to protect against most other known manifestations of vitamin $B_6$ deficiency." In other words, not only stone formers but others as well probably need five times the official RDA of $B_6$ to properly control the body's synthesis of oxalic acid.

These two nutrients, as you can see, make a great team. First, $B_6$ cuts down the amount of oxalic acid in the urine. Second, the oxalic acid that does reach the urine is made more soluble by the action of the magnesium.

If this were the whole story—if deficiency in magnesium and $B_6$ were the sole cause of kidney stones—then undoubtedly all patients in the Prien-Gershoff study would have been cured of their ailment. But kidney stones are a complex disorder with the relationships of a number of nutrients involved—calcium, phosphorus, and sulfur, for example—in addition to magnesium and vitamin $B_6$. Other factors also enter the picture—heredity, geography, metabolic disorders, and others. So the simple double-nutrient preventive approach won't help everyone. But the large proportion of kidney-stone patients who could be expected to benefit by the recommended nutritional therapy is good news indeed.

The Harvard doctors used magnesium oxide as the magnesium supplement, rather than dolomite. Since dolomite contains calcium as well as magnesium and reduced calcium intake is usually advised for stone formers, it would be best for kidney-stone patients to follow the researchers' advice. "Magnesium oxide is now available in 140 mg. capsules," said Drs. Prien and Gershoff, "and two per day should be adequate." Apart from this one caution about calcium restriction, the nutrient recommendation for chronic stone formers is sound advice for everyone.

# CHAPTER 106

# Niacin Relieves the Misery of Migraine and Meniere's Syndrome

A thorough study performed by a physician of high esteem and published in the *Archives of Otolaryngology* (vol. 75, 1962, p. 220), described a vitamin therapy successful for both migraine headaches and Meniere's disease. The physician, Dr. Miles Atkinson, an otologist, was then on the faculty of New York University, and has since retired.

Dr. Atkinson believed that Meniere's and migraine are two aspects of the same disease and that both are fundamentally related to the same metabolic disturbance. "Meniere's disease is migraine of the ear and migraine is Meniere's of the occipital lobe," Dr. Atkinson stated. The association of migraine with Meniere's is not a new observation. Meniere himself referred to it. But, according to Dr. Atkinson, the relationship has not received the recognition which is its due.

Persons with migraine often feel dizzy and some develop full-blown Meniere's disease with vertigo, ringing noises in the ears, and even loss of hearing. In some cases headaches cease when the Meniere's attack sets in. But some unfortunate victims continue to have migraine after acquiring Meniere attacks, one alternating with the other. Many a migraine patient lives the life of a recluse. "And," said Dr. Atkinson, "the physician who tells a Meniere patient he must learn to live with his attacks and prescribes phenobarbital or one of the tranquilizers quite simply does not know what he is talking about. Nor is the physician who tells his migraine patients to 'take it easy' really giving helpful advice." Those who are subject to migraine are said to be tense, rigid, perfectionist people, and such people will work just as hard at taking it easy as they ever did at ordinary living.

## Origin Is Physical, Not Psychosomatic

"In any event neither migraine nor Meniere's disease are psychosomatic in origin. Both," according to Dr. Atkinson, "are the result of a vasospasm (spasm of a blood vessel) and a subsequent vasodilation (stretched blood vessel) which leads to an increased flow of blood. In the Meniere syndrome, it is the primary vasospasm which produces the outstanding symptom, the sudden acute vertigo which comes on abruptly out of the clear sky and lays the patient low, while a secondary vasodilation, which results in the accumulation of fluid in the labyrinth of the ear, produces the secondary effects which are often by contrast relatively minor—the headache, the general malaise, the transient hearing loss of early attacks."

In the migraine syndrome, the vasospasm produces visual disturbances while the dilation produces the major symptom, the intense throbbing headache. Thus, in the Meniere's syndrome, vertigo or dizziness is the predominant manifestation, whereas in migraine, headache is the predominant manifestation. According to Dr. Atkinson, both conditions are best treated by seeking to prevent the initial cause—the spasm of the blood vessel.

How can you prevent a vasospasm? It has long been recognized that niacin is effective in controlling Meniere attacks in the vasoconstrictor group and it was assumed this effect was due to its vasodilator action. However, Dr. Atkinson suspected that some of the beneficial effects achieved with niacin were due to its properties as a vitamin. In fact, he found severe chronic deficiencies of B vitamins in both Meniere patients and in migraine patients.

"Then comes the question, routinely asked by critics and those to whom the concept of chronic vitamin deficiency is new or unacceptable—why the deficiency, particularly in a prosperous and well-fed country such as the United States? I have no certain knowledge as to why such deficiencies arise," Dr. Atkinson said, "but we do have a number of leads. For instance, it is common knowledge that the diet of a great many people is far from ideal—the rich eat too much fat, and the poor eat too little protein and the in-betweens eat too many carbohydrates. Some eat too much in order to comfort themselves; others eat too little in order to fashion themselves. The diet records of most of the patients I see in my office make dismal reading." Modern methods of food processing also contribute to deficiencies by depleting nutrients in our food.

"But intake is only one aspect of nutrition," Dr. Atkinson insisted. "What about absorption? This may be interfered with by gastrointestinal disease, for example, and by many drugs. Of the drugs, antibiotics are at the present time the most significant offenders because of their widespread use. The first Meniere attack frequently follows upon some illness in which antibiotics were liberally used. Always when antibiotics are given, vitamins should be given at the same time. How often is this done?"

Some doctors now recognize the necessity for reestablishing the colonies of bacteria (demolished by the antibiotic) which help your body to absorb the B vitamins.

When Dr. Eric Ask-Upmark, distinguished Swedish surgeon, prescribed a preparation containing lactobacillus acidophilus for one of his patients, he found that not only did her intestinal condition greatly improve, but unexpectedly her migraine disappeared almost completely. The *Lancet* (20 August 1966) report shows that Dr. Ask-Upmark tried the same treatment on ten migraine patients who had failed to respond to the ordinary regimen and he reported there was substantial improvement in eight patients—who incidentally had some degree of gastrointestinal disturbance.

Some migraine sufferers may find relief by replenishing their intestinal flora through the addition of yogurt or buttermilk to their diets—a simple expedient well worth trying. Others, however, may not. Each one of us is a metabolic individual. Those with liver disease do not utilize or store vitamins sufficiently. The incidence of gallbladder disease in patients with Meniere's is twice that of the general population, Dr. Atkinson observed. In order to overcome deficiency in these patients, high dosage, indeed, what seems to many to be excessively high dosage of vitamins over long periods of time has been found to be essential. Moreover, maintenance therapy to prevent recurrence is necessary for years, perhaps to some degree even for life, or relapses will occur.

This suggests something more than inadequate intake, but rather some defect in utilization of the B vitamins, due perhaps to a metabolic fault. Dr. Atkinson did not overlook the fact that there are other possible causes for this neurovascular dysfunction. He suggested allergy, eye strain, alcohol, tobacco, and physical and mental stress as factors which may serve as triggers in particular cases.

While such factors may trigger an attack for certain individuals, they provide no explanation of the basic cause of the neurovascular instability, and this is the crux of the matter. The acid test is, does the theory work in practice? Does the administration of vitamins overcome the deficiency which is assumed to be responsible for the dysfunction and consequently does it abolish the attacks?

## Vitamin Therapy for Other Causes

The answer, according to Dr. Atkinson, was a resounding "yes." One patient treated by Dr. Atkinson had suffered severe migraine headaches since girlhood and at the age of 45 was almost bedridden. She suffered constant headache, and all sorts of accessory symptoms. Neither ergot (a popular antimigraine drug derived from a plant fungus) nor any other drug was helpful. It took two years for vitamin therapy to make any noticeable improvement, and even at that time she was far from recovered. "That was 15 years ago," Dr. Atkinson recalled. "Today she is a fit and energetic person even though she still has a very occasional mild migraine, insufficient to put her to bed. Presumably some irreversible damage has taken place, but she regards herself as cured."

Another of Dr. Atkinson's patients was a lab technician of 35 who had to support her mother and feared she would have to give up her job because of the severity of her migraine attacks. "Again, ergot had ceased to help and," the doctor said, "was producing side effects—so usual a story. When finally she persuaded someone to give her the vitamin injections, for she lived too far away to come to see me, there was profound skepticism in the hospital where she worked. In six months her headaches were under control and it was only with great difficulty that she could be persuaded to stop injections. In 12 months, she was a new woman."

Dr. Atkinson's therapy included both injection and oral administration, in order to gain control as rapidly as possible. Injections, he pointed out, had to be intravenous because the solutions used in the dosage necessary would be painful if given intramuscularly or subcutaneously. Injections were given daily for the first one or two weeks, then three times weekly until a large measure of control had been established, usually to a total of 60 or 70 injections. Dr. Atkinson found that 60 was about the smallest amount that would produce adequate control in Meniere's disease and as many as 100 might be necessary in migraine.

Oral therapy was given together with the injections, again to the maximum dose compatible with response and tolerance. This was continued thereafter for several years.

For a period of 20 weeks or more Dr. Atkinson injected the following dosage:

|  | 1st Week Daily | 2nd Week Daily | Thereafter 3 Times Weekly |
|---|---|---|---|
| Nicotinamide ...... | 200 mg. | 400 mg. | 600 mg. |
| Riboflavin ......... | 5 mg. | 10 mg. | 15 mg. |
| Nicotinic Acid ...... | 20 mg. | 10 mg. | 100 mg. |

| For oral treatment for the first and second weeks he prescribed capsules to be taken four times daily containing: | | |
| --- | --- | --- |
| | 1st Wk. | 2nd Wk. |
| Nicotinamide .............. | 100 mg. | 250 mg. |
| Riboflavin ................ | 10 mg. | 25 mg. |
| Thiamine ................. | 10 mg. | 25 mg. |
| Ascorbic Acid ............. | 50 mg. | 100 mg. |
| Calcium pantothenate ....... | 10 mg. | 10 mg. |
| Pyridoxine hydrochloride .... | 10 mg. | 10 mg. |
| Whole dried liver or lactose .... | to fill | to fill |

Dr. Atkinson used both nicotinamide and nicotinic acid. Nicotinamide has no vasodilator action, and therefore can be used in high dosage without producing any unpleasant flushing. However, in the treatment of migraine and the vasospastic group of Meniere's cases, nicotinic acid is essential to achieve success. Nicotinic acid has a vasodilator effect and, Dr. Atkinson pointed out, this may be the reason for its effectiveness in a vasospastic condition.

## Diet Is Important

What about diet? "It would be illogical to treat a condition along nutritional lines and not give attention to eating habits," Dr. Atkinson said. "Investigation of such habits will also produce surprising results, as people who can well afford a good diet might be expected to know one but are often the worst delinquents. Perhaps the two most common faults are inadequate breakfasts and an excess, often a gross excess, of carbohydrates. Diet should be high protein, low fat, medium carbohydrate, and consideration should be paid to the possibility of allergenic foods such as chocolate and cheese as etiological factors in migraine. Tobacco in Meniere's and alcohol in migraine should be limited or preferably prohibited, as being frequent and potent causes of trouble."

Victims of migraine headaches may also be suffering from low blood sugar. The relationship between migraine and low blood sugar was brought to light in the *Journal of the American*

*Medical Association* (16 June 1951) when Dr. James A. Harrill reviewed the case histories of 72 patients complaining of headache or vertigo whose symptoms were relieved by high protein diets. In all patients the symptoms were reproduced or aggravated during a five-hour dextrose tolerance test.

Low blood sugar is usually the consequence of a diet that is overloaded with sugar and refined starches and inadequate in protein and vitamins. Not only is such a diet low in B vitamins, but the refined carbohydrates consumed tax what little B vitamins are available to the body and cause a deficiency. While low blood sugar itself can trigger a headache, it is probably the deficiency in the B vitamins, particularly niacin, which leads to the vascular weakness which makes one prone to this periodic torment.

It seems logical that a high intake of all the B vitamins which Dr. Atkinson recommended, coupled with a sensible diet, would help to prevent the kind of metabolic disturbance which can ultimately lead to the neurovascular dysfunction which triggers attacks of both Meniere's and migraine.

# CHAPTER 107

# Pioneering Megavitamin Therapy for Schizophrenia

Patients treated for mental or emotional disorders by Abram Hoffer, M.D., a psychiatrist from Saskatoon, Canada, are not restricted to such traditional therapies as electroconvulsive shock therapy, tranquilizers, and psychoanalysis. Dr. Hoffer pioneered in the use of large doses of vitamin $B_3$ (nicotinic acid and niacinamide) to treat mental illness, and it is basic to his practice.

Dr. Hoffer is convinced that, although schizophrenia manifests itself in psychiatric problems, it is really a disease caused by abnormal body chemistry. Schizophrenia is in this view actually a physical, not a mental, disease.

Dr. Hoffer has several reasons for believing this. First, symptoms can be switched on and off by regulating the drugs or vitamins used. Even if the medication is mixed into the patient's food or drink so that he does not know he is receiving it, the results still occur. This would not be true, of course, if the illness were "all in the patient's head."

Second, hallucinatory drugs such as LSD produce effects very similar to the symptoms of schizophrenia. The inference is that another chemical, this one produced in the body, causes true schizophrenia.

Third, schizophrenia seems to be hereditary. If an identical twin becomes schizophrenic, there is an 85 percent probability that the other twin will become schizophrenic too, even if they were separated at birth and reared in different families. This eliminates the possibility that the illness is the result of inability to cope with environmental factors, and suggests that it results from an inherited biologic factor.

Dr. Hoffer and his assistant, Humphrey Osmond, M.D., of the Saskatchewan Department of Public Health, have treated hundreds of schizophrenic patients metabolically with much success. In their book, *How to Live With Schizophrenia* (Secaucus, N.J.: University Books, Revised Edition, 1974), they outline the details of their megavitamin or orthomolecular therapy. For most patients, Dr. Hoffer prescribes three grams of vitamin $B_3$ and three grams of vitamin C daily. Dosages are increased if necessary. Often this is accompanied by 250 to 1,000 mg. of pyridoxine (vitamin $B_6$) and 100 to 3,000 mg. of thiamine for depression. Vitamin $B_{12}$ and folic acid may also be prescribed in some cases.

Chemical tranquilizers, antidepressants, and other conventional therapies are also used, as needed.

## Sleuthing for Chemical Clues

The scientific detective work that led these two researchers to niacin therapy makes a fascinating story. Before going to Saskatchewan in 1951, Dr. Osmond had experimented in London with mescaline. This prime hallucinatory drug, derived from a Mexican cactus plant, has a chemical structure similar to that of adrenalin. While playing back a recording of the effects produced by mescaline in a volunteer, a colleague who was a severe asthmatic remarked that when he took large doses of adrenalin for his asthma, he sometimes experienced similar effects—a feeling of unreality and distorted visions. Remembering that the writer Aldous Huxley, after taking mescaline, commented that the schizophrenic is like a man permanently under the influence of mescaline, Drs. Osmond and Hoffer picked up their first clue: if large doses of adrenalin could produce schizophrenic effects in normal people, perhaps some chemical in the body, similar to adrenalin, caused schizophrenia. They soon found a second clue. A Canadian physician told them that during World War II, a pinkish adrenalin, later identified as adrenochrome, was sometimes used during anesthesia in place of normal adrenalin. When patients recovered from surgery in which adrenochrome was used, they experienced hallucinations and other disturbances.

It is believed that the body may in some cases produce its own adrenochrome from adrenalin. Having been told that adrenochrome could produce mental disturbances, Drs. Hoffer and Osmond reasoned that abnormally large amounts of adrenochrome, produced through some metabolic defect, might be the cause of schizophrenia. The schizophrenic, they suspected, may not have the necessary body chemicals to prevent the formation of adrenochrome or to dispose of it rapidly enough to prevent intoxication and bizarre symptoms.

In an effort to see if abnormal amounts of adrenochrome would indeed cause schizophrenic tendencies in a normal person, Dr. Osmond became a guinea pig. Ten minutes after taking an injection of adrenochrome, he noticed the ceiling in the laboratory changing color. Outside, he found the corridors "sinister and unfriendly" and was unable to relate distance and time. After a second injection, he reported: "I felt indifferent toward humans and had to curb myself from making unpleasant remarks."

Speculating that inability to metabolize adrenochrome might be the culprit in schizophrenia, the two investigators began a search for some method of treatment. Their search led them to nicotinic acid. At that time, nicotinic acid had been used in what was then considered large doses for delirium and also for repression. Did the nicotinic acid neutralize adrenochrome? Would it reduce the production of adrenalin? Would it relieve the frightening symptoms of schizophrenia? It was worth a trial. The results, of course, are now history.

# CHAPTER 108

# There's Psychotherapy in the B Vitamins

A heartbreaking story of medical blundering was related by Norman Cousins, editor of *World* magazine, in his syndicated newspaper column for 10 December 1972. The true story concerned a girl Cousins called Joan, and it began in 1966, shortly after she graduated from a fashionable girls' college. Her parents noticed that she began to do strange things, such as repeating simple motions innumerable times, and endlessly wiping imaginary spots from mirrors. She became troubled by hallucinations of various kinds. A psychiatrist quickly made a diagnosis of schizophrenia, which was confirmed by several others specialists.

Joan was placed in a hospital where she was given a series of electrical shocks and put on heavy doses of tranquilizers. The result of this more or less standard treatment was that she became catatonic, a detached state of virtual immobility and speechlessness. More specialists were called in and her family tried a new hospital. But Joan's condition only deteriorated, until she was totally withdrawn from reality. Over a period of five years, she was in and out of seven hospitals, running up bills of nearly $230,000.

Finally, her parents found their way to a psychiatrist who had been experimenting successfully with treating schizophrenia as a metabolic disorder. Cousins wrote in his column, "Systematic examination revealed that Joan's mental symptoms were the result of chronic pellagra, a disease caused by malnutrition" (specifically of niacin).

It was discovered that just before she was graduated from college, Joan had decided to go on a crash diet, and a doctor had prescribed amphetamines as part of the regimen. She cut down so sharply on food that she was losing 12 pounds a week, with the result that her body was depleted of vital nutrients, including niacin, which is essential to the normal functioning of the brain.

Cousins wrote, "Joan's pellagra and her schizoid symptoms have now disappeared as a result of a carefully supervised diet, fortified with heavy doses of ascorbic acid, niacin, and other vitamins in the B complex family." But Joan's mind remains scarred by those five nightmare years in mental hospitals.

Cousins noted that Joan's family "can't help wondering how many other children like Joan may have been mistakenly committed to mental hospitals throughout the country. They hate to think that the terrible anguish they had to endure is being repeated by others." When the family confronted the doctors who treated Joan, it was explained to them that the tendency of amphetamines to produce schizophrenic symptoms was not generally known to the medical profession in 1966.

## Help Was Available But Ignored

What the psychiatrists didn't tell Joan's parents is that the link between severe psychiatric symptoms and niacin deficiency was forged 10 years before Joan was born! At that time, in the late thirties, it was discovered that niacin was the specific cure for pellagra. One of the chief symptoms of pellagra is mental disturbance, beginning with irritability and sleeplessness and progressing to a "toxic confusional psychosis with symptoms of acute delirium and catatonia," wrote M. K. Horwitt, Ph.D., in *Modern Nutrition in Health and Disease,* Wohl and Goodhart, ed., (Philadelphia, Pennsylvania: Lea and Febiger, 1964).

More pointedly, the year before Joan became ill, journalist

Gregory Stefan published *In Search of Sanity* (New Hyde Park, New York: University Books, 1966), a gripping first-hand account of how he struggled with schizophrenia for four hellish years, during which time he was treated by a dozen of America's top psychoanalysts. Like Joan, he also underwent shock treatments and took powerful tranquilizers. Nothing helped until he heard about a psychiatrist in Canada who had reported success using huge doses of niacin to treat schizophrenia. He began taking this vitamin in large amounts himself, and in short order, his symptoms vanished. For the first time in years, he said, it was no longer "a struggle to get through each day without blowing my brains out."

As if this wasn't enough to alert the psychiatric world, the same year that Joan became ill Drs. Abram Hoffer and Humphrey Osmond published *How To Live With Schizophrenia* (Secaucus, New Jersey: University Books, 1966), in which they gave numerous case histories of effective treatments with niacin, and reported on large-scale double-blind confirmation studies.

Today many people are familiar with the megavitamin therapy which Drs. Hoffer and Osmond first began using back in 1952. Dr. Linus Pauling, the brilliant biochemist and winner of two Nobel Prizes, calls it "orthomolecular psychiatry," meaning that the doctor goes about his work by adjusting nutrition so that the right molecules wind up in the right place, permitting the complex chemical reactions within the brain to proceed normally. Hundreds of psychiatrists are now using this approach, most of them reporting that when megavitamin therapy is used along with more conventional therapy, their success rate is *doubled*.

## Test Scores Reflect Improvement

One fascinating study which not too many people are familiar with was reported by Drs. George Watson and W. D. Currier in the *Journal of Psychology* (49, 1960). The study involved the use of placebo pills along with vitamin pills. Estimation of improvement was not left solely to clinical observation, but was also gauged by the standard psychological test known as the Minnesota Multiphasic Personality Inventory (MMPI). The amounts of vitamins given were much smaller than those usually administered to psychiatric patients. Whereas Dr. Hoffer ordinarily uses a niacin dose of at least three grams a day, and sometimes five or 10 times this much, Drs. Watson and Currier used a little less than one gram a day, but along with 31 other vitamins and minerals in generous amounts. *The entire B complex was used in this formula,* including thiamine, riboflavin, pyridoxine, B12, folic acid, pantothenate, inositol, and choline, along with niacin.

The patients, consisting of 30 unhospitalized emotionally disturbed subjects, were first given placebos or dummy pills. Seven improved, six got worse, and 17 showed no change. Their average reduction in total test scores on the MMPI (the higher the score, the more serious the mental disturbance) was only 4.4 points, which is not considered significant (average total score was about 220 points).

When the vitamin supplements were substituted for the placebos without the knowledge of the patients, and administered for the same length of time, 22 subjects improved, two became worse, and six were unchanged. Average reduction in the MMPI score was 17.13 points. This was considered a significant improvement. And when vitamin therapy was continued for a longer period, success was even more impressive: 24 were improved, five unchanged and only one worse. Average reduction in MMPI score was 26.77 points, considered highly significant.

# A Vitamin Dependency

Drs. Watson and Currier made this final observation: "These studies indicate that some states which are psychologically diagnosed as functional mental illness, and at the same time are not accompanied by clinical evidence of nutritional deficit, *apparently involve unsuspected nutritional deficiencies, and may be helped by appropriate nutritional therapy.*"

This is a crucial point. Generally speaking, we can distinguish between two different kinds of vitamin deficiency. The most common kind of deficiency is simply failure to eat (or sometimes, absorb) a "normal" amount of the vitamin. This amount can vary from individual to individual, but the variance is usually in the realm of requiring two or three times the amount that someone else requires for good health.

The second kind of deficiency involves a pronounced biochemical abnormality, and may require hundreds or even a thousand times the usual amount of one or more vitamins for normalization. It is really a *dependency*, rather than a deficiency. This is not to say that the individual is actually using this amount of vitamins in the normal way. In some cases, the extra amounts are required so that a faulty utilization mechanism can simply latch on to the amount it needs. It is something like pitching a thousand balls at a very clumsy batter so that he can successfully hit at least one.

In other cases, huge amounts of vitamins are needed to block a biochemical reaction which is producing toxic products. Large amounts of niacin, for example, are believed to inhibit excessive production of an adrenal hormone called adrenochrome, which can result in mental symptoms. Used in this fashion, megadoses of vitamins are something like gallons and gallons of water being poured on a fire.

## Full Range of B Complex Works Best

Niacin is the backbone of megavitamin therapy, but the related B vitamins are essential to success. Child psychiatrist Dr. Allan Cott made this clear in an article in the journal *Schizophrenia* (3; 2, 1971). Dr. Cott wrote that over a period of five years, he treated 500 children afflicted with childhood psychoses, hyperactivity, and brain injury with the orthomolecular approach and found that this treatment showed much greater promise than any other which has been tried. He noted that his results are being "duplicated by many physicians and clinics, by the Institute for Child Behavior Research and the

New York Institute For Child Development." As for the vitamins which he used, he stated: "In those cases in which positive results have been obtained, treatment included niacinamide or niacin, ascorbic acid, pyridoxine, and calcium pantothenate used in massive doses." He added that he also frequently used riboflavin, thiamine, vitamin E, and folic acid. Five of these substances, besides the niacin, are members of the B complex.

Dr. Cott pointed out that pyridoxine, or B$_6$, is involved in five different inborn vitamin dependency conditions. "Many parents and physicians reported significant changes in psychiatric cases when only pyridoxine was used in massive doses," he said.

Many investigators have reported success using pyridoxine as an anticonvulsant both for infants and adult epileptics. Dr. David Coursin reported in a 1954 issue of the *Journal of the American Medical Association* that he gave a dosage of 100 mg. of pyridoxine intramuscularly to 100 patients with various illnesses relating to the central nervous system with excellent results, especially in patients with brain disorders.

Thiamine, or vitamin B$_1$, has long been recognized as essential to a healthy nervous system. As early as 1939, it was shown that patients deprived of thiamine become confused, irritable, depressed, and fearful of impending disaster. Dr. Tom Spies in 1943 in the *Association for Research on Nervous Disorders* (vol. 22, p. 122) told of 115 patients eating a diet low in thiamine. They became timid and depressed, but within 30 minutes to 20 hours after receiving supplementary thiamine they became pleasant and cooperative.

Dr. Michael Jefferson, a British neurologist, said in the *Practitioner* (January 1964) that vitamin B-complex deficiency is responsible for many of the complaints of middle age. Dr. Jefferson mentioned that the B vitamins are all of special importance to the proper functioning of the nervous system.

## B$_{12}$ Is Valuable For Some Patients

Dr. Cott did not mention vitamin B$_{12}$ as among those which he administers, possibly because the young children he deals with have no great need for it. Older persons, however, are often in dire need of $B_{12}$ supplementation. The *Medical Journal of Australia* (11 November 1972) carried a communication by Dr. Douglas Vann concerning an 84-year-old woman who was languishing in a geriatric ward of a hospital. Her condition was "grossly psychotic and demented." Dr. Vann then gave her intramuscular injections of $B_{12}$ plus the related B vitamin, folic acid. "The response was an unexpectedly rapid return to intellectual and behavioral normality, but with almost complete amnesia for the period of psychosis and dementia," Dr. Vann said.

The New York *Herald Tribune* (17 February 1959) quoted the highly respected Dr. Victor Herbert of New York's Mount Sinai Hospital as placing the blame for many patients being committed to mental hospitals on brain damage resulting from a lack of $B_{12}$.

The *British Medical Journal* (26 March 1966) stated editorially: "It is true that vitamin $B_{12}$ deficiency may cause severe psychotic symptoms which may vary in severity from mild disorders of mood, mental slowness, and memory defect to severe psychotic symptoms . . . . Occasionally, these mental disturbances may be the first manifestations of $B_{12}$ deficiency . . . ."

A dramatic instance of how vitamin $B_{12}$ alone can sometimes help in psychiatric disorders was described by Dr. H. L. Newbold in *Orthomolecular Psychiatry* (First Quarter, 1972). The patient was a 33-year-old Ph.D. candidate who had suffered a psychotic breakdown two years before Dr. Newbold saw him. At that time, he was completely out of touch with reality, felt a kind of snapping sensation in his head, and perceived space as being greatly foreshortened, which made him feel like a midget. He was hospitalized and given tranquilizers, which controlled the worst of his symptoms, but he still felt very lethargic, lonely, and insecure, and work on his Ph.D. thesis was impossible. He underwent psychoanalysis, but it failed to help him very much.

Chemical analysis showed that his serum level of $B_{12}$ was very low. Following two injections of Hydroxocobalamin ($B_{12}$), a form of $B_{12}$ which can only be given by injection, the patient "spoke of a remarkable improvement of his condition. At that time his memory was much improved and he found that he was learning well. He was participating in class activities, and for the first time in two years, was hard at work writing his Ph.D. thesis." During the next five months, the patient maintained an excellent level of improvement. There were only two exceptions, Dr. Newbold said. They occurred when it was attempted to give injections only once every 10 days, instead of twice weekly. The result was that the patient quickly became tired and depressed. Apparently, he was not suffering from a simple deficiency, but rather a kind of dependency state.

# Vitamin C is Important in Therapy

Vitamin C plays a very special role in the mental status of the schizophrenic. According to Dr. Allan Cott, vitamin C assists in the conversion of a body substance called adrenochrome to one called leucoadrenochrome, a nontoxic substance. In persons suffering from schizophrenia, he pointed out; the adrenochrome is instead converted into a toxic substance called adrenolutin. Dr. Cott stated that " . . . vitamin C was added to the (megavitamin) treatment when it was found that the ascorbic acid retarded the oxidation of adrenalin and in this way reduced the production of adrenochrome. . . . Adrenochrome combines with vitamin C and uses it up more quickly, leaving a C deficiency in schizophrenics. VanderKamps's test shows requirements of ten to 30 grams or more in schizophrenic patients before free ascorbic acid is found in the urine."

Dr. Roger J. Williams, in his book *Nutrition Against Disease* (New York: Pitman Publishing Corp., 1971), wrote, "We cannot be absolutely certain yet that all mentally diseased individuals have ascorbic acid deficiency and are improved by massive doses. But the evidence points strongly toward the conclusion that ascorbic acid is a link in the chain and giving the brain cells an ample supply is one way to help insure healthy brain functioning."

# We Have Come A Long Way

Our present knowledge of psychiatric disorders and how they can be ameliorated by dietary means might be compared to the degree of understanding of physical illness and vitamins which existed several hundred years ago, when it was first discovered that scurvy could be cured by drinking the juice of lemons or limes. Psychiatric disorders are far more complicated than simple scurvy, but we at least know that niacin and all the related B-complex factors (along with megadoses of vitamin C) somehow bring about relief. How these vitamins do their work is not yet fully understood. Yet, this must not deter us from appreciating their effectiveness. Remember that hundreds of years passed between the time that citrus fruit was discovered to be a specific against scurvy and the eventual understanding that ascorbic acid is an essential component of collagen.

We know we have come a long way indeed when David R. Hawkins, M.D., medical director of the North Nassau Mental Health Center in Manhasset, New York, can report in *Orthomolecular Psychiatry: Treatment of Schizophrenia*, edited by David Hawkins, M.D., and Linus Pauling, Ph.D., (San Francisco, California: Freeman and Company, 1973) that after the adoption of orthomolecular methods, the number of yearly visits required per patient dropped from 150 to just 15. Dr. Hawkins further stated that by adding megavitamin treatment to other techniques used at the clinic, he has been able to double the recovery rate, halve the hospitalization rate, and virtually eliminate suicide among a group of patients whose suicide rate is ordinarily 22 times that of the general population.

# A Physician Must Guide Therapy

Megavitamin therapy is not something that you can do yourself. It must be carried out under the direction of a qualified medical psychiatrist. In most cases, these psychiatrists use megavitamin therapy along with other modalities, which may include tranquilizers and psychotherapy. In addition, the vitamins and the amounts used are generally custom-tailored to the individual. No serious side effects from megavitamin therapy have been reported, but large doses of niacin can sometimes cause a flushing syndrome. This is usually controlled by temporarily switching from niacin to niacinamide. In any case, therapy must be carried out under the watchful eye of an experienced doctor.

It is worth remembering, though, that good nutrition, particularly with respect to the B vitamins, is essential to everyone's mental health.

Depletion or even borderline deficiency, can produce a terrifying array of mental conditions, and often, the experts assure us, long before any physical symptoms appear. In some cases, as shown by the work of Drs. Watson and Currier, even relatively modest amounts of supplementation can be of significant value, if the complete range of B vitamins and other nutrients are brought to bear on the problem.

# CHAPTER 109

# Schizophrenics—How Do They Respond to Megavitamins?

Jack Burton* had worked hard all his life. His father died when he was a teenager and for years he helped support his mother. In 1964, Jack was 32 years old, married, with two youngsters of his own. He was a successful hairdresser and lived comfortably with his family in the suburbs of New York. In 1964, Jack realized a dream—he left his job and opened a beauty shop of his own.

But two months after he went into business, Jack broke down. Suddenly, the man who had driven himself all his life refused to function. The man whom friends called "Smiling Jack" cried constantly, kept to his bed, and was visibly afraid of people.

"I heard voices from nowhere. With my own eyes I would sit there and watch pictures on the wall turn into monstrous figures," Jack related.

His behavior become bizarre and his humor vicious. "Could you believe that I marked up my daughter's face with shoe polish, just for fun?" At his mother's funeral, he grinned throughout the service. He hid behind trees to avoid meeting neighbors. When he drove his car, he stopped a block away from a red light because he couldn't judge the distance.

---

*A number of patients of the North Nassau Mental Health Center were interviewed. The names used here are fictitious.

Soon Jack was in the hands of a psychiatrist and was diagnosed as schizophrenic. Kitty, his wife, sold the business and went back to work.

"He was in and out of hospitals for six years," Kitty said.

"He had shock treatment, psychotherapy, drugs . . . the works. He went from one doctor to another and they all told me he would never get well. When he was home between hospital stays, he was so heavily tranquilized that he walked around like a zombie."

In 1970, through a friend, the Burtons heard about Dr. David Hawkins and his successful treatment of schizophrenia with the use of megavitamins. In desperation, they consulted Dr. Hawkins at the North Nassau Mental Health Center in Manhasset, Long Island. The doctor advised hospitalization.

"We almost turned away. We had lost hope," said Kitty. "Then I discussed the matter with our priest who urged me to have faith. So I borrowed the money for the hospital fee and Jack entered Brunswick Hospital in Amityville for a month's stay."

## What One Month of Treatment Accomplished

While Jack was at the hospital, he submitted to a battery of physical and psychiatric tests, including tests for altered perceptual functioning, for glucose tolerance, and for cerebral allergies to food and environmental chemicals.

Megavitamin therapy was initiated immediately with heavy doses of $B_3$, $B_6$, C, and E. He was put on a high-protein, low-carbohydrate diet with caffeine and alcohol forbidden. In four weeks, he was home—happy to see his family and eager to return to work for the first time in six years.

Jack continued to consult Dr. Hawkins monthly at the clinic but these visits soon tapered off and he now sees the doctor only twice a year. He has never had a relapse but he is well aware that he will have to continue taking multiple vitamins and adhere to his diet for the rest of his life. Once or twice, he rebelled and goofed off for a few days, but when he found himself slipping into a depression, he quickly resumed his routine.

Jack is one of the thousands of schizophrenics who have been successfully treated with megavitamins at the North Nassau Mental Health Center. Patients come from all over the United States and as far away as Australia. What is this megavitamin therapy and why is traditional psychiatry skeptical?

## Schizophrenia—'A Genetic Biochemical Disturbance'

Dr. David Hawkins, director of the clinic, discussed orthomolecular psychiatry, popularly known as megavitamin therapy.

"Orthomolecular psychiatry regards schizophrenia as a genetic biochemical disturbance. The functioning of the brain is dependent on its composition and structure, on its molecular environment," he explained. "We consider biochemical defects to be primary in causing mental illness and our emphasis is on biochemistry and nutrition. Disturbed family relations and personal conflicts may contribute to the patient's illness but psychodynamics is not our primary treatment approach. First we treat the psychosis, then we help the patient adjust to life."

Orthomolecular psychiatry believes that mental illness can result from a low concentration in the brain of any of the following vitamins: thiamine, niacin, pyridoxine, $B_{12}$, biotin, ascorbic acid, or folic acid.

But the basic biochemical defect (or defects) that causes mental illness has not yet been determined. "Scientists are working on it," said Dr. Hawkins. "Maybe we'll have the answer in 10 or 20 years. Orthomolecular psychiatry is pragmatic, empirical. The point is—it works."

Why does the establishment resist the biochemical approach? It is understandable that specialists who have devoted a lifetime to psychodynamics will be hostile to change. Medicine has always been slow to accept new methods. The criticism leveled against orthomolecular psychiatry is that its claims have not been confirmed by controlled studies, but the megavitamin treatment regime does not lend itself to double-blind studies and the procedure would be costly. The controversy will probably continue until controlled studies weigh the efficacy of orthomolecular psychiatry against psychodynamic treatment. Although the opponents have the funding, Dr. Hawkins isn't worried.

## 'The Fact Is—It *Does* Work'

"We haven't discovered why it works, but we have clinical proof that it *does* work. Orthomolecular psychiatry is a promising branch of medicine and the public is making the decision in its favor," said Dr. Hawkins.

What is the recovery rate? "That's difficult to assess at this time," Dr. Hawkins stated. "When I first started practicing orthomolecular psychiatry in 1966, my recovery rate was double that of traditional psychiatry. Now that I'm getting difficult, chronic cases from all over the country, an estimate of the recovery rate would be inaccurate. However, we have received a modest grant from a foundation for an efficacy study and we will soon be making a detailed study of 50 cases."

Orthomolecular psychiatry developed during the 1960s when there was growing disillusionment with the psychodynamic approach, its cost in time and money, and its efficacy. At the same time, there was a growing interest in the relationship between diet and mental illness. The concept of biochemical individuality was developed, pointing out the enormous difference in nutritional requirements and biochemical processes in identical siblings. Research was done on the relationship among poverty, poor diet, and mental development. The importance of detecting and treating hypoglycemia in schizophrenia was studied and work was begun on the problem of cerebral allergy to food and environmental chemicals as a cause of psychiatric symptoms.

Dr. Hawkins became interested in megavitamin treatment from members of Alcoholics Anonymous. Until 1966, the Manhasset center used traditional methods of treating schizophrenia. Bill Wilson, founder of A.A., began using vitamins in treating alcoholics, especially those who were schizophrenic. Dr. Hawkins heard favorable reports, tried the vitamin therapy on his alcohol-schizophrenic patients, and got amazing results. Subsequently, he applied the treatment to all his schizophrenic patients, and dedicated himself to practicing psychiatry the orthomolecular way.

In diagnosing schizophrenia, orthomolecular psychiatrists pay particular attention to evidences of altered perceptual functioning. The use of the Hoffer-Osmond Diagnostic Test expedites appraisal of the illness far more effectively than a psychodynamic interview. It measures abnormalities of perception in sight, sound, smell, taste, and touch, and it determines thought disorders. It takes no more than 20 minutes and is self-administered. Laboratory tests include those for thyroid function, glucose tolerance, hair test analysis for trace metals, and comprehensive chemical and liver profiles. There are abnormal chemicals found in the blood or urine or tissues of schizophrenics, very much like the abnormal amount of sugar found in the blood of the diabetic.

## Nutrition and Other Therapeutic Techniques

The use of vitamins in combination and in large doses is prescribed. A typical daily dose would include four grams of B$_3$ (nicotinic acid or nicotinamide), 800 mg. of B$_6$ (pyridoxine), four grams of C, and 1,000 units of E. For the patient with low histamine level, two mg. of folic acid may be included. Zinc may be prescribed if there are high copper levels. Lithium is used in treating manic-depressives. Several grams of PABA may be included if indicated. The vitamin dosage required for the individual is determined by the physician.

Are there any toxic effects in the use of megavitamins? Side effects are rare, Dr. Hawkins explained, except in the use of niacin (one form of vitamin B$_3$) which must be monitored by a physician. Niacin produces a flushing of the skin which subsides in about an hour and usually doesn't recur after the fifth or sixth dose.

Orthomolecular psychiatry is eclectic and includes many conventional psychiatric procedures. Shock treatment has multiple biochemical effects, and supported by megavitamins, the improvement is dramatic. Hormones, antidepressants, and tranquilizers are used when necessary. Phenothiazines (tranquilizers) are often prescribed, but quickly reduced to maintenance level.

Psychotherapy is not ignored. Emotional upsets affect the brain chemistry which will aggravate the biochemical problem. While the patient is psychotic, psychotherapy is merely supportive. When the patient is no longer plagued by perceptual distortions, the orthomolecular psychiatrist will help him resolve his personal problems.

# A Life-Long Illness . . . Now At Least Under Control

Jerry Witt* is a personable young man of 27 whose psychosis has been arrested but who continues to see Dr. Hawkins weekly for psychotherapy. He had a turbulent history of mental illness which manifested itself in early childhood with nightmares, hyperactivity, and hypersensitivity to sound. Always bright, he was at the top of his class without effort until he reached sixth grade. Then he retrogressed, couldn't concentrate on his studies, and was drawn to problem kids.

"I began to have hallucinations—the Japs were always attacking me. . . . My family spent a fortune to try to help me. For years I saw psychiatrists three times a week, while I was going in and out of different private schools . . . . I was 17 when I became involved in drugs and I would just kind of disappear for weeks at a time," Jerry said.

No psychiatrist ever told his parents that he was schizophrenic, but they always believed his illness was biochemical rather than psychogenic, since their other two children functioned well.

About five years ago, Jerry's mother heard about orthomolecular psychiatry through her rabbi and after a violent episode, Jerry was admitted to Brunswick Hospital under Dr. Hawkins' care. Megavitamin therapy was initiated and Jerry was put on a high-protein, low-carbohydrate diet. When he returned home after two months, he showed considerable improvement. He got himself a job and stayed away from drugs. However, his illness is of long standing and Jerry has deep-rooted psychological problems. While the schizophrenia is definitely under control, he still finds concentration difficult and is not employed at this time.

Is the chronic patient more difficult to help? Yes, says Dr. Hawkins. A patient who has been withdrawn for years will acquire bad habit patterns and superimposed disabilities. When the disease is caught early, the response is better.

## From Visions of Terror to a Bright Future

Lilly* is an example of a schizophrenic who took ill suddenly, began orthomolecular treatment within a year, and made a dramatic recovery. Lilly, an attractive young lady with cascading dark hair and shining eyes, is now 31 years old and single.

"About six years ago," she related, "I had a romantic breakup. It broke me up, too, and I went into a deep depression. . . . . Then I began to have hallucinations. Things would seem to blow up in front of me and change colors. A white man would become black. Eerie voices were stalking me. I tried not to pay attention, but it got to the point where I couldn't concentrate, and I finally lost my job as a secretary.

"That was it . . . I panicked," said Lilly. "I went to a psychiatrist for a couple of months but psychotherapy and tranquilizers didn't help. I was so miserable, I left home. When I came back, my mother told me about megavitamin therapy and begged me to try it. She had read about it in a newspaper article."

Soon Lilly had an appointment at the clinic. Dr. Hawkins asked no psychological questions about her childhood or family. After a series of tests, he prescribed huge daily doses of vitamins $B_3$, $B_6$, C, and $B_1$, plus the high-protein, low-carbohydrate diet. In two weeks her hallucinations ended.

Lilly went back to work and is now in "the best job I ever

had." She appears confident and well integrated. She's never had a relapse and sees Dr. Hawkins only twice a year. Lilly realizes she must live with her problem all her life—like an obese person or a diabetic. She has never skipped her vitamins but when she goes off her diet, she becomes "nauseous and headachy."

Megavitamin therapy is also being successfully used in treating childhood schizophrenia, a developmental abnormality that seriously interferes with a child's functioning in all areas of his life. In the past, psychotherapy was the most common treatment and its results were questionable. The use of drugs altered the behavior disorders by sedating or tranquilizing the child, but the effect was merely stop-gap. With megavitamin therapy, the improvement in children is even more impressive than in adults. Children whose treatment begins between three and nine years of age have a fine chance of recovery.

# Dannie's Doing Fine Now

Dannie*, an alert 12-year-old who wants to be a dentist, is a schizophrenic who has made a remarkable recovery on megavitamins. Though he always had a sleeping problem, was shy, uncoordinated, and would sometimes talk to himself, his parents chalked up his increasingly erratic behavior to the stress of moving into a new neighborhood. They never thought there was anything wrong with him—just the usual problems of growing up. However, when he was eight years old in the second grade, his teacher noted the descrepancy between his obvious intelligence and his low I.Q. score. He was subnormal in abstract thinking.

"On the advice of the school psychologist, we consulted a pediatric psychiatrist, who suggested psychotherapy and said that a long-term treatment would probably be necessary," Dannie's mother, a nurse, recalled. "We turned it down.

"Then we read a newspaper article about the North Nassau Clinic, and we took Dannie there. He was immediately put on vitamins, and we noticed an improvement within a month.

"Dannie is now out-going and relaxed," his mother continued. "He's developed a sense of humor and appears to be well accepted by his classmates. He rides a two-wheeler like the other kids on the block and, best of all, his report card is sprinkled with As. Right now, he is taking vitamins, C, $B_6$, and nicotinamide."

How often does he see the doctor?

"About nine times a year."

## Megavitamin Therapy: Today and Tomorrow

What is the role of megavitamin therapy in preventive medicine? Family members who show schizoid tendencies often embark on a prophylactic regimen.

The North Nassau Mental Health Center serves as a model for the development of similar facilities throughout the country by the American Schizophrenic Association. It is licensed, non-profit, and self-sustaining. Cost to the patient is comparatively low. Because the approach is orthomolecular rather than psychoanalytic, as in most other mental health clinics, the staff composition is more economical. Ninety-five percent of all patients are seen by a psychiatrist on the first visit, in contrast to the conventional clinic where treatment may not begin until weeks after the initial visit.

The use of orthomolecular psychiatry is on the increase, both in clinics and private practice. In 1967, only 13 psychiatrists were known to use the method. By 1975 the Academy of Orthomolecular Psychiatry had over 200 members.

---

(Readers who wish to consult an orthomolecular psychiatrist in their own area should contact the Huxley Institute for Biosocial Research at 1114 First Avenue, New York, N.Y. 10021.)

# CHAPTER 110

# Adjusting Biochemistry with Vitamins

The recovery of a schizophrenic through megavitamin therapy is not a "miracle," according to Carl C. Pfeiffer, Ph.D., M.D., director of the Brain Bio Center, Princeton, N.J. He believes patients improve simply because abnormal brain chemistry has been identified and corrected by megadoses of appropriate nutrients, and with this help the brain can function normally.

A medical graduate of the University of Chicago, with a Ph.D. in pharmacology, Dr. Pfeiffer has had a long and distinguished career in acedemic medicine and research, with some 245 scientific publications to his credit. Prior to the founding of the Brain Bio Center in 1973, he was deputy director of the Bureau of Research of the New Jersey Neuropsychiatric Institute in Princeton. It was there that he began studies and treatment programs he continues to develop today.

The Center does not confine its practice to the so-called "mentally ill." Dr. Pfeiffer has found that a variety of disorders, including arthritis and headaches, can be improved by correcting biochemical imbalances. However, he is best known for his work on the group of "mental" disorders loosely characterized as schizophrenia.

In *The Schizophrenias: Yours and Mine* (New York: Pyramid House, 1970), Dr. Pfeiffer and his coauthors point out that many mental disorders once loosely categorized as "schizophrenia" have long since been rescued from the "catch-all" category.

Today, nobody disputes that the schizophrenia-like brain disorders of niacin deficiency (pellagra), brain syphillis, thyroid deficiency, vitamin $B_{12}$ and folic acid deficiency, and a number of other recognized factors affecting brain function, have a biochemical basis. Nobody suggests that such ailments are purely mental or should be treated by talk therapy. Yet, at the turn of the century, all these diversely caused yet clinically similar disorders were classified as one and the same thing.

In the future,the authors stated, "other specific entities will be separated from the hodgepodge we call the schizophrenias."

## Chemistry and Sanity

Dr. Pfeiffer is confident that he and his colleagues are further reducing the schizophrenia hodgepodge—the "cause unknown" category. Most of the schizophrenic patients coming to the Brain Bio Center show up with one of these biochemical abnormalities: (1) low serum histamine, (2) high serum histamine, (3) a metabolic abnormality that leads to a build-up of the chemical kryptopyrrole in the urine.

The early pioneers in megavitamin therapy, according to Dr. Pfeiffer, had much success with schizophrenics because their key vitamin, niacin, helps raise histamine levels, and many schizophrenics fall in the low histamine category. As these doctors began adding other vitamins to the treatment in megadoses, vitamin C with niacin strengthened this action. Vitamin $B_6$ helps counter the abnormal concentration of kryptopyrrole, so another classification of schizophrenic patients was helped when this vitamin was added to the megavitamin regime.

However, as critics were quick to point out, only a certain proportion of schizophrenics responded favorably to this "shotgun" approach. Most obviously, those with high serum histamine would require quite different and even opposite nutritional treatment from patients whose serum histamine was low. More generally, the improvement rate couldn't be truly reliable until it became possible to tailor the treatment to each individual patient's biochemical needs.

At the Brain Bio Center, patients are diagnosed through blood and urine tests and appropriate supplements and medications are prescribed. Ninety percent of diagnosed schizophrenic patients show significant improvement—the Center claims. Of these patients, some 30 to 40 percent have excess kryptopyrrole (the "mauve factor") in their urine. Dr. Pfeiffer has stated that this abnormality is not revealed by ordinary urinalysis. However, in a quite simple laboratory test, urine will turn a deep pink or mauve color when kryptopyrrole is present. Dr. Pfeiffer believes that this "mauve factor" may turn out to be "the major missing component of the schizophrenias."

Kryptopyrrole complexes with B6 and zinc, pulling them out of the blood, Dr. Pfeiffer explained, and patients with this disease are therefore severely deficient in these two essential nutrients, with consequent faulty brain chemistry. They "need *enough* B6 and zinc to compensate for the urinary loss," he emphasized. With appropriate supplements, according to Dr. Pfeiffer, "relief of symptoms is often dramatic."

# CHAPTER 111

# Vitamins Offer Hope
# for Autistic Children

Autism is a personality disease in children which inhibits them from reacting to their environment. Children who are autistic in infancy do not learn to talk—others simply stop talking. They do not respond to people and seem not to see or hear them. They are completely withdrawn. The disease has been so unresponsive to treatment that it has caused despair in medical ranks.

Until May 1973, there was little hope of a successful treatment for autism. Then, at a conference of the Canadian Schizophrenia Foundation held in Toronto, it was demonstrated that autistic children responded well to orthomolecular treatment. Bernard Rimland, Ph.D., a research psychologist from San Diego, told the Toronto meeting a compelling story of the happy results of using megavitamins to treat a group of such children. Dr. Rimland's story goes back to a 1965 *New York Times* article which described the success of Drs. Abram Hoffer and Humphrey Osmond in treating adult schizophrenics with massive doses of vitamins. A number of parents with autistic children read the article and in desperation decided to try the vitamins on their own. In most cases they had tried psychotherapy, but it proved to be useless.

# Home Treatment Sometimes Worked

"I began to get letters from parents describing the results of these experiments they had tried," said Dr. Rimland. "The *Times* article was not explicit enough to tell the parents what kinds of vitamins to use and what dosages, so there was quite a variation in vitamins and dosages. As I read these reports it became evident that some children had shown remarkable improvement on the vitamins. The parents were reporting good results when the vitamins were taken and a resumption of symptoms when they were stopped."

This sparked Dr. Rimland's interest and he decided to make a survey of all parents on his mailing list at the Institute for Child Behavior Research. About 60 parents responded and Dr. Rimland found that there were four vitamins that were outstanding in their positive effects. These were niacinamide ($B_3$), pantothenic acid, $B_6$, and vitamin C. As the megavitamin proponents steadily emphasize, vitamin C and the B vitamins are water-soluble, so there is no danger of overdose because the body simply eliminates what it doesn't use.

On the basis of these reports, Dr. Rimland and his staff designed a special vitamin formula and then enrolled about 300 children in a nationwide study. They required that any child taking part had to be under medical supervision. This created some difficulty because most physicians were less than eager to have anything to do with the vitamin therapy program.

According to Dr. Rimland, "One family with two autistic children said their doctor was adamant in his refusal to let us enroll their two children in the study. This doctor was so determined not to be taken in that he wrote to Dr. Linus Pauling, who had offered to respond with a personal letter to any physician asking about the validity and safety of our study. When the doctor got a personal reply from Dr. Pauling he reluctantly agreed to let the children take part. It turned out that the two children improved so much that the doctor wrote us a letter asking if the family's three other children could be enrolled in the same study to see if their learning disabilities would improve. It was interesting to see this extremely skeptical physician change his mind this way."

The study was designed so that the children were on the vitamins for a three-month period and then off for one month to see if there was a deterioration. Then, treatment was resumed for a short time to see if the behavior would again improve. Depending on the child's weight, dosages were one, two, or three grams a day of vitamin C, the same amount of niacinamide, 150–450 mg. of $B_6$, and 200 mg. of pantothenic acid, plus a high potency multiple B tablet.

Both parents and physicians were asked to complete a form periodically giving their observations on the child's behavior improvements relating to speech, alertness, sleeping habits, eating habits, tantrums, and other kinds of behavior. Before beginning the study, each of the parents completed a detailed form on their child's birth history and medical background and this information was recorded on a computer tape. Dr. Rimland then turned the computer tape over to several university computer centers and asked them to apply a new type of data analysis called computer cluster analysis. This was designed to learn if there were certain subgroups among these autistic children and sort each subgroup into a special cluster. In some instances there might be a genetic vitamin dependency and these children could be predicted to improve. In other cases there might be destruction of brain tissue from viral infection and these children would not improve with the vitamins.

## Results Judged Independently

After Dr. Rimland and his staff assembled all the information, they gave it to three judges who independently examined the data to decide whether or not the child had improved on a scale from 99 to zero. If the judges did not agree, that particular case was discarded. In cases where the judges were sure the child had improved a great deal the child got a score of 99. If the improvement was not spectacular he or she got an 80. Where there was probably no improvement he or she might get a 40 all the way down to zero which meant the child not only had not improved but there was some deterioration in behavior.

After the computer clustering had been completed and the scores assigned, the results showed that well over 50 percent of the children improved significantly and about three percent got worse on the vitamins. Most important from the scientific standpoint, the children differentiated by the clusters responded differently to the vitamins. "In each case," said Dr. Rimland, "these were primarily the evaluations of the parents who were observing the children every day." Improvement showed in reduced tantrums, increased alertness, improved speech, better sleep patterns, greater sociability.

One mother wrote: "We are on the 31st day of the vitamin study and I want to discuss the changes that took place these last three days. I am too excited about it to wait for the next report period. For the past two days Susan has been doing a lot of talking, initiating conversations, asking questions, commenting on everything she hears around her."

At Dr. Rimland's suggestion, some of the parents who had not seen significant changes during the study were asked to double the dosage of $B_6$. One mother who had doubled the $B_6$ wrote: "Now this has made a difference. She is very eager to do things . . . at slight suggestion ready for almost anything. Eager to play basketball in front of the house. Hasn't printed her name or numbers for over a year, but doing it now . . . . Even my husband who is a disbeliever says she has improved these past four days."

Another parent reported: "Elsie has been on the doubled $B_6$ and has shown great improvement . . . she is sharper and more aware of the outside world . . . we lit our Chanukah candles and she surprised us all by singing a Chanukah song from beginning to end."

On the other hand, when the vitamins were stopped, a parent wrote after ten days of no treatment: "William seems to have withdrawn into himself, no longer exhibiting the lively interest in the world around him that had marked the previous month. His new-found willingness to cooperate and obey such directions as he understood disappeared rapidly. His old repertoire of man-nerisms and bizarre hand motions and positions, which had been waning, reasserted itself with a vengeance.''

The three percent of the children in the study who got worse became irritable and difficult to manage. They were extremely sensitive to sound and would cover their ears when there was a loud or shrill sound. Some of the children reverted to bed-wetting. These problems were so severe that a number of the children were taken off the vitamins when the parents could no longer tolerate the behavior.

Dr. Rimland approached a number of medical people to see if they could find an answer to the problem, but it was nutritionist Adelle Davis who came upon the solution. After reviewing what nutrients the children were being given, Ms. Davis told Dr. Rim-land that magnesium should be added.

According to her, a magnesium deficiency can cause bed-wetting, sound sensitivity, and irritability.

"She hit right on the button just exactly what was happening with a segment of our study group," remarked Dr. Rimland. "This results because when you give B6 in large quantities it interacts with magnesium in such a way that magnesium is taken out of other body systems. So, if the child happens to be marginal in the amount of magnesium the body stores, then B6 takes essential magnesium and you have a magnesium-deficient child. We immediately informed the parents whose children had developed these side effects to add magnesium and they reported that the side effects went away, in some cases overnight.''

## B6 is Important

From the cases that Dr. Rimland has seen, he concluded: "It is my feeling that of these vitamins for children, B6 will be found to be the most important. Some of the children respond very well to niacin or niacinamide but in the most dramatic results we've seen, particularly the classical cases of autism, they have proven to be B6 responsive.''

There are also failures, of course. Not all behavior problems stem from vitamin dependency. There are diseases that affect the brain—allergy should be investigated as a possibility. Yet many autistic and otherwise disturbed children have responded to nutritional therapy, and that is remarkable for a disease that for decades has not responded at all to dozens of attempted treatments.

# CHAPTER 112

# Vitamin Treatment Reduces Learning Disabilities

A prominent psychiatrist has found that by administering large, therapeutic doses of certain vitamins to children with learning disabilities, he has gotten better results than have ever been claimed for the dangerous amphetamines. In effect, Allan Cott, M.D., psychiatric consultant to the New York Institute of Child Development, has found a way to improve or cure the health problem responsible for the learning disability, instead of merely masking the problem and leaving it untreated, which is what amphetamine administration does.

Hyperactivity, a major emotional problem in young children, is often treated with amphetamines or the drug Ritalin. However, Dr. Cott, who also maintains a private psychiatric practice, feels that their quieting effect wears off too soon and that they may produce dangerous side effects. But most important, Dr. Cott believes that the child's real problem is not the hyperactivity—that is but a symptom—but an internal biochemical disorder that responds to massive doses of vitamins $B_2$, $B_3$, $B_6$, C, and E, as well as to a change in diet.

While those who back behavior drugs for children claim that the problem ends with the onset of adolescence, they are speaking only about the hyperactivity. Dr. Cott found that adolescence only brings on slightly different symptoms. The real problem does not necessarily fade away with time, but just lies in wait.

"Actually," Dr. Cott related, "the first group of children I saw who had learning disabilities were adolescents who weren't doing well in junior high school or in their late elementary grades. They were perfectly normal children, in schools for normal children. They just couldn't learn and they couldn't concentrate. Their mothers remarked about them that they would try to read, but after a few mistakes would get uptight, uneasy. Taking a long history on these kids, I found that the outstanding symptom that they suffered earlier in life was hyperactivity, even though by adolescence the hyperactivity was, for the most part, gone."

Dr. Cott decided to try large doses of vitamins to reduce hyperactivity in children because of successful results with orthomolecular therapy in treating mentally ill adults.

"I've been treating psychiatric disorders, that is, mental illness, with the use of massive doses of vitamins for a number of years. I found such good results in the treatment of adults that I extended its use to the children in treating childhood mental disorders. The improvements were more marked than in adults, and produced more dramatic results."

## Strong Effect on Learning Disabilities

"One of the things that I found while I was treating these children was that as their illness began to recede and was at least under reasonable control, their hyperactivity, which is one of the major symptoms of all children who suffer from any kind of emotional disorders, subsided. As the hyperactivity subsided, the children were able to begin to learn.

"I then began to use it in children who had only learning disabilities. I saw children of all kinds and published some of the results that I had with the treatment of psychotic or grossly disturbed children."

However, it was the successful treatment of a college student that convinced Dr. Cott that his method should be applied as soon as possible to children suffering learning difficulties. Previous to that, he could only tell parents who brought their hyperactive children to him that he had no background or experience with the children who were not suffering brain injury but nevertheless had difficulties learning in school. He had found nothing in the literature of his profession to help him out. At the parents' insistence upon getting help for their children, he tried the vitamin therapy on the hyperactive children and both he and the parents were amazed by the improvement.

Then a mother brought her 19-year-old-son, a college student, to see Dr. Cott. This case was to be a turning point in the treatment of hyperactive children with vitamins.

"Again, I had to tell her I didn't know whether this was going to help because I never treated someone this age who was having learning difficulties. The boy and his mother told me that he had, with the exertion of the greatest kind of effort, gotten through high school and into his first year of college. They came to see me when he came home for the Christmas holidays.

"He said that his friends would finish their day's homework in about two hours or so, while he frequently would have to work eight hours to do the same work. Because reading, concentration, and comprehension were very difficult, he would have to read a paragraph over and over before he could absorb the meaning.

"I put him on massive doses of vitamins, those suitable for an adult of his height and weight, and about two months later received a letter from his mother. I forwarded it to the American Schizophrenia Association so that they could have it on file, if they wanted, because it was a kind of testimonial for orthomolecular therapy that I hadn't seen anywhere before.

"You see, here was a 19-year-old boy, and for the first time in his mother's memory of him, he would sit and read a book with pleasure. Up until that time reading had been almost agony for him.

"I began speaking about him to the staff of the Institute (the New York Institute for Child Development, Inc.). They began to work with the vitamins. When they had seen a sufficient number of cases in order to have a fair-sized sample, they were astonished, just as I had been, at the results that they were getting. They then set up a department for the treatment of learning disabilities, combining their standard methods of treatment with the use of the vitamins. A thirty-pound child might receive one gram of vitamin $B_3$, 200 mg. of $B_6$, one gram of C, and 400 to 800 I.U. of vitamin E. As a result, they saw a marked upswing in the rate of child development.

"In the meantime, in my own practice, I continued treating these children I saw who had learning disabilities and always got the same results. If the parents were persistent and stuck with the medication, the children began to improve. The parents who tried it and got very little results were the parents who had given it up much too early. It's not like a drug."

That is, the vitamins require a longer time to take hold because they are building up a healthy cellular foundation, step by step, and not just eliminating symptoms the way the drugs do. The slower working vitamins actually take hold where there is a demand for more of a nutrient than, perhaps, the diet is able to provide. Either the nutrient isn't in the food, or the food can't be absorbed properly by the body. The effect of the vitamins is more permanent because they encourage basic biochemical changes in the child, which may mean the reduction of hyperactivity and the ability to sit down, learn enthusiastically, and work constructively.

Don't drugs reduce hyperactivity more quickly and give the child an opportunity to learn? Drugs do indeed slow down the child's over-activity, but they eliminate only the symptoms, not the cause of the problem. Drugs also present the danger of many different side effects, and if not taken properly, may lead to drug dependencies.

## Better Diet May Be All That is Needed

While some hyperactive children need massive doses of specific vitamins in order to compensate for a metabolic disturbance which makes their digestive absorption inefficient, many other children suffer problems caused by nothing more than the foods that they eat every day, and which subside when the diet is altered.

Dr. Cott has seen many cases in which children responded favorably to the removal of sweets from their diets. According to him, hyperactive children have been found to have a high incidence of low blood sugar. Since the brain needs glucose in order to function properly, and since eating sugar will actually lower the blood sugar content, the ingestion of sweets lowers the efficiency of the brain, including its learning ability. "Even a normal child can't learn if his bloodstream doesn't carry glucose to the brain," Dr. Cott warns. Eating sweets and starches may also induce a deficiency of B vitamins, thus depriving the brain of nutrients essential for proper functioning.

# CHAPTER 113

# The Vitamin A
# Effect on Acne

Acne begins when the tiny channels or follicles leading from sebaceous (oil) glands in the skin to the skin surface become plugged up. Ordinary dirt can clog the follicles, but far more frequently skin cells themselves are responsible.

The top layer of skin is hard and horny. These outer skin cells are continually being brushed away by clothing, bathing, etc. But during adolescence, they sometimes begin adhering to each other. Then, instead of being sloughed off, they become lodged in the small follicles coming from the sebaceous glands.

Each hard little plug is known as a comedone. The plugged condition is called keratosis. When an individual has lots of comedones he or she is said to be suffering from hyperkeratosis of the sebaceous ducts or follicles.

The sebaceous glands ordinarily secrete a lubricant called sebum. Even when the follicle is plugged shut, the secretion continues. This causes swelling and irritation. A papule, or small pimple, results. If the pimple contains pus, it is called a pustule. Sometimes even a cyst forms.

In the early 1940s Jon D. Straumfjord, M.D., of Astoria, Oregon, described his study in which he treated 100 acne patients with oral doses of vitamin A. Writing in the August

1943, issue of *Northwest Medicine,* Dr. Straumfjord reported that each patient took 100,000 I.U. of vitamin A contained in halibut liver oil at bedtime. The first reaction was a definite aggravation or worsening of the condition. However, 36 of the 100 patients "became entirely free from acne while under treatment and 43 more became free except from occasional acne papule or pustule." In most cases, the responses occurred in less than nine months. "Usually definite improvement is noticeable in about three months, although at times six or more months may elapse before definite benefit is seen." Dr. Straumfjord recorded. He noted that those with severe acne recover about as quickly as those with mild cases.

In another study, reported in the *Journal of Investigative Dermatology* (April 1950), Leonard E. Savitt, M.D., of Los Angeles described his work with 35 college students suffering from acne. Each was given capsules of 100,000 units of vitamin A daily. Twenty improved, 12 experienced no change, and three became worse. Four years later Dr. K.D. Lahari observed similar results in 75 patients receiving 100,000 units of daily vitamin A. "All had previously resisted other forms of treatment, some for several years, he reported in the *Journal of the Indian Medical Association* (March 1954). The lesions disappeared in two and a half months in 30 cases, in three months in another 30 cases, and five and a half months in 10 cases. Dr. Lahari said that "All (the patients) could be regarded as cured at the end of six months."

Although these results were extremely encouraging, other studies showed that the vitamin A-acne treatment had two major drawbacks. A cure, if it occurred, could take as long as a year or more. Second, the treatment required a high dosage of the vitamin. Studies indicated that, under special circumstances, large amounts of A on a daily basis could be toxic. What was needed was a more efficient way of utilizing the vitamin's powerful anti-acne properties.

And in the past few years such a treatment has been developed. Experiments by Albert M. Kligman, M.D., Ph.D., and James E. Fulton, Jr., M.D., show that a solution containing vitamin A acid is twice as effective as previous vitamin A acne treatments. The University of Pennsylvania researchers discovered that vitamin A acid in most cases begins to clear up acne from three to five weeks after the initial treatment, and usually the skin is almost back to normal within three months. This method was discussed for the first time in June, 1968, at the American Medical Association's 117th annual convention in San Francisco. Some of the country's best-known dermatologists responded enthusiastically when Dr. Fulton read his paper, "Topical Vitamin A Acid in Acne." Dermatologists at their annual meeting in Chicago in 1971 were so impressed by the results that they awarded the University of Pennsylvania researchers a silver medal for Research in Skin Disease.

Instead of administering the vitamin orally, Drs. Kligman and Fulton applied it directly to the affected area. This required a form of vitamin A which would make the skin react in a way that enhanced the action of the vitamin. Chemically speaking, vitamin A can be an alcohol, aldehyde, acid, acetate, or palmitate ester. These various forms have slightly different properties. The researchers found that vitamin A acid was the most effective in irritating, and thus penetrating, the skin. Vitamin A acid was the material they used in their study.

A group of 229 adolescent patients at the Acne Clinic, Hospital of the University of Pennsylvania, took part in the study. The teenagers were divided into four groups: 37 underwent traditional therapy, sulfur resorcinol; 49 received benzoyl peroxide, apparently the favorite among doctors; 40 more were control subjects. Vitamin A acid was used on the remaining 103 patients. In some cases, the researchers applied a .1 percent concentration of vitamin A acid to the left side of the patient's face and one of the other substances to the right.

Every week the researchers counted the number of lesions on the patients' faces. Three or four months later the degree of improvement was evaluated. The controls showed an improvement of 8.3 percent—presumably the normal rate of improvement without therapy. Of the teenagers on the sulfur resorcinol, total improvement averaged 15.9 percent. Those receiving benzoyl peroxide had a 31.9 percent improvement.

But it was the patients treated with vitamin A acid who

improved the most. More than 75 percent of those in this group had a 50 percent or more reduction of countable lesions. More specifically, 38.8 percent of the vitamin A acid group had 75 percent or greater reduction of acne, while another 37.8 percent showed a 50 to 74 percent improvement.

Like other acne remedies, topical vitamin A works by inflaming the skin. Within a few days after the vitamin is applied, the face becomes dry and somewhat redder. The upper layer of skin—which sticks together and forms the comedones—begins to peel off.

In its early stages, the treatment aggravates the acne condition. In the first six weeks open comedones rise up from the skin. These scores of new comedones studding the skin surface can be wiped away by the fingers. Slight pimples develop into full-blown and open comedones. New pustules and papules suddenly appear.

However, the intensification of the disease really works to advantage. Dr. Fulton theorized that, "Under the influence of vitamin A acid, comedones, inert for weeks or months, suddenly 'blew up'. As a rule, these inflammatory lesions were rather small, implying that the (vitamin A) acid was exciting inflammatory explosions at an earlier stage than would occur naturally." According to Fulton, no other medication now available has this effect.

In addition to removing the dry skin plugging the follicles and shortening the life cycle of already-existing comedones, pustules, and papules, the vitamin A acid prevented the formation of new comedones. Fulton speculates that the vitamin A accelerates the production of hard skin cells, which do not stick together. Instead, the new cells flush out the old ones which form the comedones. And unlike other preparations, it doesn't lose its effectiveness after repeated use. Other remedies eventually cause the skin to harden, negating the important irritant effect. Another point in vitamin A's favor, according to Dr. Fulton, is that "even with excessive use, the skin recovers within a few days after stopping treatment. Deeply motivated patients should not be dissuaded from increasing the frequency of application, for patients with the most irritated faces achieve the most rapid improvement.''

The researchers stress the fact that vitamin A-acid therapy should not be thought of as a panacea for acne. Although some patients improve with topical application of vitamin A acid, there are some who do not. About seven percent of those patients using the therapy did not improve. Some even got worse. However, this does not discredit the outstanding record of improvement in a high percentage of adolescents studied.

The value of taking vitamin A orally should not be ignored in helping to prevent acne. The originator of vitamin A acne therapy, Dr. Jon D. Straumfjord, said that oral vitamin A supplements may keep acne away, once the condition is cleared up and the acid applications are discontinued. Daily oral doses of vitamin A and diets high in that nutrient combined with soapless face-washing several times daily may spare youngsters now entering adolescence the misery of an acne condition.

# CHAPTER 114

# Vitamin E for Special
# Skin Problems

The value of vitamin A and the B-complex vitamins in maintaining clear and healthy skin has been recognized by medical authorities all over the world, but vitamin E, a nutrient often overlooked by many dermatologists, may do more things for the skin than generally realized. Dr. Irwin I. Lubowe, clinical professor of dermatology at the New York Medical College and the author of over 100 scientific articles on cosmetics and dermatology, has successfully used topical applications of vitamin E for skin problems. " . . . in a survey I conducted, topical use of highly concentrated vitamin E has improved roughness and lines in the skin," reported Dr. Lubowe in his book *The Modern Guide to Skin Care and Beauty* (New York: E.P. Dutton and Co., 1973). Other physicians report that vitamin E is bringing about miraculous remissions in rare and ghastly skin conditions which had previously been considered incurable.

One such condition is known as *epidermolysis bullosa*, which describes a number of syndromes characterized by the formation of bullae, or fluid-filled blisters. The lesions may appear after an injury or spontaneously, and may be terribly severe. In the *Archives of Dermatology* (January 1974), Jerold D. Michaelson, M.D., and colleagues, affiliated with the Depart-

701

ments of Dermatology and Biochemistry at the Baylor College of Medicine in Houston, described the outcome in treating three patients with this condition, for which there is no recognized successful therapy.

One patient was an 11-year-old girl who developed the condition at the age of eight, and by 11, had the ugly bullae on her hands, fingers, elbows, knees, and feet. Many of these were infected, scarring was already present, and several toenails were actually absent.

For two years, the girl was treated with steroids, the anti-inflammatory drugs used for a whole host of skin problems. But no clear benefit resulted. She was then given 600 I.U. of vitamin E a day. After 15 days, the blisters stopped developing. After 30 days, her dosage was cut in half, and by the time of the medical report, the girl had been free of blisters for one year. Previously, the longest she had gone without getting blisters was six days.

Another patient was a girl only one year old, who was covered with bleeding blisters. Given 100 I.U. of vitamin E a day, she remained free of new blisters for a period of five months, at which time she began developing some more. When her dosage of vitamin E was doubled, she was again free of blisters.

Another disfiguring skin disease is known as *subcorneal pustular dermatosis*. Like *epidermolysis bullosa*, there is no satisfactory treatment for this disease, which is characterized by patches of fluid-filled vesicles which may appear widely over the body. In a recent case report, however, it was shown that vitamin E may be the answer.

Samuel Ayres, Jr., M.D., and Richard Mihan, M.D., who are respectively affiliated with the Department of Dermatology at the University of California at Los Angeles and the Department of Dermatology at the University of Southern California School of Medicine, reported the results in *Archives of Dermatology* (June 1974). Their patient was a 63-year-old woman who had been under treatment for five years without success. During this time, she had been on many drugs, not only for a skin condition, but also for diabetes, high blood pressure, and other conditions. She was begun on 100 I.U. of vitamin E and gradually worked up to 400 I.U. daily. Four weeks later, her skin was free of pustules, and only slight redness remained. Simultaneously, she was able to discontinue taking a diuretic drug for her edema, and was able to keep her urine sugar-free "with 15 to 20 units of insulin, whereas she had formerly required an average of 50 units a day." (Because of vitamin E's ability to reduce insulin requirement, patients who take insulin should be given initially a small dose of vitamin E which is increased gradually as the insulin is reduced, to avoid an insulin shock reaction, Drs. Ayres and Mihan warn.) During a two-year follow-up period, the patient remained free of the skin problem which had plagued her for five years previously.

## Another Intriguing Report From Los Angeles

The same Los Angeles doctors reported an equally dramatic case in the August 1973, issue of *Archives of Dermatology*. This one involved a rather bizarre condition known as the "yellow nail syndrome," in which the nails thicken, turn yellow, and stop growing. Simultaneously, for entirely unknown reasons, the patient usually has respiratory problems and edema, or swelling.

Drs. Ayres and Mihan were presented with a 65-year-old woman who had these symptoms and several other problems as well, notably numbness and tingling of the fingertips and frequent cramping in her legs.

Treatment with vitamin E in the form of d-alpha tocopheryl acetate, 400 I.U. twice daily before meals, was begun. Three months later, the nails were still discolored and thick, but her leg cramps were much improved. After another month, though, her nails began to grow again, and within six months, they appeared to be perfectly normal. Nearly two years after her first visit, the patient had reduced her dose of vitamin E from 800 I.U. to 400 I.U. a day, and her nails were remaining normal; she had no more puffiness of the eyelids, no numbness of the fingers, and no leg cramps. What's more, whereas she had been slated for surgery to relieve a chronic sinus condition when she was first seen, the doctors wrote that a recent x ray showed "no indication for surgery."

These last few conditions aren't common. But they were worth describing for two reasons. First, even if only a few people are so afflicted, it's still worthwhile to let them know that there is new hope for their problem. Second, these case histories illustrate that the effect of nutrients such as vitamin E on the skin can be dramatic.

# CHAPTER 115

# Psoriasis Responds to Vitamin A Applications

Vitamin A acid has also been shown to be an effective treatment for psoriasis and other skin ailments. Psoriasis is a condition which causes unsightly, scaly, and itchy splotches on its victim's skin, and has baffled skin doctors down through the ages. "Psoriasis is an antidote for the dermatologist's ego," Dr. P. Bechet, an eminent dermatologist and medical historian once remarked. Those suffering from this pesky disease usually try every treatment there is—tar or mercury Chrysarobinx ointments, phenol, x-ray therapy, or even steroids.

While some doctors still use the coal tar or mercury ointments, it is the steroids, ACTH and cortisone, and their derivatives, that are most frequently prescribed today. These can cause side effects worse than the original ailment. Cortisone causes urinary losses of calcium and phosphorus which can lead to demineralization of the bones. Steroid therapy has been known to cause ulcers and adrenal exhaustion, with a subsequent lack of recuperative powers. The steroids also break down the body's defense mechanisms.

However, psoriasis sufferers may soon be able to dispense with the more dangerous drugs. In a double-blind controlled study two researchers at the University of Miami School of

Medicine found that in its acid form, vitamin A relieved itching and unsightliness in 24 out of 26 psoriasis patients. Drs. Phillip Frost and Gerald D. Weinstein, both of the Department of Dermatology, reported that the beneficial effects were noticeable after only one week of treatment (*Journal of the American Medical Association*, 10 March 1969).

Before undertaking a clinical study of vitamin A acid, Drs. Frost and Weinstein first compared the effects of several commonly available forms of topically administered vitamin A on three patients with extensive psoriasis and three patients with lamellar ichthyosis (dry, rough, scaly skin). The doctors taped a piece of cotton gauze to four afflicted areas on the arms of each patient. Then the doctors injected each piece of gauze with either a solution of vitamin A acid, vitamin A aldehyde, vitamin A alcohol, or vitamin A acetate.

When the patches were removed 48 hours later, there was a slight softening of the skin in each of the patched areas. Drs. Frost and Weinstein marked the patch sites and checked them daily. After a week, the area which had vitamin A acid applied to it showed a marked decrease in scaling in the ichthyosis patients and less erythema (redness caused by congestion of the capillaries) in the psoriasis patients. No changes were discernible where the other forms of vitamin A had been applied.

Intrigued by the results of the patch test, the physicians began a more extensive evaluation of vitamin A acid. They chose patients with skin conditions most resistant to all types of treatment—ten with epidermolytic hyperkeratosis (in which the skin becomes hard and loose); 24 with some form of ichthyosis, and 26 with extensive psoriasis. A control preparation containing no vitamin A acid was applied to an affected area on one side of the patients' bodies. A preparation looking exactly the same but containing either .1, .2, or .3 percent vitamin A acid was applied to similarly afflicted areas on the other side of the subjects' bodies. Preparations were coded in a double-blind fashion, so that neither patients nor physicians knew which side received the "active" mixture. Both preparations were applied twice daily.

As in the patch test, vitamin A acid was responsible for a dramatic improvement in almost every patient, especially those with disorders not usually responsive to treatment. While those with a mild case of ichthyosis experienced relief on both sides of their bodies, in no case did greater improvement occur on the control side. In 24 out of 25 psoriasis patients the side treated with vitamin A acid showed a decrease in scaling and redness within a week. (Most improvement became apparent after three weeks of treatment.) Nine of the patients had complete clearing of the vitamin A-acid-treated side, but no healing on the control side. Eleven had moderate healing and four experienced a slight improvement.

Drs. Frost and Weinstein noted that, to be effective, the vitamin A acid solution had to be either a .2 or .3 percent concentration. When German investigator von Beer used only a .1 percent vitamin A acid preparation on 20 patients, there was no noticeable improvement. The Florida investigators believed the more favorable response they achieved was due to a higher concentration. Although irritation occurred in some patients, it quickly cleared up when the medication was withheld for one or two days. The irritation usually did not recur when the medication was resumed and applied only once instead of twice a day. The patients' cleared-up condition was not permanent, however. Ten to 14 days after discontinuing therapy, both the control and active ingredient-treated side began to look the same.

# CHAPTER 116

# A Vitamin for Vitiligo

Vitiligo is a painless disease that usually afflicts people between the ages of two and 30 and is characterized by the sudden appearance of light blotches on the skin. The light patches enlarge slowly, marked by a dark border. The white patches occur because the skin, for some still unknown reason, is unable to manufacture melanin, or pigment, creating an embarrassing piebald pattern on the skin surface. It afflicts people with all skin tones, although it is more pronounced in people with dark pigmentations.

There is little discussion of the disease in medical textbooks, except for detailed descriptions of it. The impression is that the medical profession sees little to be done for the victims of vitiligo except to recommend cosmetics (usually for those with light skin tones) and caution against sunbathing, since a tan only heightens the contrast between those areas with vitiligo and those that can form normal pigment.

Several years ago, Benjamin Sieve, M.D., a professor at Tufts Medical School, compiled a comprehensive history of the treatments in use dating back to the 1930s and 1940s, and the then-current thinking on the subject. Among the treatments described by Dr. Sieve was one used by Dr. H. W. Francis. He thought the disease was due to the absence of free hydrochloric acid in the stomach, since he had vitiligo and found the acid absent in himself. He took 15 cubic centimeter doses of hydrochloric acid at each meal for two years and noted that the light areas completely disappeared. He used the same therapy on three other patients and reported similar results. Dr. Sieve suggested that the effect of the hydrochloric acid might have been to aid in the processing and absorption of necessary nutrients.

Nutrition as a factor in preserving skin pigment was reported in the *Archives of Dermatology and Syphilology* (March 1937), where researchers detailed experiments using vitamin C to restore skin color. The following year a German medical journal carried an article also recommending vitamin C as a treatment for vitiligo.

Para-aminobenzoic acid (PABA), a B vitamin, has been mentioned repeatedly in connection with the treatment of vitiligo. Michael J. Costello, M.D., in the *Archives of Dermatology and Syphilology* (February 1943) reported success in treating vitiligo of the eyelids in a two-year-old child with 100 mg. of PABA daily. Dr. Sieve was impressed with the potential of PABA, and set up an experiment to observe its effect on 48 cases of vitiligo.

The group consisted of 25 females and 23 males, ranging in age from 10 to 70 years. The vitiligo condition had persisted from two to 28 years. Most of the patients showed evidence of a chronically poor diet and a history of glandular imbalance. Fatigue, irritability, and emotional instability were common among them, as were constipation, weight gain, arthritis, and various types of headaches. Physical examinations presented classic findings consistent with an underactive thyroid condition in many of the subjects. Along with these came a preponderance of brittle nails, coarse and thickened skin, and varying degrees of hypertension (high blood pressure).

After only partial success with administering a patent combination of B-complex vitamins, Dr. Sieve instituted injections of PABA coupled with monoethanolamine (to help the vitamin remain in the blood longer) twice daily—morning and evening— and a 100 mg. tablet of PABA to be taken at noon and at bedtime. He soon observed new pigmentation in the depigmented areas. Within four to eight weeks the milk white areas of vitiligo turned pinkish. In six to 16 weeks after therapy was started, small islands of brown pigment were usually noted within the areas of vitiligo. Soon streaks were thrown from these islands and the streaks reached out to join other islands. Eventually the islands disappeared and repigmentation became complete. The results of the therapy in all 48 patients were termed "striking" after six or seven months.

Dr. Sieve stressed, time and again, the important part diet plays in vitiligo. In his opinion hormonal imbalance can also cause the disease, and contributory factors can be wounds, infections, pressure points, and light rays. The problem of vitiligo is more complex than the simple lack of the B vitamin PABA. According to Dr. Sieve's research, dietary deficiencies must be corrected, hormonal imbalances righted, and local infections cleared up before a specific vitamin can be expected to have any effect. He also emphasized that the injections to supplement the tablets are essential, because the vitamin alone, taken orally, does not remain in the bloodstream for a sufficient length of time to act effectively.

# CHAPTER 117

# Warts: A Virus
# You Can Guard Against

The answer to the medical riddle of just what causes warts, according to Daniel Hyman, M.D., of New York City's Roosevelt Hospital, lies in the viral origin of warts. They disappear when the body's immune mechanism is stimulated. The patient himself produces the antibodies which interfere with viral propagation or actually destroy the viruses outright.

Nutrients found in the normal diet may have a profound influence on the cause of warts, especially those such as plantar warts that are not caused by contagious bacteria. In an article in *Modern Medicine* (1 August 1975), Dr. Hyman said that certain sulfur-containing amino acids, such as those found in desiccated liver tablets, may be involved in a yet undefined interaction in the hypothalmus which stimulates the antibodies involved in the immunity process. He noted that warts were successfully treated in a number of institutionalized patients who were put on a daily regimen of three tablets of desiccated liver. Desiccated liver is not only a good source of these essential amino acids for the immunity system but a good source of the entire B complex as well.

Most common warts are uncomfortable, unsightly, and downright painful when they appear on parts of the body which are continually rubbed and irritated by clothing or other contact irritants. They are removed in most instances by such means as surgical paring and strong caustic chemicals; however, in a number of instances, vitamin A therapy has proven effective and painless.

## Warts Successfully Treated with Vitamin A

Dr. Hyman's theory that warts appear to disappear when the body's immunologic mechanism is stimulated also brings to light the integral role that vitamin A plays in the body's immunity defenses mentioned in an earlier chapter.

B.H. Kuhn, M.D., writing in the *Southern Medical Journal,* reported treating 90 patients with various types of warts with vitamin A palmitate in a water-dispersible form averaging 25,000 units daily for one week to six months. Cure rates of 50 to 100 percent were obtained in 79 patients. There were *no* total failures. Dr. Kuhn suggested in his reports that the vitamin A exerted an *antiviral* action that has specific therapeutic usefulness in the suppression of hyperkeratosis, or warts.

Some authorities believe that a wart develops where there is a lack of vitamin A in the skin and that introducing the vitamin will bring the skin back to normal. Marvin Sandler, M.D., a podiatrist in Allentown, Pennsylvania, said that he has used an injection of vitamin A on patients with plantar warts with excellent results. Another Allentown podiatrist, Philip LeShay, M.D., said that he prescribes vitamin A systemically in conjunction with other measures in the treatment of warts on the feet.

In the July 1959, issue of *Clinical Medicine,* two researchers reported on the results achieved by 119 physicians who, among them, treated 228 cases of plantar warts with an aqueous solution of vitamin A palmitate. Substantial benefits or complete cures were achieved in 208 of the 228 cases. In only one case did the warts reappear.

In a controlled study of 25 patients at the Jewish Hospital of

Brooklyn, New York, Dr. Joel S. Freeman and his colleagues concluded that the incidence of permanent cures and permanent relief of symptoms is so high when vitamin A palmitate is used, that it is difficult to justify repeated paring and application of keratolytics (usually salicylic acids) and astringents unless vitamin A palmitate has been found to be ineffective.

# CHAPTER 118

# Shingles Treatment

Dr. Fred Klenner, a North Carolina physician, has achieved dramatic results with vitamin C treatments. He is one of the very few doctors in the United States who consistently uses vitamin C (ascorbic acid) in the truly massive doses which Linus Pauling and biochemist Irwin Stone insist are necessary for effective therapy.

Dr. Pauling cites Dr. Klenner's book, *The Key to Good Health: Vitamin C* (San Jacinto, California: Graphic Arts Research Foundation, 1969), which reports use of ascorbic acid in amounts of one to 20 grams a day in successfully treating patients with various viral and bacterial infections. In a paper published in *Southern Medicine and Surgery* (July 1949), Dr. Klenner wrote specifically about his experience in using vitamin C against the herpes zoster virus. There were eight shingles patients treated in the series he reported—all of whom were injected with two to three grams of ascorbic acid every 12 hours, plus one gram by mouth every two hours.

"Seven experienced cessation of pain within two hours of the first injection," he reported, "and remained so without the use of any other analgesic (pain-killing) medication. Seven of these cases showed drying of the vesicles (blisters) within 24 hours and were clear of lesions within 72 hours." The eighth case, a diabetic, took longer and required 14 injections (as compared to the average six injections given to the others), but she, too, cleared up within two weeks.

"One of the patients," Dr. Klenner wrote, "a man of 65, came to the office doubled up with abdominal pain and with a history of having taken *opiates* for the preceding 36 hours. He gave the impression of having an acute surgical condition. A massive array of vesicles extended from the dorsal nerve roots to the umbilicus, a hand's breadth wide. He was given 3,000 mg. (three grams) of vitamin C intravenously and directed to return to the office in four to five hours. It was difficult to convince him that his abdominal pain was the result of his having 'shingles.' He returned in four hours completely free of pain. He was given an additional 2,000 mg. of vitamin C, and following the schedule given above he recovered completely in three days."

Now, this is one physician's experience and certainly no hard-and-fast proof that vitamin C will always work so rapidly. Shingles hits with varying severity, and many patients do recover quickly without any medication at all. Nevertheless, it is very persuasive testimony that this vitamin can cut the infection short—and thereby not only relieve immediate discomfort but prevent scarring and fibrosis of the nerve which causes the lingering pain of postherpetic neuralgia.

The logic of vitamin C's usefulness against the herpes zoster virus is its general property as a detoxicant—an agent that reinforces the hundreds of defenses the body naturally possesses against poisons and infecting agents. Vitamin $B_{12}$ also has been found effective—and here we might assume that the vitamin is therapeutic because of its known importance to nerve health. Neurological damage is one manifestation of vitamin $B_{12}$ deficiency.

A number of physicians, going back to Dr. K. E. Jolles writing in the *British Medical Journal* in 1955, have reported in the medical journals on speedy response to vitamin $B_{12}$ injections given to patients with shingles. In one of the more recent studies, appearing in *The Indian Practitioner,* (July 1967), Drs. A. K. Gupta and H. S. Mital wrote that they have observed "a dramatic response to vitamin B₁₂ therapy as judged by relief of pain and the speed of disappearance of vesicles" in the cases of 21 herpes zoster patients.

Improvement usually began, they said, on the second or third day following daily injections of 500 mcg. of the vitamin. Most important, a follow-up study showed no development of postherpetic neuralgia in any of the cases. In this respect, as in the initial response to therapy, the authors pointed out, their experience confirms that of earlier experimenters.

# CHAPTER 119

# Vitamin C Relieves
# Prickly Heat

Parents usually resign themselves to the idea that prickly heat, when it develops, must be allowed to run its course. Though the baby screams and refuses to eat, though Daddy suffers a tormenting itch that can't be scratched in public, no one has known anything better to do about prickly heat than put up with it. However, a dermatologist from the British Military Hospital in sub-tropical Singapore has reported that he found and tested a safe and effective cure for this rash: large oral doses of vitamin C. The researcher is Dr. T. C. Hindson, and he made his report in *Lancet* (22 June 1968).

Prickly heat is a common summertime ailment. In temperate climates babies suffer from it more frequently than adults—but the disease is not rare in men, and often occurs on the inside of the thighs at the groin.

The rash develops very quickly as a result of excessive sweating, and can occur wherever such sweating takes place. If one side of a baby's face is pressed against the pillow or a nurse's body for any length of time, prickly heat can be expected. If a diaper is tight and warm and produces profuse sweating, the rash will probably develop. Tiny, slightly inflamed pimples develop on the skin surface accompanied by a tingling and itching sensation. Within a few days the pimples become blisters containing a milky substance. They soon disappear leaving tiny scabs which scale off.

Usually, that is. But sometimes, especially in children, the itching becomes unbearable. The youngsters scratch the irritation, infecting it, and a much more serious problem develops. No adequate treatment was known before Dr. Hindson's report. He gave convincing evidence that vitamin C can effectively treat prickly heat. He reported that "of 15 children given ascorbic acid for two weeks, 14 improved. . . ."

Dr. Hindson stumbled across his powerful treatment of prickly heat by a stroke of luck. An Australian Air Force officer came to his office one day suffering from a severe case of prickly heat (technically known as *malaria rubra papulosa*). The patient told Dr. Hindson that he had had the rash for a year, and that all forms of therapy he had tried had been ineffective.

As Dr. Hindson continued to interview the officer, the Australian remembered that the rash had suddenly disappeared for a short time while he was taking vitamin C to treat a cold. "I put him on ascorbic acid, one gram daily, as the sole treatment, and when reexamined ten days later his groin was normal," wrote Dr. Hindson.

The dermatologist felt that he was on to something important. He chose five children who were patients of his and who suffered from recurrent severe prickly heat. Each was given doses of vitamin C. The result: no further attacks of prickly heat occurred while they were taking the vitamin.

But such evidence will not win the support of the medical community. Perhaps these cases were rare coincidence. Perhaps other factors were involved. More adequate criteria were needed if Hindson's theory was to gain a hearing by other physicians. "Subsequently, I carried out a double-blind trial of ascorbic acid in the treatment of 30 cases of prickly heat," Dr. Hindson wrote.

The criterion Dr. Hindson established for selecting his 30 cases was that all patients should have suffered continuously from prickly heat for a period of eight weeks, immediately before his initial interview with them. The children were divided into two equal groups. Half were given vitamin C, and half a placebo, a tablet which looks like medication but actually has no effect whatever. Dr. Hindson guarded against unconsciously influencing the patients by having the pharmacist select each group without the physician's knowledge.

Before the experiment was begun, Dr. Hindson had to decide how much vitamin C should be administered daily. He took as his guide the amount that had been used by the Australian Air Force officer—one gram (1,000 mg.) daily for a person weighing 150 pounds.

Some children were too young to take the tablets, so Dr. Hindson instructed parents to crush the tablets thoroughly and mix them in with food. After two weeks, he tabulated the results. Two of the 15 on the placebo showed no sign of the rash. Ten on the vitamin C showed no sign. Whereas two more on the placebo showed considerable signs of improvement, four on the vitamin showed similar signs. On the placebo, nine showed no change and two grew worse. Of those taking the vitamin, only one showed no change, and none was worse.

Dr. Hindson then gave the vitamin to the 15 patients who had been on the placebo. After two weeks, six had no sign of prickly heat, and five had considerably improved.

Dr. Hindson isn't sure why the vitamin works. Past research suggests that prickly heat occurs when the sweat glands in a particular area of the body stop working. These glands usually stop functioning because of fatigue. They have been overtaxed and overworked for too long and just take a vacation.

While admitting that the exact mechanism by which vitamin C prevents prickly heat has not been established, Dr. Hindson reported that vitamin C acts as a hydrogen ion carrier for certain enzyme systems which relate to the sweat glands. When the sweat glands are overtaxed, perhaps a shortage of the vitamin develops and the enzyme does not function adequately.

Another possibility Dr. Hindson suggested is that "the vitamin in large doses might take over the action of, or replenish some essential but fatigued enzyme system such as the succinic-dehydrogenase system—which Dobson (1958) showed was the first to disappear on excess sweating. . . ."

How it works nobody knows and Dr. Hindson pointed out that vitamin C levels have never been determined in sweat collected from individuals with high ascorbic-acid intake. But what this researcher has proven rather conclusively is that, in his own words, "Ascorbic acid, when given in high doses, is effective in the treatment and prevention of prickly heat."

# CHAPTER 120

# Vitamin E for Those Unexplained Bruises

Some physicians believe that because of the increasing use of estrogens, both for birth control and as a menopausal crutch, more and more women are becoming prone to a condition known as purpura, the disease of the purple spots, a hemorrhagic disorder characterized by spontaneous bruising or bleeding, petechiae (tiny bumps) in the skin and mucous membranes, and sometimes a marked decrease in circulating platelets.

It has already been determined that estrogen is a known vitamin E antagonist. It can cause a deficiency of this important nutrient which, among other well-documented benefits to your body, can actually help to preserve the integrity of the capillary walls and prevent such spots.

Purpura, according to a study published in the *Journal of Vitaminology* (18, 125-130, 1972) could very well be just such a colorful manifestation of a vitamin E deficiency.

People with purpura, however, are still being subjected to steroid therapy with its devastating side effects. Sometimes the patient is subjected to splenectomy (removal of the spleen) before the ravages of this disease can be controlled. But now purpura can be treated without dangerous side effect medications.

721

# Japanese Study

Vitamin E was successfully tried on humans as a treatment for purpura in Japan. Dr. Takaaki Fujii of the Utsunomya Hospital used vitamin E on seven patients with purpura between the ages of 16 and 54. All of them appeared to be well nourished and showed no signs of scurvy. (Capillary fragility, sometimes a precipitating factor in purpura, can be the result of a vitamin C deficiency.) When Dr. Fujii administered vitamin E to all of these patients in dosages of 400 to 600 mg. orally every day, he noted quick recoveries and disappearance of all spots in two to four weeks.

Estrogen is not the only vitamin E antagonist. One 16-year-old boy treated by Dr. Fujii had a sore throat, cough, headache, and high fever due to an upper respiratory tract infection for five days, and then developed extensive multiple petechiae. These appeared on his arms and his legs. Physical examination revealed nothing else of significance other than a slight swelling of both tonsils. Vitamin E therapy was started two days after the petechiae developed. Four hundred mg. were given every day for one week. At the end of the week, most of the petechiae had disappeared. At the end of two weeks on the same dosage, there were no petechiae at all.

Another patient, an 18-year-old boy, had no fever or any sign of infection prior to the onset of the little purplish-red spots. His family doctor had been treating him with a series of drugs including a cortisone derivative. Despite the treatment, petechiae did not disappear completely and the young man came to Dr. Fujii's hospital where he was started on vitamin E therapy immediately. After 400 mg. of vitamin E were given daily for one week, most petechiae disappeared and two weeks after the therapy began, none remained.

Another patient, a woman of 22, had had a sore throat and fever for three days, then developed edema (swelling) around the eyelids, red colored skin eruptions accompanied by swelling on her face and extensive urticaria (elevated patches of skin that itch) and petechiae over her whole body. From the physical findings and the blood examination, the edema, eruptions, urti-caria, and petechiae were considered to be due to increased permeability of the walls of the blood vessels. Vitamin E, 400 mg. daily, was started on the day she came to the hospital, and after five days, the edema around both eyelids and the red colored eruptions of the face disappeared completely. Most of the petechiae also disappeared and in Dr. Fujii's words, "She looked to be an entirely different person." After 10 days, the urticaria and the petechiae also disappeared completely.

Of the seven patients who were treated, five of them suffered with purpura of unknown origin, and two were due to allergic reactions to drugs used in medical treatment. In one case it took 21 days for the petechiae to disappear completely. In four cases it took 14 days, and in two cases it took only five days. The dosage in every case except one was 400 mg. daily. In one case, caused by allergic reaction to phenobarbitol, 600 mg. were used daily.

While the mechanism of the antipurpuric action of vitamin E for vascular purpura is not entirely clear, Dr. Fujii feels, since vitamin E was also effective in improving local edema, urticaria or skin eruptions in addition to its effect on petechiae, that this would suggest that vitamin E has an "inhibiting action on the increased permeability of the capillary walls due to various fac-tors such as infection, drugs, and others." He notes that Dr. M. Kamimura, writing in *Vitamins* (28, 129, 1961), observed in his experiments on human skin that when he used various chemicals such as histamine, acetylcholine, and a-chymotrypsin he was able to stimulate capillary permeability and was then able to reduce this permeability by using alpha-tocopherol acetate, 300 mg. for five to seven days.

Dr. Fujii's study has a great deal of relevance not only to the treatment of purpura with vitamin E but to the whole question of how vitamin E is used in the body, and the many ways that it can be used up. Estrogen is only one of the enemies of vitamin E—the stress of medications, the stress of pollution, the stress of fever, the stress of infections, and, according to the highly respected Nutrition Institute of the Soviet Academy of Medical

Science and their Central Institute of Physical Culture, it is used up even by the stress of strenuous exercise, according to *Medical Tribune* (24 May 1972).

According to their report, the Soviets did studies of young cyclists and skiers. They divided them into groups and gave them varying dosages of vitamin E. They found that blood and urine vitamin E levels during training dropped below those found in people not doing heavy work. The athletes were then given vitamin E supplementation according to their degree of activity. Changes which they then observed were related to the dosage. The investigators found that the addition of 100 to 150 mg. of alpha-tocopherol was probably optimal "for one and one-half to two hours of training and almost twice that for three to four hours of training."

While doctors continually maintain that if you eat a well-balanced diet, you should get your estimated daily requirements of between 10 and 30 I.U., they apparently overlook the many pitfalls in calculating the E content of the diet. There are so many variations in the vitamin E content of the same food under different conditions, that we cannot rely on the food composition tables for accurate measurement. As researcher C. L. Smith and associates pointed out in the *British Journal of Nutrition* (26, 89, 1971) the analytical values obtained with different samples of the same foodstuff purchased on separate occasions showed great variability, the most remarkable being for margarine, where the concentration in the richest sample was nearly 25 times that in the lowest sample.

When Dr. Smith and his associates analyzed the diets of 40 patients in a metabolic ward, and the diets of 10 members of the staff of the hospital, they found that the average intake of vitamin E was about five mg. a day. Where does all the vitamin E go? We get nutritionally short-changed because of modern food processing. Vitamin E deteriorates in stored food, even when that food is frozen. According to a report in the *Consumer Bulletin* (January 1973), as much as 90 percent of vitamin E may be lost in the flaking, shredding, and puffing of grain in the manufacture of breakfast cereals. Substantial amounts of vitamin E are lost during the processing of cereal for consumption by infants. In fact, it has been estimated that if you could have eaten the food you are going to eat for dinner tonight 50 years ago, it would have furnished you about 50 times more vitamin E than you will get from it tonight.

Dr. Philip White of the Council on Foods of the American Medical Association, maintains that vitamin E deficiency is nonexistent in our country, but Dr. Nicholas R. DiLuzio, chairman of the Department of Physiology at Tulane University, told the American Chemical Society on 30 March 1971 that abnormal fats, which indicate the lack of vitamin E, have been detected in the blood plasma of 78 out of 81 persons examined. These fats form as a result of the oxidation of polyunsaturated fat in the body. Dr. DiLuzio said that 96 percent of all subjects studied were therefore in a state of relative antioxidant deficiency.

When you consider the many ways in which vitamin E can be used up and the shortage of this oxygen-sparing factor in the average diet, is it any wonder that we have a health crisis in our country? As Richard E. Passwater reported in *C & E News* (9 October 1972), "As vitamin E deficiency in animals leads to tissue degradation and gross changes in biochemistry, we should err on the high intake side, rather than the low." Try to calculate the many antagonists to vitamin E in your environment and then adjust your vitamin E intake accordingly. You may find yourself enjoying many health dividends.

# CHAPTER 121

# Vitamin A Hastens
# Wound Healing

Applied directly to open wounds, vitamin A hastens the healing process in cases where healing has been retarded due to the use of the steroid drugs, notably cortisone. Steroids are chemical substances of hormone origin.

Studies indicating the power of vitamin A to speed healing, disclosed at a meeting of the American Surgical Association by Dr. Thomas K. Hunt and co-workers of the University of California San Francisco Medical Center, may help to solve a widespread surgical problem, according to a report in the *Medical Tribune* (9 July 1969).

Since cortisone and the adrenocorticotropic hormone of the pituitary gland (ACTH) have found an ever-increasing field of application for the treatment of acute inflammatory and allergic diseases, it has been observed that these hormones predispose patients to infection. They also impede the healing of wounds and thus increase the risk of infection and prolong the postsurgery recovery period.

Dr. Hunt's findings that vitamin A counters this difficulty safely and effectively without taking patients off the drug or reducing its dosage, should enhance the recovery prognosis for the millions of people who might have been using steroid drugs within a period of two years prior to surgery or injury.

726

Wounds treated by Dr. Hunt and his associates ranged from large nonhealing ulcers of the limb to severe infectious lesions of the chest. In several cases, wounds that had stubbornly resisted healing for weeks, healed in a matter of days, after application of vitamin A. Dr. Hunt also reported that vitamin A, administered orally, stimulated wound healing in cortisone patients but not so well as direct application.

When the research team used vitamin A to treat ten cases of idolent (slow-healing) wounds in patients who were receiving steroids against autoimmune diseases or transplant rejection, wounds healed within three weeks, although some of the lesions had been indolent for as long as three months.

In experiments aimed at discovering where the healing effect takes place, rabbits with open wounds measuring 4.0 cm. were divided into two groups, only one of which got daily cortisone injections. Half the lesions of each group were treated daily with topical vitamin A ointment during the second week after wounding.

As reported in the *Medical Tribune* (26 June 1969), the animals without cortisone healed at the same rate (16 days) whether or not they got vitamin A. The animals who got the steroids and were treated with vitamin A healed within 25 days. Those who got the steroids and no vitamin A had not healed at the end of a month.

The cortisone, Dr. Hunt explained, suppresses the initial inflammatory response of wounding, and inhibits wound contraction, and the growth of connective tissue. While the addition of vitamin A encourages granulation tissue and tensile strength, it does nothing for wound contraction. It helps the wound to heal by fostering the growth of epithelium, the covering of internal and external surfaces of the body including the lining of vessels and other small cavities.

Dr. Hunt believes that the healing effect stems uniquely from interaction between cortisone and vitamin A at some as yet unknown point within the wound itself. This is a new role for vitamin A, already known to be necessary to many of the body's functions.

Vitamin A helps the body resist infection by maintaining the healthy structure of the membranous tissues that keep infectious agents from reaching the cells. But what is not generally known is that most drugs, including cortisone, rapidly deplete the body of its vitamin A stores while at the same time increasing the need for it (I. Clark *et al., Endocrinology* 56, 232, 1955).

The patient on cortisone, then, faces a multiple risk, especially when he is injured or after surgery. Not only does the cortisone in his body hinder the healing process, but, because of the use of cortisone, he is all but depleted of vitamin A stores which could help muster his body's natural defenses to fight infection.

# CHAPTER 122

# To Ease the Effects
of Severe Burns

Few injuries are as terrible to endure as a severe burn over a large part of the body. The agony, fear of disfigurement, and threat of massive infection make such an injury dreadful to contemplate. But all these aspects of burn damage can be alleviated by vitamin C therapy. Often, it has proven far more helpful than the most powerful drugs available. This was the conclusion of surgeon David H. Klasson, who in cooperation with the surgical staff of Greenpoint Hospital in Brooklyn treated dozens of burn victims with vitamin C according to the *New York State Journal of Medicine*, (15 October 1951).

One patient was brought to the hospital in pain after having been badly burned over 30 percent of the upper body in an airplane crash. Although he was given morphine, his pain remained severe for an hour, until his wounds were sprayed with a one percent solution of ascorbic acid. "There was almost immediate relief of pain," Dr. Klasson reported. Further, the pain did not return and no more morphine was required. The patient made an excellent and uneventful recovery in a little over a month.

In another case, two patients who had been badly burned in a gasoline explosion were brought in. The burns on their heads and necks were treated with the one percent ascorbic acid solution and daily application of a two percent ascorbic acid ointment. The burns on their hands and wrists were treated conventionally with sterile Vaseline, gauze, and Furacin ointment. Three weeks later, the wounds treated with vitamin C had healed, while those treated "conservatively" continued to exude fluid for another 30 days.

Besides direct application of vitamin C solutions, Dr. Klasson gave his patients from 200 to 500 mg. of vitamin C by mouth or injection, repeated four times daily. Summing up his clinical experience with vitamin C therapy, the surgeon said that it:

- alleviates pain in minor burns and reduces it sufficiently in major burns to keep use of dangerous morphine to a minimum;
- produces rapid and healthy healing of the wound without complications sometimes seen with use of sulfa and other drugs;
- reduces and usually eliminates the need for antibiotic treatment except in the worst cases;
- combats the accumulation of toxic protein metabolites in severe burns;
- reduces the collection of fluid under the skin in the area of the burn, permitting skin grafting at the earliest possible date, which in turn reduces chances of infection and shortens convalescence;
- saves lives.

# CHAPTER 123

# Bedsores Heal Twice as Fast with Vitamin C

Anyone who has had any experience with bedsores knows too well that they are very resistant to healing. Another unpleasant and familiar fact: medical bills skyrocket when bedsores are a complication. According to Dr. James W. Barnes, Jr., of Glenn Dale Hospital, Glenn Dale, Maryland, writing in the *Journal of the American Medical Association* (8 January 1973), the cost of healing serious bedsores ranges anywhere from $5,000 to $10,000. Worst of all, bedsores can be a serious threat to life itself.

As blood, blood protein, and other vital nutrients are lost through the sore, anemia, debility, and lowered resistance set in. Dr. Barnes noted that a study by the Veterans Administration showed that persistent bedsore ulcerations were the direct or major contributing cause of mortality in ten percent of all paraplegics who died.

The medical term for a bedsore is decubitus ulcer. Decubitus is Latin for "lying down." Those who get decubitus ulcers have disabilities which confine them to a recumbent position. There are usually two causes of the sores: unrelieved pressure, especially at bony prominences (such as the hips), and poor nutritional status, which weakens the skin and natural repair mechanisms. There's a whole catalog of medicines, physical therapy measures, and nursing-care practices designed for the comfort of the patient and the healing of the sore itself.

But the chief problem with bedsores is not so much a lack of suitable treatment as it is the poor general condition of the patients in whom such sores develop. While the sore may be initiated because of constant pressure, particularly at bony areas, the rate of development and the severity of the sores depend on other factors, more specifically nutrition.

Researchers at the Manchester Royal Infirmary, University Hospital of South Manchester in England reported in the *Lancet* (7 September 1974) on the important role of nutrition in healing bedsores. Dr. T. V. Taylor and a team of coworkers, in a double-blind trial of large doses of vitamin C for healing pressure sores, demonstrated that those patients who received supplements of vitamin C showed twice as much healing as patients who received a placebo.

Twenty surgical patients, each with a pressure sore, were included in the study. All were confined to bed with various conditions such as fractured thigh bone, stroke, and paraplegia (paralysis of the legs and lower part of the body). All the patients were using standard hospital beds and mattresses, receiving the same basic hospital diet and the same local therapy to the pressure areas. All the patients received identical-looking white tablets twice a day. Ten patients (group A) were given placebos. The other ten (group B) were given 500 mg. of ascorbic acid.

In group A the ascorbic acid levels in the blood before treatment were practically the same as those levels found in group B. After one month of treatment, however, the mean level in group B was three times greater than that of group A. With the higher levels of vitamin C came a big improvement in the pressure sores—a reduction of 84 percent in size, compared to only 42.7 percent in the unsupplemented group. Six of the 10 patients in the vitamin C group healed completely in just one month. (Three or four months is what it usually takes to heal a serious ulcer, according to Dr. Barnes.)

# Why Injuries Need Extra Vitamin C

When you understand the chemistry of vitamin C, it is not surprising at all that it should have this therapeutic effect. What is surprising is that vitamin C is not used routinely in all bedfast patients, whether at home or in the hospital.

It has been known for many years that ascorbic acid is an important factor for the normal synthesis and maintenance of collagen. Without collagen, the intercellular cement substance, no injury can heal properly because the body cannot grow strong, new tissue. Dr. W. J. McCormick of Toronto, Canada, a pioneer in the use of vitamin C, described the etiology of bedsores years ago as a deficiency of vitamin C, producing capillary fragility and impeding the development of granulation tissue which is essential to the formation of scar tissue (*Medical Record,* 19 November 1941).

Dr. McCormick noted an interesting parallel between bedsores and frostbite. Both are produced by ischemia (a deficiency of blood in a part of the body) and anoxia (a deficiency of oxygen) with consequent necrosis, or tissue death. In frostbite, the initiating cause is intense cold. In bedsores, the initiating event is, of course, constant pressure. Captain Scott, who conducted an ill-fated expedition to the South Pole in 1911 at a time when little was known of the effects of vitamins, recorded in his diary that his men had lost the ability to heal blisters and frostbite. Vitamin C could very well have changed the outcome of that expedition.

# CHAPTER 124

# Vitamin C as an Orthodontic Tool

*by Vernon A. Nord, D.D.S.*

*Dr. Nord, an orthodontist, currently resides in New South Wales, Australia. There he is studying the primitive people of the South Pacific to determine the origin of many modern dental problems. He is the author of two books on orthodontics.*

During my dental training, I was often told that many dental malocclusions (bad bite) and facial deformities were the result of heredity. It was pointed out that most modern civilized people are a mixture of many racial backgrounds. This crossbreeding supposedly led to dento-facial irregularities, making it easy to blame our ancestors for our "crooked teeth." This also shifts the responsibility: "Johnny has to have all this orthodontic work because he didn't choose the right parents."

But there have always been a few people who have not accepted this theory and have advanced ideas about more logical causative factors. For more than 20 years I, too, have been searching for the real cause of dental malocclusions.

Some years ago, during a teaching tour in the eastern states, I met Dr. Paul Elcan, who told me of his work with vitamin C in treating orthodontic cases. His claim was that regular high doses of ascorbic acid improved nasal breathing immeasurably and raised the patients' health level. In most instances he claimed more rapid orthodontic results.

It had been apparent to me for years that many orthodontic problems were associated with mouth breathing. My only attempt at a solution to this was the removal of the tonsils and adenoids in extreme cases. It had never occurred to me to use vitamin C to clear nasal airways permanently.

Incorporating vitamin C therapy into my orthodontic practice was easy, for many of my patients were mouth breathers. The problem was in trying to get them to take it regularly—as often as four to seven times a day. They usually reverted to taking one pill a day unless they were constantly reminded to take it *often*. The success of the therapy depends on spreading it out over our waking hours, because vitamin C can't be stored in the human body.

With dogged determination, I put this therapy to work and obtained fine results. One set of cases stands out in my mind above all others. The three children in one particular family were all allergic to various and sundry items. They all had severe nasal blockage, deviated nasal septum, and many other dental-facial problems. Of course, they were mouth breathers. Not only that, they had severe dermatitis with dry, scaly skin, painful, bleeding cracks in their arms, cracked and sore lips, and fissures in the corners of the mouth. These last problems often prevented or caused postponement of orthodontic treatment. It was even painful for them to wear orthodontic appliances. Needless to say, there was little progress made in correcting their dental malocclusions.

After Dr. Elcan told me of his success with ascorbic acid, I asked the mother of this family if she would try this new approach. Since she had nothing to lose by doing this, she jumped at the opportunity. We agreed the children should take 200 mg. of vitamin C at least four times daily and follow a prescribed diet.

With excellent cooperation, within a month some of the untoward symptoms had gone, and within three months most had disappeared. Now the orthodontic therapy was working too! The relief from the cracked skin alone was a "sight for sore eyes."

As the years went by, my desire to put the various pieces of the "crooked teeth" problem in their right order increased. I gave up my United States orthodontic practice in 1972 and moved to the South Pacific. Here I could study many primitive races that lived close to nature and had few or no orthodontic problems.

# Learning from Aborigines

The Australian aborigines were a perfect example. History traces their ancestry back thousands of years and there's been little change in culture or habits down through the ages. They are truly Stone Age people. They enjoyed very good health even though they lived under the most difficult circumstances nature had to offer. It was truly "survival of the fittest."

They learned to adapt to extreme conditions. But, most relevant to me, the evidence says their varied diet contained ample quantities of vitamin C. They ate almost everything raw. They had excellent teeth and very few modern illnesses. They breathed through their noses and never had colds. This was in spite of living naked, often in below freezing temperatures at night!

Unfortunately, not many of these true primitives are around today, for the white man had dispossessed them of their homeland and hunting ground. They've been forced to adopt "civilized" ways and *dietary habits*. You may already have surmised what has happened to them. They've "inherited" our modern illnesses, rampant dental decay, and the same orthodontic problems and facial deformities as the white people. This all happened in one or two generations after the aborigines accepted the impoverished foods of civilization! Their plight is a sad one.

# CHAPTER 125

# Vitamin Insurance
# Against Ulcers

The National Health Education Committee estimates that at least half the population of the country has some kind of digestive complaint. Digestive disorders are, in fact, the leading cause of hospitalization, and ulcers have to rate near the top of the list.

Almost everyone knows a hard-charging businessman or housewife who has been felled by the searing pain from an ulcer gone wild. Many have a much more intimate knowledge of the knockout power of an ulcer. In terms of personal suffering, disability, and medical expense, ulcers are an expensive plague indeed.

Is it possible to prevent ulcers? With man, no one can say positively that it is or isn't, because clinical trials would take 20 years or more and involve at least a thousand people.

Luckily, researchers interested in prevention have another course open to them. They can experiment with laboratory mice or rats whose metabolism is strangely similar to ours, except that everything is speeded up because of their much shorter life span. And if results with mice can be interpreted as being relevant to man (which they are, or no scientist would bother with them), there is good news from California.

Using large amounts of vitamin E, researchers have discovered that when mice are subjected to stress, those given this supplement develop far fewer and less serious ulcers than those who receive nothing but a standard "good" diet.

## 78 Percent More Ulceration Without Extra E

Writing in the *American Journal of Clinical Nutrition* (September 1972), Jon A. Kangas, Ph.D., K. Michael Schmidt, Ph.D., and George F. Solomon, M.D., explained that they divided rats into two groups of 12 each. The first received 50 mg. of a vitamin E solution twice daily while the second received a fluid similar to the vitamin E, but lacking the vitamin.

Special cages were built with clear plastic dividers running down the center. The dividers effectively kept the rats from their food and water but made sure that they could see it sitting there, just out of reach. The rats were permitted access to the food only once a day. Just as the constant crush of business with its high pressure gives men ulcers, seeing the food and water just out of reach gave ulcers to the rats.

After 12 days of this routine, the rats were meticulously autopsied. A panel of three pathologists then determined that the rats who didn't get vitamin E had stomach ulcers of a very strong intensity, rated 3.42 on a four-point scale. Those given vitamin E had ulcer ratings of only 1.92, far lower than the other group. Put another way, the unsupplemented rats developed fully 78 percent more ulceration.

"It was clearly demonstrated," said the authors, "that vitamin E in large doses administered at the beginning of and during a period of stress effectively retarded the production of stomach ulceration." Further: "It is possible that, because vitamin E has significant prophylactic properties in relation to the formation of ulcers, it may also facilitate the treatment of established ulcers. Further research in this area is indicated."

There is another nutritive angle to ulcers which is just as important as vitamin E, but first let's take a brief look at ulcers as a disease, and some of the "cures" which are prescribed.

# Many Theories, No Cures

Essentially, there are three types of ulcers: peptic, gastric, and duodenal. The first is a breach or erosion in the inner lining of the stomach or the part of the duodenum closest to the stomach. The second is corrosion and degeneration of the gastric organs, while a duodenal ulcer is degeneration of the duodenum, the 8-to-10 inch length of the alimentary canal that follows the stomach.

The symptoms of ulcers can be as varied as headaches and choking sensations to low back pains and itching. When pain does occur in the stomach, a person often charges it off to some dietary indiscretion. Finally, the pain becomes so intense as to be clearly recognizable as an ulcer.

Despite the fact that the medical profession has recognized ulcers for a long time, they remain an enigma. No one is willing to say for sure how they get started. Emotions have been blamed, although people with every type of personality imaginable have suffered from them. Fat people, skinny people, tall, short, meek, and aggressive people have all gotten ulcers.

When it comes to curing them, there have been just as many variations. At first, it was believed only the knife could "cure" an ulcer. Then, it was chemical treatments. The most traditional treatment is the bland diet. However, the bland diet has lately fallen into disfavor. Even the use of milk, long a staple for ulcer sufferers, has been found to be about as effective as battling a fire with an eyedropper. In an article appearing in the *American Journal of Clinical Nutrition,* February 1969, Douglas W. Piper, M.D., stated that studies showed an ulcer patient would have to drink almost a quart of milk every hour to neutralize gastric juices which were aggravating the ulcer.

Fortunately, vitamins can do more for the lining of your stomach.

# Vitamin A Is Also an Antiulcer Specific

The three researchers who reported on the vitamin E study mentioned earlier, theorized that the protective potency of vitamin E may be related to its antioxidant properties—that is, its ability to prevent bodily substances from combining chemically with oxygen compounds and thereby being degraded. But besides the general protection afforded to the tissues of the gastrointestinal system, vitamin E has a very specific protective relationship with vitamin A. In fact, had the three researchers who studied vitamin E added to their experiment a third group of animals which were given vitamins E and A together an even greater antiulcer protective action might have been observed.

Clear evidence to this effect is already part of scientific literature. The synergistic effect of vitamin E with vitamin A was observed as long ago as 1946, when J. L. Jensen published in *Science* (103, 586) his finding that alpha-tocopherol, or vitamin E, prevented stomach ulcers in rats receiving very low amounts of vitamin A.

In 1947, a kind of follow-up to this experiment was reported by T. L. Harris and associates in the *Proceedings of the Society for Experimental Biology and Medicine* (March 1947). This time, the researchers wanted to see what would happen when vitamin A was given in ample amounts, and the amount of vitamin E varied.

Forty young male rats were first placed on a diet deficient in both vitamins A and E, which is known to produce ulcers. After two weeks all rats were given 300 units of vitamin A daily, but only half the rats were also given vitamin E. Seven weeks later, the animals were examined for stomach lesions.

Fifty percent of the rats on the high-A, low-E diet had one or more ulcers in the forestomach. But not a single animal in the group which had received the vitamin E had any ulcers.

## Protective Partnership

As dramatic as this finding was, it comes as no surprise to anyone familiar with the basic physiology of vitamins A and E. Vitamin A is crucial to the health of the mucous membranes which line the body's cavities; the throat, nose, sinuses, middle ear, lungs, gallbladder, and urinary bladder. When there is adequate vitamin A, these membranes continuously secrete a liquid

or mucus which covers the cells and protects them from bacteria, acids, and other environmental assaults. Vitamin E, sparing vitamin A, assures an adequate supply of protective mucus
for the epithelial cells.

Actually, the relationship between these two vitamins is a little more complicated than that. When Harris and his colleagues
performed further experiments with these two vitamins, they
came to the conclusion that vitamin A deficiency *by itself* does
not produce ulcers. Nor can vitamin A, even in high doses,
prevent ulcers in animals under stress, they reported. This in
turn led them to the conclusion that "the action of tocopherol
(vitamin E) cannot be explained simply as a sparing of vitamin A
in the gastrointestinal tract."

In other words, vitamin E by itself affords an important kind
of protection—as was more recently reported in the California
study.

But further studies in human beings indicate that vitamin A,
by itself, is also able, "single-handedly," to fight the ulceration
process. Neil Hutcher, M.D., of the Medical College of Virginia
reported in *Medical World News* (29 October 1971) that vitamin
A helped heal ulcers brought on in people undergoing steroid
treatment.

Steroids—adrenocorticotropin and corticosteroids—are
believed to help cause ulcers by lowering the gastric defense
mechanisms. This means that the surface epithelial cells are not
renewed at the proper rate. Therefore, mucus production lags,
according to Dr. Hutcher. He and his associates believe vitamin
A retards ulcer formation by actually stimulating the epithelial
cells to reproduce normally, with the ultimate result being
increased mucus production.

## Vitamin A is a 'Must' in Serious Injury

Most of us think of ulcers as lesions which develop slowly
over the years. But they can also be produced by sudden and
severe injury. In such cases, vitamin A can be a real life-saver.

Merrill S. Chernov, M.D., and two associates reported in the

*American Journal of Surgery* (vol. 122, 1971) that when they measured the serum vitamin A levels in patients who had been hospitalized with severe burns or other major injuries, there was a dramatic reduction of this vitamin in 29 of 35 cases. It had been Dr. Chernov's experience that such patients often develop serious ulcers, and the vitamin A level finding led them to conduct an experiment.

Fourteen of 36 seriously injured patients were treated with 10,000 to 400,000 units of a special water-soluble vitamin A preparation daily. Ulcers appeared in just two cases. But of the remaining 22 patients who were treated with every resource of modern medicine—except vitamin A—stress ulcers developed in 15, and 14 of those had serious upper gastrointestinal bleeding.

Adding up all these studies, the conclusion is obvious: vitamin A and vitamin E both individually, but especially when taken together, offer a degree of protection against ulcers which is quite beyond anything else known to medical science.

The protective work of this "dynamic duo" is not limited to ulcers. Research conducted at the famous laboratories of the Battelle-Northwest Research Institute indicate that vitamins A and E also protect the lungs from the ravages of air pollution. The cells lining the lungs are, of course, different from those lining the stomach, but they are both epithelial cells, and both require the elaboration of mucus to protect them from their enemies—whether it be the sulfuric acid mist often present in smog, or the digestive acids often present to excess in our stomachs.

This does not mean that vitamins E and A should be considered a substitute for a cleaner environment. But it's reassuring to know that there's something available to help while the massive cleanup is underway.

## Protection Is Easy With Common Sense

How many units of these vitamins are needed to afford maximum protection against ulcers? This is not a question that can be answered definitively at present. The Recommended Daily Allowance (RDA) of vitamin A for an adult is 5,000 I.U., somewhat higher for growing teenagers and pregnant women, and 8,000 units for lactating mothers. For small children, of course, it is less.

It's doubtful, though, whether this amount of vitamin A is sufficient to cope with the stress of ulcer-producing acids and irritants. From a preventive point of view, anywhere from two to four times the RDA would be in order. During high-stress periods, much more can be taken on a temporary basis. Vitamin A, when not being destroyed by stress, does build up in the liver and there are a few cases of temporary toxic reactions when the vitamin has been taken to excess over a long period of time. The amounts mentioned here, though, are very conservative, and perfectly safe for any adult.

Vitamin E in amounts of 100 I.U. daily has been found to actually double the health-building effects of vitamin A. Evan Shute, M.D., famous heart specialist of London, Ontario, recommends that every adult get at least 200 I.U. of vitamin E daily—except in cases of high blood pressure. Vitamin E stimulates circulation, and the blood flowing more freely may bring about a corresponding increase in pressure. If you have high blood pressure, you should start with a small dose of vitamin E until your arteries regain elasticity, and raise the dose very gradually.

# CHAPTER 126

# Vitamins That Help Repair
# the Ravages of Smoking
# and Drinking

Despite public warnings about the hazards of cigarettes and alcohol, millions of people still flirt with cancer and heart disease, liver and brain damage, and premature death by continuing to smoke and drink. Now research has shown that certain nutrients can at least minimize the side effects of these bad habits.

"Put your drinking arm in a sling the night before and leave it there," Linus Pauling, Ph.D., once advised when asked in a newspaper poll (*Washington Post,* 1 January 1975) how to prevent or cure a New Year's Day hangover. However, the Nobel Prize winner, aware that willpower is weak at a spiritous party, offered a more practical proposal: vitamin C. "Take about six grams as a preventive before drinking," he counseled, and further advised taking extra vitamin C the next day if hangover symptoms develop despite the precaution.

Vitamin C is a powerful detoxifier and is therefore required in large amounts by anyone who courts the poisons of alcohol or tobacco. Other nutrients, too, have been experimented with and suggested as helpful to smokers or drinkers or both. These include the B vitamins, particularly $B_1$ or thiamine; certain sulfur-containing food elements; the trace mineral zinc; the fruit sugar fructose, and others.

744

## Amazing Protection

Helpful as these nutrients may be individually, animal research at the Veterans Administration Hospital, Coatesville, Pennsylvania, has shown that a trio of these nutrients—vitamin C, thiamine, and the sulfur-containing amino acid cysteine—combined, provide amazing protection against a major toxic substance found in cigarette smoke and as a primary metabolite of alcohol. This chemical, acetaldehyde, is far more toxic than alcohol itself and is implicated in many of the disease conditions common in heavy smokers and drinkers, according to VA researcher Herbert Sprince, Ph.D., and associates writing in *Agents and Actions* (vol. 5, no. 2, 1975).

The research team (composed of Dr. Sprince, who is also affiliated with Jefferson Medical College, Clarence M. Parker, George G. Smith, and Leon J. Gonzales, Ph.D.) gave rats lethal doses of acetaldehyde and then tested the protective value of various nutrients and combinations of nutrients. The trio of nutrients noted above gave "complete protection (zero percent lethality) for 72 hours in the 30 rats tested," the investigators reported.

"To the best of our knowledge," they continued, "our findings demonstrate for the first time that direct protective action against acetaldehyde toxicity and lethality can be obtained with certain naturally occurring metabolites, namely L-ascorbic acid (vitamin C), L-cysteine, and thiamine, preferably in combination at reduced dose levels."

While the researchers cautioned that further study is needed before these findings can be extrapolated for human use, they didn't hesitate to suggest that their laboratory results "point the way to a possible buildup of natural protection against chronic body insult of acetaldehyde arising from heavy drinking of alcohol and heavy smoking of cigarettes."

Smokers and imbibers could profit immediately from this therapy, for, though not yet proven in humans, the potential benefit is high and the risk nil. These are harmless food supplements.

Supplements of vitamin C and thiamine are readily available in natural food supplements. Cysteine is not, but a little care with diet can provide a good substitute. Of the sulfur-containing amino acids of protein, only methionine is called "essential" to humans, because the others can be synthesized in the body from this one product. Methionine and cystine (from which *cysteine* can be derived) are the sulfur compounds listed on charts showing amino acid content of foods. Some foods rated high in these two nutrients are peanuts, soybeans, eggs, Brazil and cashew nuts, sesame and sunflower seeds, and brewer's yeast.

It would be a good idea, too, to add vitamin $B_6$ or pyridoxine to the components of this antiacetaldehyde nutritional packet. Since pyridoxine plays a part in the metabolic conversion of amino acids, even a marginal deficiency in this vitamin might slow down the conversion of sulfur-containing amino acids.

## Why There's 'Natural' Protection Against Alcohol

When the VA researchers referred to the "natural" protection provided by their trio of nutrients, they meant that their antidote to acetaldehyde is not a foreign chemical or drug but rather a combination of ingredients that naturally belong in the body and participate in body metabolism. While the human body didn't evolve its metabolic pathways in order to cope with the bad habits of drinking and smoking, the handling of acetaldehyde (and its precursor, alcohol) is a natural and necessary function of body metabolism. This fact was vividly brought out at the First International Symposium on Alcohol and Aldehyde Metabolizing Systems, held in Stockholm, Sweden, and reported in the *New York Times* (16 July 1973).

The human intestine is a "distillery," Stockholm delegates were told by Nobel Laureate Hugo Theorell, M.D. Citing the work of another Nobel Prize winner, Sir Hans Krebs, Dr. Theorell explained that dietary sugars are fermented into ethanol before they are absorbed and reach the liver. Alcohol is thus produced to the equivalent of one quart of 3.2 (half-strength) beer each day. The alcohol our bodies make and the alcohol some of us drink is exactly the same chemical and is handled in exactly the same way by liver enzymes: the alcohol is converted to acetaldehyde and then acetaldehyde is converted to a nontoxic and, in fact, useful product, acetic acid. But, of course, this system was never designed to handle alcohol in quantity.

At the Stockholm symposium, several delegates speculated about drugs that might someday be prescribed for alcoholics to inhibit or alter the natural enzyme action so that quantities of alcohol could be metabolized less toxically. Unfortunately, such an approach would include side effects destructive in the body's normal handling of dietary sugars. A safer, wiser approach is that of the researchers at the Coatesville VA Hospital: find natural ingredients that normally help the body cope with acetaldehyde and then increase their intake to counter the abnormally high levels of the toxic substance in drinkers and smokers.

## Nutrients That Tame Deadly Acetaldehyde

In their report, Dr. Sprince and his associates discussed in some detail the biochemistry of how these nutrients might work and why there's a synergistic effect when all three are used together as a nutritional team. Here are a few of the main points they made.

In sulfur-containing molecules such as cysteine, the sulfur components can split off and bind with toxic substances and convert them to a nontoxic form.

Thiamine "is believed to complex normally with acetaldehyde to eventually form acetyl Coenzyme A (a factor important to energy production)," the researchers noted. Thiamine also contains sulfur.

As for vitamin C, the investigators pointed to "much literature evidence" suggesting this nutrient's protective role. Moreover, body levels of vitamin C are known to be depressed in alcoholics and in heavy smokers, even though their diets seem adequate. If only to restore depleted levels, smokers and drinkers need vitamin C supplementation.

The researchers found that sulfur compounds and vitamin C work best when given in their reduced (i.e., not oxidized) forms. L-ascorbic acid is the reduced form of this nutrient and is found in natural vitamin C tablets. The sulfur-containing amino acids in food proteins are primarily oxidized, but these molecules continuously undergo change from one form to the other within the body.

Vitamins A and E offer additional protection for smokers. As with any airborne pollutant, the poisons in cigarette smoke attack the respiratory tract and lungs first. The body's own defense against this assault depends on healthy mucous membranes, the moist tissues lining these passages and hollow organs. Vitamin A is essential for mucous membrane maintenance, and vitamin E (a pollutant fighter in its own right) helps preserve vitamin A levels in the body through its antioxidant activity.

# CHAPTER 127

# Powerful Virus Inactivator

The debate over vitamin C and the common cold had scarcely died down when Linus Pauling, Ph.D., speaking at the annual meeting of the California Academy of Family Physicians in late 1974, made a startling announcement. Vitamin C, said the Nobel Prize-winning scientist, has the ability to inactivate a wide range of viruses, including viral hepatitis.

In tests conducted over a period of seven years, 21 different bacterial viruses (viruses that attach themselves to bacteria inside the body) were successfully inactivated by vitamin C in test-tube experiments, reported Dr. Akira Murata of the Laboratory of Applied Microbiology in Japan's Saga University (Department of Agricultural Chemistry).

In terms of type, size, and composition, these viruses represent a wide variety of infectious agents. "Taking into consideration all of the results, the virucidal (virus-killing) activity of C seems to be a phenomenon that is accepted in all the viruses," concluded Dr. Murata (*Proceedings of the First Intersectional Congress of the International Association of Microbiological Societies,* vol. III, 1975, Tokyo University Press).

# Serum Hepatitis Prevented Absolutely

Vitamin C's antiviral activity was dramatically demonstrated in long-term studies at the Fukuoka Torikai Hospital, which Dr. Murata also described in his paper. In Japan, the attack rate for serum hepatitis is very high. This viral disease is transmitted by blood transfusions, and usually appears 60 to 120 days after a patient receives blood from an infected donor. Fukumi Morishige, M.D., chief of the hospital's surgical service, decided to investigate the effect of vitamin C on the occurrence of the disease. Over the seven-year course of Dr. Morishige's study, 11 cases of hepatitis developed among 150 transfused patients given smaller doses of vitamin C (less than two grams a day). This is an attack rate of about seven percent. But among 1,100 transfused patients given two grams (2,000 mg.) or more of vitamin C daily for a maximum of two weeks after the transfusion, there were no cases of hepatitis. Similar results using vitamin C were obtained among 1,400 transfused patients at another hospital.

As a result, "The administration of vitamin C is now routine procedure in these two hospitals," reported Dr. Murata. He and Dr. Morishige recommend giving three to six grams of vitamin C daily, divided into three doses, for a few days before and two weeks after transfusion. The vitamin is administered orally or by Intravenous drip.

In addition to hepatitis, the report stated, Dr. Morishige has used large doses of vitamin C to effectively treat measles, mumps, viral pneumonia, herpes zoster, meningitis, and other viral diseases.

All this sounds promising, but the Japanese results are likely to be challenged by the same sort of professional skepticism that initially greeted Dr. Pauling's contention that vitamin C can relieve many symptoms of the common cold. Such caution may not be a bad thing. After all, Japan is separated from us by more than 5,000 miles of ocean and even wider gaps of language and culture. Misinterpretations and reporting errors can occur. But what is to stop Western scientists from investigating for themselves vitamin C's antiviral properties? If the findings of Drs. Murata and Morishige can be verified, a safe, effective weapon against viruses will certainly be welcome.

## Viruses—As Nasty as They Are Tiny

Widespread use of antibiotic wonder drugs had dramatically brought many common bacterial infections under control. But they have been of little or no avail against illnesses caused by viruses.

Serum hepatitis, for example, strikes an estimated 20,000 people annually in the United States, according to the Food and Drug Administration (*Federal Register,* 9 July 1974). For 3,000 of them, the disease proves fatal. Those who ultimately recover suffer mental depression and extreme fatigue during the course of their illness.

In hepatitis, as in every viral disease, all this suffering is caused by minute infectious agents. Virus bodies are so small that they cannot even be seen through an ordinary microscope. Scientists had to wait for the invention of the electron microscope before they could begin to observe and study viruses. The hepatitis virus is so tiny (less than one half-millionth of an inch in diameter) it can easily pass through bacteria-tight filters.

Every virus is composed of two parts: a protective protein shell and a nucleus of either DNA or RNA, the same nucleic acids found in all living cells. (Dr. Murata reported that vitamin C inactivated the viruses under study by cutting or splitting these nucleic acid strands.)

Compared to bacteria, viruses are not only smaller but nearly inert. A virus has no life of its own. It is a parasite that can only thrive and reproduce by attaching itself to a living cell. Eventually, the "commandeered" cell bursts and dies, and the virus bodies move on to invade still other cells.

Scientists have identified more than 200 viruses capable of causing acute illness in man. Encephalitis, chicken pox, yellow fever, smallpox, hepatitis, rabies, meningitis, cold sores, influenza, and polio are all caused by viruses. Some researchers believe latent viruses are also involved in the development of cancer, diabetes, and other diseases. Any clue that can help unravel the mystery of viruses could alleviate much human suffering.

Some viruses, like polio and smallpox, can be controlled with vaccines. But because many viruses are highly adaptive, they can easily change their characteristics to become drug-resistant. Only two recently developed drugs—Ara-A and ribavirin—show much promise as antiviral agents, and both drugs cause birth defects and abortions in laboratory animals according to *Medical World News* (11 October 1974).

# Dr. Frederick Klenner—Pioneer in Using Vitamin C

That's why the news that vitamin C may be a true broad-spectrum viricidal agent is so exciting. And if the Japanese results are confirmed in controlled trials, a physician in the small town of Reidsville, North Carolina should be very pleased. Frederick R. Klenner, M.D., has been using vitamin C for more than 25 years to treat virus diseases.

In his private practice, Dr. Klenner treats many cases of viral infection usually with from 20 to 40 grams or more of vitamin C a day, administered intravenously by injection, or by mouth. Here are some of the diseases which he says have yielded to vitamin C:

Hepatitis: "Ascorbic acid (vitamin C) is the drug of choice in viral hepatitis," says Dr. Klenner. Given massive doses of the nutrient, his patients are well and back to work in from three to seven days, he says.

Viral pneumonia: One patient was unconscious, with a fever of 106.8 degrees when admitted to the hospital. After receiving vitamin C intravenously for 72 hours, she was awake and sitting up in bed. Her temperature had returned to normal.

Herpes simplex: This persistent virus is responsible for cold sores around the mouth. "In one case with five repeats of herpes virus erupting at yearly intervals and at the same site, seven to

10 grams ascorbic acid by mouth, daily, was found to eliminate the pathology," Dr. Klenner says. Many other cases were cured by applying a three percent vitamin C ointment to the lips 10 to 15 times a day.

Measles: "By 1950 we learned that we could kill the measles virus in 24 hours by giving intramuscular injections in a dose range of 350 mg. per kilogram of body weight (about 12 grams for the average child) every two hours," Dr. Klenner reports. Similar dramatic results were obtained against chicken pox.

Mononucleosis: "Large doses of vitamin C, given intravenously, will eliminate this virus in just a few days. . . ." the doctor says.

Dr. Klenner is convinced that "Vitamin C when given by needle will destroy all viruses and many can be destroyed by taking 25-30 grams each day by mouth. Lesser amounts will protect against these pathogens." The cases cited above, as well as many others, are reported in the *Journal of the International Academy of Prevention Medicine* (Spring 1974) and *Journal of Applied Nutrition* (Winter 1971).

# A Challenge to Medical Researchers

Obviously, this is not the kind of therapy that lends itself to a do-it-yourself approach. Dr. Klenner is talking about amounts of vitamin C much larger than an individual would ever use under normal circumstances. But an acute viral infection is not a normal situation. It is sometimes a matter of life or death. That's why the findings of Dr. Klenner and the Japanese investigators represent a resounding challenge to find out once and for all—in carefully designed and rigorously controlled studies—if large doses of vitamin C really can put a stop to much of the misery caused by viruses.

# APPENDICES

# Vitamins at a Glance

| VITAMIN | United States Recommended Daily Allowances | Primary Food Sources | Major Activity In The Body |
|---------|--------------------------------------------|----------------------|----------------------------|
| **A** | Infants (0-12 mo.) 1,500 IU<br>Children under 4 yrs. 2,500 IU<br>Adults and children 4 or more yrs. 5,000 IU<br>Pregnant or lactating women 8,000 IU | green and yellow vegetables (spinach, cabbage, carrots)<br>eggs<br>fish liver oils<br>organ meats (liver) | protein synthesis<br>bone growth<br>healthy skin<br>sexual functioning and reproduction |
| **B₁ (thiamine)** | Infants (0-12 mo.) 0.5 mg.<br>Children under 5 yrs. 0.7 mg.<br>Adults and children 4 or more yrs. 1.5 mg.<br>Pregnant or lactating women 1.7 mg. | whole cereal grains<br>liver<br>pork<br>fresh green vegetables<br>potatoes<br>beans<br>brewer's yeast<br>desiccated liver<br>wheat germ | cell oxidation (respiration)<br>needed for normal growth<br>appetite enhancer<br>carbohydrate metabolism<br>stimulates and transmits nerve impulses<br>heart health |

| Clinical<br>Deficiency Signs | Preventive And/Or<br>Therapeutic Applications |
|---|---|
| night blindness<br>lackluster appearance of eyeball<br>  due to dryness (xerophthalmia)<br>infection and ulceration<br>  of the eye<br>sealing and dryness<br>  of the eyelids<br>hard, dry, itching skin | infectious diseases<br>stress-induced diseases<br>impaired sense of smell<br>bleeding gums<br>hearing loss<br>night blindness<br>respiratory infections, including<br>  combatant role against ravages of<br>  environmental pollutants on the lungs<br>reported anticancer role<br>  on cellular level<br>  involving test animals |
| beriberi<br>nervous system deterioration<br>muscle tenderness and wasting | emotional stability<br>nervous disorders<br>alcoholism<br>fatigue<br>weight loss<br>heart failure<br>digestive disturbances<br>muscular disorders<br>circulatory disorders |

(cont.)

| VITAMIN | United States Recommended Daily Allowances | Primary Food Sources | Major Activity In The Body |
|---|---|---|---|
| **B₂ (riboflavin)** | Infants (0-12 mo.) 0.6 mg. <br> Children under 4 yrs. 0.8 mg. <br> Adults and children 4 or more yrs. 1.7 mg. <br> Pregnant or lactating women 2 mg. | brewer's yeast <br> desiccated liver <br> wheat germ <br> eggs <br> green leafy vegetables <br> peas <br> lima beans <br> organ meats | protein metabolism <br> lipid metabolism <br> skin, liver, and eye health |
| **B₃ (niacin)** | Infants (0-12 mo.) 8 mg. <br> Children under 4 yrs. 9 mg. <br> Adults and children 4 or more yrs. 20 mg. <br> Pregnant or lactating women 20 mg. | yeast <br> organ meats (liver, kidney) <br> poultry meat <br> fish <br> wheat germ <br> nuts <br> soybeans <br> desiccated liver <br> brewer's yeast | carbohydrate metabolism <br> circulatory system |

| Clinical<br>Deficiency Signs | Preventive And/Or<br>Therapeutic Applications |
|---|---|
| itching, burning eyes<br>cataracts<br>lesions in the corner<br>  of the mouth (cheilosis)<br>inflammation of the tongue<br>  (glossitis) | conjunctivitis<br>cataracts<br>lip and mouth cracks<br>skin lesions<br>anemia<br>personality disturbances<br>fatigue<br>stress<br>alcoholism<br>prevents birth defects |
| pellagra<br>  (diarrhea, dermatitis, dementia) | dermatitis (skin rashes)<br>diarrhea<br>dementia<br>blood cholesterol reducer<br>increases circulation<br>stress<br>weakness<br>irritability<br>mental fatigue<br>abdominal pains<br>insomnia<br>tongue sores<br>alcoholism |

(cont.)

| VITAMIN | United States Recommended Daily Allowances | Primary Food Sources | Major Activity In The Body |
|---|---|---|---|
| **B$_6$ (pyridoxine)** | Infants (0-12 mo.) 0.4 mg. Children under 4 yrs. 0.7 mg. Adults and children 4 or more yrs. 2 mg. Pregnant or lactating women 2.5 mg. | organ meats (liver) lean muscle meats fish whole grains walnuts filberts peanuts sunflower seeds buckwheat flour soybean flour wheat germ bananas | enzyme activator carbohydrate and fat metabolism protein metabolism hormone production (adrenalin and insulin) RNA and DNA synthesis antibody production |
| **B$_{12}$** | Infants (0-12 mo.) 2 mcg. Children under 4 yrs. 3 mcg. Adults and children 4 or more yrs. 6 mcg. Pregnant or lactating women 8 mcg. | yeast wheat germ liver milk eggs meat cheese | red blood cell formation healthy nervous system needed for normal growth RNA and DNA synthesis carbohydrate metabolism fertility needed during pregnancy |

| Clinical<br>Deficiency Signs | Preventive And/Or<br>Therapeutic Applications |
|---|---|
| convulsions in babies<br>eczema-like outbreaks<br>  on face and body<br>skin and mouth lesions<br>  similar to $B_2$<br>  and niacin deficiency<br>nervous system deterioration | cancer immunity<br>arteriosclerosis<br>diabetes<br>kidney stones<br>anemia<br>acne<br>seborrhea<br>tooth decay<br>rheumatism<br>asthma<br>schizophrenia<br>leg cramps<br>nausea and vomiting<br>  associated with<br>  pregnancy<br>depression<br>menstruation symptoms<br>  (puffiness and<br>  soreness)<br>menopausal symptoms |
| pernicious anemia<br>neuritis | pernicious anemia<br>nervous disorders<br>growth promoter<br>strengthens immunity system<br>mental illness |

(cont.)

| VITAMIN | United States Recommended Daily Allowances | Primary Food Sources | Major Activity In The Body |
|---|---|---|---|
| **Folic Acid** | Infants (0-12 mo.) 0.1 mg.<br>Children under 4 yrs. 0.2 mg.<br>Adults and children 4 or more yrs. 0.4 mg.<br>Pregnant or lactating women 0.8 mg. | liver<br>wheat bran<br>asparagus<br>beet greens<br>kale<br>endive<br>spinach<br>turnips | red blood cell formation<br>RNA and DNA synthesis |
| **Biotin** | Infants (0-12 mo.) 0.05 mg.<br>Children under 4 yrs. 0.15 mg.<br>Adults and children 4 or more yrs. 0.3 mg.<br>Pregnant or lactating mothers 0.3 mg. | yeast<br>liver<br>eggs<br>whole grains<br>nuts<br>fish<br>brewer's yeast<br>desiccated liver<br>wheat germ | protein metabolism<br>carbohydrate metabolism<br>unsaturated fatty acid metabolism<br>needed for normal growth<br>maintenance of skin, hair, nerves, sex glands, bone marrow, sebaceous glands |
| **Choline** | none established | brewer's yeast<br>fish<br>soybeans<br>peanuts<br>beef liver | nervous system functioning (essential ingredient of the nerve fluid acetylcholine)<br>liver functioning<br>immunity buildup |

| Clinical<br>Deficiency Signs | Preventive And/Or<br>Therapeutic Applications |
|---|---|
| anemia | toxemia of pregnancy<br>premature birth<br>megaloblastic anemia<br>birth defects<br>strengthens immunity<br>enhances wound healing<br>mental illness<br>greater demand during pregnancy |
| seborrheic dermatitis<br>desquamative erythroderma<br>muscular pains | "egg white injury"<br>seborrheic dermatitis<br>desquamative erythroderma<br>gastrointestinal symptoms<br>  (poor appetite, nausea)<br>leg cramps |
| none officially recognized | paralysis<br>cardiac arrest<br>kidney dysfunction<br>hypertension<br>liver dysfunction |

(cont.)

| VITAMIN | United States Recommended Daily Allowances | Primary Food Sources | Major Activity In The Body |
|---|---|---|---|
| **Inositol** | none established | beef heart<br>bulgur wheat<br>brown rice<br>brewer's yeast<br>molasses | found in high concentrations in the human brain, stomach, kidney, spleen, and liver |
| **Pantothenic Acid** | Infants (0-12 mo.)<br>3 mg.<br>Children under 4 yrs.<br>5 mg.<br>Adults and children 4 or more yrs.<br>10 mg.<br>Pregnant or lactating women<br>10 mg. | liver (beef, chicken)<br>kidney (beef)<br>heart (beef, chicken)<br>brewer's yeast<br>sunflower seeds<br>buckwheat flour (dark)<br>peanuts (raw) | found in human muscle adrenal gland function immunity system (antibody production) gastrointestinal tract functioning (flatulence) |

| Clinical<br>Deficiency Signs | Preventive And/Or<br>Therapeutic Applications |
|---|---|
| none officially recognized | controls cholesterol level<br>mild inhibitory effect on cancer<br>used with vitamin E to treat<br>  nerve damage in certain forms<br>  of muscular dystrophy |
| headache<br>fatigue<br>impaired motor coordination<br>gastrointestinal disturbances | lowered resistance to infection<br>muscle cramps<br>fatigue<br>appetite loss<br>constipation<br>stress<br>arthritis<br>protects against radiation injury<br>bruxism (tooth grinding) |

(cont.)

| VITAMIN | United States Recommended Daily Allowances | Primary Food Sources | Major Activity In The Body |
|---|---|---|---|
| **PABA** (para-amino-benzoic acid) | none established | liver<br>eggs<br>molasses<br>brewer's yeast<br>wheat germ | coenzyme in the metabolism of protein<br>blood cell formation<br>stimulates intestinal bacteria to produce folic acid<br>utilization of pantothenic acid |
| **C** | Infants (0-12 mo.) 35 mg.<br>Children under 4 yrs. 40 mg.<br>Adults and children 4 or more yrs. 60 mg.<br>Pregnant or lactating women 60 mg. | citrus fruits<br>rose hips<br>green peppers<br>broccoli<br>spinach<br>tomatoes | antioxidant<br>healthy sex organs<br>healthy adrenal glands<br>collagen (connective tissue) formation<br>tooth formation<br>bone cartilage<br>skin<br>enhances iron absorption<br>infection fighter<br>tissue repair (heart)<br>mental health<br>strengthens capillary tissue |

| Clinical<br>Deficiency Signs | Preventive And/Or<br>Therapeutic Applications |
|---|---|
| none officially recognized | digestive disorders<br>nervousness<br>depression<br>prevents sunburn<br>  by acting as a sunscreen<br>possible preventive for skin cancer |
| scurvy<br>bleeding gums and loose teeth<br>skin lesions and bruises | prevents cholesterol buildup<br>  in blood vessels<br>aging symptoms<br>  (wrinkles, stoop, easy hemorrhaging)<br>transformation of nitrite<br>  into nitrosamines<br>anemia<br>scurvy<br>atherosclerosis<br>arthritis<br>  (to avoid the side effects of aspirin)<br>lead poisoning<br>mercury poisoning<br>cadmium poisoning<br>prevents recurrence of bladder cancer<br>burns and bruising<br>leg cramps during pregnancy<br><br>(cont.) |

| VITAMIN | United States Recommended Daily Allowances | Primary Food Sources | Major Activity In The Body |
|---|---|---|---|
| **C** <br> *(cont.)* | | | |
| **D** | Infants (0-12 mo.) <br> 400 IU <br> Children <br> under 4 yrs. <br> 400 IU <br> Adults <br> and children <br> 4 or more yrs. <br> 400 IU <br> Pregnant or <br> lactating women <br> 400 IU | cod liver oil <br> halibut liver oil <br> eggs (yolk) <br> milk <br> (vitamin D <br> enriched) <br> salmon <br> tuna | bone health <br> and growth <br> calcium <br> metabolism <br> regulator <br> nerve health <br> helps regulate <br> heartbeat |
| **E** | Infants (0-12 mo.) <br> 5 IU <br> Children <br> under 4 yrs. <br> 10 IU <br> Adults <br> and children <br> 4 or more yrs. <br> 30 IU <br> Pregnant or <br> lactating women <br> 30 IU | green leafy <br> vegetables <br> (cabbage, spinach, <br> asparagus, <br> broccoli) <br> whole grains <br> (rice, wheat, oats) <br> safflower oil <br> wheat germ <br> vegetable oils <br> peanuts | dissolves fibrin <br> reduces thrombin <br> formation <br> antioxidant <br> (keeps oxygen <br> from combining <br> with wastes <br> to form toxic <br> compounds) <br> red blood <br> cell health |

| Clinical<br>Deficiency Signs | Preventive And/Or<br>Therapeutic Applications |
|---|---|
|  | hemorrhaging<br>diabetes<br>enhances wound healing<br>  following surgery<br>bed sores<br>bleeding gums |
| rickets<br>osteomalacia<br>osteoporosis | rickets<br>osteomalacia<br>osteoporosis<br>multiple sclerosis<br>combats harmful effects<br>  of steroid therapy |
| fat absorption defects<br>anemia (premature infants)<br>metabolic dysfunction<br>  in the muscles | blood clots (antithrombotic agent)<br>aging process<br>  (prolongs the life of human cells)<br>wrinkled skin<br>cancer development<br>  (breast and ovarian)<br>lung damage caused by smog<br>lowers cholesterol in conjunction<br>  with polyunsaturated fatty acids<br>vitamin E-deficiency anemia<br>  (premature infants)<br>heart disease<br>aging (senility)<br>menopause symptoms<br>varicose veins |

(cont.)

| VITAMIN | United States Recommended Daily Allowances | Primary Food Sources | Major Activity In The Body |
|---------|-------------------------------------------|---------------------|---------------------------|
| E (cont.) | | | |
| K | none established | green leafy vegetables (spinach, cabbage) pork liver egg yolk tomatoes wheat germ soybeans potatoes | blood clotting or coagulation factor |

| Clinical<br>Deficiency Signs | Preventive And/Or<br>Therapeutic Applications |
|---|---|
| | skin ailments (eczema, ulcers)<br>endurance (athletic performance)<br>reproductive failures<br>  (sterility or habitual abortion) |
| hemorrhaging<br>delayed blood coagulation | hemorrhaging<br>bruising<br>offsets the risks associated<br>  with anticoagulant drugs<br>hypoprothrombinemia<br>  (low thrombin levels in blood)<br>often given to mothers<br>  before delivery and to newborn infants,<br>  to protect against hemorrhages |

# THE FUTURE ROLE
# OF NUTRITION
# IN HEALTH CARE

**Editor's Note:** Few areas of science can claim a development as spectacular and meaningful as nutrition has in the past generation. Just what we have learned, how far we have come, where we are headed, needs to be defined for those of us who are not working in the laboratories and the treatment rooms. Will degenerative diseases such as heart disease and cancer respond to nutritional therapy? Do humans need concentrations of specific nutrients at certain stages of life? Can we get all of our vitamin needs from a balanced diet? Should we be concerned about overdosing with vitamins?

To answer these and other questions on the current and potential role of nutrition in health, we have prevailed upon some of the most distinguished figures in the fields of scientific research and clinical medicine to join in a symposium. Among them are a Nobel Prize winner, several practicing physicians, a biochemist, and a famous nutritional researcher. You will see that their attitudes vary from unbounded enthusiasm for the value of massive doses of nutritional supplementation, to an insistence that we should get all our nutrition from food and nowhere else.

But finding truly nutritional foods in today's marketplace is a real challenge. For that reason most of the participants recommend vitamin supplementation as one way to insure adequate nutrition when the quality of food sources is doubtful. Of course, those who use nutrients therapeutically must rely on manufactured vitamins, since that is the only way to get the required quantities.

It makes no difference whose side you are on in this controversy—the participants present ideas that are sure to stimulate and inform you. Prior to the actual debate, several of the contributors present general statements which provide a useful framework for what follows.

# The Participants

**Irwin Stone:**
Author of *The Healing Factor, "Vitamin C" Against Disease,* (New York: Grosset and Dunlap, 1975). Over a 40-year period he has published more than 60 papers in professional journals on various aspects of ascorbic acid. He is a member of the New York Academy of Sciences and the American Chemical Society. In 1965 Mr. Stone identified the genetic liver enzyme disease, hypoascorbemia.

**Roger J. Williams, Ph.D., D.Sc.:**
Pioneer in the field of vitamin research and discoverer of the B vitamin, pantothenic acid. From 1941 to 1963 he was director of the Clayton Foundation Biochemical Institute at the University of Texas where more vitamins and their variants have been discovered than in any other laboratory in the world. Dr. Williams is the author of several important books on organic chemistry and biochemistry as well as numerous books for the layman, including *Nutrition Against Disease* (New York: Pitman Publishers, 1972).

**John Yudkin, M.D., Ph.D.:**
Physician, biochemist and professor of nutrition emeritus at London University. He is the author of *Sweet and Dangerous* (New York: P. H. Wyden, 1972), about the damaging effects sugar has on the body, and he is the author or coauthor of five other books and 30 papers published in American and British scientific journals.

**Albert Szent-Gyorgyi, M.D., Ph.D.:**
Winner of the Nobel Prize in medicine and physiology in 1937, he served as professor of biochemistry at the University of Budapest from 1945 to 1947. He is now Director of Research at the Institute of Muscle Research of the Marine Biological Laboratories, Woods Hole, Massachusetts. Noted for the discoveries concerning ascorbic acid and the bioflavonoids and for his investigations of actin, a muscle protein, he is the author of several books, including *The Living State* (New York: Academic Press, 1972).

**Frederick R. Klenner, M.D., F.C.C.P., A.A.F.P.:**
General practitioner, specializing in diseases of the chest, Dr. Klenner has published 28 scientific papers on the action of ascorbic acid against disease. He is a Fellow of the American Association for the Advancement of Science, Diplomate of the International College of Applied Nutrition, Fellow of the Royal Society of Health, London, England, and member and Fellow of many other medical and scientific organizations.

**Abram Hoffer, M.D., Ph.D.:**
President of Huxley Institute for Biosocial Research in New York City, Fellow, Academy of Orthomolecular Psychiatry, editor of the *Journal of Orthomolecular Medicine* and author of many scientific papers on megavitamin therapy, Dr. Hoffer is perhaps best known as coauthor, with Humphrey Osmond, of one of the first books for the layman on nutritional treatment for mental illness, *How to Live with Schizophrenia* (Secaucus, New Jersey: University Books, 1974).

**Allan Cott, M.D., F.A.P.A.:**

Medical Director, Churchill School for Learning Disabilities, New York City, consultant to New York Institute for Child Development and president of the Academy of Orthomolecular Psychiatry. Dr. Cott practices psychiatry in New York City, and frequently speaks and writes for scientific journals on the subject of orthomolecular medicine for the treatment of emotional disorders. He was guest lecturer at the First World Congress on Biological Psychiatry in Buenos Aires, Argentina in 1974, and is the author of *Fasting, the Ultimate Diet* (New York: Bantam Books, 1975).

**Wilfrid E. Shute, M.D., F.I.A.P.M.:**

Cofounder and codirector of the Shute Institute for Laboratory and Clinical Medicine in London, Ontario, Canada, where he was chief cardiologist. Dr. Shute has been responsible for treating more than 35,000 cardiac patients. He is the world's foremost authority on vitamin E and he has contributed numerous medical reports to various scientific and professional journals. He is the author of several books including *Dr. Wilfrid E. Shute's Complete Updated Vitamin E Book* (New Canaan, Connecticut: Keats Publishing Co., 1975).

# Preliminary Statements

**Allan Cott:**

The importance of the role of nutrition in maintaining physical health was clarified earlier in the century by those who pioneered in the discovery of the vitamin-deficiency diseases and their cure. The understanding of the role of nutrition in mental health began as a ripple early in the third quarter of our century, rapidly built to a groundswell, and is now attracting the attention of our populace as a whole and of the scientific community.

"We are what we eat" no longer refers only to our physical being, but to our mental health as well. The state of our nutrition affects our behavior, our mood, and can affect our sanity. The need to relate the advances in the nutritional sciences to the body of medicine will be realized in this last quarter of our century. Until the present, neither medical education or medical practice has kept abreast of these advances. Medical teaching and thinking adhered to the narrow focus of nutritional deficiency diseases and missed the importance of diet, the maintenance of physical health, and the creation of an optimum molecular environment for the mind. The following generations will experience the ultimate benefits of the growing awareness that nutrition operates on all levels of biochemical and metabolic functioning.

### Albert Szent-Gyorgyi:

I am deeply convinced that our bodies are much more perfect than we believe, and that the majority of diseases are due to our abusing and mistreating our bodies. Food is only part of the picture, perhaps the most important one. There is no such thing as "good food" or "bad food." The question is what food is the human body made for? It is no use telling a rabbit to eat more meat or telling a shark to eat more vegetables. We must eat what is natural to our systems. Such foods, if they are not tampered with, naturally contain the vitamins and minerals and other nutrients we need.

### Abram Hoffer:

I would like to emphasize that one judges the future from the past. In watching the trends as they have developed over the past twenty years it is clear that we have gradually moved from a study of vitamin deficiencies where small quantities only are required, to a study of dependency where a few individuals out of our population require very much larger quantities or megadosages of certain of the vitamins.

It has been discovered that certain diseases, up till now considered as having no known origin, are being related to these vitamin dependencies. For example, in a recent publication Irwin Stone has shown that hypodysplasia, considered a genetic disease of dogs, is simply a manifestation of scurvy and can be prevented completely by giving vitamin C to the mother and to the puppies. A projection into the future therefore suggests that more and more of this kind of recognition will take place.

# Question

In your opinion, what is the most promising area for vitamin therapy in the future?

**Roger J. Williams:**

I do not regard vitamins as magic bullets comparable to medicines, each of which is given to cure a specific disease. I do not think "vitamin therapy" can or should be separated from "mineral therapy" or "amino-acid therapy." The most promising fields for nutritional therapy are, in my opinion, birth defects and mental retardation, mental disease, alcoholism, and heart disease.

**Allan Cott:**

The treatment of illnesses in which there is a demonstrated disorder of brain chemistry is particularly hopeful. Vitamins $B_3$ and $B_6$ show great promise as substances which can affect, in a beneficial way, the levels of neuro-transmitters.

**Abram Hoffer:**

I believe the most promising area will be the exploration of diseases of unknown origin for the presence of single or multiple vitamin dependencies as well as single or multiple mineral dependencies. As an example, there is increasing information that the rare muscular wasting diseases such as muscular dystrophy, Huntington's Chorea, and perhaps multiple sclerosis may be manifestations of a dependency on certain of the B vitamins, especially thiamine and vitamin B₃. I have seen a patient with Huntington's Chorea who had been degenerating for a period of twenty years when it was halted and near normal functioning was restored by large quantities of vitamin E, that is, 3,200 units per day, and vitamin C, six grams per day. The patient now receives nicotinic acid in smaller dosages in order to maintain a normal mental state. I think that this is the most promising area and I hope that it will be greatly expanded.

**Frederick R. Klenner:**

Control of virus pathology. I believe this will lead in many cases to control of cancer, since it is my opinion that some types of cancer are virus-based. I also see hope for prevention and/or reversal of neurological syndromes.

# Question

If you were asked to design a nutrition curriculum for a medical school, what areas would you emphasize as most useful to a practicing physician?

**John Yudkin:**

The present, largely inadequate, curriculum in nutrition in medical schools fails because it tends to be excessively academic and inadequately practical. For example, great store is laid upon the biochemical reactions in which vitamins are involved, but almost none on the foods that contain them, especially how much of the vitamin is in how much of the food. The same is true for other aspects of diet, so that there is no understanding of how the biochemistry of the nutrients in food is related to the food that people eat.

**Abram Hoffer:**

I would set up a Department of Clinical Nutrition which would have equal status with the Department of Surgery, the Department of Medicine, and the Department of Psychiatry. It should be one of the major divisions of any medical college. I would be opposed to the standard type of teaching by biochemists who merely enumerate the vitamins, give their structure, and list their properties, because this has no relevance to the average medical student. I would teach the elements of clinical nutrition by demonstrating with actual patients how disease can be relieved when proper nutrition is established.

It would be important to define nutritional individuality, to promote the concept of vitamin and mineral dependency, and to establish Dr. Roger William's concept that no single nutrient is of any value by itself since all must play their role together. This he calls the "orchestra principle."

I would also teach the principles of food allergy since this may have a direct impact in producing mineral and vitamin dependencies. Finally, I would spend a good deal of time teaching the impact of modern food technology using a book entitled *Food for Nought: The Decline of Nutrition* by Ross H. Hall (New York: Harper & Row, Inc., 1974).

Currently, there are about a dozen different textbooks that could be used in teaching clinical nutrition, most of them in the field of orthomolecular psychiatry, with a few coming along in the field of orthomolecular medicine. *The Saacharin Disease* by T. L. Cleave (New Canaan, Connecticut: Keats Publishing, Inc., 1975) which discusses the impact of fiber-free foods would be extremely pertinent.

I would start out in first-year medicine with the basic principles of clinical nutrition and then gradually throughout each year keep hammering home the impact of nutrition upon every disease which appears in the hospital.

**Allan Cott:**

A nutrition curriculum in any medical school should emphasize the importance of altering medical thinking about the doses of vitamins, minerals, and amino acids. These essential nutrients must be used in much larger doses than the minimal or Recommended Daily Allowance doses, for in the larger doses they have an action which is over and above their action as a food supplement. It is only in the larger doses that these nutrients can alter the body chemistry in a beneficial way and alleviate symptoms of disease.

Greater emphasis must be placed on the research findings which indicate that we really are what we eat. For example, eating a meal which contains a high content of tryptophane results in an increase in the brain levels of tryptophane. Missing protein in one meal is sufficient to lower the level of neuro-transmitters in the brain. It is logical to expect this level to be reflected in the brain's activity.

**Roger J. Williams:**

The facts of nutritional science should be woven into every aspect of physiology, biochemistry, and pathology. I doubt that "courses" in nutrition as such will ever be introduced into medical schools.

**Wilfrid E. Shute:**

Medical students should learn to discover, evaluate, and recommend foods that contain the essential amino acids, vitamins, and minerals. At the same time, they should be informed enough to discourage their patients from excessive sugar use and the use of all unnecessary chemicals, especially artificial colorings and flavors.

# Question

What are the three most underrated nutrients in terms of preventive or therapeutic potential and why?

**Frederick R. Klenner:**

Ascorbic acid, thiamine HCI, and pyridoxine in that order. Ascorbic acid is the number one and antifatigue vitamin. It works to increase the IQ and keeps us in peak health if adequate amounts are taken daily by mouth. Thiamine HCI is the number two antifatigue vitamin. It is essential in maintaining proper nutrition for nerve tissue. Eighty percent of our population lacks sufficient thiamine in the diet. Pyridoxine has gained widespread attention for its value in such pathological conditions as arthritis, heart disease, nervous disorders, and rheumatism. Pyridoxine phosphate plays an exceptional role among the coenzymes.

I would, however, be hard pressed to exclude vitamin E which I hold, along with vitamin C, to be the great protector of the cardiovascular system. Unfortunately, these chemicals have never been exploited to their real potential because of the insignificant dose schedule adopted by most physicians.

## John Yudkin:

I believe we are unnecessarily concerned about nutrition and not enough about food. A good diet contains all the nutrients we need; a bad diet not only is likely to be deficient in ways we cannot easily assess (in terms of what nutrients are lacking and by how much), but also is likely to contain items that are unwholesome.

## Abram Hoffer:

In my opinion the most underrated vitamins are vitamins $B_3$, C, and E.

$B_3$ (nicotinic acid and nicotinamide) has a role not only in arthritis but in perceptual disturbances, schizophrenia or allied conditions, and in treating a large number of children with learning and behavioral disorders. It is also very effective in the treatment and prevention of senility especially if diagnosed early.

Vitamin C's value as a preventive and treatment has been amply described by Irwin Stone and has been given worldwide attention by Dr. Linus Pauling.

Finally, I think vitamin E has been grossly neglected in terms of its enormous potential for healing and for treating cardiovascular disease, as well as for its action in preventing senility.

**Wilfrid Shute:**

I must address myself here to the nearly total removal from food of our natural supply of a substance which everyone must have for normal function—vitamin E. If it is not present in adequate amounts a wide variety of conditions can result, including the number one killer, heart disease, thrombophlebitis, and much else.

# Question

Do you see a major role for topically applied vitamins? Have you personally had any experience in this area?

**Irwin Stone:**

The topical use of ascorbate is a therapeutic measure of wide usefulness. Ascorbic acid can be used to remove warts and a mixture of sodium ascorbate and ascorbic acid is a valuable topical treatment of skin cancers such as epitheliomas. Topical sodium ascorbate will regress the lesions of herpes on the skin and mucous membrane. Various eye pathologies and irritations respond well to bathing the eye in a soothing five percent to 10 percent sodium ascorbate solution. The use of topical sodium ascorbate solution was one step in a procedure developed many years ago by Dr. Klenner for the treatment of severe burns. It prevents infection, reduces the pain, promotes healing, and tends to replace the needed sodium normally lost in severe burns. It would appear that many other uses are possible for this versatile material which is only limited by the imagination and inventiveness of the investigator.

**Allan Cott:**

Experience in my practice shows a rather limited use for topically applied vitamins. The results of the use of vitamin E for burns, however, has indeed been dramatic.

**John Yudkin:**

I see even less a role for the topical application of vitamins, in conditions in which there is no demonstrable and specific deficiency, than for their oral administration.

**Frederick R. Klenner:**

I consider ascorbic acid to be the main drug or chemical for the treatment of burns. A three percent solution should be sprayed over the burn area at least every four hours, along with massive doses administered intravenously and by mouth. By massive doses I mean at least 500 mg. per kg. body weight given repeatedly so that an adult weighting 54 kg. would receive at least 100 grams during the first 24 hours. I have had extremely beneficial results using this schedule with no scarring. Most patients are completely healed in 30 days or less—and I have never had to resort to skin grafting.

**Roger J. Williams:**

I think topically applied vitamins have no *major* role.

**Wilfrid E. Shute:**
    Topically applied vitamin E does fantastic things to burn cases, and as one of the originators of its use, I must suggest that my experience with it is meaningful. Vitamin C ointment is also recommended by men I trust and admire.

# Question

Which of the major degenerative diseases has the greatest potential for improvement through nutrition?

**Frederick R. Klenner:**
    Heart disease would rate number one. Ascorbic acid, at least 10 grams a day taken orally, with between 4,000 and 6,000 I.U.s of vitamin E are needed for optimum results. Arthritis would rate number two and cancer number three. We have had some results using massive doses of thiamine HCl against deafness and ascorbic acid and vitamin E have shown value in treating vision problems.

**Roger J. Williams:**
    While all degenerative diseases can probably be prevented eventually by nutritional means, heart disease, some types of arthritis, and cataracts seem to be most promising. We have quite a way to go before all types of arthritis are controlled and probably even longer before cancer incidence can be markedly diminished.

**John Yudkin:**

The major defect in our current diets lies not in the adequacy or inadequacy of particular nutrients, but in its distortion *in toto* by the consumption of food for palatability rather than for nutritional value. The most important result of this attitude is the vastly excessive consumption of sugar, which not only (or not even most importantly) dilutes the nutrient content of the diet, but actually causes a range of untoward actions on the tissues of the body.

**Albert Szent-Gyorgyi:**

It is very difficult to connect any disease directly with a vitamin. For example, say you have too little vitamin C, your next cold may be more severe and you may get pneumonia and end up in a mortuary. But the cause of death will not be listed as "too little ascorbic acid," it will be "pneumonia." It will be difficult to prove that death would not have occurred if you had gotten enough vitamin C in the first place.

There are too many other factors besides vitamins that can have an influence on any disease. Though nutrition is important, it is only one of the possible causes.

**Allan Cott:**

Heart disease, arteriosclerosis, arthritis, hearing loss, and the aging process have the greatest potential for improvement through nutrition.

**Abram Hoffer:**

In my opinion heart disease, arthritis, and cancer could best be dealt with by nutritional methods. With respect to heart disease I would recommend that the incidence could be greatly reduced by following a sugar-free diet which is high in fiber and which does not contain excessive quantities of the unsaturated fatty acids. I would suggest an increase in the amounts of vitamin $B_3$ and $B_6$, vitamin E (to compensate for what has happened to our food), and an increase in the amount of vitamin C. In addition it would be important not to be overweight and to increase one's exercise.

With respect to arthritis, I believe it will respond to increased intake of vitamin $B_3$, either nicotinic acid or nicotinamide. This was first established by Professor William Kaufman who published two books on the subject, *The Common Form of Niacin Amide Deficiency Disease: Aniacinamidosis* (Bridgeport, Connecticut: W. Kaufman, 1943) and *The Common Form of Joint Dysfunction* (Boston, Massachusetts: Eugene Hildreth Publishing, 1949). Unfortunately, his work came out just before the "wonder drugs" such as cortisone came along and since that time rheumatologists have paid no attention whatever to the use of vitamins for these conditions.

The treatment of cancer with nutrients has been amply described by Irwin Stone and Dr. Linus Pauling. I think it deserves a major expenditure of funds to research this area properly. I also think that there is enough information with respect to vitamin $B_{17}$ to warrant further examination of this area. The hostility of the establishment against this vitamin is not warranted if one looks at it scientifically.


**Wilfrid E. Shute:**

I see the greatest possibility in the treatment of heart disease, blindness, and all peripheral vascular lesions whether in kidney, brain, eye, or extremity, through vitamin E plus C.

# Question

At some stages in life humans are said to be particularly vulnerable to vitamin deficiencies. Which vitamins are most likely to be needed when, and what quantities of supplementation do you consider reasonable? Would you suggest vitamin supplementation at such times as a rule?

**Frederick R. Klenner:**

We are diet poor in the United States and a great majority of the people are vitamin deficient. Naturally, the geriatric group suffers most. A very high potency B complex capsule or tablet taken before meals and bed hour is most helpful. Older people also need high vitamin A, therefore, the toxicity scare on vitamin A must be removed. Only 65 cases of toxicity to A have been reported in the world medical literature (a very small percentage out of a population of billions). All people over 30 should have some vitamin supplement.

**Roger J. Williams:**

All vitamins are needed at all times. During gestation possibly the vitamins most likely to be in short supply in the environment of growing fetuses (in the U.S.A.) are vitamin A, pantothenic acid, and vitamin B6. This is largely guesswork. Expert vitamin supplementation is very often desirable.

**Allan Cott:**

At those stages in life when humans are particularly vulnerable to vitamin deficiencies they are most likely to need the B complex group of vitamins, vitamins A and D, and vitamin C. One cannot say what quantities of supplementation are reasonable or adequate since this varies from person to person. An adequate amount is that quantity which fulfills the requirement of each person's biochemical structure.

### Abram Hoffer:

I think humans are particularly vulnerable when they are under great stress, either from rapid growth or as a result of bacterial or viral invasions, or near the end of life when senility is imminent.

The vitamins that are required throughout life should be given in increased quantity during these times. I think it would be a good idea to provide a general vitamin supplement which would provide most of the vitamins, especially vitamin C, and, for elderly people, vitamin E.

### Wilfrid E. Shute:

I recommend vitamin E to be used by both parents before conception and steadily thereafter.

### John Yudkin:

There is a little evidence, though not very impressive to me, that pregnant and nursing mothers are likely to suffer from deficiency of folic acid and perhaps $B_6$, and that the elderly are prone to deficiency of vitamin D. There is, however, good evidence that, in colder climates, or in large cities, or where social custom leads to children being kept away from sunlight, deficiency of vitamin D occurs, so that it is reasonable in these circumstances for young children to take some special source of vitamin D.

**Irwin Stone:**

I believe humans at *all* stages of life are vulnerable to deficiencies of ascorbate and the other vitamins and minerals. This is a "conception-to-grave" proposition and deficiencies must be avoided throughout one's entire lifetime. A critical period is the time spent "in utero" where full correction of maternal deficiencies should be maintained throughout pregnancy. After birth, the full correction should be maintained throughout life. The daily quantities I regard as necessary are: for children, one gram of ascorbate per year of age up to 10, then 10 grams a day thereafter. For the vitamins I believe it is reasonable to use (except for vitamin D) several or more times the present RDAs. I believe that all of us who depend solely upon our foodstuffs as the sole source of ascorbate and the vitamins and minerals, are fighting a losing battle.

# Question

How do you respond to the argument that eating a balanced diet provides sufficient vitamin intake? Do you think the present direction of our dietary habits leads to an improvement in our individual nutrition levels?

**Abram Hoffer:**

The concept of the balanced diet that provides all necessary nutrition is no longer valid. It might have been useful twenty-five years ago, before foods were so thoroughly emasculated, but since that time it is impossible to obtain everything we should have by eating modern foods. However, I do agree with the principle of "balanced," in terms of eating the right quantities of protein, carbohydrate and fat, vitamins and minerals. To do this, there is no substantial evidence that a large number of foods is required; many animals live perfectly well on single foods or just a small variety of foods. The important thing is to consume the right combination of whole foods, benefiting from the balance which is provided by nature.

**Roger J. Williams:**

A "balanced diet" is a most indefinite entity and has no scientific meaning. Vitamin (and other nutrient) needs vary greatly from individual to individual, and what might be balanced for one might be severely unbalanced for another. "Balanced diets" as often recommended by naive physicians frequently contain large amounts of highly unbalanced foods—sugar, starch, alcohol, milled grains, etc.—and the diets cannot be balanced. Improvement in balance can be attained by avoiding these unbalanced foods.

**Allan Cott:**

I generally respond to the argument that eating a balanced diet provides sufficient vitamin intake by stating that this may have been true a hundred years ago, but I doubt that it has been true for the past 50 years. A deterioration of our diet became accelerated after World War II when food processing and food additives entered the kitchen of nearly every home in this country.

I feel greatly encouraged by the present direction of our dietary habits, since there are indications of great improvement in our individual nutrition levels. Many more millions of people in the United States each year are refusing to buy foods which have been adulterated with artificial colors and artificial flavors, preservatives, and other chemicals.

It is my opinion that the current officially recommended dosages for the various vitamins are not sufficient for the needs of most people. As the aging process continues, there is a need for increased amounts of vitamins and minerals. I doubt that these doses will be increased officially, but there is no doubt in my mind that they should be increased.

**Albert Szent-Gyorgyi:**

On the whole one could say that the vitamin content of our foods is too low. The average human diet even in the "have" countries is far from ideal. We eat too much of some things and not enough of others. For this reason, many people probably die as the long-range consequence of eating too much meat or too much ice cream or all sorts of pastry and sugar and alcohol, while, at the same time, eating too little of fruits and vegetables. Or, if they do eat the fruits and vegetables, they do so after eliminating (through storage and processing) some of their most valuable constituents, such as nutrients and roughage.

**John Yudkin:**

The usual concept of a balanced diet is one that includes a mixture of the foods to which we have become accustomed in the Western world. But not all of these foods are good, nor is it axiomatic that we take our foods in the correct proportion. In order to gain an insight into the diet best suited to the human species, we have to look at how preneolithic man ate over the millions of years of evolution, before the development of agriculture, and certainly before the very recent developments in food technology. We shall then find that the nearer we get to eating foods that are not man-made, the better our diets will be, not only in vitamin content but in all other respects.

The USDA findings are that our diets are deteriorating rather than improving, because of the increased consumption of "junk foods."

**Wilfrid E. Shute:**

We have all seen adequate evidence showing that the hope of getting sufficient vitamins in the diet is a false one. Our food is full of unnecessary substances and many essential elements are removed before or during manufacture. Television and radio programs are full of beautiful, persuasive, (and deceptive) ads to get mothers and children to substitute convenience foods for natural ones—think of the millions spent during the Olympics broadcasts to advertise diet colas and substitutes for mayonnaise and eggs. I see our dietary habits deteriorating, not improving.

# Question

What is your opinion of the current officially recommended dosages for the various vitamins? Do you think they will—or should—be increased in the near future? What about the danger of vitamin overdose?

**Allan Cott:**

The danger of vitamin overdose is more a myth than a reality. I have not seen a single case of vitamin overdose.

**Frederick R. Klenner:**

It is a travesty the way the officially recommended doses of vitamins are listed. In many cases labeling proclaiming "100 percent of the daily recommended requirement" has no meaning. Every individual differs in his or her requirements for ascorbic acid; with some individuals, requirements change by the hour and by the day.

If we are to continue to use animals in gauging the amounts humans need, then let us see what an ever-increasing amount will show in these animals, not just the amount that will keep them from contracting disease or help them to hold their own!

I contend that, except for unusual cases, there is no danger in vitamin overdosage. No one has ever shown just what the levels of threshold for excess really are, even with ascorbic acid. Individual variations are too great.

I do think that such warnings as the loss of appetite or loss of hair, indicating possibly too much vitamin A, and pain and weakness at the hamstring muscle attachment of the legs, suggesting too much vitamin D, should appear on the labels of these products.

If we are to be a healthy nation we'd better quickly increase the suggested amounts of vitamin supplements recommended for daily use.

**Albert Szent-Gyorgyi:**

The official recommended allowances are generally too low. This is especially true for ascorbic acid. The toxic levels for most vitamins are so high that there is little chance of overdosing. The only exception may be vitamin D, which is very active and easy to produce in unlimited quantity.


**Abram Hoffer:**

It is my opinion that the officially recommended dosages for the various vitamins have no logical basis and are totally unreal. I think they should be completely eliminated and replaced with a range of optimum requirements so that people can decide for themselves what range fits them best.

With respect to vitamin overdosages, it is possible to overdose with vitamins just as it's possible to overdose with water. Recently, I saw medical reports of patients who made themselves sick by consuming huge quantities of water. The term "overdose" has no value unless it is properly related to the quantity which was taken. To state therefore that it is harmful to take a vitamin overdose has no meaning whatever.


**Wilfrid E. Shute:**

Dr. M. K. Horwitt is responsible for the RDA allowance for vitamin E—which, depending on the source, may have none of the potent alpha portion in it. The RDA of five to 20 (or even) 30 I.U. per day is probably $1/20$th to $1/8$th of a sensible average (if such there be) RDA. Dr. Horwitt now admits this, many years too late. He now advises that the RDA be revised, and that up to 800 units daily is probably safe. Dr. Menzel, because of industrial air pollution, its damaging effects on the lungs, and the proven protection of vitamin E, suggests that every American should take a supplement of 200 I.U. daily!

Vitamin C is in the same category.

**Roger J. Williams:**

The current officially recommended dosages for vitamins and other nutrients cannot be justified scientifically because sufficient knowledge of individual needs is not at hand. If these needs are formulated so as to include the whole population, the recommendations must be increased in many areas. Vitamin overdose is not a serious threat as long as some degree of moderation is practiced. Even megadoses of some of the vitamins appear to be tolerated well by a large number of individuals.

**John Yudkin:**

There have been recent revisions of tables of recommended allowances in many countries, after careful sifting and assessment of all the evidence. I have no reason to suppose that these allowances should be increased, since they already contain a margin of safety. There is certainly danger from overdose of vitamins A and D, and increasing evidence of possible danger from overdose of vitamins C and E.

In general, I do not see the logic of trying to persuade people to eat good (natural) foods by avoiding bad (man-made) foods, while at the same time saying that they need to take vast doses of man-made concentrates or synthetic preparations.

**Irwin Stone:**

The current RDAs for ascorbate and the water-soluble vitamins are tragically low. The present RDA for ascorbate is 45 mg. for a human adult. The closely related mammal, the goat, is capable of producing 13,300 mg. ascorbate per 150 pounds of body weight, per day, in its liver to satisfy its daily needs for this vital metabolite. This is nearly 300 times more than is recommended for Man. I wish the Food and Nutrition Board would explain this great discrepancy between the needs of a goat and their idea of the needs of humans for ascorbate.

The Food and Nutrition Board has been reducing the RDA for ascorbate with each new edition of their book, *Recommended Dietary Allowances*. In 1958, the adult RDA for ascorbate was 75 mg., in 1968 it went down to 60 mg., and in their latest exploit in 1975, it lost another 25 percent and became 35 mg. If the Food and Nutrition Board continues whittling away at its present rate, the RDA will be zero by the year 2000.

Except for vitamin D, I think the RDAs for vitamins should be increased, but I do not think this will happen in the near or far future with our present Food and Nutrition Board.

With regard to the danger of vitamin overdose, this is a subject that has been highly exaggerated by orthodox medicine. With ascorbate this is practically nonexistent. The water-soluble vitamins, at many times their RDAs, are generally nontoxic and harmless and the risk of overdosing is remote.

In the case of the fat-soluble vitamins, D and A, the story may be different, but orthodox medicine has a tendency to indict *all* vitamins on the basis of these fat-soluble ones. I believe that the present RDAs for vitamin A of 4,000 to 5,000 I.U. for adults are low and several times this RDA would prove beneficial and not be "overdosing." Vitamin D is different and amounts beyond the RDA should be avoided.

# Index

vitamin C and, 509–516
Ascorbic acid, *See* Vitamin C
Aspirin, as cold remedy, 293–294
    effect on vitamin C, 302, 509–512
    vitamin deficiency and, 50
Asthma, pyridoxine and, 543–546
Atherosclerosis, 63
    cadmium and, 344
    polyunsaturated fats and, 440, 442
    pyridoxine and, 198
    vitamin C and, 82, 279, 314–324, 325–332, 616–617
    vitamin E and, 472
Autism, megavitamin therapy and, 685–690
    pyridoxine and, 689

—B—

Backache, vitamin C and, 534–537
Bacteria, body's defense against, 283–285
Bedsores, vitamin C and, 731–733
Beriberi, 154, 160
    *See also* Thiamine
Bile acids, 329–330, 333–334
Biochemical individuality, Roger Williams and, 94–95
Bioflavonoids, 46, 363–375
    capillaries and, 363–366, 368
    food sources, 367, 374, 375
    hemorrhoids, 368–370
    interaction with vitamin C, 374
    menstruation and, 367–368
    pregnancy problems and, 368–370
    thrombosis and, 371–373
Biotin, 253–256
    antagonists, 51, 256
    dosages, 43, 254, 761
    food sources, 256, 761
    growth and, 254

Birth defects, pantothenic acid and, 240
    riboflavin and, 176–177
    vitamin A and, 145–146
Bladder cancer, *See* Cancer
Bladder stones, 103
Bleeding, internal, alcohol and, 350
    vitamin C and, 349–352, 512
Blindness, diabetes and, 628
    night, vitamin A and, 21, 99, 102, 129–132
    tobacco, 634–636
    vitamin A and, 106
Blood, vitamin $B_{12}$ and, 216–217
    vitamin C and, 282–287, 314–324
    vitamin E and, 407–408, 466–470, 472–473
    vitamins for, 601–602
Blood clots, 318, 425, 471–472, 598
    *See also* Thrombosis
Blood pressure, choline and, 265
    high, *See* Hypertension
Blood vessels, *See* Arteries, Capillaries, Veins
Bone, marrow, vitamin $B_{12}$ and, 216
    vitamin A and, 135, 136–137
    vitamin D and, 538, 542
    *See also* Osteomalacia, Osteoporosis, Rickets
Bone meal, 44–45
Brain, inositol in, 258
    vitamin C and, 336, 340
    *See also* Mental Ability, Mental Disturbance
Brain damage, thiamine deficiency and, 161–162
Bread, enriched, 26–27
Breastfeeding, 255, 267
Breast cancer, *See* Cancer
Brewer's yeast, 43–44
Bronchial asthma, *See* Asthma
Bronchitis, vitamin A and, 115
Bruises, 366, 370
Bruxism, 248–251